T0314282

Guide to Canine and Feline Electrocardiography

Guide to Canine and Feline Electrocardiography

Ruth Willis

BVM&S DVC MRCVS
RCVS Recognised Specialist in Veterinary Cardiology
Holter Monitoring Service
Dick White Referrals
Newmarket
Cambridgeshire, UK
and
Honorary Associate Professor
University of Nottingham
Nottingham, UK

Pedro Oliveira

DVM, Diplomate ECVIM-CA (Cardiology), MRCVS
RCVS Recognised Specialist in Veterinary Cardiology
Davies Veterinary Specialists
Higham Gobion
Hertfordshire, UK

Antonia Mavropoulou

DVM, PhD, Diplomate ECVIM-CA (Cardiology), MRCVS
RCVS Recognised Specialist in Veterinary Cardiology
Davies Veterinary Specialists
Higham Gobion
Hertfordshire, UK

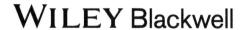

Registered Offices
John Wiley & Sons, Inc., 111 River Street, Hoboken, NJ 07030, USA
John Wiley & Sons Ltd, The Atrium, Southern Gate, Chichester, West Sussex, PO19 8SQ, UK

Editorial Office
9600 Garsington Road, Oxford, OX4 2DQ, UK

For details of our global editorial offices, customer services, and more information about Wiley products visit us at www.wiley.com.

Wiley also publishes its books in a variety of electronic formats and by print-on-demand. Some content that appears in standard print versions of this book may not be available in other formats.

Library of Congress Cataloging-in-Publication Data

Names: Willis, Ruth, 1973– author. | Oliveira, Pedro, 1980– author. | Mavropoulou, Antonia, author.
Title: Guide to canine and feline electrocardiography / Ruth Willis, Pedro Oliveira, Antonia Mavropoulou.
Description: Hoboken, NJ : John Wiley & Sons, Inc., [2018] | Includes bibliographical references and index. |
Identifiers: LCCN 2018007638 (print) | LCCN 2018009442 (ebook) | ISBN 9781119254300 (pdf) | ISBN 9781119254317 (epub) |
   ISBN 9781119253846 (cloth)
Subjects: | MESH: Arrhythmias, Cardiac–veterinary | Electrocardiography–veterinary | Dog Diseases–diagnosis | Cat Diseases–diagnosis
Classification: LCC SF772.58 (ebook) | LCC SF772.58 (print) | NLM SF 992.C37 | DDC 636.089/61207543–dc23
LC record available at https://lccn.loc.gov/2018007638

Cover Design: Wiley
Cover Images: (Dog photo) Steve Magennis, Working Dogs in Action photography; (ECG report) Pedro Oliveira

Set in 10/12pt Warnock by SPi Global, Pondicherry, India

10 9 8 7 6 5 4 3 2 1

Contents

List of Contributors

Erin L. Anderson
VMD, MSc, DACVIM (cardiology)
Associate Cardiologist
Pittsburgh Veterinary Specialty and Emergency Center
Pittsburgh, USA

Domingo Casamian-Sorrosal
DVM, Cert SAM, DVC, Diplomate ECVIM-CA, MRCVS
RCVS Diplomate and Recognised Specialist in
Veterinary Cardiology
ECVIM Diplomate and Specialist in Small Animal
Internal Medicine
Southfields Vet Specialists
Laindon
Essex, UK

Louise Clark
BVMS, Cert VA, Diplomate ECVAA, MSc (Clinical
Management of Pain), MRCVS
Davies Veterinary Specialists
Higham Gobion
Hertfordshire, UK

Frances Downing
BVSc, MSc, Diplomate ECVAA, MRCVS
Davies Veterinary Specialists
Higham Gobion
Hertfordshire, UK

Martin Lowe
BSc, MB, BS, PhD, FRCP
Cardiology Consultant
BARTS Heart Centre
London, UK

Antonia Mavropoulou
DVM, PhD, Diplomate ECVIM-CA (Cardiology), MRCVS
RCVS Recognised Specialist in Veterinary Cardiology
Davies Veterinary Specialists
Higham Gobion
Hertfordshire, UK

Pedro Oliveira
DVM, Diplomate ECVIM-CA (Cardiology), MRCVS
RCVS Recognised Specialist in Veterinary Cardiology
Davies Veterinary Specialists
Higham Gobion
Hertfordshire, UK

Romain Pariaut
DVM, Diplomate ACVIM and ECVIM-CA
(Cardiology)
Associate Professor of Cardiology, Section Chief of
Cardiology
Cornell University, College of Veterinary Medicine,
Department of Clinical Sciences
Ithaca, USA

Thibault Ribas
DVM, Diplomate ECVIM-CA (Cardiology)
Azurvet
Cagnes-Sur-Mer, France

Joel Freitas da Silva
DVM, Diplomate ECVIM-CA (Cardiology), MRVC
RCVS Recognised Specialist in Cardiology
North Downs Specialist Referrals
Bletchingley
Surrey, UK

Simon Swift
MA, VetMB, CertSAC, DipECVIM-CA (Cardiology),
MRCVS
Clinical Associate Professor – Cardiology
Department of Small Animal Clinical Sciences
University of Florida
Gainesville, USA

Marin Torti
DVM, PhD
Clinic for Internal Diseases, Faculty of Veterinary
Medicine, University of Zagreb
Zagreb, Croatia

Gerhard Wess
DVM, Dr. med. vet., Dr. habil., Diplomate ACVIM
(Cardiology), Diplomate ECVIM-CA (Internal
Medicine and Cardiology)
Clinic for Small Animal Medicine, Ludwig-Maximilian
University
Munich, Germany

Ruth Willis
BVM&S, DVC, MRCVS
RCVS Recognised Specialist in Veterinary Cardiology
Holter Monitoring Service
Dick White Referrals
Newmarket
Cambridgeshire, UK

Jon Wray
BVSc, CertVC, Diplomate ECVIM-CA (Internal
Medicine), MRCVS
Holter Monitoring Service
Dick White Referrals
Newmarket
Cambridgeshire, UK

Preface

To many veterinary students, veterinarians and veterinary nurses, electrocardiography (ECG) can seem like a daunting challenge and somewhat of a mystery. Arrhythmias can be life threatening and anti-arrhythmic drugs may have the potential to be pro-arrhythmic, factors which often intimidate clinicians and can instill a fear of possibly harming rather than helping a patient. However, for those who master this challenge, they find ECG thoroughly rewarding as it is one of the more logical fields in veterinary medicine and it appeals to the puzzle solver in us.

The authors of this *Guide to Canine and Feline Electrocardiography* have undertaken the challenge of bringing together their expertise in understanding the pathophysiology, but also diagnosing and managing arrhythmias in an outstanding, extensive review of cardiac ECG.

The reader is taken systematically through the basics of ECG generation: the required equipment for ECG acquisition, detailed explanation of the mechanisms underlying arrhythmias as well the evaluation of the arrhythmia substrate. The book provides advanced, up-to-date description of all important arrhythmias encountered in dogs and cats, highlighting both the main characteristics and breed-specific differences and in-depth therapeutic considerations. The authors have taken a highly visual approach, where all phenomena described are illustrated with original colour figures and beautiful ECG traces. Examples of normal ECG recordings, practice electrocardiograms and a diagnostic approach to real-life electrocardiograms of many clinically important arrhythmias will help the reader to feel comfortable and confident to interpret even the most complex arrhythmias. Valuable review questions, self-assessment sections as well as recommended reading are also built-in, and a comprehensive list of references are provided at the end of each chapter.

This book is a first of its kind in veterinary medicine as it also includes chapters on arrhythmia interpretation using long-term ambulatory ECG (Holter or event recorder) monitoring; provides insight into interpretation of heart rate variability parameters and detailed description of pacemaker therapies, including surgical implantation techniques and programming instructions; and delivers valuable information on abnormal ECGs encountered in veterinary patients under anesthesia.

For those interested in advanced, interventional arrhythmia therapies, a large chapter is dedicated to cutting-edge techniques of radiofrequency ablation, and the reader is presented with practical tips on how to set up an electrophysiology laboratory and taught the step-by-step approach on interpretation of intracardiac electrograms.

For all these reasons, this comprehensive veterinary ECG book is worth the highest merit, and undoubtedly deserves to be in every personal library of veterinary students, residents, veterinarians and veterinary nurses.

Anna Gelzer, Dr.med.vet. PhD
LDACVIM & ECVIM-CA-Cardiology
Associate Professor of Cardiology
School of Veterinary Medicine
University of Pennsylvania, USA

Acknowledgements

The decision to write a book was relatively straightforward but then, as the enormity of the task became apparent, we were incredibly fortunate to have so many people willing to help us achieve our objective.

Firstly I would like to remind my family – Greg, Sophie and Josh – that you are, and always will be, the most important part of my life. Thank you is such a small phrase to encompass the sacrifices you have all made over the last two years, and I could not have completed this project without your support, patience and encouragement.

Secondly I would like to thank Pedro and Antonia who have patiently filtered my ideas. You have both been an invaluable source of knowledge and reassurance on this journey, and your attention to detail is reflected in the quality of this book.

Also thanks to all the chapter authors for giving us your precious time and expertise to improve the quality and breadth of this book. Thanks too to numerous colleagues who have assisted us by supplying figures and providing constructive criticism and encouragement along the way.

A special thanks is due to Paul Wotton for his mentorship throughout my career and to the team at Dick White Referrals, who ask good questions and are constantly striving to improve the care we provide for our patients. I am privileged to have such inspiring colleagues.

I would like to thank Wiley for believing in us, their commitment to this project and the hard work of all involved.

Last but not least, thanks to my parents Helen and Ray. You are the people who taught me to work hard and persevere. Thanks also to our extended family and all our friends – I am immensely grateful for the support, company and humour you bring to my life.

December 2017 **Ruth Willis**

To my family, friends and colleagues for all their support.

Pedro Oliveira

To my family, friends and mentors for their love, support and encouragement.

Antonia Mavropoulou

About the Companion Website

Don't forget to visit the companion website for this book:

www.wiley.com/go/willis/electrocardiography

There you will find valuable material designed to enhance your learning, including:

- Self-assessment questions
- Figures from the book
- Appendices.

Scan this QR code to visit the companion website:

Anatomy of the Conduction System

Pedro Oliveira

Introduction

The heart possesses a specialised conduction system that is responsible for generating and transmitting electrical stimuli to the whole heart in a specific and ordered fashion. It is composed of the sinoatrial node (SA), internodal and inter-atrial pathways, atrioventricular junction, bundle branches and Purkinje fibres (Figure 1.1). The SA contains specialised 'pacemaker' cells that have the ability to spontaneously depolarise, generating electrical impulses. The remainder of the conduction system is composed mainly of cells organised in bundles that allow conduction of the electrical stimuli. These structures are present in the walls of the heart and are interwoven with the myocardial tissue itself. It is not possible to distinguish them from the rest of the myocardium (working myocardium) with the naked eye, only with certain stains under the microscope.

The anatomy of these structures is presented in this chapter. To avoid confusion, the use of human anatomical terminology is avoided, and terminology commonly used in veterinary medicine for quadruped patients is preferred. Given the different orientation of the heart within the chest of dogs and cats in comparison to humans, the following terms are used: cranial instead of anterior; caudal instead of posterior; dorsal instead of superior; and ventral instead of inferior. However, since some terms are so widespread in veterinary literature (e.g. left anterior or posterior fascicles), it is difficult to avoid the use of such terms even though they are not entirely appropriate.

Sinoatrial Node

Anatomy

The SA, also known as the sinus node, is found in the wall of the right atrium at its junction with the cranial vena cava in the upper portion of the terminal groove (sulcus terminalis) (Figure 1.1).

In dogs, it lies less than 1 mm beneath the epicardium and occupies almost the entire thickness of the atrial wall from epicardium to endocardium.[1] The total size of the canine node was described as being approximately 5 mm^3 with an oblong shape, although with significant variation observed amongst individuals.[1,2] Other reports suggest a more extensive location of up to 3–4 cm between both venae cavae.[3,4]

In cats, according to one study including five male and five female domestic shorthair cats, the SA node was located 0.06–0.11 mm beneath the epicardium with an almost triangular shape.[5] In males the reported size was 2.78 × 2.80 × 0.54 mm, and in females it was 2.75 × 2.64 × 0.45 mm.[5] A different study involving 12 cats produced different results.[6] A reconstruction of the SA node based on histological and electrophysiological data was performed in five of these cats, revealing an ellipsoid shape with a total area of 10.5 ± 0.76 mm^2, a maximum length of 7.4 ± 0.74 mm, a maximal width of 2.2 ± 0.10 mm and a thickness of 0.41 ± 0.060 mm.[6]

Histology

Histologically, the SA is composed of specialised muscle fibres arranged in a network.[7] Many small bundles are present with irregular courses interspersed with connective tissue accompanied by capillary vessels and nerve cells. The surface of the SA is covered by epicardium, and the remaining areas are surrounded by atrial muscle. Each nodal fibre shows a smooth transition to ordinary atrial muscle fibres at the periphery of the SA.

Three different types of cells are present: normal working myocardial cells, transitional cells and P (pacemaker) cells.

The P cells are responsible for the ability of the SA to spontaneously generate electrical stimuli. They represent approximately 50% of the cells in the SA and are also present in other areas of the conduction system

Guide to Canine and Feline Electrocardiography, First Edition. Ruth Willis, Pedro Oliveira and Antonia Mavropoulou.
© 2018 John Wiley & Sons Ltd. Published 2018 by John Wiley & Sons Ltd.
Companion website: www.wiley.com/go/willis/electrocardiography

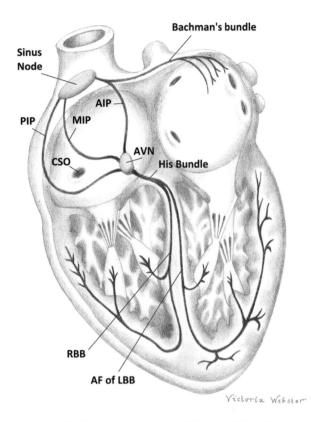

Figure 1.1 Cardiac conduction system. The sinoatrial node, also known as the sinus node, is found in the wall of the right atrium at its junction with the cranial vena cava in the upper portion of the terminal groove (sulcus terminalis). It is connected to the atrioventricular node (AVN) located on the floor of the right atrium via the anterior (AIP), middle (MIP) and posterior (PIP) internodal pathways. Connections also exist between the right and left atria, of which Bachmann's bundle and the inferior interatrial pathway (not illustrated) are the most important. Bachmann's bundle runs in the upper portion of the atrial septum towards the left auricle. The inferior interatrial pathway is composed of fibres that are continuous with the right atrial myocardium at the level of the ostium of the coronary sinus (CSO) and with the left atrial myocardium from which they separate approximately 20–30 mm from the CSO. The AVN is continued by the Bundle of His that penetrates the fibrous skeleton of the heart and ramifies into the right (RBB) and left (LBB) bundle branches. The LBB is composed of anterior (AF) and posterior ramifications (not illustrated). The bundle branch subdivisions give rise to numerous small branches that spread all over the subendocardium of both ventricles, forming the Purkinje network that connects the conduction system to the working myocardium.

(e.g. atrioventricular node [AVN]) in fewer numbers. They are organised in small groups of approximately five cells surrounded by connective tissue that function as a unit.

The transitional cells are also present in other parts of the conduction system (e.g. internodal tracts and the atrioventricular junction) and seem to provide a link between the specialised cells and the normal working myocardium.

Sinoatrial Exit Pathways

The existence of discrete exit sites has been described at the cranial and caudal ends of the canine sinus node.[8] Ablation of these sites resulted in sinoatrial block, suggesting that the SA was not anatomically continuous with the atrial myocardium.[8,9] It was suggested that vessels and connective tissue around the SA tissue were responsible for anatomical and physiological blocks on both sides of the node with the exception of the exit sites.[9] These findings, together with the reports of a length of up to 3–4 cm,[3,4] provide a plausible explanation for the occurrence of 'wandering pacemaker' in this species (see chapter 5).

Internodal Pathways

The presence of preferential pathways that connect the SA and AVN has been the subject of debate for the past century, and there is still disagreement about their existence and significance. In the dog, there is anatomical and electrophysiological evidence to support the presence of three distinct pathways in the right atrium, with cells that possess characteristics similar to those of Purkinje cells.[10] However, these pathways are not insulated from neighbouring atrial muscle and are not composed of specialised conduction cells only. This raises questions about their role, and some argue that they should not be termed *bundles* for this reason.[11] Nonetheless, surgical resection of these pathways was shown to result in a junctional rhythm in dogs, supporting their role as internodal pathways.[10]

The *anterior internodal pathway* originates in the sinus node and courses through the cranial aspect of the cranial vena cava, at which point it bifurcates into Bachman's bundle (see the 'Inter-atrial pathways' section) and a branch that courses ventrally through the cranial inter-atrial septum to join the cranial aspect of the AVN (Figure 1.1).

The *middle internodal pathway* originates in the sinus node and travels downwards cranially to the fossa ovalis towards the AVN (Figure 1.1).

The *posterior internodal pathway* originates in the sinus node, then it courses along the crista terminalis and downwards through the caudal aspect of the inter-atrial septum, past the coronary sinus (CS) ostium and joining the caudal aspect of the AVN (Figure 1.1).

Inter-atrial Pathways

At least four distinct inter-atrial electrical connections have been identified in dogs.

Bachman's bundle, or the inter-atrial band, originates close to the SA and traverses the upper portion of the inter-atrial septum towards the left auricle (Figure 1.1).

It is composed of normal atrial muscle and of specialised conducting fibres capable of rapid conduction, similar to the Purkinje fibres in the ventricles.[12]

Another connection is present ventrally via striated muscle fibres identical to atrial myocardium that surround the CS.[13] These fibres are continuous with the right atrial myocardium at the level of the CS ostium and with the left atrial myocardium from which they separate approximately 20–30 mm from the CS ostium.[14] A tract of atrial muscle that terminates blindly within the ligament or vein of Marshall (a remnant of the left cranial vena cava) has been proposed as the terminal end of this pathway in the left atrium, and the term *inferior inter-atrial pathway* was used to describe it.[15]

Additional connections exist at the level of the atrial septum craniodorsally, in the proximity of the fossa ovalis, and caudoventrally, possibly via the subepicardial band that connects the left atrium and cavoatrial junction ventrally.[16,17]

Bachman's bundle and the CS musculature are believed to be the major connections and the preferred pathways for conduction of electrical stimuli between the atria.[16]

The Atrioventricular Junction

The atrial and ventricular myocardium are separated by a fibrous skeleton that consists of the distinct valve annuli and intervening fibrous trigones. This structure provides attachment for the valve leaflets and the myocardium itself. As a consequence, the atrial and ventricular myocardium are electrically isolated, which is important to ensure that atrial and ventricular contractions occur in a coordinated fashion. The only point of electrical connection is provided by a specialised conduction structure that traverses the central portion of the fibrous skeleton (the *central fibrous body*), commonly described as the *atrioventricular node* or *junction* (Figures 1.1 and 1.2). It is located approximately 1 mm beneath the epicardium on the floor of the right atrium in an area known as the *triangle of Koch* (Figure 1.2).[11,18] The CS ostium limits the base of this triangle, and the apex is formed by the junction between the fibrous tendon (tendon of Todaro) and the septal leaflet of the tricuspid valve (Figure 1.2). In the dog, the AVN has an elongated shape with a concave surface facing the central fibrous body. It averages approximately 2–4 mm in length, 2 mm in width and 0.5–1 mm in thickness.[19,20] In the cat, an elongated oval shape has also been reported that is approximately 1.2–1.8 mm in length, 0.2–0.5 mm in width and 0.4–0.6 mm in thickness.[21] Male cats appear to have a larger AVN than females.[21]

The AVN can be divided into an atrionodal region formed by atrionodal bundles that converge into a proximal atrioventricular bundle, the compact node and the distal atrioventricular bundle (DAVB; Figure 1.2).[20] This division is based on histological differences between each area. The remainder of this section focuses on canine anatomy.

Atrionodal Bundles and the Proximal Atrioventricular Bundle

Three distinct atrionodal bundles have been described in the dog and are thought to be the continuation of the internodal pathways (Figure 1.2).[20,22,23] They are associated

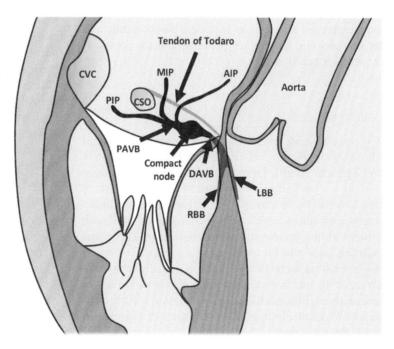

Figure 1.2 The atrioventricular junction. The atrioventricular junction may be divided into the proximal atrioventricular bundle (PAVB), the compact node and the distal atrioventricular bundle (DAVB). It is located on the floor of the right atrium in a triangular-shaped area (triangle of Koch) formed caudally by the coronary sinus ostium (CSO) and with the tendon of Todaro and the tricuspid valve rim as its lateral boundaries. The posterior (PIP), middle (MIP) and anterior (AIP) internodal pathways join the atrioventricular junction via distinct atrionodal bundles forming the PAVB. The DAVB extends from the compact node approximately 3 mm to a branching point at the cranial edge of the tricuspid septal leaflet. Here, it penetrates the septum fibrosum of the cardiac fibrous skeleton bridging the atria and ventricles. The DAVB divides into the left (LBB) and right (RBB) bundle branches at the level of the upper portion of the interventricular septum beneath the non-coronary and the right aortic leaflets. CVC, Caudal vena cava.

with epicardium of the medial right atrial wall and the crest of the ventricular septum, approximately 1 cm away from the annulus fibrosus.[20] The cells are organised into small fascicles of myofibres surrounded by collagen without connection to ordinary atrial myocardium. The myofibres run in a parallel fashion.

The *superior (dorsal) atrionodal bundle* is located beneath the epicardium of the dorsal-cranial aspect of the medial right atrial wall, closely apposed to the crest of the interventricular septum.

The *middle atrionodal bundle* is located beneath the epicardium on the dorsal-caudal aspect of the medial right atrial wall, opposed to the medial aspect of the tendon of Todaro, associated with the dorsal-medial aspect of the CS ostium.

The *lateral atrionodal bundle* input is located beneath the epicardium on the caudal-ventral aspect of the medial right atrial wall, subjacent to the lateral aspect of the CS ostium.

The presence of additional atrionodal bundles has not been proved but was suggested.[24] Remnants of bundles extending into the left atrium have been described, but further studies are necessary to determine their significance.[20]

The atrionodal bundles converge into the *proximal atrioventricular bundle* (PAVB) that is continuous with the compact node (Figure 1.2). It is located beneath the epicardium of the right atrial medial wall, cranially to the floor of the CS ostium, medially to the tendon of Todaro and approximately 1 cm away from the hinge point of the tricuspid leaflet at the annulus fibrosus. At this level, the myofibres are tightly coiled in single strands that form fascicles running in parallel.[20,25] A small number of intercalated discs are present in comparison to the atrionodal bundles. The PAVB is also characterised by numerous ganglia nestled amongst its fascicles, blood vessels and fat vacuoles and particularly prominent at the ventricular septal apposition.[25]

Compact Node

The *compact node* rests on the atrial aspect of the central fibrous body (Figure 1.2). In the dog, it is approximately 1–1.5 mm in length. From caudal to cranial, it appears initially as two half-ovals separated by the nodal artery that become fused cranially.[26] It is composed of closely interwoven fibres which frequently connect with each other within a sparse collagen framework.[7] The nodal cells are small and are arranged in a parallel fashion on the caudal aspects of the node. Cranially, they are arranged in interweaving fascicles on the left margin, and on the right the cells become larger and are arranged in a more parallel fashion. This arrangement is also seen in the proximal part of the DAVB.[11]

Distal Atrioventricular Bundle

The DAVB extends cranially from the compact node approximately 3 mm to a branching point at the cranial edge of the tricuspid septal leaflet (Figure 1.2).[20] It resides in the cranial part of the central fibrous body, where it penetrates the septum fibrosum bridging the atria and ventricles. The myocytes are larger in the DAVB, and the myofibres and fascicles run in a parallel fashion as in the atrionodal bundles. Given that the initial part of the DAVB is often histologically similar to the compact node, some authors only consider the bundle where it becomes surrounded by the tissues of the fibrous body.[11] The term *bundle of His* is commonly used for this structure, named after Wilhelm His Jr., who described it for the first time. In dogs, it is approximately 8–10 mm long and has a width of 1.5–2.0 mm.[27] The presence of two distinct functional strands within the common trunk of the canine His bundle has been described.[27] According to this report, a dorsal strand extends from the dorsal part of the compact node and continues ventrally with the right bundle branch, and a ventral strand extends from the ventral part of the compact node to continue with the left bundle branch. The electrophysiological properties of both strands are similar, with the exception of the conduction velocity which seems to be faster in the ventral strand.[27] Traversing bridges are present between the strands and ensure their activation as a single conducting structure.

The Bundle Branches

The DAVB divides into several branches that supply the Purkinje network of the right and left ventricles (Figures 1.1 and 1.3). A division into right and left bundle branches is common, although variations exist amongst individuals.[7] This division occurs at the level of the upper portion of the interventricular septum beneath the non-coronary and the right aortic leaflets.

The *right bundle branch* courses in the subendocardium of the right side of the interventricular septum.[7] Proximally, it branches from the DAVB approximately 2–3 mm away from the insertion of the septal leaflet of the tricuspid valve and runs as a single chord until it reaches the cranial (anterior) papillary muscle. At this level, it divides into three branches:

1) *Ramification for the conus pulmonalis*: These branches separate from the right bundle at the level of the base of the papillary muscle and spread over the cranial part of the interventricular septum with an irregular pattern to supply the Purkinje fibres in the area of the conus pulmonalis.

2) *Ramification for the free wall*: After the branching for the conus, the right bundle courses around the base of the papillary muscle and proceeds downward, giving

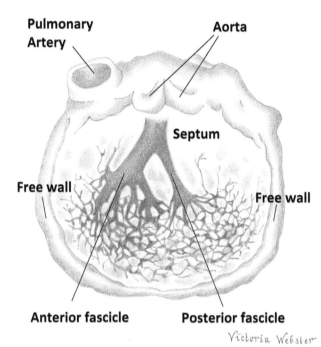

Pulmonary Artery

Aorta

Septum

Free wall

Free wall

Anterior fascicle

Posterior fascicle

Victoria Webster

Figure 1.3 The divisions of the left bundle branch. The left bundle branch and its ramifications are illustrated in this picture with the left ventricle open as if cut across its free wall and looking into the septum. The left bundle branch runs in the subendocardium on the left side of the interventricular septum in close proximity to the aortic valve. The initial part (or trunk) is brush-like in shape, approximately 4–7 mm in width and 2–6 mm in length. It ramifies into two main groups of peripheral branches: the *cranial group*, commonly referred to as the anterior fascicle, and the *caudal group* or posterior fascicle. The cranial group splits into a few small branches that run beneath the endocardium for approximately 10–15 mm until they change into bands that project into the ventricular cavity – pseudotendons. Once they reach the base of the cranial (anterior) papillary muscle, they spread to the cranial area of the left ventricle in a mesh pattern. The caudal group gives off a few small branches that run approximately 10–15 mm beneath the endocardium in parallel with each other like a chord until they change into pseudotendons projecting into the ventricular cavity towards the caudal (posterior) papillary muscle. From this point, the Purkinje fibres from the pseudotendons spread over the caudal area of the left ventricle.

off wide and short pseudotendons of approximately 2–3 mm in length and <4 mm in width. These form bridges from the septum to the free wall.

3) *Ramification for the septum*: After the ramifications for the conus and for the free wall, the right bundle gives rise to a few small branches supplying the caudal half of the right side of the interventricular septum.

The *left bundle branch* runs in the subendocardium on the left side of the interventricular septum in close proximity to the aortic valve (Figure 1.3). The initial part (or trunk) of the left bundle is brush-like in shape and approximately 4–7 mm in width and 2–6 mm in length.[7] Its width increases gradually until it ramifies into two main groups of peripheral branches:

1) *Cranial (anterior) group*: The first branch to divide from the trunk splits into a few small branches that run cranially beneath the endocardium for approximately 10–15 mm until they change into bands that project into the ventricular cavity – 'pseudotendons'. Once they reach the base of the cranial (anterior) papillary muscle, they spread to the cranial area of the left ventricle in a mesh pattern.

2) *Caudal (posterior) group*: Another few small branches run approximately 10–15 mm beneath the endocardium in parallel with each other like a chord until they change into pseudotendons, projecting into the ventricular cavity towards the caudal (posterior) papillary muscle. From this point, the Purkinje fibres from the pseudotendons spread over the caudal area of the left ventricle.

Another small subendocardial network of branches from the left bundle has been described between the cranial and caudal groups spreading directly over the septum without giving off pseudotendons – the *intermediate group*.[7]

The terms *anterior* and *posterior fascicles* are often used to describe the cranial and caudal divisions of the left bundle, respectively.

The Purkinje Fibres

The bundle branch subdivisions give rise to numerous small branches that spread all over the subendocardium of both ventricles.[7] These branches are composed of Purkinje cells and form a network connecting the conduction system to the ventricular myocardium. They are more abundant over the base of the papillary muscles and apical regions of the heart. A similar density of Purkinje fibres has been reported in the free wall of both ventricles, but it is higher in the left side of the interventricular septum due to the existence of the intermediate group. As a consequence, the peripheral ramifications are denser in the left ventricle, which makes sense due to its larger dimensions and higher contractile force.

Blood Supply

Sinus Node

The canine SA artery has been reported to derive in most instances (90%) from the distal right atrial branch, a terminal branch of the right coronary artery, and less commonly from a branch of the left coronary artery.[1,28–30] However, other reports showed that the blood supply to the sinus node was instead derived from branches of the left circumflex coronary artery either alone or in combination with distal branches of the right coronary artery.[31,32] This highlights the high degree of variation possible in this species. The venous return occurs via tiny valveless veins – *Thebesian veins* – that are present in the endocardium and empty directly into the right atrium.

The blood supply of the feline SA also shows a high degree of variation. In most instances, the supply was seen to originate from collaterals of the right circumflex or right coronary arteries, and less frequently from the proximal left atrial branch originating from the left coronary artery.[33]

Atrioventricular Junction

The blood supply to the atrioventricular junction in the dog has been described as originating from two branches from the right coronary artery and one from the left, as well as anastomoses of these vessels in the septum.[34] The DAVB is supplied by the septal artery and the dorsal left artery which are both branches from the left coronary artery. Additionally, perfusion is provided in part by the accessory ventral right atrial branch of the right coronary artery. The venous return occurs via Thebesian veins.

Innervation

The SA and AVN regions of the canine heart are richly innervated by the autonomic nervous system.[35] The SA is especially responsive to parasympathetic stimulation, whereas the AVN is preferentially sensitive to sympathetic tone. The effects of both are discussed in chapter 2.

Sympathetic innervation of both the SA and AVN is provided by sympathetic efferents from the ansae subclaviae via branches of the cervicothoracic ganglia and the middle cervical ganglia.[36] Parasympathetic innervation of the SA is provided by the right vagus, whilst the AVN is innervated by both the right and left vagus nerves. The parasympathetic fibres synapse in ganglia located in the heart and short postsynaptic fibres, then supply the relevant cardiac structures (e.g. the SA and AVN). These ganglia are located in fat pads at the level of the junction between the cranial vena cava and aorta, the caudal vena cava and left atrium and the junction of the right pulmonary vein with the atrium.[37,38] The bundle branches and its ramifications do not seem to be innervated, although autonomic fibres have been identified in close proximity to the subendocardial Purkinje fibres.[39]

References

1 James TN. Anatomy of the sinus node of the dog. Anat Rec. 1962;143:251–265.

2 Nabipour A. Comparative histological structure of the sinus node in mammals. Turk J Vet Anim Sci. 2012;36:463–469.

3 Monfredi O, Dobrzynski H, Mondal T, Boyett MR, Morris GM. The anatomy and physiology of the sinoatrial node: a contemporary review. Pacing Clin Electrophysiol. 2010;33:1392–1406.

4 Kalman JM, *et al.* Radiofrequency catheter modification of sinus pacemaker function guided by intracardiac echocardiography. Circulation. 1995;92:3070–3081.

5 Ghazi SR, Tadjalli M, Baniabbas A. Anatomy of the sinus node of domestic cats (*Felis catus*). J Appl Animal Res. 1998;14:57–64.

6 Opthof T, Dejonge B, Massonpevet M, Jongsma H, Bouman L. Functional and morphological organization of the cat sinoatrial node. J Molec Cell Cardiol. 1986;18:1015–1031.

7 Hara T. Morphological and histochemical studies on the cardiac conduction system of the dog. Archiv Histolog Japon. 1967;28:227–246.

8 Bromberg BI, Hand DE, Schuessler RB, Boineau JP. Primary negativity does not predict dominant pacemaker location: implications for sinoatrial conduction. Am J Physiol. 1995;269:H877–H887.

9 Fedoro VV, *et al.* Structural and functional evidence for discrete exit pathways that connect the canine sinoatrial node and atria. Circ Res. 2009;104:915–923.

10 Holsinger JW, Wallace AG, Sealy WC. The identification and surgical significance of the atrial internodal conduction tracts. Ann Surg. 1968;167:447–453.

11 Ho SY, *et al.* The architecture of the atrioventricular conduction axis in dog compared to man: its significance to ablation of the atrioventricular nodal approaches. J Cardio Electrophysiol. 1995;6:26–39.

12 Wagner ML, Lazzara R, Weiss RM, Hoffman BF. Specialized conducting fibers in the interatrial band. Circ. Res. 1966;18:502–518.

13 Antz M, *et al.* Electrical conduction between the right atrium and the left atrium via the musculature of the coronary sinus. Circulation. 1998;98:1790–1795.

14 Arruda M, *et al.* Dispersion in ventricular repolarization in the human, canine and porcine heart. J Am Coll Cardiol. 2016;120:222–235.

15 Scherlag BJ, Yeh BK, Robinson MJ. Inferior interatrial pathway in the dog. Circ Res. 1972;31:18–35.

16 Sakamoto S, *et al.* Interatrial electrical connections: the precise location and preferential conduction. J Cardio Electrophysiol. 2005;16:1077.

17 Ott P, *et al.* 1014-210 Coronary sinus Os and fossa ovalis ablation: effect on interatrial conduction and inducibility of atrial fibrillation. J Am Coll Cardiol. 2004;43:A105.

18 Meijler FL, Janse MJ. Morphology and electrophysiology of the mammalian atrioventricular node. Physiol Rev. 1988;68:608–647.

19 James TN. Anatomy of the A–V node of the dog. Anat Rec. 1964;148:15–27.

20 Racker DK. The AV junction region of the heart: a comprehensive study correlating gross anatomy and direct three-dimensional analysis. Part II. Morphology and cytoarchitecture. Am J Physiol Heart Circ Physiol. 2004;286:H1853–H1871.

21 Tadjalli M, Ghazi SR, Shahri AB. Anatomy of the atrioventricular node in the heart of cat. J Appl Anim Res. 1999;15:35–40.

22 Racker DK. Atrioventricular node and input pathways: a correlated gross anatomical and histological study of the canine atrioventricular junctional region. Anat Rec. 1989;224:336–354.

23 Moïse NS, Gladuli A, Hemsley SA, Otani NF. 'Zone of avoidance': RR interval distribution in tachograms, histograms, and Poincaré plots of a Boxer dog. J Vet Cardiol. 2010;12:191–196.

24 Antz M, Scherlag BJ, Otomo K, Pitha J. Evidence for multiple atrio-AV nodal inputs in the normal dog heart. J Cardio Electrophysiol. 1998;9:395.

25 Racker DK, Kadish AH. Proximal atrioventricular bundle, atrioventricular node, and distal atrioventricular bundle are distinct anatomic structures with unique histological characteristics and innervation. Circulation. 2000;101:1049–1059.

26 Ho SY, *et al.* The architecture of the atrioventricular conduction axis in dog compared to man: its significance to ablation of the atrioventricular nodal approaches. J Cardio Electrophysiol. 1995;6:26–39.

27 Alanis J, Benitez D. Two preferential conducting pathways within the bundle of His of the dog heart. Jap J Physiol. 1975;371–385. doi:10.2170/jjphysiol.25.371

28 Moore RA. The coronary arteries of the dog. Am Heart J. 1930;5:743–749.

29 Amaral RC, Borelli V, Didio L. The blood supply of the sinu-atrial node of Dobermann dogs. Arch Ital Anat Embriol. 1985;1985.

30 Izumisawa N, Machida N, Kiryu K, Kitayama T. Blood supply of the sinus node artery in beagle dogs. Heart Vess. 1994;9:96.

31 Biasi C, Borelli V, Prazeres RF, Favaron PO. Análise comparativa entre a vascularização arterial ventricular e do nó sinoatrial em corações de cães. Pesq Vet Bras. 2013;33:111–114.

32 Pina JA, Pereira AT, Ferreira SA. [Arterial vascularization of the sino-auricular node of the heart in dogs]. Acta Cardiol. 1975;30:67–77.

33 Biasi, C, Borelli, V, Benedicto HG, Pereira MR. Análise comparativa entre a vascularização ventricular e do nó sinoatrial em gatos. Pesq Vet Bras. 2012;32:78–82.

34 Halpern MH. Blood supply to the atrioventricular system of the dog. Anat Rec. 1955;121:753–762.

35 Randall WC, Ardell JL, O'Toole MF, Wurster RD. Differential autonomic control of SAN and AVN regions of the canine heart: structure and function. Prog Clin Biol Res. 1988;275:15–31.

36 Yuan BX, Ardell JL, Hopkins DA, Losier AM, Armour JA. Gross and microscopic anatomy of the canine intrinsic cardiac nervous system. Anat Rec. 1994;239:75–87.

37 Randall WC, Ardell JL, Wurster RD. Vagal postganglionic innervation of the canine sinoatrial node. J Auton Nerv Syst. 1987;20:13–23.

38 Chiou CW, Eble JN, Zipes DP. Efferent vagal innervation of the canine atria and sinus and atrioventricular nodes: the third fat pad. Circulation. 1997;95:2573–2584.

39 Tcheng KT. Innervation of the dog's heart. Am. Heart J. 1951;41:512–524.

2

Cardiac Electrophysiology
Antonia Mavropoulou

Introduction

As described in chapter 1, the heart possesses a specialised conduction system responsible for the spontaneous generation and transmission of electrical impulses to the whole heart in a specific manner. This is possible due to the presence of different cardiac cells, each with a specific purpose and characteristics. In this chapter, we will discuss the mechanisms that allow the various cardiac cells to generate and transmit electricity. The aim is to cover the basic electrophysiological principles of normal cardiac cell function that are essential to understand how cardiac arrhythmias are generated and how they can be influenced by antiarrhythmic drugs. For the interested reader, a more detailed discussion on cardiac physiology may be found in the textbooks listed under the 'Recommended Reading' section.

Cardiac Cell Types

Cardiac cells may be broadly divided into *pacemaker cells*, *specialised conduction cells* and the *working myocardium*. Throughout this chapter, the differences between each of these cells will become apparent. As the name suggests, the pacemaker cells are responsible for spontaneous generation of electrical impulses. They are prevalently located in the sinus node, although cells in the atrioventricular node (AVN) and His–Purkinje are also capable of performing this task.[1,2] The specialised conduction cells are responsible for rapid (e.g. Purkinje cells) or slow (e.g. AVN) propagation of the electrical impulse that ultimately reaches the working myocardial cells, triggering muscle contraction.

The Cardiac Action Potential

The ability of cells to generate and propagate electrical impulses is linked to the presence and movement of particles (ions or electrolytes) with positive or negative charges between both sides of the cell membrane. Mammalian cells are rich in potassium (K^+ = 150 mmol/L) and magnesium (Mg^{2+} = 12 mmol/L) and are bathed by fluid in the extracellular space that is rich in sodium (Na^+ = 140 mmol/L), calcium (Ca^{2+} = 1 mmol/L), chloride (Cl^- = 110 mmol/L) and bicarbonate (HCO_3^- = 30 mmol/L).[3] If these ions are allowed to move across the cell membrane, they will flow towards the less concentrated area and by doing so will create differences in electrical potential. This flow depends largely on the presence of ion channels, exchangers or pumps in the cell membrane. The various ionic currents across the membrane influence the resting membrane potential (RMP) and the cardiac action potential, as described in the remainder of this section.

Resting Membrane Potential

In the resting state, the inside of the cell is negatively charged, in contrast to the outside in which positive charges prevail. This is mainly due to different concentrations of Na^+ and K^+ molecules on both sides of the cell membrane. As mentioned in the last paragraph, the cell interior is rich in K^+ and the extracellular space is rich in Na^+. Numerous sodium–potassium pumps in the cell membrane constantly remove sodium from the cell (three Na^+ molecules) in exchange for potassium (two K^+ molecules), and this accounts for the accumulation of K^+ in the cell and of Na^+ in the extracellular space. It is apparent from this exchange that more positive charges leave the cell than enter it, leaving the inside of the cell with a deficit of positive charges. Additionally, the cell membrane is semipermeable to K^+, thereby allowing it to leak back into the extracellular space along its concentration gradient, causing an even greater loss of positive charges. By contrast, inward movement of Na^+ occurs to a much lesser extent, as the cell membrane is less permeable to Na^+ in comparison to K^+. Ultimately, these mechanisms are responsible for an imbalance of positive charges on both sides of the cell membrane, accounting for cell polarisation. The RMP of the various cardiac cells varies from –50 to –95 mV (Table 2.1).

Guide to Canine and Feline Electrocardiography, First Edition. Ruth Willis, Pedro Oliveira and Antonia Mavropoulou.
© 2018 John Wiley & Sons Ltd. Published 2018 by John Wiley & Sons Ltd.
Companion website: www.wiley.com/go/willis/electrocardiography

Table 2.1 Properties of membrane potentials in canine heart

	Sinus node cell	Atrial cardiomyocyte	Atrioventricular node cell	Purkinje fibre	Ventricular cardiomyocyte
Resting membrane potential (mV)	−56±7 mV[a]	−73 mV[b,c]	−50 to −60 mV[d]	−90 mV[e]	−84.2±2.7 mV[f]
Action potential duration (ms)	100–300 ms[g]	138±18 ms[h] 100–300 ms[g]	100–300 ms[g]	300–500 ms[i]	226.5±11 ms[f]
Propagation velocity	1.2–14 cm/s[h]	80 cm/s[j]	5.6±0.7 cm/s[k] 33–50 mm/s[l]	200–250 cm/s[m]	20–48 cm/s[n]
Fibre diameter (um)	5–10 μm[o]	15–20 μm[o]	7 μm[m]	50 μm[m]	20–33 μm[f]

References

a. Woods WT, Urthaler F, James TN. Spontaneous action potentials of cells in the canine sinus node. Circ Res. 1976;39:76–82.

b. Feng J, Yue L, Wang Z, Nattel S. Ionic mechanisms of regional action potential heterogeneity in the canine right atrium. Circ Res. 1998;83:541–551.

c. Li D, Zhang L, Kneller J, Nattel S. Potential ionic mechanism for repolarization differences between canine right and left atrium. Circ Res. 2001;88:1168–1175.

d. Bartos DC, Grandi E, Ripplinger CM. Ion channels in the heart. Compr Physiol. 2015;5:1423–1464.

e. Gadsby DC, Cranefield PF. Direct measurement of changes in sodium pump current in canine cardiac Purkinje fibers. Proc Natl Acad Sci USA. 1979;76:1783–1787.

f. Tseng GN, Robinson RB, Hoffman BF. Passive properties and membrane currents of canine ventricular myocytes. J Gen Physiol. 1987;90:671–701.

g. Britton OJ, Bueno-Orovio A, Van Ammel K, Lu HR, Towart R, Gallacher DJ, *et al.* Experimentally calibrated population of models predicts and explains intersubject variability in cardiac cellular electrophysiology. Proc Natl Acad Sci USA. 2013;110:E2098–E2105.

h. Fedorov VV, Schuessler RB, Hemphill M, Ambrosi CM, Chang R, Voloshina AS, *et al.* Structural and functional evidence for discrete exit pathways that connect the canine sinoatrial node and atria. Circ Res. 2009;104:915–923.

i. Aslanidi OV, Stewart P, Boyett MR, Zhang H. Optimal velocity and safety of discontinuous conduction through the heterogeneous Purkinje-ventricular junction. Biophys J. 2009;97:20–39.

j. Spach MS, Miller WT3, Dolber PC, Kootsey JM, Sommer JR, Mosher CEJ. The functional role of structural complexities in the propagation of depolarization in the atrium of the dog: cardiac conduction disturbances due to discontinuities of effective axial resistivity. Circ Res. 1982;50:175–191.

k. Woods WT, Sherf L, James TN. Structure and function of specific regions in the canine atrioventricular node. Am J Physiol. 1982;243:H41–H50.

l. Spach MS, Lieberman M, Scott JG, Barr RC, Johnson EA, Kootsey JM. Excitation sequences of the atrial septum and the AV node in isolated hearts of the dog and rabbit. Circ Res. 1971;29:156–172.

m. Meijler FL, Janse MJ. Morphology and electrophysiology of the mammalian atrioventricular node. Physiol Rev. 1988;68:608–647.

n. Linnenbank AC, De Bakker JMT, Coronel R. How to measure propagation velocity in cardiac tissue: a simulation study. Front Physiol. 2014;5:267.

o. Boyett MR, Honjo H, Kodama I. The sinoatrial node, a heterogeneous pacemaker structure. Cardio Res. 2000;47:658–687.

Ion Channels, Exchangers and Pumps

To understand the mechanisms that lead to cell depolarisation, it is important to first highlight the differences between the various types of ion carriers involved and how they work. Ion movement across the cell membrane depends on the presence of ion channels, exchangers or pumps:

Ion channels are pore-forming membrane proteins that allow passage of ions along an electrical or concentration gradient when in the open state.[4] Each channel is guarded by one or more gates that control its opening and closing in response to different triggers. Most ion channels involved in cell depolarisation and repolarisation are *voltage-gated*, which means that they open and close in response to differences in voltage across the membrane. Other triggers include ligands (e.g. acetylcholine) and stretch (which is detected by mechanoreceptors).[5]

Ion pumps move ions continuously against their concentration gradients and use energy (in the form of adenosine triphosphate [ATP]) in the process. They are responsible for maintaining the ion gradients across the cell membrane (e.g. a $3Na^+/2K^+$ pump).[4]

Ion exchangers are similar to pumps but exploit the energy stored in ion gradients rather than ATP hydrolysis to move ions against their concentration gradient. For example, the $3Na^+/1Ca^{2+}$ exchanger removes Ca^{2+} from inside the cell against its concentration gradient by moving Na^+ into the cell along its concentration gradient as its driving force. The excess Na^+ is then removed from the cell in exchange for K^+ by the $3Na^+/2K^+$ pump.[4]

Table 2.2 lists the various ion currents involved in cell depolarisation and correspondent carriers and characteristics.

Table 2.2 Ion currents and correspondent carriers involved in cardiac cell depolarisation and repolarisation

Ion current	Activation kinetics	Influenced by

I_{Na} – Fast inward sodium[5,6]	*Voltage-gated*
	Activation: –70 to –60 mV
	<1 ms
	    Overshoot: +20 to +35 mV
	    Inactivation: <1 to 4 ms
	    100% until <–40 mV
		• Increases with β-adrenergic stimulation
		• Blocked by class 1 anti-arrhythmics
		• Inhibited by hyperkalaemia

$I_{Ca(T)}$ – Transient calcium current[5,6]	*Voltage-gated*
	Activation: 10–20 ms
	    SA node: –60 to –50 mV
	    Atria: –50 mV
	    Ventricles: Absent
	    –40 mV in cats with HCM[7]
	Mean open time: 1–2 ms
	Inactivation: Rapid
		• No change with β-adrenergic stimulation
		• Blocked by nickel and amiloride

$I_{Ca(L)}$ – Long-lasting calcium current[5,6]	*Voltage-gated*
	Activation: 10–20 ms
	    SA node: –40 mV
	    Atria: –30 mV
	    Ventricles: –30 to –35 mV
	Mean open time: <1 ms
	Inactivation: Slow
	    100% until <0 mV
		• Increases with β-adrenergic stimulation
		• Blocked by class IV anti-arrhythmics (e.g. verapamil and diltiazem), amlodipine and nifedipine

I_{to1} – Transient outward potassium currents[6]
I_{to2} – Transient outward calcium-activated chloride current[6]
	Voltage-gated
	Activation: <10 ms
	    Inactivation:
	    Variable and voltage-dependent
		• Reduced expression with chronic adrenergic stimulation and angiotensin II

I_{Kur}, I_{Kr}, I_{Ks} – Delayed rectifier potassium currents[6]	*Voltage-gated* Activation: Slow, 100% at –10 mV Inactivation: Slow, deactivated by full repolarisation	• I_{Ks} increases with β-adrenergic stimulation • Blocked by class III anti-arrhythmics (e.g. amiodarone and sotalol)
I_{K1} or I_{Kir} – Inward rectifier potassium currents[5,6]	Above RMP: Outward current Below RMP: Inward current Inactivated with depolarisation	• Modified by ethanol and acetaldehyde[8]
$I_{Na/Ca}$ – Sodium-calcium exchange[5]	$3Na^+$ exchanged with $1Ca^{2+}$ Na^+ out if membrane potential is positive Ca^{2+} out if membrane potential is negative	
$I_{Na/K}$ – Sodium–potassium ATPase pump	$3Na^+$ driven out of cell whilst $2K^+$ are driven in 1 ATP molecule used per cycle	• Inhibited by digoxin
I_{Cl} – Chloride current	Inward flow of chloride	• Increases with β-adrenergic stimulation, shortening action potential
Additional currents (sinus node and atrioventricular node cells)		
I_f – Inward sodium (and potassium) current[5,9]	Activated with hyperpolarisation: –90 to –50 mV Pacemaker cells	• Increases with β-adrenergic stimulation • Blocked by ivabradine
I_{ACh} – Acetylcholine-activated potassium channel[6]	G protein-coupled inward potassium channels activated by acetylcholine Prevalent in sinus and atrioventricular nodes	• Parasympathetic stimulation

ATP, Adenosine triphosphate; HCM, hypertrophic cardiomyopathy; RMP, resting membrane potential; SA, sinoatrial node.

Relevant Aspects of Cardiac Cell Structure and Function

The cardiac muscle is organised as a syncytium of cells that are tightly interlinked by the presence of special junctions between adjacent cells called *intercalated disks* (Figure 2.1).[3] These are composed of specialised structures – *desmosomes* and *fascia adherens* – that form tight junctions, creating a strong mechanical link between each cell. Additionally, another structure is present in the intercalated disks that provides a functional connection between cells; it is called the *nexus* or *gap junction*.[5] Gap junctions allow the passage of ions from the cytoplasm of one cell to the next through aqueous pores, making it possible for the depolarisation wave to be transmitted from cell to cell. For this reason, when one cell becomes depolarised, the impulse is transmitted to all adjacent cells, resulting in a depolarisation wave that sweeps the entire myocardium until all cells become depolarised. The number and position of the intercalated disks influence the direction and velocity of the depolarisation wave. In cardiac muscle, they are more prevalent in the direction of the long axis of myocardial fibres, ensuring that the depolarisation wave is propagated in this direction rather than transversally.[10,11] This arrangement is logical as the myocardial fibres are oriented in specific ways that allow the heart to function effectively as a pump. Conduction in the myocardium is therefore *anisotropic* with a conduction velocity that is faster in the direction of the long axis of the myocardial fibres than it is transversally. This property of myocardial conduction has implications for

the genesis of arrhythmias, as given the right conditions (e.g. slower conduction in areas with damaged cells), it may allow re-entry to occur (see chapter 6).[12] There are protective mechanisms to prevent this from happening, such as the fact that gap junctions are able to change their electrical resistance in response to various conditions. For example, with myocardial infarction, there is an increase in intracellular calcium levels in damaged cells that causes the gap junctions with neighbouring cells to close in an attempt to protect them from the effects of the injured cells.[13] Changes in pH also have an effect on gap junctions: acidosis causes an increase in electrical resistance, slowing the rate of propagation of the action potential and possibly leading to conduction delay or block; alkalosis has the opposite effect.[14,15] These are some examples of cardiac cell physiology facts that are relevant to the genesis of cardiac arrhythmias in our patients. This topic will be developed further in chapter 6.

Cell Depolarisation and the Action Potential

Normally, the pacemaker cells in the sinoatrial node are responsible for initiating the depolarisation wave, which is then transmitted to all the cardiac myocytes. There are substantial differences between the depolarisation of conduction system cells (e.g. pacemaker cells, compact node cells and Purkinje cells) and working myocardial cells (e.g. atrial and ventricular). The RMP, and the shape and duration of the action potential, are shown in Figures 2.2 and 2.3.

The action potential in cardiac myocytes is generated by a series of ion movements, as described in the remainder of this section, which focuses on working myocardial and specialised conduction cells. The action potential of the pacemaker cells will be discussed in a separate section later in the chapter.

Stage 0 (rapid depolarisation due to inward flow of Na⁺)

In diastole, the RMP of a ventricular cell is close to −85 mV. An action potential triggered in a neighbouring cell causes a slight increase in potential to around −70 to −60 mV, which is the activation threshold for sodium channels, resulting in an inward current of Na⁺ (I_{Na}) that effectively causes depolarisation.[10,16] The membrane potential increases to above 0 mV. These channels are characterised by rapid activation (<1 ms) and inactivation (from <1 to 4 ms), which accounts for the very rapid depolarisation and steep upstroke of the action potential. This process is both time- and voltage-dependent, and the Na⁺ channels can exist in either of three states: when *activated*, they open; shortly after, they close, becoming *inactivated*; and, once the RMP has been restored, they enter a *resting state* and are ready to open again.

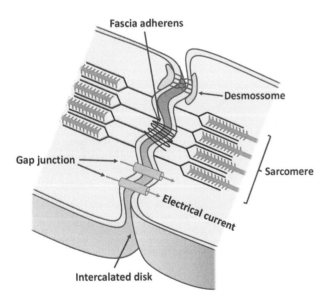

Figure 2.1 The intercalated disk. The intercalated disk is composed of specialised structures – *desmosomes* and *fascia adherens* – that form tight junctions creating a strong mechanical link between cells. The *gap junctions* provide a functional connection between cells that allows passage of ions.

Figure 2.2 Stages of the cardiac action potential and ionic currents. (A) Ventricular myocyte. (B) Pacemaker cell. Note that in ventricular myocytes, the action potential has five stages – 0, 1, 2, 3 and 4 – whereas in pacemaker cells stages 1 and 2 are absent.

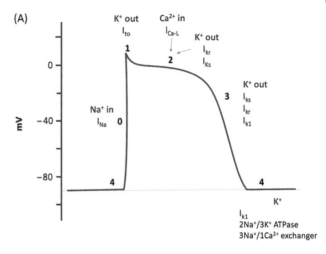

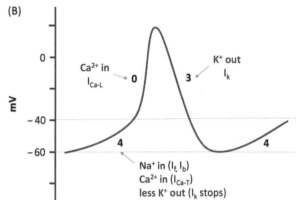

Figure 2.3 The cardiac action potential of the various cardiac cells.

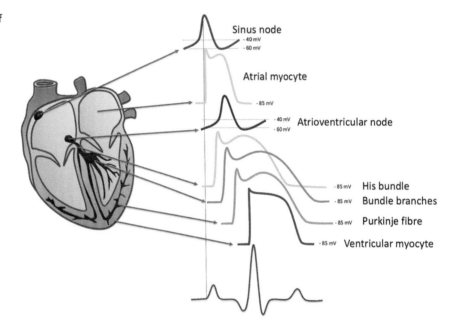

Stage 1 (rapid repolarisation)

With the increase in membrane potential above 0 mV, another type of voltage-gated channels (I_{to}) become activated, allowing the exit of K^+ from the cell.[17,18] At the same time, the Na^+ channels have entered the inactivated state, and the inward Na^+ current has stopped. The combination of these two events leads to a net decrease in membrane potential to approximately 0 mV. This is stage 1 of the action potential. I_{to} channels are present in higher densities in Purkinje cells, atrial cells, epicardial cells and mid-myocardial ventricular cells in comparison to endocardial ventricular cells, resulting in a more prominent phase 1, as shown in Figure 2.3.[19]

Stage 2 (plateau phase)

During this stage, there is a combination of several ion currents involving a balance between entry of Ca^{2+} in the cell (I_{Ca-L}) and exit of K^+ (I_K and I_{to}).[10,16] During stage 0 of depolarisation, voltage-gated calcium channels (L subtype) become activated when the voltage reaches −35 to −30 mV. They open quickly (<1 ms) but inactivation is slow, accounting for the duration of stage 2 (Figure 2.2). During this period, the inward Ca^{2+} flow will trigger release of Ca^{2+} from the sarcoplasmic reticulum, causing muscle contraction in working myocardial cells. The outward flow of K^+ during this stage is due to activation of several channels, of which the most important are the voltage-gated I_{Kr} (*r* for rapid) and I_{Ks} (*s* for slow) currents. They become fully active during depolarisation when the membrane potential reaches −10 mV, and their function is enhanced with the increased internal calcium levels.[20] The activity of I_{to} channels also has an influence on the duration and amplitude of stage 2.[21] As mentioned in this chapter, they are more prevalent in atrial cells and epi-/mid-myocardial ventricular cells, contributing to a lower plateau phase and shorter action potential (see Figure 2.3).

Stage 3 (repolarisation)

As the L-type calcium channels become inactivated and the I_{ca-L} current stops, the outward currents of K^+ continue until the RMP is restored once again. In addition to the I_{Kr} and I_{Ks} currents, a background K^+ current (I_{K1} or I_{Kir}) contributes to late phase 3 repolarisation.[10,16] These channels aim to maintain the RMP by allowing the exit of K^+ from the cell if the potential is above the RMP and allowing entry of K^+ into the cell if the membrane potential is below the RMP. During depolarisation, they are briefly shut and open again during the repolarisation stages.

Stage 4 (resting state)

During this stage, the changes that occurred during depolarisation are rectified. The $3Na^+/2K^+$ ATPase pumps and the $3Na^+/1Ca^{2+}$ exchanger work to remove the excess Na^+ and Ca^{2+} from the cell and restore the K^+ levels. It is important to highlight that the ionic movements driving cell depolarisation and repolarisation involve only minute amounts of ions and the cell content of these ions remains virtually unchanged.[16]

Cell Excitability and Refractoriness

The ability to generate an action potential following an electrical impulse of sufficient magnitude represents the *excitability* of the cell. This is proportional to the intensity of the electrical stimulus propagated from cell to cell that is able to trigger depolarisation (stage 0 of the action potential). This will also depend on the RMP and how close it is to the activation threshold which is the membrane potential above which cell depolarisation occurs. If cells are more or less excitable than normal, this will have significant implications on heart rate, conduction velocity and likelihood of arrhythmias.[12,16]

Once depolarisation is triggered, the cell is unable to generate another action potential until repolarisation occurs (from stage 0 until the end of stage 3). The cell becomes *refractory* to additional stimuli during this period because the fast sodium channels become inactivated at membrane potentials above −50 mV. Until the membrane potential falls below this threshold during stage 3 of repolarisation, the cell is incapable of generating another action potential regardless of the intensity of the triggering stimulus. This is the *effective refractory period* (ERP) (Figure 2.4). Whilst the membrane potential is between −50 mV and the resting membrane potential (−85 to −90 mV, which is reached at the end of stage 3), it may be possible for a stimulus of sufficient magnitude to trigger an early depolarisation. The resulting action potential will have a slower stage 0 and will achieve lower voltages which result in a slower conduction velocity, as a proportion of fast sodium channels are still inactive at this stage. This is the *relative refractory period* (RRP). By the end of the RRP, there is a period called the *vulnerable period* in which a stimulus of sufficient intensity may cause a repetitive response. A relevant example would be the triggering of ventricular fibrillation when a premature beat (an ectopic or paced beat) happens to occur during the vulnerable period, which on the electrocardiogram corresponds to the peak of the T wave. The vulnerable period for the atrial myocardium occurs during the descending R wave or during the S wave of the

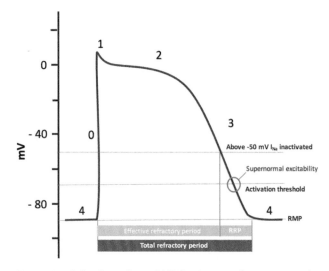

Figure 2.4 Cell refractoriness. RMP, Resting membrane potential; RRP, relative refractory period.

electrocardiogram. By the end of stage 3, but before the cell is fully repolarised, the membrane potential is close to the activation threshold for depolarisation, and it may be possible for depolarisation to be triggered by weaker stimuli. The cell is in a *period of supernormal excitability*.

The sum of the ERP and RRP is the *total refractory period* (TRP). It lasts from the beginning of stage 0 until the end of stage 3 of the action potential which on the electrocardiogram corresponds to the beginning of the QRS to the end of the T wave.

Differences in the Action Potential Between Different Areas of the Heart – Purkinje Fibres Compared to Working Myocardial Cells

The action potential of cardiac cells varies according to the cell type and function, as is illustrated in Figure 2.3. Conduction system cells such as the Purkinje cells are capable of rapid transmission of the cardiac impulse, and to facilitate this they display more pronounced stages 0 and 1 of the action potential, reaching a higher positive membrane potential and rapid depolarisation. This occurs due to a larger inward flow of Na^+ (I_{Na}) and a larger early outward potassium current (I_{to}). The action potential is also longer due to slower repolarisation (a longer stage 3) in comparison to normal working cells. This is important as it ensures that Purkinje cells stay refractory for a longer period, thereby preventing re-entry of the impulse back up the conduction system after the ventricles have been depolarised.[16,22–24]

Pacemaker Cells

The pacemaker cells in the sinoatrial node have the important task of spontaneously generating electrical impulses that effectively initiate the heartbeat. This is made possible by spontaneous depolarisation currents during stage 4 of the action potential – the *voltage clock*.[2,5,16] Figure 2.5 illustrates these currents and the resulting action potential that differs from the other cardiac cells.

The RMP of pacemaker cells, at around –65 mV, is higher than that of working myocardial cells. During stage 4 of the action potential, the membrane potential increases to approximately –40 mV, at which point rapid depolarisation is triggered. This spontaneous increase is due to a combination of the following ionic currents.

Outward K^+ Current (I_k)

It was mentioned in this chapter that constant leakage of K^+ ions from the cells is a major contributor to the RMP. In pacemaker cells, the K^+ currents have an important influence on the spontaneous increase in the RMP

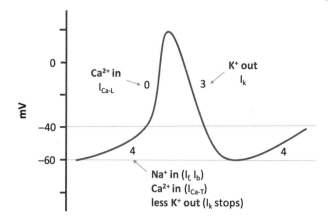

Figure 2.5 Pacemaker currents and action potential. During the resting state (stage 4), there is a spontaneous increase in membrane potential due to a combination of inward flow of Na^+ (I_f, I_b) and Ca^{2+} (I_{Ca-T}), and a reduction in outward flow of K^+ (I_k). When the depolarisation threshold is reached at approximately –40 mV, L-type Ca^{2+} channels open, allowing Ca^{2+} to enter the cell causing cell depolarisation (stage 0) until they become inactivated less than 1 ms later. Cell repolarisation then follows via outward flow of K^+ (I_k).

during stage 4. The major potassium current in these cells is the I_K (also called the *delayed rectifier*), whereas the background current (I_{K1} or I_{Kir}) does not exist.[5] The reduction in outward K^+ current during stage 4 together with the other pacemaker currents make it possible for the cell to spontaneously depolarise, as shown in Figure 2.5. I_k is activated by depolarisation and then contributes to repolarisation during stage 3 before stopping, as this current is time dependent.

Inward Ca^{2+} Currents (I_{Ca}) – the Calcium Clock

In contrast to cardiac myocytes, the depolarisation of pacemaker cells occurs via inward Ca^{2+} currents (I_{Ca}) rather than fast sodium currents (I_{Na}). This explains the slower upstroke of the action potential during stage 0.

Two types of currents can be identified mediated by different channels (Figure 2.5). The relatively rapid depolarisation (stage 0) is due to activation of L-type channels causing long-lasting calcium current. These channels are activated when the membrane potential reaches approximately –40 mV. During stage 4, a transient calcium current occurs via T-type channels that become activated when the membrane potential is around –60 to –50 mV. This current contributes to the spontaneous depolarisation of pacemaker cells.

$I_{Na/Ca}$ exchange is also involved in normal pacemaker activity. During late stage 3 and stage 4 of the action potential, the $I_{Na/Ca}$ channel is active, exchanging three extracellular Na ions with one intracellular calcium ion, resulting in a net intracellular charge gain. $I_{Na/Ca}$ is activated by spontaneous rhythmic calcium release from the sarcoplasmic reticulum in a process that is highly regulated by cyclic adenosine 3′,5′-monophosphate (cAMP) and the autonomic nervous system.[25] Delayed afterdepolarisations and triggered activity may occur via abnormal $I_{Na/Ca}$ activation.[26]

Inward Na⁺ Current (I_f) – the 'Funny Channels'

Pacemaker cells possess channels that allow Na⁺ and K⁺ currents (I_f) depending on the membrane potential. They are activated during stage 4 at membrane potentials below −40 to −45 mV and lead to inward flow of Na⁺ and K⁺, causing a progressive increase in membrane potential during stage 4 until the activation threshold is reached.[27] I_f is effectively a pacemaker current that increases with sympathetic stimulation, leading to a more rapid stage 4 and therefore an increase in heart rate.[28]

Inward Background Na⁺ Current (I_b)

Another sodium current has been proposed to be involved in spontaneous depolarisation of pacemaker cells.[29] This current was termed I_b for background or I_p for pacemaker. It is not time-dependent and is thought to rely on entry of Na⁺ ions into the cell.

Other Pacemaker Currents

Other ion currents may contribute to the spontaneous depolarisation of the pacemaker cells.[16] They are all thought to contribute, and the absence of one does not completely stop the process (e.g. the I_f may be blocked by the drug ivabradine and, despite causing a reduction in heart rate, it does not stop the pacemaker cells from depolarising).

Interestingly, genetic mutations that affect a single pacemaker current do not always result in severe symptomatic bradycardia – for example, many human patients with reduced I_f are asymptomatic and can increase their heart rate to >150 beats/min during exercise.[25] However, in situations such as atrial fibrillation and heart failure, more than one current may be affected and significant sinus dysfunction can occur as a complication of the disease.[25]

Autonomic Control of the Pacemaker Cells

Sympathetic stimulation leads to an increase in heart rate, whereas an increase in parasympathetic tone has the opposite effect. Additionally, an increase in sympathetic tone is accompanied by a decrease in parasympathetic tone, and vice versa. Their effects on the pacemaker cells are discussed in this section and are illustrated in Figure 2.6.

Sympathetic Stimulation

During periods of sympathetic stimulation, the I_f current is increased, leading to an increase in heart rate.[27,30,31] This is influenced by the production of cAMP, which increases the probability of opening of I_f channels and also of the long-lasting calcium channels (I_{Ca-L}). The end result is a faster rate of depolarisation during stage 4, ultimately resulting in a faster heart rate. Additionally, under adrenergic stimulation, there is a shift from the dominant P cells in the centre of sinus node to the more peripheral T cells (see chapter 1).[32] The latter have a lower diastolic resting membrane potential (they are more polarised) which favours maximal activation of the I_f current.

β-adrenergic stimulation results in increased levels of intracellular cAMP and cAMP-dependent protein kinase A (PKA), which in turn leads to activation of proteins that regulate intracellular calcium balance and spontaneous sarcoplasmic reticulum calcium cycling (phospholamban and L-type calcium channels).[25,33] The PKA-dependent phosphorylation of these proteins determines the phase and size of subsarcolemmal sarcoplasmic reticulum calcium release and its influence on the sinoatrial depolarisation rate.[33]

Parasympathetic Stimulation

During parasympathetic stimulation, acetylcholine is released and activates acetylcholine–ligand potassium channels that allow an outward flow of K⁺ (I_{KACh}).[16,30] This reduction in intracellular K⁺ leads to a lower resting membrane potential (hyperpolarisation), making it more difficult for the activation threshold to be reached and effectively lowering the heart rate.

Overdrive Suppression of Pacemaker Cells

In normal conditions, the pacemaker cells of the sinus node are dominant, but other cells capable of spontaneous depolarisation exist lower down the conduction system. The cells in the AVN, bundle of His and Purkinje fibres are possible subsidiary pacemakers that may become active if the sinus node fails. Spontaneous depolarisation during stage 4 is slower in these cells, accounting for a lower discharge rate. Since the depolarisation rate of sinus node cells is normally higher, these subsidiary pacemakers do not have time to reach the activation threshold and, in other words, never get a chance to act as dominant

Figure 2.6 Effect of sympathetic and parasympathetic stimulation on pacemaker cells. Sympathetic stimulation results in an increase in inward sodium (I_f) and calcium (I_{Ca-L}) currents via increased levels of cAMP inside the cell. The end result is a faster rate of depolarisation during stage 4, ultimately resulting in a faster heart rate. Additionally, under adrenergic stimulation there is a shift from the dominant P cells in the centre of the sinus node to the more peripheral T cells that have a lower diastolic resting membrane potential (they are more polarised), favouring maximal activation of the I_f current. Parasympathetic stimulation causes an increase in outward K^+ currents during stage 4 via activation of acetylcholine–ligand potassium channels (I_{KACh}). This reduction in intracellular K^+ leads to a lower resting membrane potential (hyperpolarisation), making it more difficult for the activation threshold to be reached and effectively lowering the heart rate.

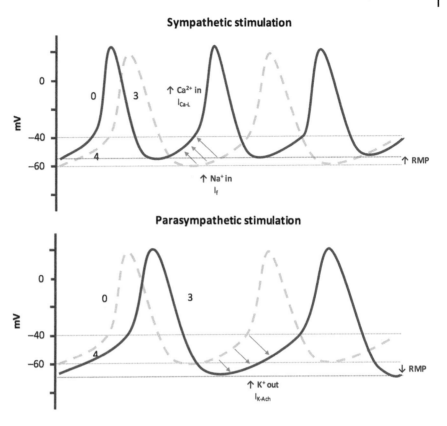

pacemakers. This is mainly due to the fact that when the latent pacemakers are depolarised at a higher rate by the dominant pacemaker, they tend to accumulate intracellular Na^+ as a result of the increased depolarisation rate. The increased Na^+ stimulates the $3Na^+/2K^+$ pump that leads to hyperpolarisation of the cell, making it more difficult to reach the threshold potential.[34] This phenomenon is called *overdrive suppression*, and it is an important concept in the study of electrocardiography and cardiac arrhythmias.[16,35] If for some reason the sinus node fails or is suppressed, the activity of a subsidiary pacemaker may become apparent. A typical example occurs during anaesthesia when the sinus rate is lowered (e.g. during opioid influence) and a junctional or ventricular rhythm is seen competing with the sinus rhythm (see chapter 24).

Atrioventricular Node Cells

The AVN acts as a filter for impulses arriving from the atria towards the ventricles. One of its main purposes is to cause a slight delay in impulse transmission to allow the atria to contract just before the ventricles to ensure ventricular filling is optimised. This is possible due to different conduction properties of the cells in the

compact node. These cells are similar to the transitional cells in the sinus node and display the same electrophysiological characteristics (Figure 2.3).[11,36,37] The rapid depolarisation stage of the action potential relies on an inward Ca^{2+} (I_{Ca-T} and I_{Ca-L}) current rather than Na^+ which means that the impulse propagation is slower in comparison to the rest of the conduction system and even normal working myocardial cells. This characteristic is often used to our advantage when treating supraventricular tachyarrhythmias with calcium channel blockers (e.g. diltiazem and verapamil). The aim is to further reduce the velocity of conduction through the AVN and the number of impulses that actually reach the ventricles.

The AVN cells also display spontaneous depolarisation during stage 4 of the action potential, albeit at a slower rate, and therefore are normally overdrive suppressed by the sinus node.[38] As described for the sinus node, the AVN is heavily influenced by the autonomic nervous system. Sympathetic stimulation increases conduction velocity of the AVN (positive dromotropic effect), whereas parasympathetic stimulation has the opposite effect (negative dromotropic effect). This effect is mediated by increasing (sympathetic) or decreasing (parasympathetic) the long-lasting Ca^{2+} current (I_{Ca-L}).[31,39]

Recommended Reading

Cunningham JG, Bradley GK. Textbook of veterinary physiology (4th ed.). Amsterdam: Saunders Elsevier; 2007.

Katz AM. Physiology of the heart (5th ed.). Philadelphia: Lippincott Williams & Wilkins; 2011.

Opie LH. Heart physiology: from cell to circulation (4th ed.). Philadelphia: Lippincott Williams & Wilkins; 2004.

References

1 Laske TG, Shrivastav M, Iaizzo PA. In Handbook of cardiac anatomy, physiology, and devices (ed. Iaizzo PA, pp. 159–175). New York: Springer; 2009. doi:10.1007/978-1-60327-372-5_11

2 Dobrzynski H, Boyett MR, Anderson RH. New insights into pacemaker activity: promoting understanding of sick sinus syndrome. Circulation. 2007;115:1921–1932.

3 Heideman SR. In Textbook of veterinary physiology (eds. Cunningham JG, Klein BG). New York: Elsevier; 2007.

4 Gadsby DC. Ion channels versus ion pumps: the principal difference, in principle. Nat Rev Mol Cell Biol. 2009;10:344–352.

5 Opie LH. In Heart physiology: from cell to circulation (ed. Opie LH, pp. 73–118). Philadelphia: Lippincott Williams & Wilkins; 2004.

6 Grant AO. Cardiac ion channels. Circ Arrhythm Electrophysiol. 2009;2:185–194.

7 Nuss HB, Houser SR. T-type Ca^{2+} current is expressed in hypertrophied adult feline left ventricular myocytes. Circ Res. 1993;73:777–782.

8 Horakova Z, Matejovic P, Pasek M, Hosek J, Simurdova M, Simurda J, *et al.* Effect of ethanol and acetaldehyde at clinically relevant concentrations on atrial inward rectifier potassium current IK1: separate and combined effect. J Physiol Pharmacol. 2016;67:339–351.

9 DiFrancesco D, Borer JS. The funny current: cellular basis for the control of heart rate. Drugs. 2007;67:15–24.

10 Kleber AG, Rudy Y. Basic mechanisms of cardiac impulse propagation and associated arrhythmias. Physiol Rev. 2004;84:431–488.

11 Opie LH. In Heart physiology: from cell to circulation (ed. Opie LH, pp. 42–69). Philadelphia: Lippincott Williams & Wilkins; 2004.

12 Gaztañaga L, Marchlinski FE, Betensky BP. Mechanisms of cardiac arrhythmias. Revista Española de Cardiología (Engl ed). 2012;65:174–185.

13 Vila J, Pariaut R, Moïse NS, Oxford EM, Fox PR, Reynolds CA, *et al.* Structural and molecular pathology of the atrium in boxer arrhythmogenic right ventricular cardiomyopathy. J Vet Cardiol. 2017;19:57–67.

14 Takamatsu T. Arrhythmogenic substrates in myocardial infarct. Pathol Int. 2008;58:533–543.

15 Vorperian VR, Wisialowski TA, Deegan R, Roden DM. Effect of hypercapnic acidemia on anisotropic propagation in the canine ventricle. Circulation. 1994;90:456–461.

16 Opie LH. In Heart physiology: from cell to circulation (ed. Opie LH, pp. 119–156). Philadelphia: Lippincott Williams & Wilkins; 2004.

17 Furukawa T, Myerburg RJ, Furukawa N, Bassett AL, Kimura S. Differences in transient outward currents of feline endocardial and epicardial myocytes. Circ Res. 1990;67:1287–1291.

18 Tseng GN, Hoffman BF. Two components of transient outward current in canine ventricular myocytes. Circ Res. 1989;64:633–647.

19 Litovsky SH, Antzelevitch C. Transient outward current prominent in canine ventricular epicardium but not endocardium. Circ Res. 1988;62:116–126.

20 Nitta J, Furukawa T, Marumo F, Sawanobori T, Hiraoka M. Subcellular mechanism for Ca(2+)-dependent enhancement of delayed rectifier K^+ current in isolated membrane patches of guinea pig ventricular myocytes. Circ Res. 1994;74:96–104.

21 Greenstein JL, Wu R, Po S, Tomaselli GF, Winslow RL. Role of the calcium-independent transient outward current I(to1) in shaping action potential morphology and duration. Circ Res. 2000;87:1026–1033.

22 Verkerk AO, Veldkamp MW, Abbate F, Antoons G, Bouman LN, Ravesloot JH, *et al.* Two types of action potential configuration in single cardiac Purkinje cells of sheep. Am J Physiol. 1999;277:H1299–H1310.

23 Li P, Rudy Y. A model of canine purkinje cell electrophysiology and Ca(2+) cycling: rate dependence, triggered activity, and comparison to ventricular myocytes. Circ Res. 2011;109:71–79.

24 Vassalle M, Bocchi L. Differences in ionic currents between canine myocardial and Purkinje cells. Physiol Rep. 2013;1:1–34.

25 Chen P-S, Joung B, Shinohara T, Das M, Chen Z, Lin S.-F. The initiation of the heart beat. Circ J. 2010;74:221–225.

26 Mangoni ME, Nargeot J. Genesis and regulation of the heart automaticity. Physiol Rev. 2008;88:919–982.

27 DiFrancesco D. The role of the funny current in pacemaker activity. Circ Res. 2010;106:434–446.

28 Brown HF, DiFrancesco D, Noble SJ. How does adrenaline accelerate the heart? Nature. 1979;280:235–236.

29 Dokos S, Celler B, Lovell N. Ion currents underlying sinoatrial node pacemaker activity: a new single cell mathematical model. J Theor Biol. 1996;181:245–272.

30 Brown H, DiFrancesco D, Noble S. Cardiac pacemaker oscillation and its modulation by autonomic transmitters. J Exper Biol. 1979;81:175–204.

31 Randall WC, Ardell JL, O'Toole MF, Wurster RD. Differential autonomic control of SAN and AVN regions of the canine heart: structure and function. Prog Clin Biol Res. 1988;275:15–31.

32 Goldberg JM. Intra-SA-nodal pacemaker shifts induced by autonomic nerve stimulation in the dog. Am J Physiol. 1975;229:1116–1123.

33 Vinogradova TM, Lyashkov AE, Zhu W, Ruknudin AM, Sirenko S, Yang D, *et al.* High basal protein kinase A-dependent phosphorylation drives rhythmic internal Ca^{2+} store oscillations and spontaneous beating of cardiac pacemaker cells. Circ Res. 2006;98:505–514.

34 Vassalle M. The relationship among cardiac pacemakers: overdrive suppression. Circ Res. 1977;41:269–277.

35 Neely BH, Urthaler F, Hageman GR. Differences in the determinants of overdrive suppression between sinus rhythm and slow atrioventricular junctional rhythm. Circ Res. 1985;57:182–191.

36 McGuire MA, DeBakker JM, Vermeulen JT, Moorman AF, Loh P, Thibault B, *et al.* Atrioventricular junctional tissue: discrepancy between histological and electrophysiological characteristics. Circulation. 1996;94:571–577.

37 Meijler FL, Janse MJ. Morphology and electrophysiology of the mammalian atrioventricular node. Physiol Rev. 1988;68:608–647.

38 Mesirca P, Marger L, Torrente A, Striessnig J. Pacemaker cells of the atrioventricular node are Ca v 1.3 dependent oscillators. Biophys J. 2010;98:339a.

39 Geis WP, Kaye MP, Randall WC. Major autonomic pathways to the atria and S-A and A-V nodes of the canine heart. Am J Physiol. 1973;224:202–208.

3

Cardiac Vectors and the Genesis of the Electrocardiogram

Pedro Oliveira

The electrocardiogram (ECG) is a graphic representation of the electrical impulses generated within the heart during the different stages of the cardiac cycle. As mentioned in chapter 2, specialised cells in the sinoatrial node can spontaneously generate electrical impulses that are subsequently transmitted in an ordered fashion to the working myocardium and trigger contraction. These impulses are transmitted from cell to cell, generating electrical currents that travel through the heart with a certain direction and energy. The electrocardiograph senses these currents by detecting electrical changes between two electrodes positioned in the body and displays them graphically as a series of deflections (waves) known as the ECG.

The normal flow of electrical currents through the heart and how it translates into the ECG will be discussed in this chapter.

Basic Principles

The Electrocardiograph

The electrocardiograph is a galvanometer – an instrument that is able to detect the presence, direction and strength of electrical currents.[1,2] It uses two electrodes that conduct the electricity from the skin surface to the galvanometer. The strength (voltage) of the electrical current is measured over time and is displayed on the ECG. One of the electrodes acts as the positive pole (exploring electrode), whilst the other is the negative pole (indifferent or reference electrode). If the electrical current moves towards the exploring electrode, a positive deflection will be recorded (Figure 3.1A). Movement in the opposite direction will result in a negative deflection (Figure 3.1C). If the exploring electrode is perpendicular to the direction of the electrical current, a positive deflection followed by a negative

deflection will be seen (Figure 3.1B), as the current moves towards the electrode initially and then away from it.[3]

The Electric Dipole

Imagine a single cardiac cell undergoing depolarisation (Figure 3.2).

In the resting state, there is a prevalence of negative charges inside the cell in contrast to the outside compartment (see chapter 2). As depolarisation starts, an area of the cell will start to fill up with positive charges (positive pole), whilst in the other end negative charges still prevail (negative pole). This creates an electrical dipole with a potential difference between both extremities of the cell. If two electrodes were positioned on each end of the cell and then attached to a galvanometer, this potential difference (voltage) could be recorded and displayed graphically over time. This is depicted in Figure 3.2. Before depolarisation, a flat line (baseline) is seen (Figure 3.2A). Upon the start of depolarisation and creation of a potential difference, a deflection is registered with its peak at maximal potential difference (Figure 3.2B) and then a return to baseline as the whole cell is depolarised (Figure 3.2C).

Given that all cardiac cells are interconnected with free passage of the action potential from one cell to the other, the same principle can be applied to the whole myocardium.[4,5]

Cardiac Vectors

A vector is a diagrammatic way to represent the direction and strength of an electrical impulse (Figure 3.3).[6,7] In the example given in 'The electric dipole' section, the electrical impulse caused by depolarisation of a single cardiac cell can be represented as a small vector

Guide to Canine and Feline Electrocardiography, First Edition. Ruth Willis, Pedro Oliveira and Antonia Mavropoulou.
© 2018 John Wiley & Sons Ltd. Published 2018 by John Wiley & Sons Ltd.
Companion website: www.wiley.com/go/willis/electrocardiography

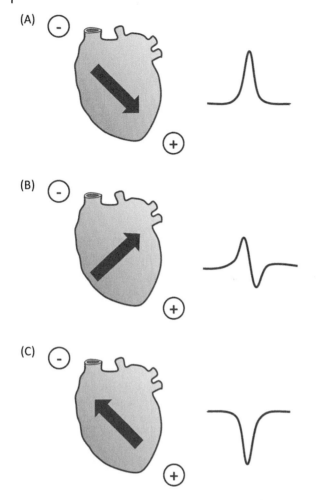

Figure 3.1 Appearance of the electrocardiographic deflections depending on the direction of the electrical current in relation to the exploring electrode (+). (A) If the electrical current moves towards the exploring electrode, a positive deflection is recorded. (B) If the exploring electrode is perpendicular to the direction of the electrical current, a positive deflection followed by a negative deflection is seen as the current moves towards the electrode initially and then away from it. (C) If the electrical current moves away from the exploring electrode, a negative deflection is recorded.

pointing in the direction of depolarisation (Figure 3.3A). Now imagine that the cells to the left, to the right and in front of that cell are depolarised. This creates three new vectors with different directions (Figure 3.3B). These three individual vectors can be added or subtracted. Vectors going in the same direction add up, whilst vectors travelling in opposite directions cancel each other out (Figure 3.4). Vectors at an angle add or subtract energy and change direction when they meet (Figure 3.4). As the depolarisation wave travels from one myocardial cell to the next, millions of individual vectors are created until the whole myocardium has been depolarised. The sum of these vectors represents the general direction and energy of the electrical impulse as it flows through the myocardium. The energy (voltage) is proportional to the mass of myocardium involved, and the direction depends on where the impulse originated and the direction of travel. The different vectors that represent atrial and ventricular depolarisation as well as repolarisation will be discussed later in this chapter, when the genesis of the ECG is described.

Electrocardiographic Leads

Several sets of electrodes are used in clinical electrocardiography to study the flow of electricity through the heart in the different anatomical planes (Figure 3.5). These are called the *electrocardiographic leads*. Each lead interrogates the flow of electricity in a specific direction as if we were 'viewing the heart from different perspectives'. By combining the information given by all leads, the propagation of electricity can be studied in all three dimensions.

Two main lead systems are used:

- Hexaxial system
- Precordial system.

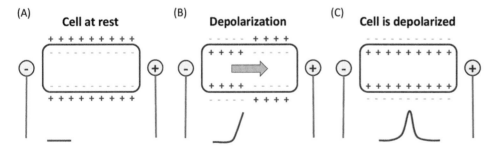

Figure 3.2 Illustration of the deflections recorded on the electrocardiogram during cell depolarisation. A cell is depicted with electrocardiographic electrodes on each extremity with the corresponding electrocardiographic trace below. (A) In the resting state, there is a prevalence of negative charges inside the cell in contrast to the outside compartment. Since there is no movement of electrical charges, the electrocardiograph records a flat line (baseline) without any positive or negative deflections. (B) As depolarisation starts, an area of the cell starts to fill up with positive charges (positive pole), whilst in the other end negative charges still prevail (negative pole). This creates an electrical dipole with a potential difference between both extremities of the cell. The electrocardiograph records this potential difference (voltage) as a deflection with its peak at maximal potential difference. (C) Once the entire cell is depolarised, there is no longer a potential difference between the cell extremities, and the electrocardiograph displays a return to baseline.

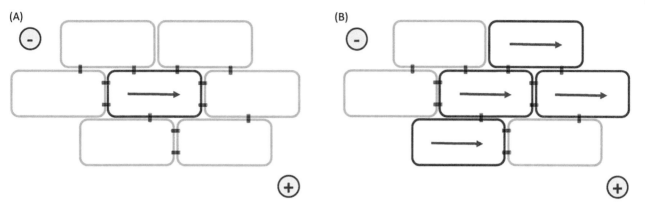

Figure 3.3 Depolarisation of neighbouring cells and respective individual depolarisation vectors (arrows).

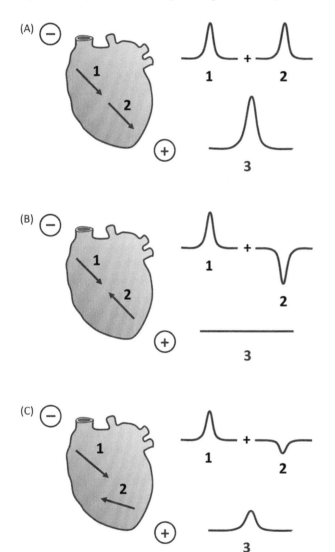

Figure 3.4 Vector summation and subtraction and its effect on the electrocardiographic deflections. (A) Two vectors travelling in the same direction add up (1 + 2), resulting in a larger electrocardiographic deflection (3) than they would individually. (B) Two vectors of the same amplitude travelling in the exact opposite direction cancel each other out and do not cause a deflection on the electrocardiogram. (C) Two vectors travelling at an angle add or subtract energy.

The Hexaxial System

The hexaxial system is the most commonly used lead system. It allows the assessment of electrical activity in the frontal plane, which is why they are often referred to as the frontal leads. As the name indicates, it includes six distinct leads (Figures 3.6, 3.7 and 3.8).

Bipolar, or Standard, Limb Leads

Leads I, II and III were the first leads to be used in clinical practice in the early 1900s. They were devised by the Dutch physiologist Willem Einthoven and have been in use ever since.[8–10] By positioning one electrode on each forelimb and a third electrode on one of the hindlimbs, three bipolar leads are obtained forming an inverted triangle with the heart at the centre – *Einthoven's triangle* (Figure 3.6). In a biped patient, the shape of this triangle is roughly equilateral if the arms are held apart and the feet are kept together. In our quadruped patients, this is not exactly the case, and therefore some assumptions are not entirely correct (e.g. lead III in humans points downwards and to the right whereas in dogs it points caudally); however, this detail is normally overlooked, and this lead system is considered adequate for clinical purposes.[11]

Lead I: Lead I uses the left forelimb electrode as the exploring electrode (positive) and the right forelimb electrode as the reference electrode (negative). A depolarisation wave travelling from right to left will cause a positive deflection on the ECG, and the opposite will cause a negative deflection.

Lead II: Lead II uses the left hindlimb electrode as the exploring electrode (positive) and the right forelimb electrode as the reference electrode (negative). A depolarisation wave travelling 'downwards and to the left' (cranial-to-caudal and right-to-left) will cause a positive deflection on the ECG, and the opposite will cause a negative deflection.

Lead III: Lead III uses the left hindlimb electrode as the exploring electrode (positive) and the left forelimb electrode as the reference electrode (negative).

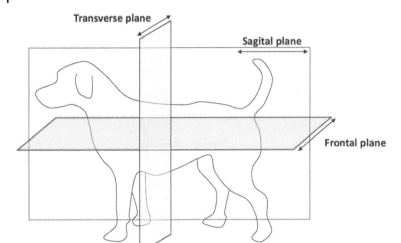

Figure 3.5 The anatomical planes.

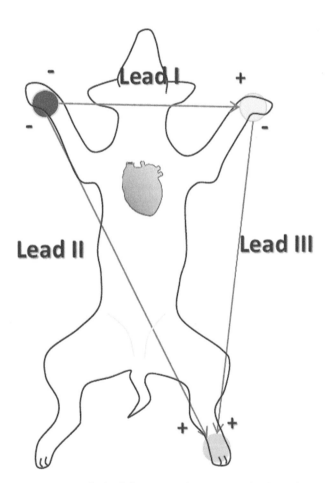

Figure 3.6 Bipolar leads forming Einthoven's triangle. Electrodes are placed in the forelimbs and the left hindlimb to record leads I, II and III.

A depolarisation wave travelling 'downwards' (cranial-to-caudal) will cause a positive deflection on the ECG, and the opposite will cause a negative deflection. Assuming an equilateral triangle, depolarisation from left to right would also cause a positive deflection.

Unipolar Limb Leads

To increase the number of 'viewing perspectives' available, three additional leads were integrated with Einthoven's bipolar lead system to create the hexaxial system. These are the augmented unipolar leads and use the same limb electrodes as described in this chapter, although they do not use two dedicated electrodes like the bipolar leads (Figure 3.7). They were introduced by Emanuel Goldberger in 1942.[12,13] The term *unipolar* was popularised by Frank Wilson and colleagues, who a few years earlier had suggested the measurement of unipolar potentials with respect to a remote reference (indifferent electrode) formed by all three limb electrodes interconnected, which is called *Wilson's central terminal* (WCT).[14,15] However, by using WCT as the reference electrode (negative) and each limb electrode (R for right arm, L for left arm and F for foot) as the exploring electrode (positive), only low-amplitude waves and thick-lined (>2 mm) ECG traces were obtained. Goldberger suggested disconnecting the electrode of the unipolar lead being recorded from the indifferent electrode.[13] This resulted in a 50% augmentation of the recorded limb leads and gave rise to the augmented unipolar leads: aVR, aVL and aVF.

Lead aVR: Lead aVR uses the right forelimb electrode as the exploring electrode (positive). A depolarisation wave travelling 'upwards and to the right' (caudal-to-cranial and left-to-right) will cause a positive deflection on the ECG, and the opposite will cause a negative deflection.

Lead aVL: Lead aVL uses the left forelimb electrode as the exploring electrode (positive). A depolarisation wave travelling 'upwards and to the left' (caudal-to-cranial and right-to-left) will cause a positive deflection on the ECG, and the opposite will cause a negative deflection.

Lead aVF: Lead aVF uses the left hindlimb electrode as the exploring electrode (positive). A depolarisation wave travelling 'downwards' (cranial-to-caudal) will cause a positive deflection on the ECG, and the opposite will cause a negative deflection.

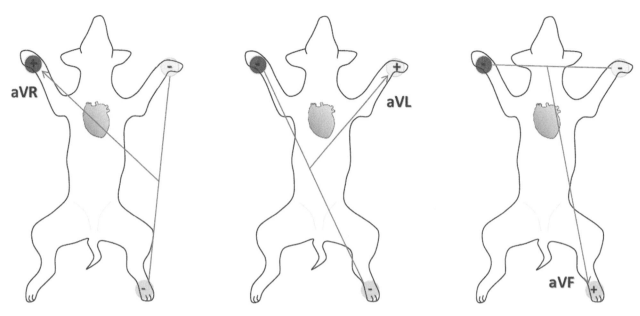

Figure 3.7 The unipolar leads. (See text for explanation.)

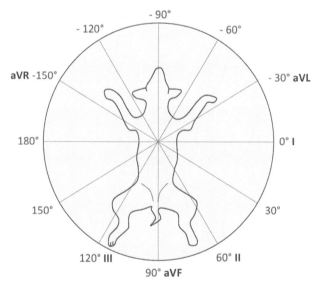

Figure 3.8 The hexaxial lead system. The combination of the bipolar and unipolar augmented leads forms the hexaxial system that allows the study of the electricity flow in the frontal plane. Taking the heart as the central point, the diagram illustrates the possible directions of electricity flow measured in angles. The location of the name of the lead corresponds to the position of the exploring electrode (+). This diagram is used to calculate the mean electrical axis of the heart that represents the average of the sum of all vectors during ventricular (or atrial) depolarisation (see chapter 4).

The Precordial System

The precordial lead system assesses the flow of electricity on the transverse or horizontal plane. The exploring electrode (positive) is positioned in specific locations on the chest, and the WCT is used as the reference electrode (negative). More than one precordial lead system has been described in dogs; however, the large variation in chest conformation among breeds makes it difficult to find a system that offers repeatable results for all individuals of this species. A precordial lead system for cats has not been described.

The precordial lead systems most commonly used in dogs are: Lannek's system modified by Detweiler and Patterson, and Wilson's system modified by Kraus *et al*. Another more complex system was proposed by Takahashi in 1964 and modified in 1966. More recently, another precordial system was proposed by Nunes and colleagues.[16] These will not be discussed here, as they are not commonly used in clinical practice.

Lannek's Precordial System Modified by Detweiler and Patterson
The first precordial system applied to the dog was proposed by Nils Lannek in 1949.[17] It included three unipolar leads:

CR_{6L}: With the exploring electrode positioned at the left 6th intercostal space at the level of the junction between the rib and the sternum
CR_{6U}: With the exploring electrode positioned at the left 6th intercostal space at the level of the costochondral junction
CR_5: With the exploring electrode positioned at the right 5th intercostal space at the level of the junction between the rib and the sternum.

In 1965, Detweiler and Patterson proposed a modification by adding an additional lead – V_{10} – with the exploring electrode positioned dorsally at the level of

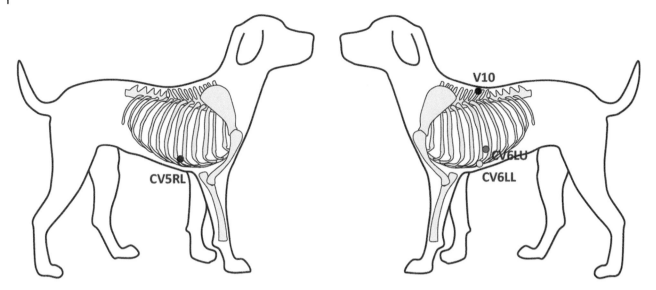

Figure 3.9 Lannek's precordial lead system modified by Detweiler and Patterson. On the right side of the chest, an electrode is positioned at the 5th intercostal space at the level of the junction between the rib and the sternum (CV5RL). On the left side of the chest, an electrode is positioned at the 6th intercostal space at the level of the junction between the rib and the sternum (CV6LL), and another is positioned at the 6th intercostal space over the costochondral junction (CV6LU). A fourth electrode is positioned over the spinous process of the 7th thoracic vertebra (V10).

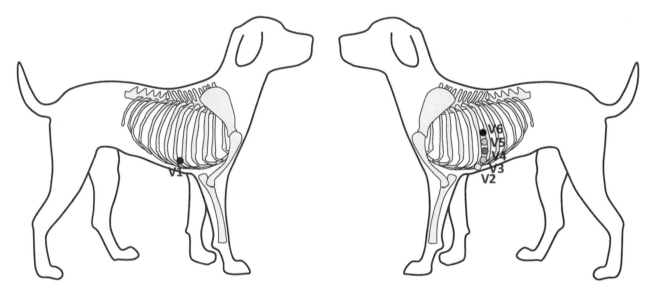

Figure 3.10 Wilson's precordial lead system modified by Kraus *et al.* On the right side of the chest, an electrode is positioned at the 5th intercostal space at the level of the junction between the rib and the sternum (V1). On the left side of the chest, an electrode is positioned at the 6th intercostal space at the level of the junction between the rib and the sternum (V2); another is positioned at the level of the costochondral junction (V4), and another further up the same intercostal space at approximately the same distance between V2 and V4 (V6). Additional electrodes are then positioned approximately halfway between V2 and V4 (V3) and between V4 and V6 (V5).

the spinous process of the 7th thoracic vertebra (Figure 3.9).[18] The leads were also renamed CV_5RL (CR_5), CV_6LL (CR_{6L}) and CV_6LU (CR_{6U}).

Wilson's Precordial System Modified by Kraus et al.

Frank Wilson introduced a precordial lead system in 1944 that is still used in human medicine.[19] This was adapted for use in dogs in 2002 by Marc Kraus and colleagues (Figure 3.10).[20] It includes six unipolar leads:

V_1: The exploring electrode is positioned at the right 5th intercostal space at the level of the junction between the rib and sternum.

V_2: The exploring electrode is positioned at the left 6th intercostal space at the level of the junction between the rib and sternum.

V_3: The exploring electrode is positioned at the left 6th intercostal space between V_2 and the costochondral junction, where V_4 will be positioned.

V_4: The exploring electrode is positioned at the left 6th intercostal space at the level of the costochondral junction.

V_5: The exploring electrode is positioned at the left 6th intercostal space above V_4 using the same distance between V_3 and V_4.

V_6: The exploring electrode is positioned at the left 6th intercostal space above V_5 using the same distance between V_4 and V_5.

The ECG tracings in this text were obtained with this precordial system.

Genesis of the Electrocardiogram

Now that we have discussed the concepts of cardiac vectors and the various electrocardiographic leads, we can see how the electrocardiographic waves are generated. Each event of the cardiac cycle produces a deflection or *wave* on the ECG (Figure 3.11). Atrial depolarisation is represented by the P wave (Figures 3.12 and 3.13), and ventricular depolarisation by the QRS complex (Figure 3.15). It is important to point out that the waves seen on the ECG are the result of depolarisation or repolarisation of the working myocardium and not the specialised conduction system. The depolarisation of the sinus node and impulse travelling through the conduction system are not seen on the surface ECG. Between events, there is a return to baseline, producing a *segment* (e.g. PR and ST segments). The distance between two events represents the time – *interval* – elapsed between them.

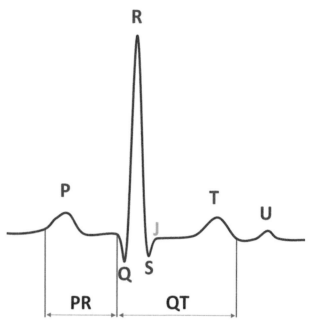

Figure 3.11 Illustration of the electrocardiographic waves as seen in lead II of the electrocardiogram. The P wave represents atrial depolarisation. The Q, R and S waves together form the QRS complex that represents ventricular depolarisation. The J point represents the return to baseline after the QRS. The T wave is the result of ventricular repolarisation, and the U wave (normally not visible) is attributed to delayed repolarisation of the Purkinje or M cells of the myocardium. Between each wave, there is a return to baseline called a *segment*. The PR segment, from the end of the P wave to the beginning of the QRS, represents the time the impulse spends travelling through the AVN and His-Purkinje. During the ST segment, from the end of the QRS to the beginning of the T wave, the myocardial cells are in stage 2 of the action potential, and actual contraction is occurring. The PR interval starts from the beginning of the P wave to the beginning of the QRS, and the QT interval from the beginning of the QRS until the end of the T wave.

Figure 3.12 Atrial depolarisation. The arrows represent the direction of the depolarisation wave which is recorded as a positive deflection in lead II of the electrocardiogram called the P wave.

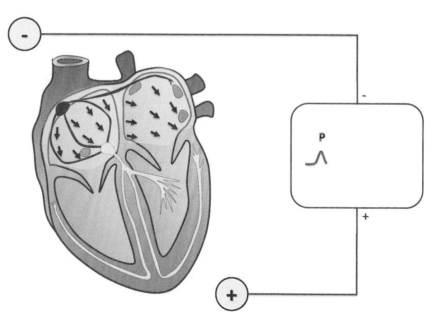

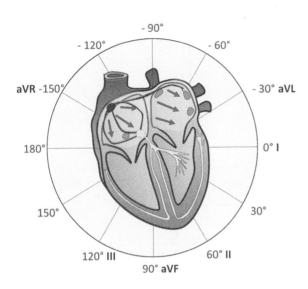

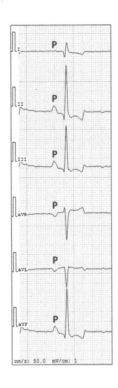

Figure 3.13 Atrial depolarisation and the appearance of the P wave in all six leads. The P wave is positive in leads II, III and aVF (inferior leads) and negative in leads aVL and aVR. In lead I, it may appear as a positive, biphasic or isobiphasic wave.

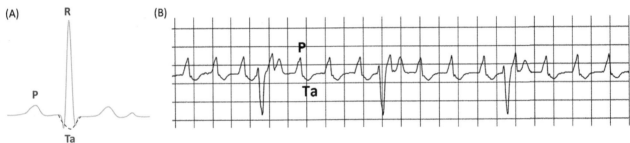

Figure 3.14 T$_a$ wave. (A) Atrial repolarisation occurs at the same time as the QRS, and therefore the T$_a$ is not normally visible. (B) Holter recording showing non-conducted P waves where the T$_a$ can be seen. [10-year-old, female neutered Greyhound dog with third-degree atrioventricular block]

The individual components of the ECG complex

The P wave

The P wave represents atrial depolarisation. The impulse starts in the sinus node on the roof of the right atrium and travels "downwards" and towards the left (figure 3.12). Its appearance on the 6 limb leads may be seen in figure 3.13. It will appear as a positive wave in leads II, III and aVF (inferior leads) and as a negative wave in leads aVL and aVR; in lead I it may appear as a positive, biphasic or isobiphasic (see chapter 4). The duration of the P wave represents the time it takes for both the right and left atrial myocardium to be completely depolarised. Its amplitude is directly proportional to the atrial mass which is why the P wave is smaller in comparison to the QRS and why an increase in amplitude suggests atrial enlargement (see Chapter 4).[21]

The T$_a$ Wave (or T$_P$)

The T$_a$ wave represents atrial repolarisation.[22] Since this occurs at the same time as the ventricles are undergoing depolarisation (during the QRS complex), the T$_a$ wave is not normally seen on the ECG. However, T$_a$ waves can sometimes be seen in cases with atrial enlargement as a PR or ST segment depression depending on the heart rate,[23,24] and they may also be seen occasionally if a QRS does not follow the P wave (e.g. atrioventricular block) (Figure 3.14).

The PR Segment

The PR segment starts at the end of the P wave and finishes at the start of the QRS complex. This return to baseline occurs whilst the impulse is travelling through the atrioventricular node (AVN) and the His–Purkinje between the end of atrial depolarisation and just before ventricular depolarisation. If the PR segment is not seen, it may indicate atrioventricular dissociation (see chapter 10) or the presence of ventricular pre-excitation via an accessory pathway (see chapter 10). In humans, PR segment depression (below baseline) has been described with pericarditis or an atrial infarct.[25,26] It is possible that this could also occur in our patients.

The PR Interval

The PR interval is the time from the start of atrial depolarisation (beginning of P wave) to the start of ventricular depolarisation (beginning of QRS). The term *PQ interval* is used by some authors if the Q wave is the initial component of the QRS. It represents the time it takes for an impulse to originate in the sinus node, depolarise the atria, reach the AVN and travel through it until it finally reaches the ventricles. Since the impulse reaches the AVN quickly and most of the time is spent travelling through the compact node, the PR interval is an indicator of AVN function. A prolonged PR interval indicates a longer delay than normal through the AVN and suggests the presence of first-degree atrioventricular block (see chapter 7).

The QRS Complex

The QRS complex represents ventricular depolarisation. The ventricular myocardial cells are experiencing stages 0 and 1 of the action potential, and the depolarisation wave sweeps the whole myocardium. Once all cells have depolarised, there is a return to baseline. The ramifications of the bundle branches deliver the impulse to the ventricles via the Purkinje network, and, since the Purkinje fibres are located beneath the endocardium, the depolarisation wave travels from the endocardium to the epicardium. The distribution of the impulse to the working myocardium occurs in a very specific way designed to trigger contraction directed from the apex to the base, effectively pushing blood towards the semilunar valves. This sequence of events will now be described, including the resulting vectors of depolarisation and how they are recorded on the ECG.

Q, R and S

Before we proceed, a brief discussion on the nomenclature of the Q, R and S waves is necessary. The designation *QRS* derives from its typical appearance in lead II of the electrocardiogram in humans where three distinct waves – Q, R and S – may be seen. However, not all three waves are always visible, and different QRS morphologies are possible (see Figure 4.20). By convention, the first positive deflection of the QRS complex is called *R*. If a negative wave is present before an R wave, it is named *Q*; and a negative wave that occurs after an R wave is named *S*. If a second positive wave exists, it is named an *R' wave*. The point where the QRS ends and the ST segment begins is called the *J-point*.

Q

The impulse reaches the left side of the interventricular septum first ($\approx$5 ms) via divisions of the left bundle branches, and it is followed by the right side of the septum ($\approx$12 ms). This results in an initial depolarisation front travelling 'upwards' (caudal-to-cranial/ventral-to-dorsal) and towards the right (Figure 3.15A; vector 1 in Figure 3.16). In leads I, II, III and aVF of the ECG, this appears as an initial negative deflection called the *Q wave*, although it is not always visible. In aVR, it appears as a small positive wave (R instead of Q). In aVL, it may not be visible or may appear as either a small negative or positive wave (Figure 3.17).

R

The impulse then reaches the apex of the ventricles ($\approx$15–25 ms) and the base ($\approx$40–45 ms) via the right and left bundle branches (Figure 3.15B and 3.15C). The depolarisation wave travelling through the right ventricle has an 'upwards' (caudal-to-cranial/ventral-to-dorsal) direction and towards the right (vector 2 in Figure 3.16). Activation of the left ventricle occurs via the branches of the cranial (anterior) and caudal (posterior) fascicles. Synchronous activation of the left ventricular areas supplied by both fascicles results in a depolarisation vector travelling with a 'downwards' (cranial-to-caudal/dorsal-to-ventral) direction and towards the left (vector 3 in Figure 3.16). Given that both ventricles are depolarised at the same time, the next wave recorded on the ECG corresponds to the sum of vectors 2 and 3. Since the mass of the left ventricle greatly exceeds that of the right ventricle, the resulting vector is directed 'downwards' (cranial-to-caudal/dorsal-to-ventral) and towards the left. In leads I, II, III and aVF, this results in a positive deflection – an R wave (Figure 3.17). In leads aVR and aVL, it appears as a negative deflection (S instead of R).

S

The base of the ventricles is the last to be depolarised, resulting in a fourth vector directed 'upwards' (caudo-dorsally). In humans, this may result in a small negative deflection on the ECG called the *S wave*. However, in quadruped animals, the direction of this vector is perpendicular to the frontal plane and is often not recorded on the hexaxial system.

The ST Segment

The ST segment starts at the end of the QRS complex and finishes at the start of the T wave (Figure 3.11). During this period, the ventricular cardiomyocytes are in stage 2 of the action potential, and actual myocardial contraction is occurring. The point where the QRS complex ends and the ST segment starts is called the *J point*, but it is often difficult to distinguish. Since during this

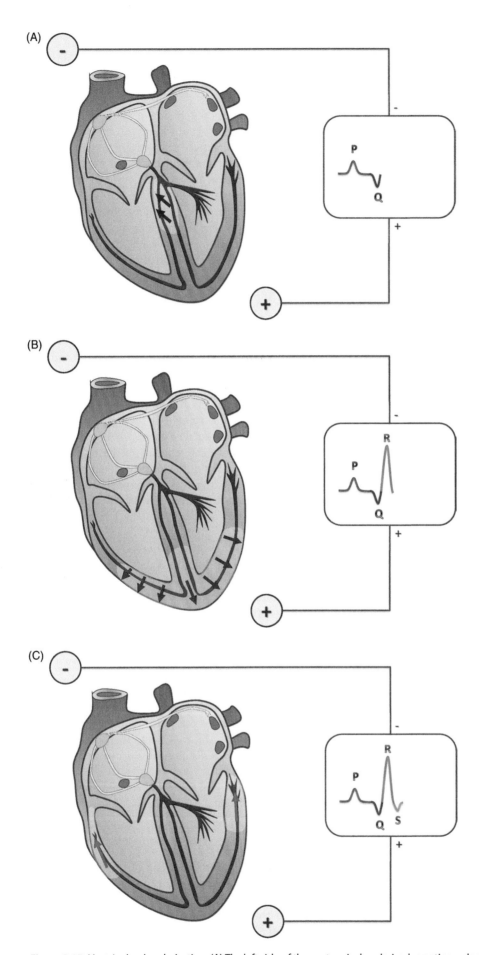

Figure 3.15 Ventricular depolarisation. (A) The left side of the septum is depolarised, creating a depolarisation wave upwards towards the right (arrows). This is recorded as negative deflection in lead II – the *Q wave*. (B) The free walls of both ventricles are depolarised next from the apex towards the base. The sum of the depolarisation vectors is recorded as a positive deflection in lead II – the *R wave*. (C) Finally, the base of the ventricles is activated with a depolarisation vector directed upwards. This may be recorded as a negative deflection in lead II – the *S wave*. (See text for more details.)

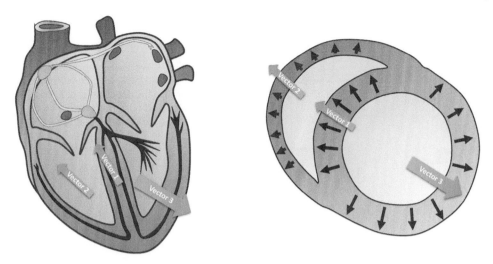

Figure 3.16 Representation of the main cardiac vectors resulting from the propagation of the wavefronts through the ventricles. Vector 1: The left side of the interventricular septum is depolarised first (≈5 ms) via divisions of the left bundle branches, and is followed by the right side of the septum (≈12 ms). This results in an initial depolarisation front travelling 'upwards' (caudal-to-cranial/ventral-to-dorsal) and towards the right. Vector 2: The impulse then reaches the apex of the ventricles (≈15–25 ms) and the base (≈40–45 ms) via the right and left bundles. The depolarisation wave travelling through the right ventricle has an 'upwards' (caudal-to-cranial/ventral-to-dorsal) direction and towards the right. Vector 3: Activation of the left ventricle occurs via the branches of the cranial (anterior) and caudal (posterior) fascicles. Synchronous activation of the left ventricular areas supplied by both fascicles results in a depolarisation vector travelling with a 'downwards' (cranial-to-caudal/dorsal-to-ventral) direction and towards the left. See text for a more detailed description. Please note that this illustration is very simplified and has the sole purpose of making it easier to understand these concepts.

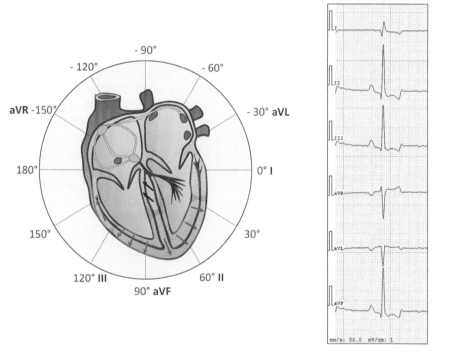

Figure 3.17 Appearance of the QRS in all six leads. The appearance of the QRS in all six surface leads may be seen on the electrocardiographic trace on the right. On the left, the three ventricular depolarisation vectors discussed in Figures 3.15 and 3.16 are represented in the heart in the context of the hexaxial system to understand the appearance of the QRS waves on each lead. Depolarisation of the interventricular septum (vector 1 – red arrows) results in an initial depolarisation front travelling 'upwards' (caudal-to-cranial/ventral-to-dorsal) and towards the right. In leads I, II, III and aVF of the electrocardiogram (ECG), this appears as an initial negative deflection called the *Q wave*, although it is not always visible. In aVR it appears as a small positive wave (R instead of Q). In aVL it may not be visible or may appear as either a small negative or positive wave. It is followed by depolarisation of the right and left ventricles from apex to base. The depolarisation wave travelling through the right ventricle has an 'upwards' (caudal-to-cranial/ventral-to-dorsal) direction and towards the right (vector 2 in Figure 3.16), and synchronous activation of the left ventricle results in a depolarisation vector travelling with a 'downwards' (cranial-to-caudal/dorsal-to-ventral) direction and towards the left (vector 3 in Figure 3.16). Given that both ventricles are depolarised at the same time, the next wave recorded on the ECG corresponds to the sum of vectors 2 and 3, and since the mass of the left ventricle greatly exceeds that of the right ventricle, the resulting vector is directed 'downwards' (cranial-to-caudal/dorsal-to-ventral) and towards the left. In leads I, II, III and aVF, this results in a positive deflection – the R wave. In leads aVR and aVL, it appears as a negative deflection (S instead of R). The base of the ventricles is the last to be depolarised, resulting in a fourth vector directed 'upwards' (caudo-dorsally; upward blue arrows at ventricle base). In humans, this may result in a small negative deflection on the ECG called the S wave. However, in quadruped animals, the direction of this vector is perpendicular to the frontal plane and is often not recorded on the hexaxial system.

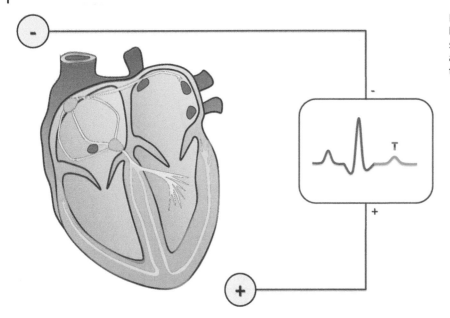

Figure 3.18 Ventricular repolarisation. Epicardial cells achieve full repolarisation sooner than the endocardial cells, creating an electrical dipole that is registered on the electrocardiogram as the T wave.

period all cells have a similar membrane potential, an electrical dipole is not present and the ECG shows a return to baseline. In cats, the ST segment should appear as a flat line at the level of the baseline (isoelectric).[27] In dogs, an upwards or downwards deviation of up to 0.20 mV in the limb leads and of 0.25 mV in the precordial leads may be seen in normal subjects.[11] A more pronounced ST deviation is considered abnormal and may be caused by the presence of areas of myocardium in different stages of depolarisation or repolarisation, effectively creating an electrical dipole that is recorded by the electrocardiograph. This may occur in cases of early repolarisation of parts of myocardium (repolarisation abnormalities), left bundle branch block and supraventricular tachycardia with a 1:1 ventriculo-atrial retrograde activation. The ST deviation in these cases is real. Alternatively, a deviation of the TP and PR segments also creates an apparent deviation of the ST segment on the ECG. This is commonly observed with acute myocardial infarction, in which damaged cells are in a state of partial depolarisation accounting for the change in TP and PR segments. The causes of ST deviation (elevation and depression) are discussed in chapter 4.

The J Wave

Occasionally, a small deflection may be seen following the QRS called the *J wave* or Osborn wave. It is most commonly seen with hypothermia, but may occasionally be seen under baseline conditions and has been reported in normal dogs.[28–32] Its origin is poorly understood, but evidence suggests that it is caused by the presence of a prominent action potential notch (spike and dome morphology) in the epicardium in contrast to the endocardium, leading to a voltage gradient that manifests as a J wave or an elevated J point.[30]

The T Wave

The T wave represents ventricular repolarisation. During this period, cells are undergoing stage 3 of the action potential with a progressive return to the resting membrane potential. The epicardial cells achieve full repolarisation before the endocardial cells, creating an electrical dipole that is recorded as a deflection on the ECG – a *T wave* (Figure 3.18). The overall direction of repolarisation is from the apex to the base and from the epicardium to endocardium.[33] In both dogs and cats, the appearance of the T wave is variable and can occur as a positive, negative or biphasic deflection in normal subjects.[11,34] Commonly, the two branches of the T wave are asymmetric. A small and flat T wave may also be seen in normal subjects, particularly in leads I, aVR, aVL and V_1.

The U Wave

A small wave may be seen after the T wave in some cases (Figure 3.11). It is termed a *U wave* and is thought to be due to delayed repolarisation of the Purkinje or mid-myocardial 'M' cells.[35,36] When visible, it normally appears approximately 40 ms after the T wave and with the same polarity as the T. It is most visible in the precordial leads (V_1, V_2, V_4, CV_5RL, CV_6LL and CV_6LU).

The QT Interval

The period of time from the beginning of the QRS to the end of the T (or U) wave represents the entirety of ventricular depolarisation and repolarisation from stages 0 to 4 of the action potential.

Further discussion on the electrocardiographic waves and intervals can be found in chapter 4, which will include how to perform measurements of amplitude and duration, and how to interpret the ECG.

References

1 Fye WB. A history of the origin, evolution, and impact of electrocardiography. Am J Cardio. 1994;73:937–949.

2 Rivera-Ruiz M, Cajavilca C, Varon J. Einthoven's string galvanometer. Tex Heart Inst J. 2008;35(2):174–178.

3 Barker JM. The unipolar electrocardiogram: a clinical interpretation. Am J Med Sci. 1954;227(1).

4 Wilson FN, Johnston FD, Rosenbaum FF. On Einthoven's triangle, the theory of unipolar electrocardiographic leads, and the interpretation of the precordial electrocardiogram. Am Heart J. 1946;32:277–310.

5 Geselowitz DB. Dipole theory in electrocardiography. Am J Cardio. 1964;14:301–306.

6 Burger HC, Van Milaan JB. Heart-vector and leads. Br Heart J. 1946;8:157–161.

7 Mann H. A method of analysing the electrocardiogram. Arch Intern Med (Chic). 1920;25:283–294.

8 Einthoven W. Die galvanometrische Registrirung des menschlichen Elektrokardiogramms, zugleich eine Beurtheilung der Anwendung des Capillar-Elektrometers in der Physiologie. Pflüger, Archiv Ges Physiol Mensch Thiere. 1903;99:472–480.

9 Barold SS. Willem Einthoven and the birth of clinical electrocardiography a hundred years ago. Card Electrophysiol Rev. 2003;7:99–104.

10 Einthoven W. Weiteres über das Elektrokardiogramm. Pflügers Archiv Eur J Physiol. 1908;122:517–583.

11 Detweiler DK. Comprehensive electrocardiology 1861–1908. London: Springer; 2010. doi:10.1007/978-1-84882-046-3_41

12 Goldberger E. A simple, indifferent, electrocardiographic electrode of zero potential and a technique of obtaining augmented, unipolar, extremity leads. Am Heart J. 1942;23:483–492.

13 Goldberger E. The aVL, aVR, and aVF leads: a simplification of standard lead electrocardiography. Am Heart J. 1942;24(3):378–396.

14 Wilson FN, Macleod AG, Barker PS. The potential variations produced by the heart beat at the apices of Einthoven's triangle. Am Heart J. 1931;7:207–211.

15 Wilson FN, Johnston FD, Macleod AG, Barker PS. Electrocardiograms that represent the potential variations of a single electrode. Am Heart J. 1934;9:447–471.

16 Nunes AA, Moffa PJ, Iwasaki M. Standardization of a new precordial chest leads system in the dog. Braz J Vet Res Anim Sci. 1990;27:233–246.

17 Lannek N. Clinical and experimental study on the electrocardiogram in dogs. Stockholm: I. Haeggstrom; 1949.

18 Detweiler DK, Patterson DF. The prevalence and types of cardiovascular disease in dogs. Ann NY Acad Sci. 1965;127:481–516.

19 Wilson FN, *et al*. The precordial electrocardiogram. Am Heart J. 1994;27:19–85.

20 Kraus MS, Moïse NS, Rishniw M, Dykes N, Erb HN. Morphology of ventricular arrhythmias in the boxer as measured by 12-lead electrocardiography with pace-mapping comparison. J Vet Intern Med. 2002;16:153–158.

21 O'Grady M, DiFruscia R, Carley B, Hill B. Electrocardiographic evaluation of chamber enlargement. Can Vet J. 1992;33:195–200.

22 Hayashi H. The experimental study of normal atrial T wave (Ta) in electrocardiograms. Japanese Heart J. 1970;11:91–103.

23 Ihara Z, van Oosterom A, Hoekema R. Atrial repolarization as observable during the PQ interval. J Electrocardiol. 2006;39:290–297.

24 Tranchesi J, Adelardi V, Oliveira JMD. Atrial repolarization – its importance in clinical electrocardiography. Circulation. 1960;22:635–644.

25 Bruce MA, Spodick DH. Atypical electrocardiogram in acute pericarditis: characteristics and prevalence. J Electrocardiol. 1980;13:61–66.

26 Nielsen FE, Andersen HH, Gram-Hansen P, Sørensen HT, Klausen IC. The relationship between ECG signs of atrial infarction and the development of supraventricular arrhythmias in patients with acute myocardial infarction. Am Heart J. 1992;123:69–72.

27 Harpster NK. In Diseases of the cat: medicine and surgery (ed. Holzworth J). Philadelphia: W.B. Saunders; 1987.

28 Agudelo CF, Schanilec P. The canine J wave. Vet Medicina. 2015;60:208–212.

29 Santos EM, Kittle CF. Electrocardiographic changes in the dog during hypothermia. Am Heart J. 1958;55:415–420.

30 Yan G-X, Antzelevitch C. Cellular basis for the electrocardiographic J wave. Circulation. 1996;93:372–379.

31 West TC, Frederickson EL, Amory DW. Single fiber recording of the ventricular response to induced hypothermia in the anesthetized dog: correlation with multicellular parameters. Circ Res. 1959;7:880–888.

32 Rudling EH, *et al*. The prevalence of the electrocardiographic J wave in the Petit Basset Griffon Vendéen compared to 10 different dog breeds. J Vet Cardiol. 2016;18:26–33.

33 van Dam RT, Durrer D. The T wave and ventricular repolarization. Am J Cardio. 1964;14:294–300.

34 Mukherjee J, *et al*. Electrocardiogram pattern of some exotic breeds of trained dogs: a variation study. Vet World. 2015;8:1317–1320.

35 Sicouri S, Fish J, Antzelevitch C. Distribution of M cells in the canine ventricle. J Cardiovasc Electrophysiol. 1994;5:824–837.

36 Watanabe Y. Purkinje repolarization as a possible cause of the U wave in the electrocardiogram. Circulation. 1975;51:1030–1037.

4

Electrocardiography
Ruth Willis

Introduction

As described in chapter 3, electrocardiography is the recording of the electrical activity of the heart at the body surface using electrodes placed on the limbs or chest. The resulting recording, plotted against time, is then shown as a visual trace on paper or a screen to facilitate further assessment of heart rate and rhythm. The electrocardiograph is the machine used to obtain the recording. Electrical activity is generated in cardiac tissue by changes in the transmembrane electrical potential as a result of ion movement, as explained in chapters 2 and 3.

The aims of this chapter are to demonstrate how to:

- Obtain a diagnostic electrocardiogram (ECG) from cats and dogs.
- Identify common artefacts.
- Understand methods used to calculate heart rate.
- Assess heart rate and rhythm.
- Measure wave amplitude and intervals.
- Calculate the mean electrical axis (MEA).

Procedure

How to Obtain a Diagnostic Resting ECG Trace in a Dog

The ECG will detect electrical activity in skeletal muscle as well as in cardiac tissue, and therefore it is important to have the patient as still and calm as possible. Conventionally, patients are gently restrained in right lateral recumbency, with forelimbs perpendicular to the long axis of the body and hindlimbs slightly flexed (Figure 4.1).

The ECG cables are attached to the skin using either pre-gelled self-adhesive electrodes attached to the digital pads or metacarpal and metatarsal pads, or crocodile clips with the ends smoothed or slightly bent to avoid them pinching the patient (Figures 4.1A and 4.2).[1] If crocodile clips are used, electrical contact is generally achieved using alcohol (*Caution – flammable!*) on the clips or, less commonly, an ECG gel.

On the forelimbs, the clips are placed over the olecranon, and on the hindlimbs the clips are placed over the patellar tendon (Figure 4.1B). These areas are chosen as there is relatively little underlying muscle, thereby minimising electrical interference of muscle activity, as described by Tilley.[2]

How to Obtain a Diagnostic Resting ECG Trace in a Cat

Ideally, cats are also gently restrained in right lateral recumbency for ECG recording, as shown in Figure 4.3. In cats adhesive, electrodes on the digital or metatarsal/metacarpal pads may be better tolerated than crocodile clips.[1]

Purring can be a cause of baseline artefact, and, depending on the temperament of the cat, methods suggested to minimise purring include avoiding stroking the cat during the procedure, turning on a tap in the room and also holding a small piece of cotton wool soaked in alcohol or antiseptic hand gel close to the cat's face.[3]

Non-Standard ECG Positioning

Sometimes in large, uncooperative or dyspnoeic dogs, it is necessary to obtain the recording with the dog standing or in sternal or left lateral recumbency, and the effects of this on the ECG trace have been described.[4] ECGs recorded from dogs in a standing position showed increased Q and R wave amplitudes in leads I and II, and increased R and S wave amplitudes in lead III. Dogs in left lateral recumbency showed increased R wave amplitude in leads II, III and aVF; increased S wave amplitude in lead aVL; but decreased R wave amplitude in aVR. The MEA shifted to the left in the standing position but remained within the normal range in the left lateral position.[4–6]

Combative cats or cats with moderate-severe dyspnoea may necessitate making the ECG recording with the cat in sternal or left lateral recumbency. ECGs

Guide to Canine and Feline Electrocardiography, First Edition. Ruth Willis, Pedro Oliveira and Antonia Mavropoulou.
© 2018 John Wiley & Sons Ltd. Published 2018 by John Wiley & Sons Ltd.
Companion website: www.wiley.com/go/willis/electrocardiography

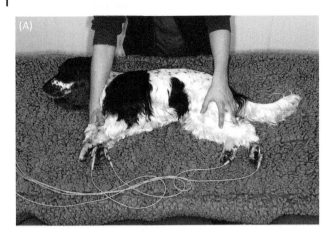 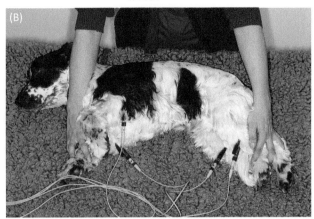

Figure 4.1 Patient positioning for electrocardiography (dog). (A) Adhesive electrodes can be attached to the digital pads or metacarpal/metatarsal pads. (B) If 'crocodile' clips are used, they can be placed on the skin over the olecranon in the forelimbs and over the patellar tendon in the hindlimbs. During a standard examination, the patient should always be in right lateral recumbency.

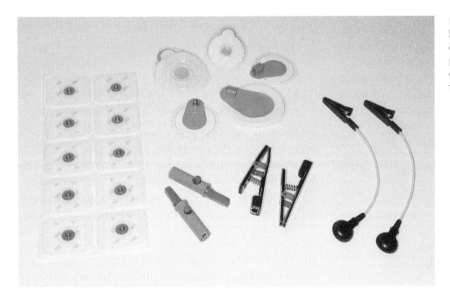

Figure 4.2 Examples of different types of ECG electrodes. Pre-gelled self-adhesive electrodes are more comfortable for the patient. If crocodile clips are used, their ends should be smoothed or slightly bent to avoid pinching the patient.

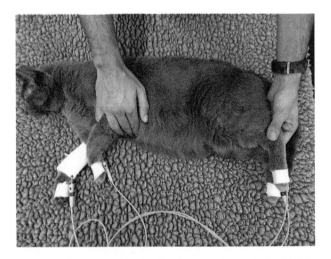

Figure 4.3 Patient positioning for electrocardiography (cat). With the cat in right lateral recumbency, adhesive electrodes are placed on the digital pads or metatarsal/metacarpal pads depending on their size.

obtained with cats restrained in left lateral or sternal recumbency will generally show a lower R wave amplitude.[7] The MEA will be affected by restraining the cat in left lateral recumbency.[7]

One, Three or Six Leads?

If each lead is compared to a camera looking at the heart from a different direction, then it becomes logical that the more 'cameras' we use, the more complete a picture we will obtain of the complex pattern of electrical activity in the heart.

As described more fully in chapter 3, leads I–III are sometimes called the *bipolar leads*, and the electrode positions are:

- Lead I records the potential difference between the right forelimb (negative electrode) and the left forelimb (positive electrode).

- Lead II records the potential difference between the right forelimb (negative electrode) and the left hindlimb (positive electrode).
- Lead III records the potential difference between the left forelimb (negative electrode) and left hindlimb (positive electrode).

As described more fully in chapter 3, there are also three augmented unipolar leads – aVR, aVL and aVF – which combine or average the ECG potentials from two limbs and compare this to the third point:

- *Lead aVR*: The right forelimb forms the positive electrode, and the combined left forelimb and left hindlimb leads form the negative electrode.
- *Lead aVL*: The left forelimb is the positive electrode, and the combination of the right forelimb and left hindlimb forms the negative electrode.
- *Lead aVF*: The left hindlimb is the positive electrode, and the combined left and right forelimbs form the negative electrode.

See Figures 3.6, 3.7 and 3.8 for a more detailed explanation. Table 4.1 shows the standard limb lead positions and colours.

Table 4.1 Standard limb positions and various electrode colour codes

Electrode	Lead colour in Europe	Lead colour in the USA	Position
Right forelimb	Red	White	On skin over right olecranon
Left forelimb	Yellow	Black	On skin over left olecranon
Left hindlimb	Green	Red	On skin over left patellar tendon
Right hindlimb	Black	Green	On skin over right patellar tendon

---

Example illustrating the importance of multiple leads

Issues such as poor electrode contact and also patient conformation will sometimes result in low-complex amplitudes in some of the leads, as illustrated in the trace in Figure 4.4, where leads II and aVR show low-amplitude complexes in comparison to the other leads. In such cases, it may be difficult to distinguish and measure the P, QRS and T waves accurately. If all leads are recorded, then the picture becomes much clearer.

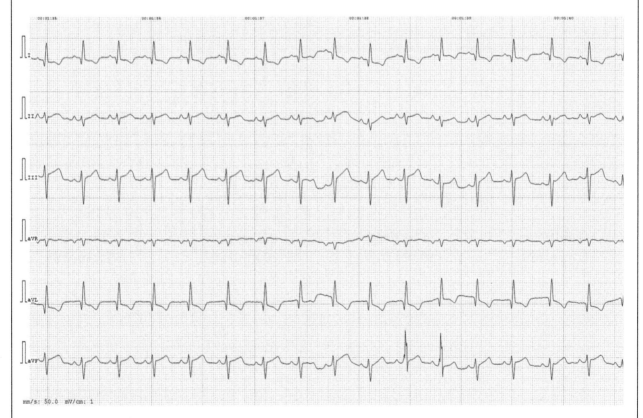

Figure 4.4 Multiple ECG leads.

Should I Use Chest Leads?

The use and positioning of chest leads are described in chapter 3. The incorporation of further leads allows the directions of the electrical impulse to be mapped in more detail – to return to the camera analogy, having more cameras makes it possible to look at an object, in this case the heart's three-dimensional electrical field, from more directions. Cardiac mapping is the process of identifying the temporal and spatial distribution of electrical potentials generated by the myocardium during arrhythmias. Chest leads can be useful in the evaluation of supraventricular tachyarrhythmias and also the mapping of ventricular arrhythmias in dogs (see chapters 8–11).[8,9]

The number of leads recorded may depend on the clinical setting. For example, if the purpose of the ECG recording is to monitor for malignant arrhythmias in real time in an intensive care setting, then a single lead may be sufficient. However, three and six-lead traces will provide more information about the way that electrical activity is moving across the heart and would be routine in the setting of investigating cardiac disease, especially narrow-QRS complex tachycardias (see chapters 8, 9, 10 and 13).

What to Record?

In a patient undergoing evaluation of heart rhythm, it would be typical for a good quality trace showing 6 or 12 leads with a paper speed of 50 mm/s to be obtained, before a longer rhythm strip is recorded, often using just a single lead, over 1 to 5 min. The sensitivity (or gain) settings should be adjusted on traces with multiple leads to maximise the ECG amplitude without allowing adjacent lead recordings to overlap.

ECG Machine Settings

The Vertical Axis – Sensitivity

The vertical axis of the ECG trace shows voltage, generally measured in millivolts, and 10 mm/mV is the default setting. The sensitivity (or gain) setting on the ECG allows adjustment of the scale. For example, 5 mm/mV may be useful if the R wave amplitude is high to avoid superimposition of multiple leads; conversely, 20 mm/mV may be useful for ECGs with low amplitudes, as often seen in cats. Figure 4.5 shows examples of different sensitivity settings.

Calibration

At the start of a recording, many ECG machines will insert a calibration spike (Figure 4.6). The purpose of this spike is to show that the data conform to a standard format. The standard box varies between machines but is often 1 mV high and 200 ms wide. If the R wave is very tall, then it may be necessary to halve the sensitivity, and this may be represented by the calibration spike containing a step on the left side. If the paper speed is set to 50 mm/s, then the calibration spike will still be 200 ms wide.

ECG Filters

Most ECG machines will have the option of using a filter. Some understanding of signal processing can help in appropriate use of the filter. The frequency or cycle rate of any signal is measured in Hertz – for example, a heart rate of 60 beats per minute (bpm) has a frequency of 1 cycle per second that can be expressed as 1 Hz. As the P, QRS and T components of the signal all occur during each cycle, the frequency of each individual component will occur at or above this frequency, and these individual waves are called *harmonics*. The QRS complex forms the high-frequency component, and the P wave, ST segment and T wave form the lower frequency components. The process of breaking the ECG signal down into a series of sine waves is called *Fourier analysis*, and, if these waves are superimposed, then the original signal is recreated.

Each harmonic has several inherent properties:

1) *Amplitude*: The magnitude of the signal is the height of the wave and, in the context of an ECG, is measured in millivolts.

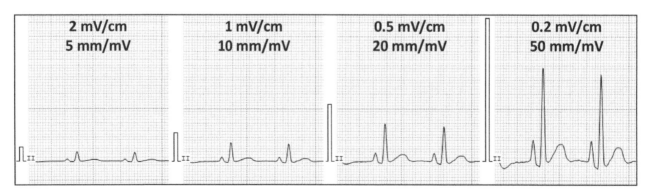

Figure 4.5 Different sensitivity settings, and effect on the ECG trace. [6-year-old, female neutered, Birman cat without evidence of heart disease] (50 mm/s)

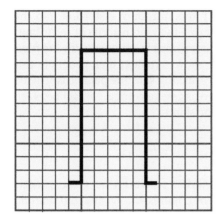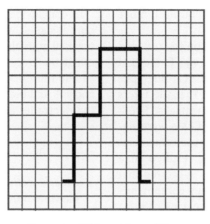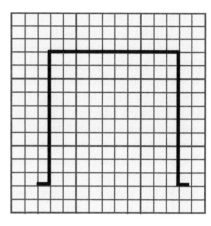

Figure 4.6 Calibration spikes. At the start of a recording, many ECG machines will insert a calibration spike. The purpose of this spike is to show that the data conform to a standard format. The standard box varies between machines but is often 1 mV high and 200 ms wide (example at left: five small squares at 25 mm/s). If the R wave is very tall, then it may be necessary to halve the sensitivity, and this may be represented by the calibration spike containing a step on the left side (example in the middle). If the paper speed is set to 50 mm/s, the calibration spike will still be 200 ms wide (example at right: ten small squares at 50 mm/s).

2) *Frequency*: The repetition rate of the signal; in the context of an ECG, this is influenced by heart rate, and higher heart rates give higher frequencies. In normal dogs, heart rate will vary from 40 bpm (0.67 Hz) at rest to 240 bpm (4 Hz) during intense exercise.

3) *Phase*: The delay before the signal begins; for example, during sinus rhythm, the harmonics making up the QRS complex will occur after the P wave signal.

Low-frequency harmonics have higher amplitudes and therefore have the largest effect on the resulting ECG trace. Naturally, the ECG is capable of detecting electrical activity from sources outside the heart, and the resulting signal(s) superimposed on the myocardial activity are called *interference*.

The frequencies of common sources of interference are:

- Muscle: 5–50 Hz
- Respiration: 0.3–0.67 Hz (assuming 20–40 breaths/min)
- External electrical circuits: 50–60 Hz (mains interference)
- Skin–electrode interface interference: Varies according to the type of electrode (size, adhesive and electrolyte used) and the thoroughness of skin preparation, but interference from this source tends to be low frequency and high amplitude – sometimes as high as 200–300 mV. Given that the myocardial activity is typically in the range of 0.1–2 mV, this form of interference can have a massive result on the resulting ECG trace.

Manipulation of the ECG signal is performed to remove the elements of the trace caused by interference, ideally with minimal distortion of the myocardial signal. There are multiple methods for achieving this, including:

1) High-pass filters that remove low-frequency signals such as motion artefact, respiratory movement and baseline drift.

2) Low-pass filters that remove high-frequency signals such as high-frequency muscle artefact and external interference, and consequently will also have an effect on the QRS complex and late potentials such as epsilon (ε a small positive signal at the end of the QRS complex) and J waves.

   If high and low-pass filters are used together, this is known as a *bandpass filter* which will only allow signals in the range between the low and high filters to pass.

3) Notch filtering combines high and low-pass filters to create a small range of frequencies to be removed. This form of filtering is useful for removing mains interference.

4) Common-mode rejection is a system whereby an inverse signal of leads I, II and III is sent back to the ECG machine through the right leg electrode. This technique reduces the incoming level of the common-mode signal. The source of common-mode signal is typically the alternating current (AC) mains frequency of 50–60 Hz.[10,11]

Diagnostic quality ECGs are typically processed with a bandwidth of 0.05–100 Hz, whereas monitor quality ECGs may be limited to 0.5–40 Hz. The advantage of the lower cut-off of 0.05 Hz is better reproduction of the ST segments, with the trade-off being more baseline drift. The advantage of the higher cut-off of 100 Hz is that rapid changes in the QRS complex are reproduced well even at higher heart rates; however, this higher upper limit makes the trace susceptible to mains interference with a frequency of 50–60 Hz. To counteract this, many machines will contain a notch filter to specifically remove mains interference frequencies.[12]

The effect of manual frequency filters on the ten-lead ECG of 33 cats has been assessed, and it was found that the voltages recorded by all three electrocardiographs were greatest when filters were off and that the filters had the greatest effect on R and S wave voltages. The R wave amplitudes of high-fidelity lead II ECGs were significantly decreased, with digital filters set at frequencies of <150 Hz. Although manual filtering resulted in a reduction in baseline artefact, this study suggested that feline ECGs contain substantial frequency components >150 Hz, and therefore filters with frequencies <150 Hz markedly attenuate the R wave in cats.[13]

Signal averaged electrocardiograms (SAECGs) also provide some insight into the frequency components of the ECG. Signal-averaged electrocardiography is a diagnostic technique that averages multiple QRS complexes over several minutes to reveal small variations in the QRS complex not apparent on the standard ECG. SAECGs are used to highlight ventricular late potentials (LPs). LPs are low-amplitude electrical signals that may indicate slow conduction in areas of damaged myocardium, and they have been used to investigate if these signals can be a predictive factor for sudden death in dogs at risk of sustained ventricular tachycardia. In Boxers, a high-pass frequency cut-off of 25–40 Hz was used to optimise detection of LPs.[14] In another study using Dobermans, a 40 Hz low-frequency filter was used in conjunction with a 250 Hz high-frequency cut-off to highlight LPs.[15]

In conclusion, all filters introduce distortion into the output signal, and during the vast majority of recordings in small animals a better trace is obtained with the filter off. If the trace still shows artefact, then generally this can be minimised by making sure the patient is relaxed and still and that there is good electrical contact between the electrodes and the skin.[13,16]

Troubleshooting Common Artefacts

1) *Muscle activity* (EMG) results in irregular, chaotic baseline movement (Figures 4.7, 4.8 and 4.9). In mild cases, this can obscure the baseline, making it difficult to identify P waves; but, if more severe, even the QRS complexes may be completely obscured, and the trace may not be of any diagnostic value. This can be minimised by ensuring that the patient is calm, relaxed and in a comfortable position. Placement of a hand on the chest wall may help to reduce the effects of respiratory movement, and changing the sensitivity of the trace may dampen the artefact sufficiently to make the trace easier to read. On ambulatory traces, a degree of movement artefact is unavoidable but can be minimised by diligent skin preparation, as discussed in chapter 15.

2) *Electrical interference* results in regular sharp undulations of the ECG trace which occur at a frequency of 50–60 Hz (depending on country) (Figure 4.10). To minimise or correct this issue, it is important to ensure that there is good electrical contact with the

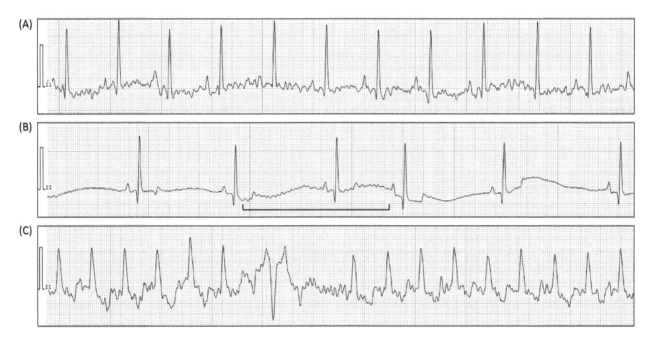

Figure 4.7 Artefacts. (A) Muscle tremor. [10-year-old, female neutered, Schnauzer dog] (50 mm/s; 20 mm/mV) (B) Shivering artefact (red bracket). [10-year-old, female neutered, Schnauzer dog] (50 mm/s; 20 mm/mV) (C) Purring artefact. [10-year-old, male neutered, Tonkinese cat] (50 mm/s; 20 mm/mV)

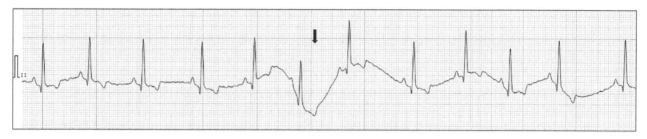

Figure 4.8 Movement artefact. A sudden baseline shift is seen (arrow) due to limb movement. [11-year-old, male neutered, West Highland White Terrier dog] (50 mm/s; 10 mm/mV)

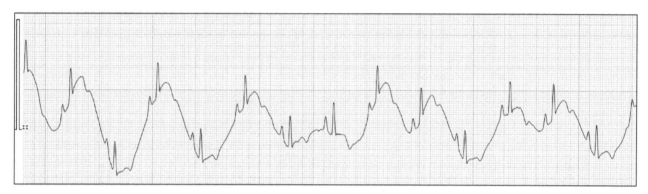

Figure 4.9 Breathing movement artefact. Oscillation of the baseline due to breathing movement. [9-year-old, male neutered, Ragdoll cat] (50 mm/s; 50 mm/mV)

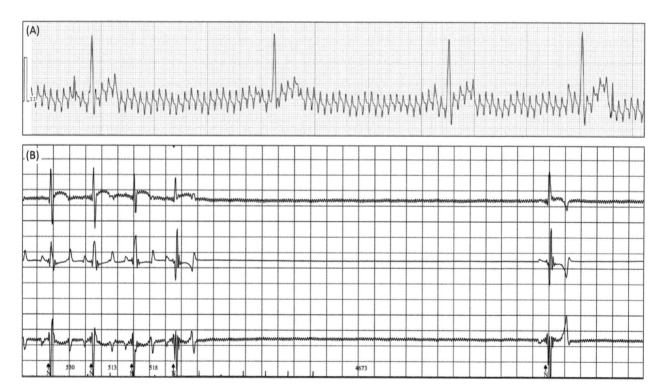

Figure 4.10 Electrical interference. Regular, high-frequency, sharp deflections of the baseline may be seen on electrocardiographic (A) and ambulatory ECG (Holter) (B) recordings due to electrical interference. The QRS complexes are visible in all leads, but P waves are not discernible on the electrocardiographic trace (A) and the first channel of the ambulatory ECG (Holter) trace. (A) [8-year-old, female neutered, Hungarian Vizsla dog] (50 mm/s; 20 mm/mV) (B) [2-year-old, male Lurcher dog]

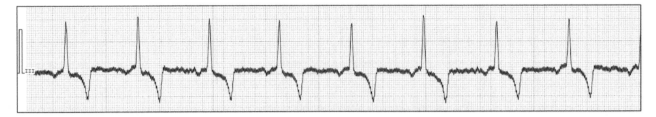

Figure 4.11 Poor electrode contact. The baseline appears thicker with poor detail. [15-year-old, male neutered, Border Terrier dog] (50 mm/s; 20 mm/mV)

skin (especially the right leg electrode which is the ground electrode) by placing the patient on an insulated blanket, ensuring that the ECG machine is earthed and, most importantly, turning off other electrical appliances in the room.

3) *Poor electrode contact* results in a trace of reduced quality, with smaller R waves and baseline artefact (Figure 4.11). The artefact may result in complete obliteration of the ECG trace.

The Normal ECG

The components of a normal ECG complex, as discussed in chapter 3, are illustrated in Figure 4.12 and are as follows:

- *P*: Depolarisation of the atria
- *Ta*: Repolarisation of the atria – often superimposed on or hidden within/by the QRS complex

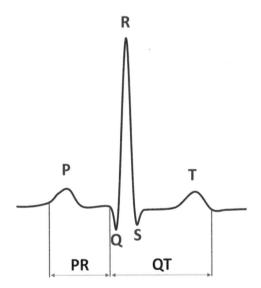

Figure 4.12 Normal electrocardiographic complex in lead II. The normal electrocardiographic complex is formed of a P, a QRS and T waves corresponding to atrial and ventricular depolarisations as well as ventricular repolarisation, respectively. The interval between the beginning of the P and QRS is the PR interval that corresponds to the time the impulse spends travelling through atria, the atrioventricular node and His–Purkinje before reaching the ventricular working myocardium. The QT interval represents the time necessary for ventricular depolarisation and repolarisation. The sections of return to baseline between the P and QRS and the QRS and T are the PR and ST segments.

- *PR*: Trace returns to baseline as the electrical impulse traverses the AV node.
- *QRS*: Depolarisation of the ventricles
- *ST*: Time during which electrical activity is translated into mechanical contraction
- *T*: Repolarisation of the ventricles.

Before setting the ECG to record, ensure that the trace on the screen is of good quality with clear complexes and minimal artefact. If a rhythm disturbance is present, then it is possible that not all components of a normal ECG trace will be visible. Always ensure that the trace is clearly labelled with patient name, a unique patient identification number and the time and date of recording; also note any drugs administered prior to or during the recording and the timing of any other interventions such as vagal manoeuvres that were performed during the recording. Also note whether the filter was used and the body position if non-standard.

Interpretation of the ECG

In this section, a systematic approach to ECG interpretation is described which can be summarised as:

1) Calculate heart rate.
2) Assess whether the heart rhythm is regular or irregular.
3) Assess the relationship (synchrony) between P waves and QRS complexes – is there consistent coupling between the P waves and the ensuing QRS complexes?
4) Evaluate the QRS complexes – are they upright in lead II and narrow, or are they wide and bizarre?
5) Take measurements, and know how to interpret them.
6) Calculate the MEA, and know how to interpret it.
7) Formulate a rhythm diagnosis.
8) Most importantly, interpret the ECG findings in light of patient history, clinical findings and the results of other tests.

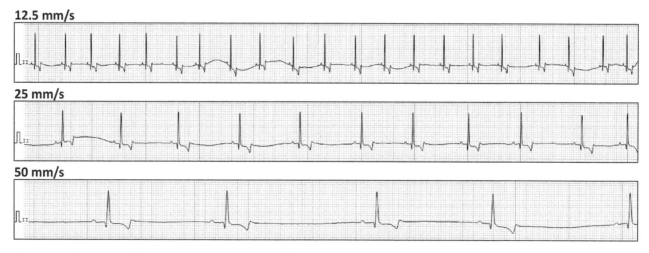

12.5 mm/s

25 mm/s

50 mm/s

Figure 4.13 Examples of different paper speeds. [2-year-old, female neutered, Border collie dog] (5 mm/mV)

1. Calculating Heart Rate

The ECG trace plots time on the horizontal axis against voltage on the vertical axis. To calculate the heart rate, we will first focus on the horizontal axis. Most ECG machines produce traces at 25 mm/s or 50 mm/s, and some at the slower rates of 12.5 mm/s or 5 mm/s (Figure 4.13). The grid on the ECG paper is divided into small squares, each measuring 1 × 1 mm, usually with a slightly thicker line every 5 mm. Therefore, at 25 mm/s, each 1 mm box = 1/25 s = 0.04 s = 40 ms. At 50 mm/s, each 1 mm box = 1/50 s = 0.02 s = 20 ms. (See Table 4.2).

Calculating Instantaneous Heart Rate Using a Machine-Generated R-R Interval

The instantaneous (beat-to-beat) heart rate is the heart rate calculated from a single R-R interval. If the rhythm is regular, then the instantaneous heart rate will be a good representation of the mean heart rate.

The instantaneous heart rate can be calculated in several ways:

1) Some ECG machines will display the R-R interval in milliseconds (ms) between each beat. Alternatively, the distance between two consecutive beats can be measured, and the R-R can be calculated using the principal that there are 60,000 ms in each minute; therefore, the heart rate in bpm is 60,000/R-R interval (see Figure 4.14).

Table 4.2 Time measurements according to paper speed

Paper speed (mm/s)	1 mm in seconds	1 mm in milliseconds
5	0.2	200
25	0.04	40
50	0.02	20

Calculating Instantaneous Heart Rate Using an ECG Ruler

An ECG ruler can be used to measure instantaneous heart rate more easily. The key is to ensure that the scale used on the ruler (25 mm/s or 50 mm/s) corresponds to the scale on the ECG (see Figure 4.15). Alternatively, the ruler scale for 50 mm/s can be used on a 25 mm/s ECG trace by counting two cycles instead of one.

The arrow on the ruler is placed against an R wave, and the position of the following R wave on the scale will show the instantaneous heart rate.

Calculating Mean Heart Rate

To account for variations in heart rate (e.g. in cases with sinus arrhythmia), it is often more useful to look at the mean heart rate over several beats rather than calculating the instantaneous rate. As distance is the product of speed × time, we can calculate the distance that 3 and 6 s intervals will occupy at different paper speeds, as shown in Table 4.3.

Using this method, a ruler is placed on the trace, and the number of beats occurring in 6 s is counted. To calculate the number of beats per minute, this figure is multiplied by 10. As should be intuitive, if we are using a 3 s interval, then we multiply by 20 to calculate the mean 1 min heart rate. See Figure 4.16.

2. Assess the Heart Rhythm

Callipers or a ruler can be useful to determine whether the rhythm is regular or irregular.

In dogs, the normal heart rhythms are sinus rhythm and sinus arrhythmia. Sinus arrhythmia is a regular variation in heart rate often associated with the breathing movements (respiratory sinus arrhythmia). The heart

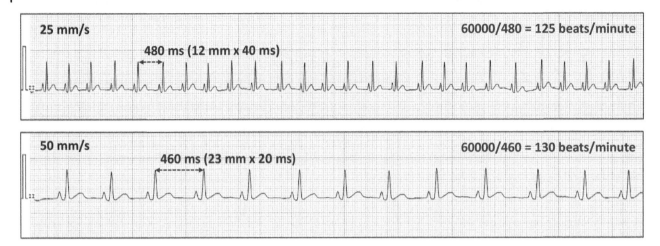

Figure 4.14 How to calculate the instantaneous heart rate. The instantaneous heart rate may be calculated by determining the RR interval in milliseconds, and then dividing 60,000 by that number. This may be appropriate if the rhythm is regular, but with irregular rhythms the final result will be inaccurate in terms of how many beats actually happen in 1 min. [6-year-old, female, neutered Birman cat] (20 mm/mV)

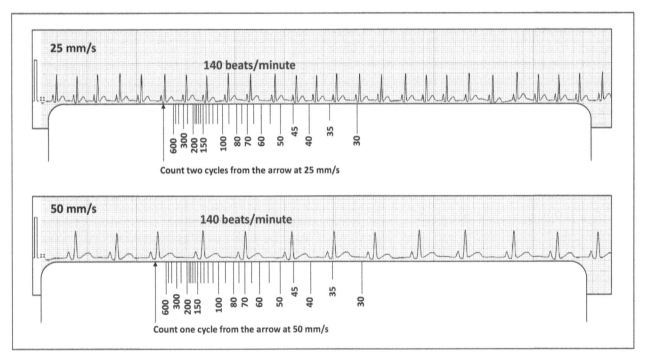

Figure 4.15 How to calculate the heart rate with an ECG ruler. Many ECG rulers have two different scales, one for use at 25 mm/s and another for 50 mm/s. If that is the case, one cycle (one beat) should be counted from the arrow using the corresponding scale. In the example here, the scale on the ruler is for use with 50 mm/s but can still be used on a 25 mm/s trace by counting two cycles from the arrow instead of one. [6-year-old, female neutered, Birman cat] (20 mm/mV)

Table 4.3 Distance occupied by 3 and 6 s intervals at different paper speeds

Paper speed (mm/s)	3 seconds	6 seconds
5	1.5 cm	3 cm
25	7.5 cm	15 cm
50	15 cm	30 cm

rate increases during inspiration and decreases during expiration.[17] For further information, see chapter 5.

In cats, sinus rhythm and sinus tachycardia are the most common rhythms encountered on the resting ECG. When ambulatory ECGs are used to monitor cats in their home setting, slight sinus arrhythmia may be observed.[18]

Premature beats are beats that occur earlier than the normal R-R interval, and these can occur singly or as

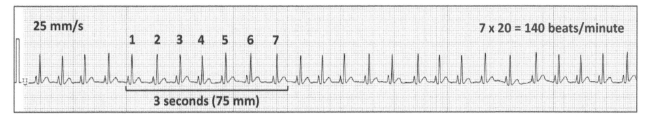

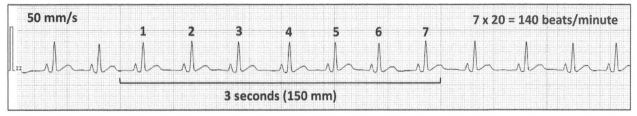

Figure 4.16 How to calculate the mean heart rate. To calculate the mean heart rate, one should count the number of beats in 3 s (75 mm at 25 mm/s and 150 mm at 50 mm/s) and multiply them by 20. Alternatively, count the number of beats in 6 s and multiply by 10 instead of 20. [6-year-old, female neutered, Birman cat] (20 mm/mV)

multiple consecutive beats. If these beats have a QRS complex similar to the sinus beats, they are likely to originate above the atrioventricular node. If these beats have a wide QRS that appears different from the sinus beats, then they are more likely to be either ventricular in origin or supraventricular with aberrant conduction. Escape beats are beats originating outside the sinoatrial node after a longer than normal R-R – premature and escape beats are discussed more fully in chapters 8, 10 and 11.

3. P:QRS

In normal sinus rhythm and sinus arrhythmia, there will be a P wave preceding every QRS complex, and the coupling interval between the P waves and QRS complexes will be consistent (constant PR interval). If there is baseline artefact, it may be difficult to see every P wave, so efforts should be made to keep the patient as still and quiet as possible and also to ensure that the clips or electrodes have good electrical contact with the skin.

With supraventricular premature beats, a P (or P' if the focus is outside the sinoatrial node) wave may or may not be visible prior to the premature QRS. With ventricular ectopy, a P wave may be seen but is not coupled to the ectopic QRS complex.

4. QRS Complex

As discussed in this chapter, a normal QRS complex is upright and narrow in leads I, II, III and aVF. There are several potential mechanisms by which a QRS complex can have a wide, bizarre morphology, contrasting with the sinus beats. Examples would include:

- Ventricular ectopic beats (see chapter 11)
- Intraventricular conduction disturbances, for example bundle branch block (see chapter 7)

- Notched QRS, for example in tricuspid dysplasia
- Accessory pathway with antegrade conduction from atria to ventricles (see chapter 10).

5. P-QRS-T Measurements

Measurements of the ECG complex are usually made from lead II, with the paper speed set at 50 mm/s. (See Table 4.4). The amplitude is recorded in millivolts, and measurements of upward deflections are made from the upper edge of the baseline to the peak of the wave. For downward deflections, measurements are taken from the lower side of the baseline to the lowest point of the wave. The duration of a wave or segment of the complex is taken from start to finish (Figure 4.17). The amplitude of biphasic waves is calculated by adding the amplitudes above and below the baseline.

Whilst inferences regarding cardiac chamber size were commonly made from ECGs in the past, echocardiography is more sensitive, specific and accurate in this regard and has now largely superseded electrocardiography as the means of assessing cardiac chamber dimensions. The increase in the availability of echocardiography means that cardiologists of this generation will use the ECG primarily for assessing heart rate and rhythm rather than for assessing heart size, although this aspect is discussed in more detail in this chapter.

P Wave

The P wave represents atrial depolarisation. It normally appears as a positive wave in leads II, III and aVF (inferior leads) and as a negative wave in leads aVL and aVR. In lead I, it may appear as positive, biphasic or isobiphasic (see Figure 4.18 for different P wave nomenclature). The duration and amplitude of the P wave are measured on the ECG, as illustrated in Figure 4.17.

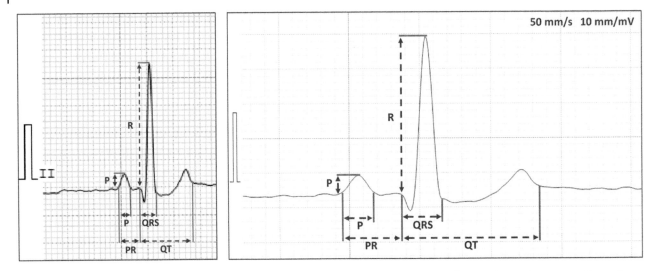

Figure 4.17 Where measurements are taken from a normal ECG complex. Measurements of the ECG complex are usually made from lead II, with the paper speed set at 50 mm/s and with the patient in right lateral recumbency. The amplitude is recorded in millivolts, and measurements of upward deflections are made from the upper edge of the baseline to the peak of the wave. For downward deflections, measurements are taken from the lower side of the baseline to the lowest point of the wave. The duration of a wave or segment of the complex is taken from start to finish. Measurements of duration are not influenced by patient position.

Table 4.4 Normal reference ranges for cat and dog electrocardiographic measurements

Parameter	Dog	Cat
Heart rate (bpm)	Adult: 70–160 Puppy: 70–200	Adult: 140–220
P wave amplitude (mV)	<0.4	<0.2
P wave width (ms)	Adult: <40 Giant breed: <50	<40
PR interval (ms)	60–130*	50–90
R wave amplitude (mV)	<3 mV	<0.9
QRS width (ms)	<70	<40
QT duration (ms)	150–250**	120–180
QTc (ms)	150–240	70–200
ST segment	Elevation and depression <0.2 mV	
T wave amplitude	Positive, negative or biphasic. No more than 25% height of R wave.	Positive, negative or biphasic

*The PR interval is inversely correlated to heart rate.[19]
**The QT interval also decreases at high heart rates (see the section on corrected QT intervals in this chapter).
Note: Measurements are taken from lead II, with a paper speed of 50 mm/s and the patient in a standard right lateral recumbency.
Source: Adapted from Tilley LP. Essentials of canine and feline electrocardiography. St Louis: Mosby; 1980.[2]

Duration: The duration of the P wave represents the time it takes for both the right and left atrial myocardium to be completely depolarised. An increase in duration may occur in case of atrial enlargement (particularly left) or with a delay in interatrial conduction such as with Bachman's bundle block (Figure 4.19). Interatrial conduction blocks have been described in humans and may precede the development of atrial arrhythmias, including atrial fibrillation.[20] Naturally occurring partial interatrial conduction block has been reported in a Boxer dog.[21]

Amplitude: The amplitude of the P wave is directly proportional to the atrial mass. An increase in amplitude suggests atrial enlargement, particularly affecting the right atrium (Figure 4.19).

Changes in the P Wave
Right atrial enlargement

- P wave amplitude >0.4 mV, duration <40 ms in lead II in dogs; amplitude >0.2 mV, duration <40 ms in cats
- P wave tall and peaked in leads II, III and aVF
- This change is sometimes known as *P pulmonale*.
- A Ta wave may be visible.
- Associated conditions include respiratory disease[22] and also congenital cardiac defects, resulting in right atrial enlargement such as tricuspid dysplasia.[23]
- Increases in heart rate will sometimes cause a subtle increase in P wave amplitude as a result of a change in the site of impulse generation in the sinoatrial node.

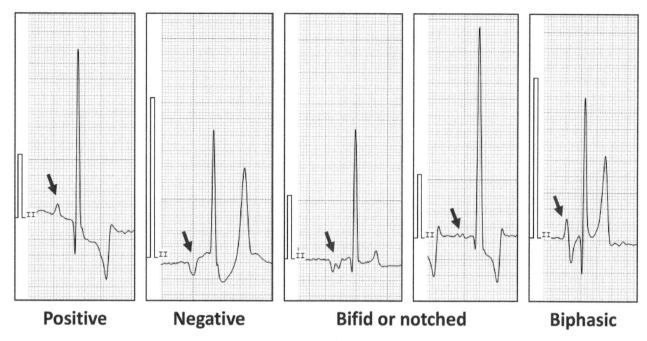

Positive　　**Negative**　　**Bifid or notched**　　**Biphasic**

Figure 4.18 Variations in P wave morphology. (Positive) A P wave entirely above the baseline. (Negative) A P wave entirely below the baseline. (Bifid or notched) This describes a notch in the complex which does not cross the baseline. (Biphasic) This describes a P wave with unequal sections above and below the baseline, resulting in a wave that can be predominantly positive or negative; if equal components are seen above and below the baseline, the term *isobiphasic* may be used.

Right　　**Left**　　**Biatrial**

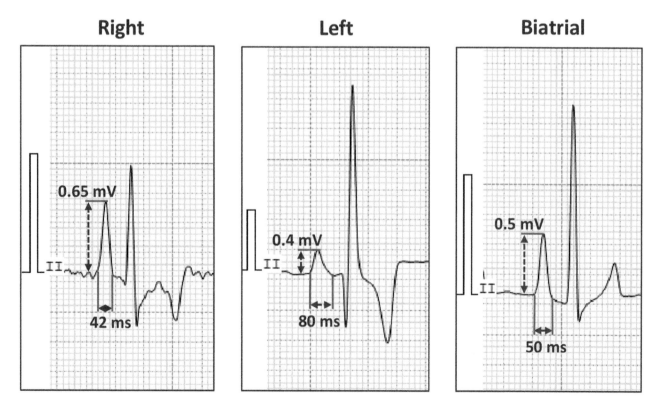

Figure 4.19 Changes in P wave amplitude and width suggestive of atrial enlargement. An increase in P wave amplitude (>0.4 mV in dogs and >0.2 mV in cats) is suggestive of right atrial enlargement, whereas an increase in P wave duration (>40 ms in dogs and in cats) suggests left atrial enlargement. If both are present, bi-atrial enlargement may be suspected. It is important to note that, although these findings are suggestive of atrial enlargement, they are not always reliable and should not replace echocardiography for this purpose. If anything, they should prompt further investigation with echocardiography. [The examples here are from dogs.]

Left atrial enlargement

- Sinus impulses traverse the atria from right to left; therefore, left atrial enlargement may result in prolongation of the P wave >40 ms in lead II in dogs or cats.
- Notching may result from simultaneous left and right atrial activation and is only considered abnormal if the P wave is also wide.
- Interatrial conduction disturbances in human patients will also cause P wave widening without left atrial enlargement.[24]
- In dogs, conditions causing left atrial enlargement include myxomatous mitral valve disease, dilated cardiomyopathy and mitral valve dysplasia/stenosis.[25]
- In cats, cases with various forms of cardiomyopathy may have left atrial enlargement, and this is also seen with mitral valve dysplasia.[26]

Other causes of variation in P wave morphology

- Negative P waves may be seen in cases with junctional or ectopic atrial rhythms (see chapters 8 and 10); or they may be positional.
- Wandering pacemaker is a regular variation in P wave amplitude associated with variations in vagal tone (see chapter 5).
- Multifocal atrial tachycardia
- Small or absent P waves can be seen with sinus node and atrial disease and also secondary to electrolyte abnormalities, including hyperkalaemia[27] (see chapters 7 and 23).

Biatrial enlargement

- The diagnosis of atrial enlargement from an ECG is unreliable and should always be supported by echocardiographic findings.
- Biatrial enlargement may be seen in feline hypertrophic and restrictive cardiomyopathy and also dilated cardiomyopathy in both dogs and cats.
- In dogs, biatrial enlargement is also commonly seen in dogs with advanced myxomatous atrioventricular valve disease.

PR Interval

The PR interval reflects the time taken for the depolarisation wave to be conducted through the atria, atrioventricular node and bundle of His.

Lengthening of the PR interval

- A long PR is defined as >130 ms in dogs or >90 ms in cats.
- A prolonged PR interval is known as first-degree atrioventricular block (1AVB) (see chapter 7).
- The PR interval tends to increase with decreasing heart rate,[28] and therefore a long PR interval may be seen in cases with sinus arrhythmia and also wandering pacemaker.

- Lengthening of the PR interval may occur secondary to:
  - Physiologically or pathologically raised vagal tone
  - Conduction system disease, for example sick sinus syndrome
  - Electrolyte abnormalities, such as hyper- or hypokalaemia[29]
  - Drugs, for example digoxin and β-blockers
  - Chagas' myocarditis[30]
  - After intravenous atropine administration, the PR interval will initially lengthen.[31]

Shortening of the PR interval

- A short PR interval is defined as <60 ms in dogs or <50 ms in cats.
- The PR interval will naturally shorten as heart rate increases.[19]
- Shortening of the PR interval occurs with pre-excitation antegrade conduction via an accessory pathway (see chapter 10).
- Dystrophin deficiency (Duchenne's cardiomyopathy) may result in deep Q waves and also a short PR interval (see chapter 23).[32]

Variable PR interval

This may occur secondary to:

- Multifocal atrial tachycardia
- Atrioventricular dissociation with an accelerated junctional rhythm (see chapter 10)
- Second-degree atrioventricular block (2AVB) results in some P waves without an ensuing QRS complex. Occasional examples of low-grade 2AVB with single unconducted P waves can be seen in normal dogs during periods of low heart rate (e.g. during sleep), but would not be expected during normal sinus rhythm when alert.[33]
- Complete or third-degree atrioventricular block (3AVB).

QRS Complex

The QRS complex is generated by depolarisation of ventricular tissue. It is normally upright and narrow in leads I, II, III and aVF; and negative in leads aVR and aVL. As shown in Figure 4.17, the amplitude of the R wave is measured from the top edge of the baseline to the peak of the R wave. The depth of Q or S waves is measured from the lower edge of the baseline to the lowest part of the deflection. QRS duration is measured from the point when the trace leaves until it returns to baseline.

Terminology for Describing QRS Complex Morphology

Variations in QRS morphology may occur as illustrated in Figure 4.20. If the deflection amplitude is >0.5 mV, then it is designated with an uppercase letter (Q, R and S); and, if <0.5 mV, then lowercase (q, r and s) is used for the respective components (Table 4.5).

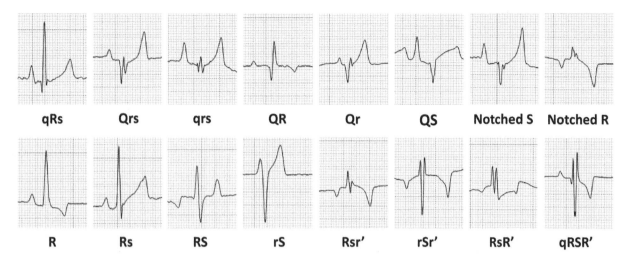

Figure 4.20 Examples of different QRS complex configurations and nomenclature. The first deflection of the QRS is termed Q, if it is negative and R if positive; a negative deflection after an R is termed S. A second positive deflection after an S is termed R′ (*R prime*). Additionally, if the amplitude of a deflection is less than 0.5 mV, a lowercase letter is used (q, r and s); if the amplitude is greater than 0.5 mV, capital letters are used (Q, R and S). This nomenclature is illustrated in the examples given here. Please note that this is not an extensive list and other conformations are possible.

Table 4.5 The normal QRS morphologies in different leads in order of frequency

Lead	Normal morphology
I	QR, qR, qRS
II	qR, qRs, Rs, QrS
III	qRs, qR, Rs, rS
aVR	rS, rSr′, qrS
aVL	Qr, QR, qRs
aVF	qR, Rs, QrS

Chapter 41: The Dog Electrocardiogram: A Critical Review. Pages 1877–1908. Published by Springer, 2010. *Source*: With permission from Comprehensive Electrocardiology. Edited by Peter W. Macfarlane *et al.*

Variations in QRS Morphology with Possible Causes

1) Tall QRS (>2.5 mV if <20 kg and >3 mV if >20 kg)
   - LV enlargement; also seen normally in athletic, narrow-chested breeds such as Greyhounds and Whippets
2) Low-amplitude QRS
   - Effusions (pleural, pericardial)
   - Intrathoracic mass
   - Broad chest conformation
   - Poor electrode contact
   - Hyperkalaemia[29]
   - Obesity
   - Hypothyroidism.
3) Wide QRS (>70 ms in dogs, >40 ms in cats)
   - Ventricular beats and rhythms are characterised by a wide, bizarre QRS complex without an associated P wave.

- Intraventricular conduction disturbance, such as bundle branch block (see chapter 7) or 'splintered QRS' with tricuspid valve dysplasia
- Supraventricular ectopic/premature beats with aberrant conduction result in a wide QRS.
- Hyperkalaemia.[29]

4. Variation in R Wave Amplitude

The term *electrical alternans* is used when P, QRS or T segments alter their configuration and/or magnitude in a rhythmic pattern, such as every other beat, or even every third or fourth complex (see chapter 8). Whilst any of the components can be affected, it is usually the QRS complex which varies by >1 mm in at least one lead.[9] In dogs with pericardial effusion, electrical alternans is likely to be due to the swinging movement of the heart within the fluid-filled pericardial sac, and the phenomenon is also sometimes seen with movement. In dogs with tachycardia, it may reflect varying refractory periods at high heart rates.[34]

Hypocalcaemia has been reported as a cause of T wave alternans *in vitro*.[35]

Changes in body position associated with exercise may result in changes in QRS complex amplitude and morphology.

5. Ventricular Enlargement

1. Right Ventricular Enlargement

If the following criteria are met, then there is a reasonable probability of right ventricular enlargement being present (see Figure 4.21):

- MEA shifted to the right (see Figure 4.22)
- S waves in leads I, II, III and aVF

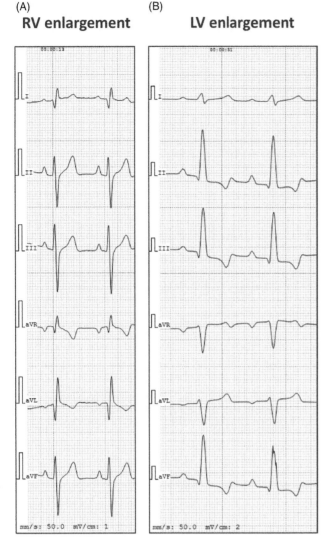

(A) RV enlargement

(B) LV enlargement

Figure 4.21 Ventricular enlargement. (A) Electrocardiographic findings in a case with right ventricular enlargement (hypertrophy) due to severe pulmonary hypertension. The QRS complex shows deep S waves in leads II, III and aVF. The mean electrical axis (MEA) using either the quadrant or calculation method is −71° and therefore would be classified as a left axis deviation despite echocardiography demonstrating right-sided enlargement. [7-month-old, male entire, German Shepherd dog] (50 mm/s; 10 mm/mV) (B) Electrocardiographic findings in a case with left ventricular enlargement (hypertrophy) secondary to severe subaortic stenosis. The QRS is wide (80 ms; >70 ms) with tall R waves in leads II (3.8 mV; >3.0 mV), III (3.4 mV) and aVF (3.4 mV; >3.0 mV); the MEA is normal (+90°). [7-month-old, male entire, German Shepherd dog] (50 mm/s; 5 mm/mV)

- S wave in lead I >0.05 mV
- S wave in lead II >0.35 mV.[36,37]

As conditions causing right ventricular enlargement (e.g. tricuspid valve dysplasia) will also cause right atrial enlargement, tall P waves may also be present.

Possible causes include:

- Congenital heart disease (e.g. pulmonic stenosis, tetralogy of Fallot)[38]
- Dirofilariasis in endemic areas[39]
- Cor pulmonale.

2. Left Ventricular Enlargement

Left ventricular enlargement can be due to either concentric hypertrophy (in response to pressure overload) and/or eccentric hypertrophy (in response to volume overload). It is important to note that young, athletic individuals with a slim chest confirmation may also have high-amplitude QRS complexes.[40]

Left ventricular enlargement is likely if there is:

- Increased R wave amplitude (>3 mV in leads II and aVF)
- Wide-QRS complex with severe enlargement (>70 ms)
- ST segment depression or coving (thought to be associated with myocardial ischaemia)
- Altered T wave morphology, for example T wave amplitude >25% R wave amplitude
- Abnormal left axis deviation <40° (see Figure 4.22).[41]

3. Biventricular Enlargement

This is more accurately diagnosed using echocardiography than the ECG. Features of biventricular enlargement include:

- Increased R wave amplitude (>3 mV in leads II and aVF)
- Wide QRS complex with severe enlargement (>70 ms)
- ST segment depression or coving (thought to be associated with ischaemia)
- Altered T wave morphology, for example T wave amplitude >25% of R wave amplitude
- Abnormal left axis deviation <40°.

ST Segment

This is measured from the end of the QRS complex to the onset of the T wave and represents the time taken for ventricular contraction and then the early part of ventricular repolarisation. It can be above or below the baseline but is considered abnormal if it is depressed by 0.2 mV or elevated by 0.15 mV in leads I, II, III and aVF.

The ST segment may be abnormal in cases with:

- Hyperkalaemia
- Myocardial ischaemia and hypoxia
- Trauma
- Artefact – a wandering baseline
- Pseudo-depression due to a prominent Ta wave (see chapter 3's section on the Ta wave).

Figure 4.22 Mean electrical axis (MEA) in the horizontal ('frontal') plane in dogs. The normal MEA in dogs varies from +40° to +100°. Any dog with a MEA less than +40° is said to have a left axis deviation, whereas a right axis deviation is present if the MEA is greater than +100°.

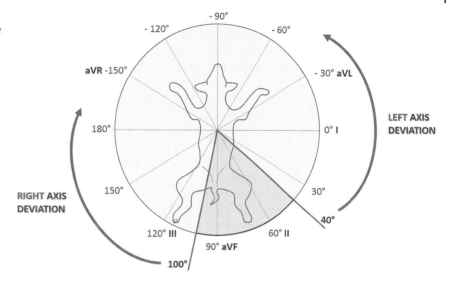

QT Interval

The QT interval is measured from the onset of the QRS to the end of the T wave. It represents the time it takes for ventricular depolarisation and repolarisation to occur. In dogs, the end of the T wave and return to baseline may be difficult to distinguish in lead II and is best appreciated in leads aVF and V3.

An excessively long QT interval (e.g. due to the effect of class III anti-arrhythmic drugs) may predispose to life-threatening ventricular arrhythmias (see chapter 6).

Corrected QT Interval (QTc)

The duration of the QT interval varies with the heart rate, being shorter during tachycardia and longer during low heart rates. To take this into account, several correction formulae have been suggested and are listed in Table 4.6, although none is perfect. Bazett's and Fridericia's formulae tend to overestimate the QT during tachycardia and underestimate during bradycardia. The linear Hodges formula seems to provide a better correlation than these and the Framingham formula.[42] When investigating congenital QT prolongation in English Springer Spaniels, Van de Water's correction formula was used, with the mean R-R interval calculated from the mean heart rate (over 6–10 s) to normalise the QT interval to an R-R interval of 1000 ms.[43] However, this formula tends to underestimate the QT during bradycardia. The logarithmic formula seems to be the most reliable for use in dogs.[44] In cats, these formulae have not been tested.

Causes of Long QT

- Hypokalaemia
- Hypocalcaemia (e.g. associated with primary hypoparathyroidism in dogs)[49]
- Hypercalcaemia and hypomagnesaemia[50]
- Anti-arrhythmic drugs such as sotalol and amiodarone
- Ethylene glycol toxicity

Table 4.6 Formulae for correcting QT interval for heart rate

Formulae for correcting the QT interval:

Logarithmic (Matsunaga):[44]

$QTc = \log 600 \times QT / \log RR$, with QT and RR in ms

Van de Waters:[45]

$QTc = QT - 0.087(RR-1000)$, with QT and RR in ms

Bazett:[46]

$QT_c = QT/RR^{0.5}$ with QT in ms and RR in s

Fridericia:[47]

$QT_c = QT/RR^{0.33}$ with QT in ms and RR in s

Framington:[48]

$QT_c = QT + 0.154*(1000/RR-1)$ with QT and RR in ms

Hodges:[42]

$QT_c = QT + 105*(1/RR-1)$ with QT in ms and RR in s

- Strenuous exercise
- Hypothermia
- Central nervous system (CNS) disease
- KCNQ1 gene mutation.[43]

QT Prolongation and Sudden Death in English Springer Spaniels

A syndrome of QT prolongation associated with a KCNQ1 gene mutation has been reported in a family of English Springer Spaniels with a high incidence of sudden death.[43] Prolongation of the QT interval suggests a heterogeneous pattern of ventricular repolarisation, which may provide a substrate for arrhythmias. Affected puppies had prolonged QT intervals of 260–270 ms with a QTc of 304–314 ms and also large biphasic T waves.

Causes of Short QT

- Hypercalcaemia (e.g. primary hyperparathyroidism)[51]
- Digoxin toxicity

T Wave

In dogs and cats, the T wave may be positive, negative or biphasic. On ambulatory ECGs, the T wave may change polarity with movement and changes in body position.

The normal T wave should be <25% of the R wave amplitude and is often slightly asymmetrical.

Causes of T wave change:[2]

- Myocardial hypoxia
- Abnormal intraventricular conduction
- Electrolyte abnormalities, especially potassium.[52] This is described in more detail in chapter 23.
- Severe systemic disease (e.g. septicaemia, bacteraemia anaemia)
- Drug toxicity.

6. Mean Electrical Axis

The electrical axis of the heart is the total sum of the many electrical vectors generated by the action potentials of individual ventricular myocytes (see chapter 3). We cannot measure the electrical axis directly, but it can be inferred from looking at the QRS complex amplitude in multiple leads using the hexaxial lead system.

The ventricular electrical axis, sometimes also known as the MEA, is the average direction of ventricular depolarisation during the whole of the QRS, and this may be clinically relevant in cases where we suspect abnormal conduction through the ventricles – for example, due to an area of the conduction system being diseased or blocked. The electrical axis can also be useful when evaluating some supraventricular tachycardias, especially those with an abnormal pathway connecting the atria and ventricles, as this pathway changes how the ventricle depolarises.

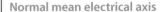

Normal mean electrical axis
Dogs: +40° to +100°
Cats: 0° to +160°
In neonates (<4 weeks of age), the MEA is directed towards the right but normalises by 12 weeks of age.[53]

Key point
It is important to note that, despite being useful, the MEA must be interpreted with care in our patients. The fact that the Einthoven's triangle is not equilateral in quadruped patients was highlighted in chapter 3. This limits the reliability of the MEA in our patients in comparison to humans. Additionally, different breeds of dogs possess very different chest conformations with varying effects on the orientation of the heart inside the chest. Narrow-chested dogs (e.g. collies, poodles and German Shepherds) tend to have an MEA closer to +90°, and conversely round-chested dogs (e.g. spaniels) have a more horizontal axis closer to +40°. For these reasons, the MEA should be used with care, and the various ranges provided in this text to describe different abnormalities should be interpreted as guidance rather than absolute measurements.

An explanation for the very variable MEA in cats is lacking.

Three ways to calculate the MEA are described:

1) *Estimation using quadrants*: The quadrant method is a recognised means of approximating the MEA. When calculating the MEA, it is important to realise that if the vector of depolarisation is moving predominantly in the plane of one lead, then the impulse recorded in the perpendicular lead is likely to be of low amplitude or isoelectric – see Figures 4.22 and 4.23. Key points:

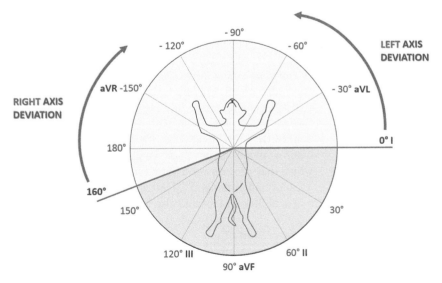

Figure 4.23 Mean electrical axis (MEA) in the frontal plane in cats. The normal MEA in cats varies from 0° to +160°. A MEA less than 0° is said to be deviated to the left, whereas a right axis deviation is present if the MEA is greater than +160°.

- Lead I is perpendicular to lead aVF.
- Lead II is perpendicular to aVL.
- Lead III is perpendicular to aVR.

In any given lead, the impulse may be positive, negative or isoelectric. Positive indicates that most of the complex is above the baseline, and negative indicates that most of the complex is below the baseline. Isoelectric indicates that the sum of the deflections in that lead is zero.

To calculate the quadrant of the MEA, we will concentrate on leads I and aVF.

If lead I is predominantly positive, then the MEA must lie between −90° and +90°.

If lead aVF is predominantly positive, then the MEA must lie between 0° and +180°.

If the trace shows a predominantly positive deflection in leads I and aVF, then the MEA is likely to be between 0° and 90°. (See Table 4.7).

2) *Tall or small QRS lead*: A rapid but very approximate way; if one of the six leads has a larger R wave than all the other leads, then the MEA will be approximately in the direction of that lead. For example, if the R wave is largely positive in lead II (and therefore approximately isoelectric in aVL), then the MEA will be approximately along the plane of lead II (+60°).

The converse way of applying the same principal is to find a lead which is isoelectric and the MEA will be perpendicular to this lead. Whether the MEA is positive or negative in the perpendicular lead is influenced by the net deflection in that lead.

3) A third method is to measure the net amplitudes of the QRS complex in leads I and III and plotting these on the hexaxial lead system (see Figure 4.24). Whilst this method will yield a number rather than a quadrant, care should be taken not to over-interpret the result obtained. The red line is projected from the centre outwards to the intersection of the perpendicular lines from leads I and III, and this gives the MEA.

> As plotting these values can be cumbersome, tables are provided in appendix 3 to facilitate rapid calculation of the MEA. However, given the underlying assumptions behind the accuracy of the hexaxial reference system, this could create a false impression of accuracy.

Forming a Rhythm Diagnosis

In the preceding sections of this chapter, we have discussed:

1) How to calculate heart rate
2) Assessing whether the heart rhythm is regular or irregular.
3) Assessing the relationship between P waves and QRS complexes: Is there consistent coupling between the P waves and the ensuing QRS complexes?
4) Evaluate the QRS complexes: Are they upright and narrow, or wide and bizarre?

Table 4.7 Using the quadrant method to approximate the mean electrical axis

−ve in leads I and aVF	+ve in lead I, −ve in aVF
MEA between −180° and −90°	MEA between −90° and 0°
MEA 'right cranial'	MEA 'left cranial'
−ve in lead I, +ve in aVF	**+ve in leads I and aVF**
MEA between +180° and +90°	MEA between 0° and +90°
MEA 'right caudal'	MEA 'normal or left caudal'*

*Note that the normal MEA in dogs is 40–100° and therefore can lie slightly outside this quadrant.

Figure 4.24 The R wave amplitude in lead I is +0.8 mV, but the Q wave is −0.2 mV, so the net deflection is +0.6 mV. This is plotted on the positive arm of lead I, and a line drawn perpendicular to the measurement. This process is then repeated in lead III, where the R wave amplitude is +1.85 mV and the Q is −0.2 mV. This distance is plotted on the positive arm of lead III, and then a line is drawn perpendicular to this measurement and extended until it intersects the first line. The red line is projected from the centre outwards to the intersection of the perpendicular lines from leads I and III, and this gives the mean electrical axis.

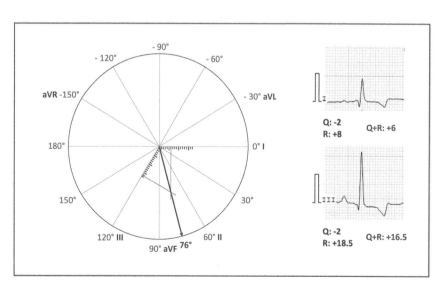

Table 4.8 Quick guide to making a rhythm diagnosis

Rhythm	Heart rate	P waves present?	Is there P:QRS coupling?	Narrow or wide QRS?	Possible rhythm diagnosis
Predominantly regular	Slow	Yes	Yes	Narrow	Sinus bradycardia Intermittent 2AVB
			No	Wide	3AVB
		No	No	Wide	Atrial standstill Hyperkalaemia
	Normal	Yes	Yes	Narrow	Sinus rhythm Intermittent 2AVB
			No	Wide	Accelerated idioventricular rhythm
				Narrow	Isorhythmic atrioventricular dissociation
		No	No	Wide	Atrial standstill Hyperkalaemia
	Fast	Yes	Yes	Narrow	Sinus tachycardia Supraventricular tachycardia (FAT) Atrial flutter
			No	Wide	Ventricular tachycardia
				Narrow	Junctional tachycardia
		No	No	Narrow	Supraventricular tachycardia*
Predominantly irregular	Slow	Yes	Yes	Narrow	Sinus arrhythmia Sick sinus syndrome 2AVB
			No	Wide	3AVB
		No	No	Narrow	Slow atrial fibrillation
	Normal	Yes	Yes	Narrow	Sinus arrhythmia 2AVB Atrial flutter
		No	No	Narrow	Atrial fibrillation
	Fast	Yes	Yes	Narrow	Sinus tachycardia Atrial flutter Supraventricular tachycardia
			No	Wide	Ventricular tachycardia
				Narrow	Junctional tachycardia
		No	No	Narrow	Atrial fibrillation

*In cases with supraventricular tachycardia caused by an ectopic atrial focus, P' waves may be superimposed on the preceding ST segment, making them difficult to see. 2AVB, Second-degree atrioventricular block – see chapter 7; 3AVB, third-degree or complete atrioventricular block – see chapter 7.

5) Take measurements, and know how to interpret them.
6) Calculate the MEA, know how to interpret this and be aware of its limitations.

We have now arrived at the final stage:

7) Formulate a rhythm diagnosis: Table 4.8 provides some guidelines that may be useful in arriving at a rhythm diagnosis. The features of each arrhythmia are described more fully in subsequent chapters of this book, and it is also important to note that excep-

tions exist to the generalisations made in this table – for example, atrial fibrillation with an intraventricular conduction disturbance will have a wide-QRS complex.

Sample Form for ECG Report

The ECG findings should be recorded an stored as part of the clinical record. A sample report form is shown in appendix 5.

References

1   Ferasin L, Amodio A, Murray JK. Validation of 2 techniques for electrocardiographic recording in dogs and cats. J Vet Intern Med. 2006;20:1–4.

2   Tilley LP. Essentials of canine and feline electrocardiography. Hoboken: John Wiley & Sons, Inc.; 1995.

3   Little CJL, Ferasin L, Ferasin H, Holmes MA. Purring in cats during auscultation: how common is it, and can we stop it? J Small Anim Pract. 2014;55:33–38.

4   Rishniw M, Porciello F, Erb HN, Fruganti G. Effect of body position on the 6-lead ECG of dogs. J Vet Intern Med. 2002;16:69–73.

5   Coleman MG, Robson MC. Evaluation of six-lead electrocardiograms obtained from dogs in a sitting position or sternal recumbency. Am J Vet Res. 2005;66:233–237.

6   Hulin I. Why does the electrocardiogram of the dog change with a change in the foreleg position? Am Heart J. 1970;79:143.

7   Harvey AM, Faena M, Darke PGG, Ferasin L. Effect of body position on feline electrocardiographic recordings. J Vet Intern Med. 2005;19:533–536.

8   Kraus MS, Moïse NS, Rishniw M, Dykes N, Erb HN. Morphology of ventricular arrhythmias in the boxer as measured by 12-lead electrocardiography with pace-mapping comparison. J Vet Intern Med. 2002;16:153–158.

9   Santilli RA, et al. Utility of 12-lead electrocardiogram for differentiating paroxysmal supraventricular tachycardias in dogs. J Vet Intern Med. 2008;22:915–923.

10   Winter BB, Webster JG. Driven-right-leg circuit design. IEEE Trans Biomed Eng. 1983;30:62–66.

11   Spinelli EM, Martinez NH, Mayosky MA. A transconductance driven-right-leg circuit. IEEE Trans Biomed Eng. 1999;46:1466–1470.

12   Venkatachalam KL, Herbrandson JE, Asirvatham SJ. Signals and signal processing for the electrophysiologist: part I: electrogram acquisition. Circ Arrhythm Electrophysiol. 2011;4:965–973.

13   Schrope DP, Fox PR, Hahn AW, Bond B, Rosenthal S. Effects of electrocardiograph frequency filters on P-QRS-T amplitudes of the feline electrocardiogram. Am J Vet Res. 1995;56:1534–1540.

14   Spier AW, Meurs KM. Use of signal-averaged electrocardiography in the evaluation of arrhythmogenic right ventricular cardiomyopathy in boxers. J Am Vet Med Assoc. 2004;225:1050–1055.

15   Calvert CA, Jacobs GJ, Kraus M. Possible ventricular late potentials in Doberman pinschers with occult cardiomyopathy. J Am Vet Med Assoc. 1998;213:235–239.

16   Luo S, Johnston P. A review of electrocardiogram filtering. J Electrocardiol. 2010;43:486–496.

17   Darke PG. The interpretation of electrocardiograms in small animals. J Small Anim Pract. 1974;15:537–552.

18   Ware WA. Twenty-four-hour ambulatory electrocardiography in normal cats. J Vet Intern Med. 1999;13:175–180.

19   Osborne BE, Leach GD. The beagle electrocardiogram. Food Cosmet Toxicol. 1971;9:857–864.

20   Chhabra L, Devadoss R, Chaubey VK, Spodick DH. Interatrial block in the modern era. Curr Cardiol Rev. 2014;10:181–189.

21   Gouvea de Almeida GL, Esteves CH, Barbosa de Almeida M, et al. Intermittent advanced Bachmann's bundle block in a Boxer dog. Acta Scientiae Veterinariae. 2010;38:439–442.

22   Miller MS, Tilley LP, Calvert CA. Electrocardiographic correlations in pulmonary heart disease. Semin Vet Med Surg (Small Anim). 1986;1:331–337.

23   Liu SK, Tilley LP. Dysplasia of the tricuspid valve in the dog and cat. J Am Vet Med Assoc. 1976;169:623–630.

24   van Dam I, Roelandt J, Robles de Medina EO. Left atrial enlargement: an electrocardiographic misnomer? An electrocardiographic-echocardiographic study. Eur Heart J. 1986;7:115–117.

25   Brownlie SE, Cobb MA. Observations on the development of congestive heart failure in Irish wolfhounds with dilated cardiomyopathy. J Small Anim Pract. 1999;40:371–377.

26   Moise NS, et al. Echocardiography, electrocardiography, and radiography of cats with dilatation cardiomyopathy, hypertrophic cardiomyopathy, and hyperthyroidism. Am J Vet Res. 1986;47:1476–1486.

27   Coulter DB, Duncan RJ, Sander PD. Effects of asphyxia and potassium on canine and feline electrocardiograms. Can J Comp Med. 1975;39:442–449.

28   Hanton G, Rabemampianina Y. The electrocardiogram of the Beagle dog: reference values and effect of sex, genetic strain, body position and heart rate. Lab Anim. 2006;40:123–136.

29   Klein SC, Peterson ME. Canine hypoadrenocorticism: part I. Can Vet J. 2010;51:63–69.

30   Anselmi A, Gurdiel O, Suarez JA, Anselmi G. Disturbances in the A-V conduction system in Chagas' myocarditis in the dog. Circ Res. 1967;20:56–64.

31   Muir WW. Effects of atropine on cardiac rate and rhythm in dogs. J Am Vet Med Assoc. 1978;172:917–921.

32   Fine DM, et al. Age-matched comparison reveals early electrocardiography and echocardiography changes in

dystrophin-deficient dogs. Neuromuscul Disord. 2011;21:453–461.

33 Ulloa HM, Houston BJ, Altrogge DM. Arrhythmia prevalence during ambulatory electrocardiographic monitoring of beagles. Am J Vet Res. 1995;56:275–281.

34 Morady F, DiCarlo LAJ, Baerman JM, de Buitleir M, Kou WH. Determinants of QRS alternans during narrow QRS tachycardia. J Am Coll Cardiol. 1987;9:489–499.

35 Navarro-Lopez F, Cinca J, Sanz G, Magrina J, Betriu A. Isolated T wave alternans elicited by hypocalcemia in dogs. J Electrocardiol. 1978;11:103–108.

36 Boineau JP, Hill JD, Spach MS, Moore EN. Basis of the electrocardiogram in right venricular hypertrophy: relationship between ventricular depolarization and body surface potentials in dogs with spontaneous RVH-contrasted with normal dogs. Am Heart J. 1968;76:605–627.

37 Brown FK, Brown WJJ, Ellison RG, Hamilton WF. Electrocardiographic changes during development of right ventricular hypertrophy in the dog. Am J Cardiol. 1968;21:223–231.

38 Trautvetter E, Detweiler DK, Bohn FK, Patterson DF. Evolution of the electrocardiogram in young dogs with congenital heart disease leading to right ventricular hypertrophy. J Electrocardiol. 1981;14:275–282.

39 Miller MS, Hadlock DJ, Brown J, Calvert CA, Cohn SR. The electrocardiogram in dogs with heartworm infection: clinical report and review of the literature. Semin Vet Med Surg (Small Anim). 1987;2:28–35.

40 Constable PD, Hinchcliff KW, Olson J, Hamlin RL. Athletic heart syndrome in dogs competing in a long-distance sled race. J Appl Physiol. 1994;76:433–438.

41 Hamlin RL. Electrocardiographic detection of ventricular enlargement in the dog. J Am Vet Med Assoc. 1968;153:1461–1469.

42 Patel PJ, *et al*. Optimal QT interval correction formula in sinus tachycardia for identifying cardiovascular and mortality risk: findings from the Penn Atrial Fibrillation Free study. Heart Rhythm 2016;13:527–535.

43 Ware WA, Reina-Doreste Y, Stern JA, Meurs KM. Sudden death associated with QT interval prolongation and KCNQ1 gene mutation in a family of English Springer Spaniels. J Vet Intern Med. 2015;29:561–568.

44 Matsunaga T, *et al*. QT corrected for heart rate and relation between QT and RR intervals in beagle dogs. J Pharmacol Toxicol Meth. 1997;38:201–209.

45 Van de Water A, Verheyen J, Xhonneux R, Reneman RS. An improved method to correct the QT interval of the electrocardiogram for changes in heart rate. J Pharmacol Meth. 1989;22:207–217.

46 Bazett HC. An analysis of the time-relations of the electrocardiogram. Heart. 1920;7:353–370.

47 Fridericia LS. The duration of systole in an electrocardiogram in normal humans and in patients with heart disease. 1920. Ann Noninvasive Electrocardiol. 2003;8:343–351.

48 Sagie A, Larson MG, Goldberg RJ, Bengtson JR, Levy D. An improved method for adjusting the QT interval for heart rate (the Framingham Heart Study). Am J Cardiol. 1992;70:797–801.

49 Russell NJ, Bond KA, Robertson ID, Parry BW, Irwin PJ. Primary hypoparathyroidism in dogs: a retrospective study of 17 cases. Aust Vet J. 2006;84:285–290.

50 Kadar E, Rush JE, Wetmore L, Chan DL. Electrolyte disturbances and cardiac arrhythmias in a dog following pamidronate, calcitonin, and furosemide administration for hypercalcemia of malignancy. J Am Anim Hosp Assoc. 2004;40:75–81.

51 Drazner FH. Hypercalcemia in the dog and cat. J Am Vet Med Assoc. 1981;178:1252–1256.

52 Tag TL, Day TK. Electrocardiographic assessment of hyperkalemia in dogs and cats. J Vet Emerg Crit Care. 2008;18:61–67.

53 Trautvetter E, Detweiler DK, Patterson DF. Evolution of the electrocardiogram in young dogs during the first 12 weeks of life. J Electrocardiol. 1981;14:267–273.

5

Sinus Rhythms
Ruth Willis

Introduction

This family of heart rhythms all originate from the sinoatrial node and, assuming that the rate is appropriate, represent the normal heart rhythms of dogs and cats.

This group of rhythms includes:

- Sinus rhythm
- Sinus arrhythmia
- Sinus bradycardia
- Sinus tachycardia.

The key features of sinus rhythms are:

- A normal P wave originating from the sinus node in the roof of the right atrium
- Consistent coupling between the P wave and the ensuing QRS complex
- Generally, the QRS complexes are narrow and upright in leads II, III and aVF. The exception to this would be if there is aberrant intraventricular conduction which results in a wide-QRS complex (for further information, see chapter 7).

Sinus Rhythm

Sinus rhythm is a normal heart rhythm seen in cats and dogs. The distinction between sinus rhythm, sinus bradycardia and sinus tachycardia depends on the heart rate (see Table 5.1). Sinus rhythms originate from the sinoatrial node located in the roof of the right atrium, as described in chapter 1. The electrophysiological properties of the sinoatrial node are described in chapter 2.

Cardiac Structure and Function

Cardiac anatomy is designed to facilitate conduction of electrical impulses across the myocardium in a consistent and efficient manner. As discussed in chapter 1,

cardiac anatomy provides both bridges and barriers to conduction – for example, Bachmann's bundle facilitates rapid and coordinated atrial depolarisation,[2] whereas the atrioventricular node slows conduction (also known as *decremental conduction*), thereby allowing time for atrial contraction and ventricular filling prior to ventricular contraction. Atrial fibre orientation and cell coupling are also integral to conduction of the impulse, with the impulse being conducted more rapidly in the longitudinal direction parallel to fibre orientation rather than in a transverse direction perpendicular to fibre orientation.[3] For further information on the electrophysiological properties of myocardial and pacemaker cells, see chapter 2.

Key point

During sinus rhythms, the P-QRS-T morphology is consistent because the anatomy of the heart favours the electrical impulse being conducted in a consistent fashion.

Sympathetic and Parasympathetic Influence on Sinus Node Depolarisation

The sinoatrial node is innervated by both parasympathetic and sympathetic efferent fibres, as described in chapter 1. There is a continual 'tug of war' between the sympathetic fibre discharge which increases heart rate and vagal nerve activity which lowers heart rate – see chapter 2 and Figure 2.6. Vagal effects are almost instantaneous, and they are mediated via the synaptic release of acetylcholine which is rapidly recycled, resulting in a short duration of effect (short latency). In contrast, sympathetically mediated increases in heart rate are stimulated by synaptic release of noradrenaline that is resorbed and metabolised more slowly (long latency).[4]

Guide to Canine and Feline Electrocardiography, First Edition. Ruth Willis, Pedro Oliveira and Antonia Mavropoulou.
© 2018 John Wiley & Sons Ltd. Published 2018 by John Wiley & Sons Ltd.
Companion website: www.wiley.com/go/willis/electrocardiography

Table 5.1 Guide to heart rates for sinus rhythm, sinus bradycardia and sinus tachycardia in dogs and cats

Parameter	Dog	Cat
Sinus rhythm	Adult: 70–160 bpm Puppy: 70–200 bpm	Adult: 140–220 bpm
Sinus bradycardia	Adult: <60 bpm Puppy: <70 bpm	<100–120 bpm
Sinus tachycardia	Adult: >180 bpm Puppy: >200 bpm	>220 bpm

Note: As heart rate is a highly labile parameter, it is understandable that wide fluctuations are possible in normal individuals, and therefore the numbers quoted should be used only as a guide rather than interpreted rigidly.
Source: Data from Tilley (1995).[1]

Table 5.2 Sinus rhythm

Rate	*Dog*: A rate appropriate for temperament and level of activity, usually around 120 bpm *Cat*: A rate appropriate for temperament and level of activity, usually around 150 bpm
Regularity	Regular
Onset/offset	Changes in heart rate are gradual.
P wave	P waves are present and positive in leads II, III and aVF; they are negative in aVL and aVR, with an electrical axis suggesting that the origin is in the roof of the right atrium (+18° to +90° in dogs, 0 to +90° in cats).
P:QRS ratio	P:QRS is 1:1 with consistent coupling and normal duration unless there is atrioventricular block.
QRS	A QRS is present after each P wave with a normal appearance (R wave in leads II, III and aVF; S wave in leads aVL and aVR) and duration <70 ms in dog, and <40ms in cat, indicating normal intraventricular conduction and activation.

Sinus Rhythm

Sinus rhythm is regular with a rate of approximately 70–160 bpm in adult dogs and approximately 140–220 bpm in cats; the features of sinus rhythm are summarised in Table 5.2. The rate of sinus node discharge is influenced by numerous factors including breed, fitness, drugs and whether there is underlying cardiac or systemic disease. Heart rate in healthy dogs is related to their demeanour – for example, nervous individuals will tend to have higher heart rates.[5] Individuals who are <12 months old have higher heart rates than adults.[6,7] In dogs >12 months of age, heart rate is poorly correlated to body size but remains correlated totemperament.[5] Therefore, whether the heart rate is appropriate depends on history and clinical findings. It is also important to remember that resting heart rate whilst the patient is relaxing at home is likely to be lower than the heart rates observed when animals are in the clinic.[8] For normal heart rates and complex dimensions in cats and dogs, see chapter 4 and appendix 1.

Figures 5.1 and 5.2 show sinus rhythms on electrocardiograms (ECGs) from a dog and cat, respectively.

Sinus Arrhythmia

Sinus arrhythmia is a regularly irregular rhythm commonly seen in normal dogs, especially in the brachycephalic breeds, and it describes a rhythmic variation in heart rate (see Figure 5.3 and Table 5.3 for a summary of the features of sinus arrhythmia). The mechanisms for sinus arrhythmia include respiratory and non-respiratory factors.

Respiratory Sinus Arrhythmia

During sinus arrhythmia, the R-R interval shortens with inspiration and lengthens with expiration, and this is a well-recognised feature of healthy heart function.

Driving mechanisms for sinus arrhythmia:[4]

- Arterial pressure fluctuations
  - Arterial baroreceptor reflex is the fastest and most powerful regulator of blood pressure.[9]
  - As the thorax expands during inspiration, intrathoracic pressure decreases. As fluids move from areas of high to low pressure, this has the effect of increasing venous return to the heart (like opening a set of billows).
  - The increase in venous return results in increased right ventricular filling and right heart output into large capacitance pulmonary blood vessels. Whilst this blood is pooled in the pulmonary circuit, there is a temporary decrease in left heart filling and output, and this slight reduction in arterial blood pressure results in modulation of vagal stimulation and an increase in heart rate during inspiration to offset the drop in blood pressure.[10]
  - These fluctuations in arterial pressure stimulate the baroreceptors, thereby generating small changes in vagal activity.
- Vagal cardiomotor neurons – inhibited during inspiration, and activated during expiration by stimulation of arterial chemoreceptors and baroreceptors.

> **Respiratory sinus arrhythmia summary**
>
> The heart rate **INCREASES** during inspiration and **DECREASES** during expiration.

Non-respiratory Sinus Arrhythmia

A cyclical variation in heart rate may also be seen without being associated with the respiratory movements, and it is thought to be due to Mayer waves. Mayer

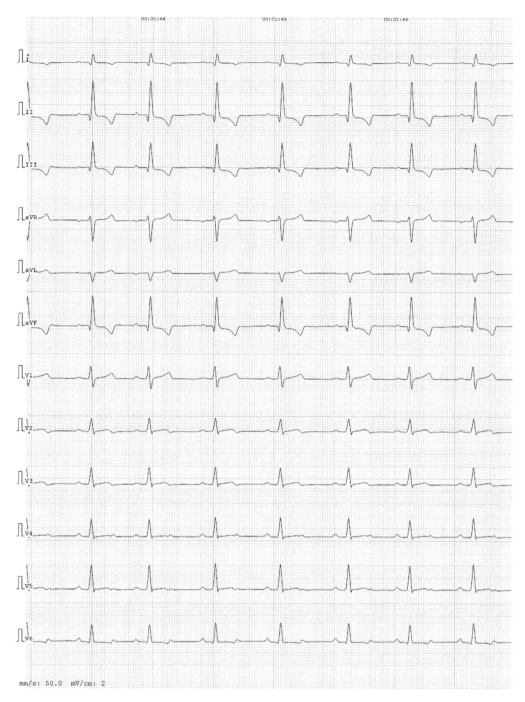

Figure 5.1 Twelve-lead electrocardiogram during sinus rhythm in a dog. A normal (sinus) P wave is seen in all beats with an electrical axis of approximately 60°, consistent with an origin in the roof of the right atrium (+18° to +90°; positive wave in leads II, III and aVF; negative wave in leads aVL and aVR). The PR interval is consistent for all beats and within normal limits for a dog (≈100 ms; normal: 60–130 ms), suggesting normal atrioventricular conduction. A QRS is present after each P wave with a normal appearance (R wave in leads II, III and aVF; S wave in aVL and aVR) and duration (60 ms; normal: <70 ms), indicating normal intraventricular conduction and activation. [2-year-old, male neutered, Boxer] (50 mm/s, 5 mm/mV)

waves are oscillations of sympathetic vasomotor tone with a frequency of around 0.1 Hz (therefore, a 10 s cycle) that have been studied in dogs and other mammalian species.[11] Mayer waves account for the regular, rhythmic, slight fluctuations in arterial blood pressure that occur with a frequency lower than the respiratory rate, and these waves are enhanced by sympathetic stimulation.[12] Mayer waves were thought to originate in the brainstem and spinal cord, but, more recently, studies investigating the effects of sino-aortic baroreceptor denervation have challenged this theory.[12] Therefore, current thinking is that the amplitude of

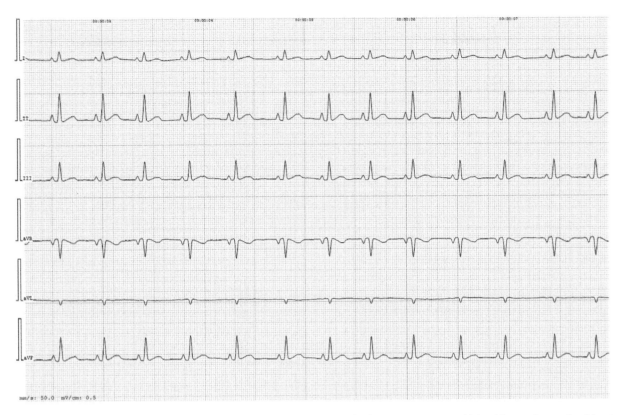

Figure 5.2 Sinus rhythm in a cat. Six-lead electrocardiogram during sinus rhythm in a cat. A normal (sinus) P wave is seen in all beats with an electrical axis of approximately 65°, consistent with an origin in the roof of the right atrium (0 to +90°; positive wave in leads II, III and aVF; negative wave in leads aVL and aVR). The PR interval is consistent for all beats and within normal limits for a cat (≈70 ms; normal: 50–90 ms), suggesting normal atrioventricular conduction. A QRS is present after each P wave with a normal appearance (R wave in leads II, III and aVF; S wave in leads aVL and aVR) and duration (40 ms; normal: <40 ms), indicating normal intraventricular conduction and activation. [8-year-old, female neutered, Birman cat] (50 mm/s, 20 mm/mV)

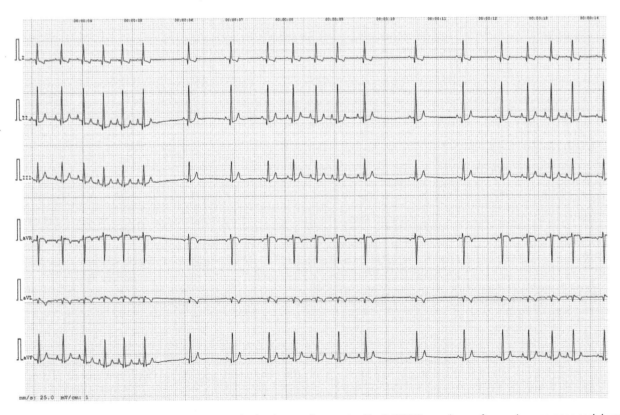

Figure 5.3 Respiratory sinus arrhythmia. A sinus rhythm is seen characterised by P-QRS-T complexes of normal appearance and duration. A cyclical variation of the heart rate is seen with an acceleration and deceleration of the rate that were associated with inspiratory and expiratory movements, respectively. [5-year-old, male neutered, Staffordshire Bull Terrier dog] (25 mm/s, 10 mm/mV)

Table 5.3 Sinus arrhythmia

Rate	*Dog*: A rate appropriate for temperament and level of activity, usually 60–120 bpm *Cat*: Rare in healthy cats in the clinic
Regularity	Regularly irregular
Onset/offset	Changes in heart rate are gradual.
P wave	P waves are present and positive in leads II, III and aVF; they are negative in aVL and aVR, with an electrical axis suggesting that the origin is in the roof of the right atrium (+18° to +90° in dog, 0 to +90° in cat). Wandering pacemaker may be present.
P:QRS ratio	P:QRS is 1:1 with consistent coupling and normal duration unless there is atrioventricular block.
QRS	A QRS is present after each P wave with a normal appearance (R wave in leads II, III and aVF; S wave in leads aVL and aVR) and duration <70 ms in dogs and <40 ms in cats, indicating normal intraventricular conduction and activation.

Mayer waves is determined by the strength of triggering impulses and sensitivity of the sympathetic component of the baroreceptor reflex.[12]

In cats, sinus arrhythmia is less common than in dogs (Table 5.3). If sinus arrhythmia is present in a cat in the consulting room, then it usually accompanies conditions altering autonomic tone (e.g. respiratory disease) or occurs after administration of drugs such as beta-adrenergic antagonists or opioids. Mild sinus arrhythmia is sometimes seen on ambulatory ECGs from cats that are relaxed and in familiar surroundings.[13,14]

Ventriculophasic Sinus Arrhythmia

Ventriculophasic sinus arrhythmia is another example of a non-respiratory sinus arrhythmia that may be seen in cases of second or third-degree atrioventricular block. The sinus discharge rate increases whenever ventricular contraction occurs, causing a shorter PP interval when a QRS complex is included than the PP interval not enclosing a QRS complex (see Figure 5.4). The exact mechanism is not fully understood, although the most plausible explanation consists of two-phase chronotropic effects causing acceleration and deceleration of the sinus discharge rate.[15]

The negative chronotropic effect is attributed to arterial baroreceptor–mediated changes in vagal tone.[15] A sensed increase in arterial blood pressure following ventricular contraction may elicit an increase in vagal tone lowering sinus node discharge rate for the next beat(s). As this surge in vagal tone then subsides, the P-P interval shortens prior to the next ventricular systole.[15] The positive chronotropic effect could be explained by the mechanical effects of ventricular systole enhancing sinus node perfusion.[16,17] In humans, this phenomenon has been reported in up to 40% of cases with third-degree atrioventricular block, and less commonly in 2:1 second-degree atrioventricular block.[15,18,19] Less information is available in veterinary literature, although it has been described in dogs.[20,21]

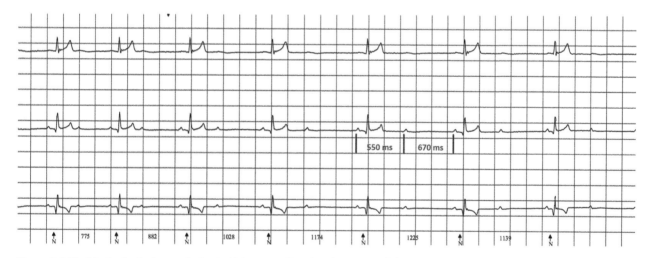

Figure 5.4 Ventriculophasic sinus arrhythmia. Holter recording showing a second-degree atrioventricular block with 2:1 conduction. The interval between the P wave of the beat including the QRS and the blocked P (550 ms) is shorter than the interval between the blocked P and the following P (670 ms). This is suggestive of ventriculophasic sinus arrhythmia. The underlying mechanism is not fully understood; however, a positive chronotropic effect caused by the effects of atrial stretch during ventricular systole, and an increase in sinus node perfusion, are thought to elicit an earlier sinus depolarisation following ventricular contraction. A sensed increase in pressure by arterial baroreceptors following ventricular contraction is thought to elicit an increase in vagal tone, lowering the sinus node discharge rate in the subsequent beat. [11-year-old, male Labrador Retriever with second-degree atrioventricular block]

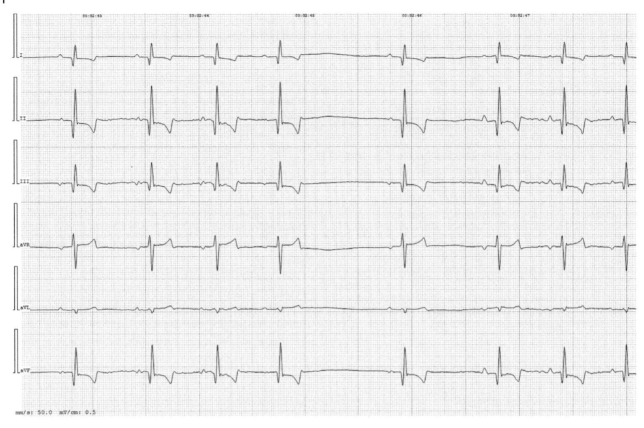

Figure 5.5 Respiratory sinus arrhythmia with wandering pacemaker. A slightly irregular rhythm is seen due to respiratory sinus arrhythmia in this patient. The QRS appearance and duration are normal, suggesting a normal intraventricular conduction and activation. The P wave morphology is variable: during periods of higher heart rate (such as in the last three beats), it is normal, with origin in the roof of the right atrium (positive wave in leads II, III and aVF; negative wave in leads aVL and aVR); during periods of lower heart rate, the P wave amplitude is progressively reduced, with a shift in origin to areas lower in the right atrium (negative in leads III and aVR, whilst positive in aVL). The P wave duration (≈40 ms) and PR interval (≈120 ms) remain similar in all beats. This variation of the P wave morphology associated with the heart rate is described as *wandering pacemaker*. It is due to a shift in atrial activation via impulses originating in the dorsal areas of the sinus node during higher heart rates, and ventral areas of the sinus node during periods of lower heart rates. [9-year-old, female neutered, Boxer dog] (50 mm/s, 20 mm/mV)

Wandering Pacemaker

As described in chapter 1, the sinoatrial node is not a single cell but a collection of cells, and the size of the node can reach several centimetres in length. The P wave can be generated from anywhere in the node and, at higher heart rates, the site of impulse generation tends to move proximally to a more dorsal location. In contrast, during periods of lower heart rates, the site of impulse generation moves distally to a more ventral portion of the node. As a result of the change in the site of impulse generation, the P wave as seen on the surface ECG will appear slightly different, and this is termed *wandering pacemaker*. Wandering pacemaker may also be accompanied by a slight variation in the PR interval (Figure 5.5).

Whilst sinus arrhythmia has been described as a regularly irregular rhythm, it may be interrupted by supraventricular or ventricular ectopic beats as discussed in chapters 8 and 11.

Sinus Bradycardia

Sinus bradycardia is a rhythm originating from the sinoatrial node with a slower rate than sinus rhythm; the features of sinus bradycardia are summarised in Table 5.4. Sinus bradycardia may be appropriate if it occurs during periods of rest, and this rhythm is also commonly seen during or after general anaesthesia, especially if opioid medications have been administered. Assuming that blood pressure and perfusion are adequate, then this may be a normal physiological rhythm; but, if seen in a patient where high sympathetic tone would be expected (e.g. in a situation where the patient is painful), then it would be considered inappropriate.

As physiological sinus bradycardia is mediated by high resting vagal tone, it is common to simultaneously see first-degree atrioventricular block (lengthening of the PR interval) and wandering pacemaker.

Table 5.4 Sinus bradycardia

Rate	*Dog*: A rate slower than appropriate for temperament and level of activity, usually <60 bpm in adult dogs and <70 bpm in puppies *Cat*: Rare in healthy cats in the clinic, usually <100 bpm
Regularity	Regular or regularly irregular rhythm if combined with sinus arrhythmia
Onset/offset	Changes in heart rate are gradual.
P wave	P waves are present and positive in leads II, III and aVF; and negative in aVL and aVR, with an electrical axis suggesting that the origin is in the roof of the right atrium (+18° to +90° in dog, 0 to +90° in cat). Wandering pacemaker may be present.
P:QRS ratio	P:QRS is 1:1 with consistent coupling and normal duration unless there is concurrent atrioventricular block.
QRS	A QRS is present after each P wave with a normal appearance (R wave in leads II, III and aVF; S wave in leads aVL and aVR) and duration <70 ms in dogs and <40 ms in cats, indicating normal intraventricular conduction and activation.

Clinical Significance

Whilst sinus bradycardia is usually well tolerated, if there is a sudden decrease in heart rate (as may be seen during an episode of neurally mediated syncope), then this can result in hypotension (see chapters 7 and 12).

Causes of Sinus Bradycardia

Causes include:

- Physiological – for example, during periods of rest or as a response to athletic training
- Electrolyte abnormalities – for example, hyperkalaemia (see chapter 23)
- Drugs – for example, opioids, beta-adrenergic antagonists, calcium channel blockers, sotalol, amiodarone and digoxin (see chapters 17, 23 and 24)
- Concurrent disease altering autonomic tone – for example, increased intracranial pressure, gastrointestinal disease and respiratory or ocular conditions (see chapter 23)
- Pathology of the sinus node – for example, sick sinus syndrome and sinus node dysfunction (see chapter 7)
- Hypoxia (see chapters 23 and 24)
- Hypothermia
- Hypothyroidism (see chapter 23)
- Toxicity (see chapter 23)
- Idiopathic.

Athletic Heart

Athletic training results in physiological changes in the heart, including a reduction in resting heart rate, as shown in Figure 5.6.[22,23] A study to investigate electrocardiographic parameters from 105 healthy whippets was used to establish reference intervals for the breed. The most important differences compared to published

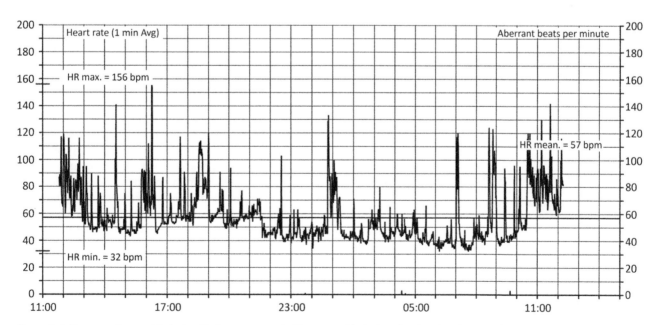

Figure 5.6 Heart rate in an athletic dog. Tachogram recorded from an athletic dog showing that the mean heart rate was 57 bpm and therefore below the accepted range of 65–90 bpm. The resting heart rate was between 30 and 40 bpm. [6-year-old, male neutered, German short-haired pointer]

reference values were the higher median R wave amplitudes in leads II, CV_6LL and CV_6LU. For some parameters (P wave amplitude, ST segment deflection and T wave amplitude in lead II; R wave amplitude in CV_5RL), a marked percentage of the whippet values were above the published maximum reference data. The results confirmed that whippets have electrocardiographic characteristics similar to those reported in athletic heart syndrome in humans. Some of these characteristics could be erroneously taken as evidence of cardiac disease, and clinicians should be aware of the possibility of athletic change in healthy breeds.[24]

Changes associated with athletic training in heavily trained sled dogs include a prolonged QRS duration (66.1 ± 7.4 ms) and QT interval (236 ± 20 ms), and also a rightward shift in the mean electrical axis was observed in the horizontal ('frontal') plane.[25] Another study, involving 319 Alaskan sled dogs, replicated these findings and also reported tall R waves (median: 3.02 mV).[26] The increase in QRS may be due to the increase in heart mass associated with endurance training.[27]

Sinus Tachycardia

Sinus tachycardia is a heart rhythm originating from the sinoatrial node with a faster rate than sinus rhythm; the features of this rhythm are summarised in Table 5.5. Sinus tachycardia is an appropriate and common physiological response to sympathetic stimulation – for example, during periods of excitement, exercise, pain or fear. Dogs are phenomenal athletes

Table 5.5 Sinus tachycardia

Rate	*Dog*: A rate faster than appropriate for temperament and level of activity, usually >180 bpm *Cat*: >220 bpm
Regularity	Regular
Onset/offset	Changes in heart rate are gradual.
P wave	P waves are present and positive in leads II, III and aVF; and negative in aVL and aVR, with an electrical axis suggesting that the origin is in the roof of the right atrium (+18° to +90° in dog, 0 to +90° in cat).
P:QRS ratio	P:QRS is 1:1 with consistent coupling.
QRS	A QRS is present after each P wave with a normal appearance (R wave in leads II, III and aVF; S wave in leads aVL and aVR) and duration <70 ms in dogs and <40 ms in cats, indicating normal intraventricular conduction and activation.
T wave	Morphology of T wave may be variable.

and show marked increases in heart rate during periods of exercise and excitement. A fit dog at rest may have a heart rate of around 30 bpm; however, during exercise this increases to around 240 bpm. Short periods of >300 bpm are observed in some individuals with excitable temperaments performing intense exercise, and whether this is physiological or pathological is debatable.

QT Segment and T Waves Changes During Sinus Tachycardia

During periods of sinus tachycardia, there is often a change in T wave morphology which may occur for several reasons (see Figures 5.7 and 5.8). At higher heart rates the PR, RR and QT intervals shorten, and this may result in the atrial repolarisation wave (Ta) being superimposed on the ST segment instead of the QRS complex. Another potential reason for ST segment change during exercise is relative endocardial ischaemia.

Causes of Sinus Tachycardia

- Physiological (e.g. exercise, excitement, pain and fear)
- Hypovolaemia
- Hypotension
- High cardiac output states (e.g. pyrexia, anaemia, septicaemia, bacteraemia and hyperthyroidism)
- Drugs (e.g. sympathomimetics)
- Congestive heart failure.

As sinus tachycardia generally occurs secondary to another condition, treatment is aimed at addressing the underlying cause of sinus tachycardia.

Inappropriate Sinus Tachycardia

This condition is recognised in human patients and can be challenging to diagnose and treat.[28] In humans, the syndrome of inappropriate sinus tachycardia is defined as a resting heart rate of >100 bpm and a mean heart rate of >90 bpm with no obvious underlying cause, resulting in distressing symptoms of palpitations.[28] An experimental model of this condition has been created in dogs to study treatment interventions.[29] It is difficult to determine if a similar, naturally occurring condition occurs in veterinary patients, but marked, and perhaps inappropriately high, maximum and mean heart rates are sometimes documented on ambulatory ECGs from young dogs with excitable temperaments and exercise intolerance. Figure 5.9 illustrates an example of a young dog with suspicion of inappropriate sinus tachycardia.

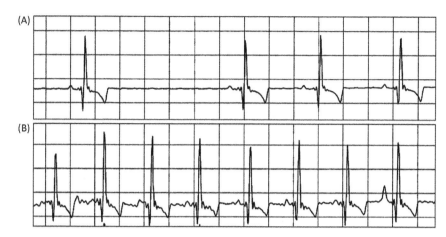

Figure 5.7 P-QRS-T changes with tachycardia. Ambulatory ECG traces from the same dog during (A) sinus rhythm and (B) sinus tachycardia. During tachycardia, note:

- Shortening of RR, PR and QT intervals.
- Slight depression of the early part of the ST segment that may reflect superimposition of a Ta wave. At slower heart rates, this atrial repolarisation wave would be superimposed on the QRS complex, but at higher heart rates, it moves into the early part of the ST segment.
- Electrical alternans due to rapid mechanical movement of the heart during tachycardia changing the net vector of cardiac conduction.

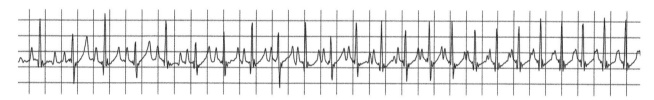

Figure 5.8 P and T wave superimposition during tachycardia. Ambulatory ECG trace from a dog during sinus tachycardia showing superimposition of the P and T waves as the heart rate increases. [6-year-old, female, neutered Greyhound dog]

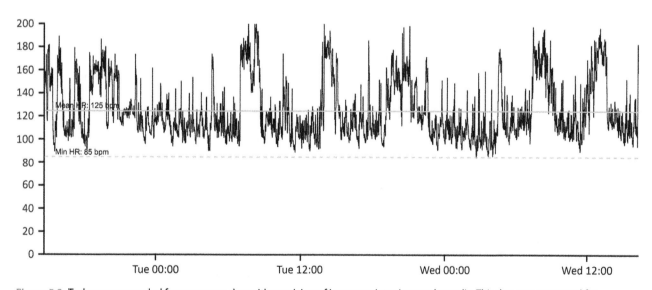

Figure 5.9 Tachogram recorded from a young dog with suspicion of inappropriate sinus tachycardia. This dog was presented for suspicion of persistent tachycardia even during sleep. A 12-lead electrocardiogram was consistent with sinus tachycardia, and a 24 h Holter monitor revealed tachycardia with P waves that had the same conformation during periods of higher and lower rates, also suggestive of a sinus rhythm. The minimum heart rate (95 bpm) and the average heart rate (125 bpm) were both above the expected range. [5-month-old, female Rhodesian Ridgeback dog]

References

1 Tilley LP. Essentials of canine and feline electrocardiography. Philadelphia: Lea & Febiger; 1995.

2 Nikolaidou T, Aslanidi OV, Zhang H, Efimov IR. Structure-function relationship in the sinus and atrioventricular nodes. Pediatr Cardiol. 2012;33:890–899.

3 Spach MS, Miller WT3, Geselowitz DB, Barr RC, Kootsey JM, Johnson EA. The discontinuous nature of propagation in normal canine cardiac muscle: evidence for recurrent discontinuities of intracellular resistance that affect the membrane currents. Circ Res. 1981;48:39–54.

4 Draghici AE, Taylor JA. The physiological basis and measurement of heart rate variability in humans. J Physiol Anthropol. 2016;35:22.

5 Ferasin L, Ferasin H, Little CJL. Lack of correlation between canine heart rate and body size in veterinary clinical practice. J Small Anim Pract. 2010;51:412–418.

6 Adelman RD, Wright J. Systolic blood pressure and heart rate in the growing beagle puppy. Dev Pharmacol Ther. 1985;8:396–401.

7 Piccione G, Giudice E, Fazio F, Mortola JP. The daily rhythm of body temperature, heart and respiratory rate in newborn dogs. J Comp Physiol B. 2010;180:895–904.

8 Abbott JA. Heart rate and heart rate variability of healthy cats in home and hospital environments. J Feline Med Surg. 2005;7:195–202.

9 Cooke WH, Cox JF, Diedrich AM, Taylor JA, Beightol LA, Ames JE4, Hoag JB, Seidel H, Eckberg DL. Controlled breathing protocols probe human autonomic cardiovascular rhythms. Am J Physiol. 1998;274:H709–H718.

10 Hayano J, Yasuma F, Okada A, Mukai S, Fujinami T. Respiratory sinus arrhythmia: a phenomenon improving pulmonary gas exchange and circulatory efficiency. Circulation. 1996;94:842–847.

11 Kollai M, Koizumi K. Cardiovascular reflexes and interrelationships between sympathetic and parasympathetic activity. J Auton Nerv Syst. 1981;4:135–148.

12 Julien C. The enigma of Mayer waves: facts and models. Cardiovasc Res. 2006;70:12–21.

13 Hanas S, Tidholm A, Egenvall A, Holst BS. Twenty-four hour Holter monitoring of unsedated healthy cats in the home environment. J Vet Cardio. 2009;11:17–22.

14 Ware WA. Twenty-four-hour ambulatory electrocardiography in normal cats. J Vet Intern Med. 1999;13:175–180.

15 Rosenbaum MB, Lepeschkin E. The effect of ventricular systole on auricular rhythm in auriculoventricular block. Circulation. 1955;11:240–261.

16 Hashimoto K, Tanaka S, Hirata M, Chiba S. Responses of the sino-atrial node to change in pressure in the sinus node artery. Circ Res. 1967;21:297–304.

17 de Marchena E, Colvin-Adams M, Esnard J, Ridha M, Castellanos A, Myerburg RJ. Ventriculophasic sinus arrhythmia in the orthotopic transplanted heart: mechanism of disease revisited. Int J Cardiol. 2003;91:71–74.

18 Parsonnet AE, Miller R. Heart block: the influence of ventricular systole upon the auricular rhythm in complete and incomplete heart block. Am Heart J. 1944;27:676–687.

19 Roth IR, Kisch B. The mechanism of irregular sinus rhythm in auriculoventricular heart block. Am Heart J. 1948;36:257–276.

20 Strickland KN. ECG of the month: third degree atrioventricular block and ventriculophasic sinus arrhythmia in a dog. J Am Vet Med Assoc. 1998;212:28–29.

21 Erlanger J, Blackman JR. Further studies in the physiology of heart block in mammals: chronic auriculoventricular block in the dog. Heart. 1910;1:177–230.

22 Wyatt HL, Mitchell JH. Influences of physical training on the heart of dogs. Circ Res. 1974;35:883–889.

23 Stepien RL, Hinchcliff KW, Constable PD, Olson J. Effect of endurance training on cardiac morphology in Alaskan sled dogs. J Appl Physiol. 1998;85:1368–1375.

24 Bavegems V, Duchateau L, Ham LV, Rick AD, Sys SU. Electrocardiographic reference values in whippets. Vet J. 2009;182:59–66.

25 Constable PD, Hinchcliff KW, Olson J, Hamlin RL. Athletic heart syndrome in dogs competing in a long-distance sled race. J Appl Physiol. 1994;76:433–438.

26 Hinchcliff KW, Constable PD, Farris JW, Schmitt KE, Hamlin RL. Electrocardiographic characteristics of endurance-trained Alaskan sled dogs. J Am Vet Med Assoc. 1997;211:1138–1141.

27 Constable PD, Hinchcliff KW, Olson JL, Stepien RL. Effects of endurance training on standard and signal-averaged electrocardiograms of sled dogs. Am J Vet Res. 2000;61:582–588.

28 Sheldon RS, Grubb BP2, Olshansky B, Shen W-K, Calkins H, Brignole M, et al. 2015 heart rhythm society expert consensus statement on the diagnosis and treatment of postural tachycardia syndrome, inappropriate sinus tachycardia, and vasovagal syncope. Heart Rhythm. 2015;12:e41–e63.

29 Zhou X, Zhou L, Wang S, Yu L, Wang Z, Huang B, Chen M, Wan J, Jiang H. The use of noninvasive vagal nerve stimulation to inhibit sympathetically induced sinus node acceleration: a potential therapeutic approach for inappropriate sinus tachycardia. J Cardiovasc Electrophysiol. 2016;27:217–223.

6

Pathogenesis and Classification of Arrhythmias
Antonia Mavropoulou

Introduction

In this chapter, the mechanisms responsible for cardiac arrhythmias will be discussed. They include abnormalities of impulse formation (e.g. abnormal automaticity), conduction (e.g. block or re-entry) or a combination of both. In some cases, the mechanism may be apparent from the electrocardiogram (ECG) (e.g. atrial flutter is caused by re-entry); however, it must be highlighted that in the majority of cases, the exact arrhythmia mechanism is not possible to determine based on electrocardiographic findings alone. The classification of arrhythmias and their haemodynamic effects will also be discussed.

Pathogenesis of Arrhythmias

Abnormal Impulse Formation

Normally, the sinus node generates impulses at a rate that is appropriate to the current physiological needs of the individual (e.g. exercise versus rest). If the sinus rate is inappropriately slow or fast, or if the impulse originates from an ectopic pacemaker located outside the sinoatrial node, the resulting rhythm is abnormal.

Subsidiary Pacemakers
There are cells capable of spontaneous discharge in areas of the specialised conduction system outside the sinus node (see chapter 2). Normally, the discharge rate of these cells is lower than the sinus rate, so they succumb to overdrive suppression (see chapter 2). However, if for some reason the sinus rate is low or there is a block preventing the sinus impulse from reaching these cells, then they may reach threshold potential. An example of this is seen during complete atrioventricular block, in which the sinus impulse does not reach the ventricles and a subsidiary pacemaker further down the conduction system takes over at a lower rate of around 20–60 bpm. The discharge rate of the ectopic pacemaker is determined by interactions between the maximum diastolic potential, the threshold potential for depolarisation and the slope of stage 4 depolarisation.[1]

Reduced Automaticity
The sinus node discharge rate may be lower than normal in response to electrolyte abnormalities (see chapter 23), elevated vagal tone (e.g. with airway obstructive disorders – see chapter 23), abnormal pacemaker currents (e.g. gene mutations altering potassium and calcium currents), structural disease including degenerative disease of the conduction system (e.g. sick sinus syndrome) or damage caused by acquired or congenital heart disease. When there is reduced automaticity of the sinus node, a subsidiary pacemaker generally takes over with a junctional or a ventricular escape rhythm. The surface ECG cannot distinguish reduced impulse generation by the sinus node P cells from an exit block of the impulse from the sinus node to the atrial myocardium (sinoatrial block – see chapter 7).

Enhanced Normal Automaticity
Occasionally, the discharge rate of the sinus node or a subsidiary pacemaker may become abnormally high and cause tachycardia, a phenomenon called *enhanced normal automaticity*. The underlying mechanisms include a reduction in the activation threshold, a higher diastolic membrane potential and an increase in the rate or slope of stage 4 depolarisation (Figure 6.1). Enhanced normal automaticity can occur with excessive sympathetic stimulation or low potassium levels (see chapter 23). Normally, sympathetic stimulation of the sinus node would not increase the heart rate above 300 bpm in dogs and cats. Tachycardia above these levels is likely due to another arrhythmia mechanism. Low potassium levels (hypokalaemia) or hypoxia may lead to inhibition of the $3Na^+/2K^+$ pumps, reducing the background repolarising current and enhancing stage 4 diastolic depolarisation.[1]

Examples of arrhythmias caused by enhanced normal automaticity include accelerated junctional or idioventricular rhythms, and some forms of atrial tachycardia (e.g. digitalis toxicity).

Guide to Canine and Feline Electrocardiography, First Edition. Ruth Willis, Pedro Oliveira and Antonia Mavropoulou.
© 2018 John Wiley & Sons Ltd. Published 2018 by John Wiley & Sons Ltd.
Companion website: www.wiley.com/go/willis/electrocardiography

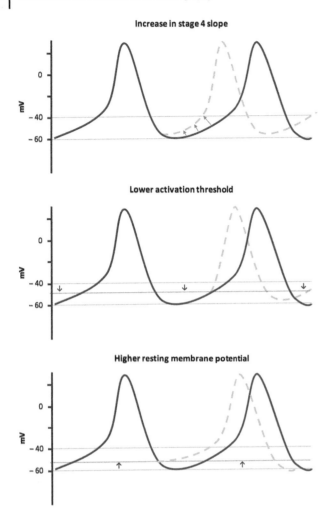

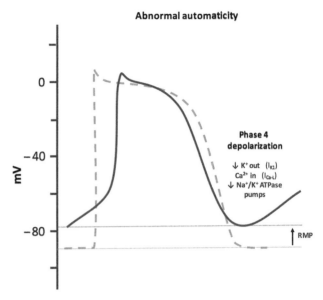

Figure 6.2 Mechanisms of abnormal automaticity. Occasionally, cardiac cells that are not normally capable of spontaneous depolarisation such as the working myocardium acquire the ability to depolarise spontaneously. This can occur with cell damage that impairs cell membrane function (especially the $3Na^+/2K^+$ ATPase pumps), causing an increase in the resting membrane potential (RMP) illustrated here. If the RMP increases to around −50 mV, inactivation of I_k and activation of I_{Ca-L} currents may occur, leading to spontaneous cell depolarisation.

Figure 6.1 Mechanisms of enhanced normal automaticity. As the name suggests, *enhanced normal automaticity* refers to an increase in the discharge rate of pacemaker cells in the sinus node or subsidiary pacemakers above the expected range. The underlying mechanisms include an increase in the rate or slope of stage 4 depolarisation (top picture), a reduction in the activation threshold (middle picture) and a higher diastolic membrane potential (bottom picture). Enhanced normal automaticity can occur with excessive sympathetic stimulation or low potassium levels.

Abnormal Automaticity

In some cases, cardiac cells that are not normally capable of spontaneous depolarisation (e.g. working myocardium) acquire the ability to depolarise spontaneously. This can occur with cell damage (e.g. infarction) that impairs cell membrane function (especially the $3Na^+/2K^+$ ATPase pumps) such that the normal resting membrane potential is no longer maintained (Figure 6.2). If the resting membrane potential increases to around −50 mV, inactivation of I_k and activation of I_{Ca-L} currents may occur, leading to spontaneous cell depolarisation. The less negative the membrane diastolic potential, the faster the firing rate.[2] Abnormal automaticity is less sensitive to overdrive suppression than enhanced normal automaticity.[3]

Examples of abnormal automaticity include ectopic atrial, junctional or ventricular rhythms, particularly when associated with acute ischaemia and reperfusion.

Triggered Activity

This type of abnormality is caused by premature depolarisation of the cell before full repolarisation from the preceding depolarisation event has occurred (Figure 6.3). This is due to oscillations of the membrane potential during stages 2 or 3, or the beginning of stage 4, of the action potential and is not truly due to spontaneous cell depolarisation.[1] For this reason, the commonly used term *triggered automaticity* is not correct. If premature depolarisation occurs during stages 2 or 3 of the preceding action potential, the term *early afterdepolarisation* (EAD) is used. If this occurs during early stage 4, the term *delayed afterdepolarisation* (DAD) is used instead. If the right conditions are present, an afterdepolarisation can trigger another, thereby self-perpetuating and causing tachycardia.

Early Afterdepolarisations

A variety of abnormalities can lead to EADs, all of which contribute to a higher than normal membrane potential during stages 2 and 3 of the action potential and also an increase in the action potential duration.[1] Torsades de pointes is an example of an arrhythmia caused by EADs, but the exact mechanisms are unclear.

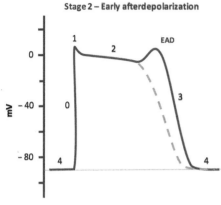

Stage 2 – Early afterdepolarization

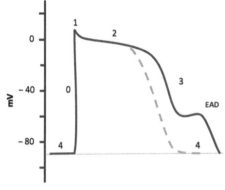

Stage 3 – Early afterdepolarization

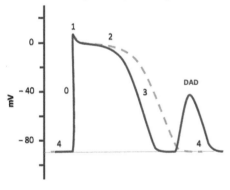

Stage 4 – Delayed afterdepolarization

Figure 6.3 Representation of triggered activity. Triggered activity is characterised by premature depolarisation of the cell before it is fully repolarised. This occurs due to oscillations of the membrane potential during stages 2 or 3, or the beginning of stage 4, of the action potential. A premature depolarisation that occurs during stages 2 or 3 is termed an *early afterdepolarisation* (EAD), and during stage 4 is referred to as a *delayed afterdepolarisation* (DAD). EADs are caused by abnormalities that contribute to a higher than normal membrane potential during stages 2 and 3 of the action potential and also an increase in the action potential duration. DADs occur in circumstances where the cardiomyocyte cytoplasm is overloaded with Ca^{2+}, such as intense sympathetic stimulation, ischaemia or digoxin toxicity. Intracellular hypercalcaemia stimulates oscillatory release of more Ca^{2+} from the sarcoplasmic reticulum that subsequently favours a transient inward current of Na^+, by either exchange with Ca^{2+} ($3Na^+/1Ca^{2+}$ exchanger) or activation of a non-selective cation channel. This transient inward Na^+ current (I_{TI}) results in premature depolarisation of the cell.

For EADs that occur at voltages close to the plateau of the action potential (stage 2), reactivation of time- and voltage-dependent I_{Ca-L} currents is thought to be involved.[4] This may occur preferentially in Purkinje cells and M cells of the ventricular myocardium. EADs that occur at lower voltages (stage 3) may be due to electric currents during repolarisation or the result of low I_{k1} currents.[5]

EADs occur in human patients with long QT syndrome which may be congenital (e.g. abnormal outward potassium currents or inward calcium currents) or acquired (e.g. due to use of quinidine, class III anti-arrhythmics, procainamide, erythromycin etc.). Sympathetic stimulation and/or catecholamine administration may also lead to EADs, resulting in ventricular tachyarrhythmias. Magnesium supplementation may be used to suppress arrhythmias caused by EADs.

An important aspect of arrhythmias triggered by EADs is that they are rate dependent, and, in general, the amplitude of EADs increases at slower heart rates.[6] These arrhythmias are therefore not expected to be triggered by premature stimulation, with the exception of a long compensatory pause following a premature stimulus. This phenomenon is commonly seen with torsades de pointes (see chapter 11).

Delayed Afterdepolarisations

DADs occur in circumstances where the cardiomyocyte cytoplasm is overloaded with Ca^{2+}, such as during intense sympathetic stimulation, ischaemia or digoxin toxicity. This intracellular hypercalcaemia stimulates oscillatory release of more Ca^{2+} from the sarcoplasmic reticulum that subsequently favours a transient inward current of Na^+, by either exchange with Ca^{2+} ($3Na^+/1Ca^{2+}$ exchanger) or activation of a non-selective cation channel. This transient inward Na^+ current (I_{TI}) results in premature depolarisation of the cell. Drugs that reduce the diastolic Ca^{2+} currents (e.g. calcium channel blockers or β-blockers), inhibit Ca^{2+} release from the sarcoplasmic reticulum (e.g. caffeine) or block Na^+ currents (e.g. class I anti-arrhythmics) can abolish DADs.

In contrast to EADs, the amplitude and rate of DADs increase with shorter cycle lengths (i.e. higher heart rates). In most cases of DAD-induced arrhythmias, the shorter the coupling interval of the initiating stimulus (i.e. the R-R from sinus to premature beat), the shorter the coupling interval of the arrhythmia.[1] This is in contrast with re-entrant mechanisms where the shorter the coupling interval of the initiating stimulus, the longer the coupling interval of the first arrhythmia beat. Unfortunately, this is not always the case and cannot be used as the only electrophysiologic feature to distinguish between these types of arrhythmia mechanism.

Abnormal Impulse Conduction

A delay or block of impulse conduction may result in bradyarrhythmias (e.g. sinoatrial and atrioventricular block) or tachyarrhythmias by allowing re-entry to occur.

Block

Conduction through cardiac tissue depends on both passive and active membrane properties. These include the stimulating efficacy of the propagating impulse, the excitability and the geometry of the tissue into which the impulse is being conducted.[1] Additionally, the gap junctions between cells play a crucial role in impulse conduction.[7] A delay or block of impulse conduction may occur during periods of tachycardia or bradycardia. Tachycardia-dependent block (or phase 3 block) is the most common type of block and is due to incomplete recovery of tissue refractoriness.[1] At higher rates, there may not be enough time for complete voltage- or time-dependent recovery of excitability, causing a conduction delay or block. Clinical examples of this type of block include Ashman's phenomenon during atrial fibrillation (see chapter 9), and functional bundle branch block during tachycardia (see chapter 7) or after a premature beat with a short coupling interval (see Figure 7.11).

Bradycardia or deceleration-dependent block (or phase 4 block) is thought to be due to a reduction in action potential amplitude and excitability at long diastolic intervals.[8]

Re-entry

Normally, an impulse generated in the sinus node propagates through the conduction system to the whole heart until all cells have become depolarised. The refractory period that follows depolarisation ensures that once all cells have been depolarised, the impulse cannot propagate any further and is extinguished. Normally, another impulse cannot be propagated until cell repolarisation has occurred. However, if an area of tissue is able to recover excitability sooner than expected, the impulse could be allowed to propagate in a re-entrant path, causing repeated stimulation of the myocardium (Figure 6.4). Re-entry can occur around an anatomical structure – *anatomical re-entry* – or can occur in contiguous fibres with different electrophysiological properties – *functional re-entry*. Both forms of re-entry can coexist.[9]

The following pre-requisites must be met for re-entry to occur:[1]

1) A substrate is necessary: adjacent myocardial tissue with different electrophysiological properties, conduction and refractoriness
2) An area of block (anatomical, functional or both) around which the wavefront may travel
3) A unidirectional conduction block
4) An area of slowed conduction that allows sufficient delay in wavefront conduction to enable the recovery of the refractory tissue proximal to the site of the unidirectional block
5) A critical tissue mass to sustain re-entry
6) An initiating trigger (e.g. a premature beat).

Anatomical Re-entry

Anatomical re-entry occurs around an anatomical barrier of unexcitable tissue. It can occur in a very small area of myocardium (micro re-entry) or may involve several structures in the heart (macro re-entry).

Micro Re-entry

Let's imagine a cat with hypertrophic cardiomyopathy who suffered a myocardial infarction causing a small area of unexcitable tissue in the ventricular myocardium (blue area in Figure 6.4). The depolarisation wave travels around that area on both sides until the wavefronts meet on the other end and cancel each other out (Figure 6.4A). There are effectively two pathways for the impulse to travel around the area of unexcitable tissue that correspond to pathways a and b in Figure 6.4. Now imagine that the cells around the infarcted area on the side of pathway b, despite being still alive, are damaged and have a higher resting membrane potential. As a consequence, they display slower conduction velocity and a shorter refractory period in comparison to the cells in pathway a. A properly timed impulse (e.g. a premature beat) reaches pathway a when it is still refractory and is therefore blocked (purple arrow in Figure 6.4B). However, at the same time, pathway b is ready to depolarise and allows the impulse to propagate to the other end of the anatomical barrier (blue arrow in Figure 6.4B). By the time it gets there, pathway a has had time to repolarise, and the impulse can travel retrogradely back to the initial point where pathway a meets with pathway b (green arrow in Figure 6.4B). Since pathway b has a shorter refractory period, it is ready to depolarise again, and re-entry is sustained. For this to occur, the refractory period of one of the pathways must be substantially shorter than the other (to recover quickly enough) with a slower conduction velocity (to allow time for the tissue ahead to recover). Enough time must be allowed so that, as the impulse propagates within the re-entrant circuit, it continues to encounter excitable tissue. The excitable myocardium between the head and the tail of the wavefront is called the *excitable gap*.[9] The length of the re-entrant pathway must be long enough to allow the wavefront to continue encountering excitable tissue. This depends on the *wavelength* of re-entry which is determined by the product of the conduction velocity and the refractory period of each pathway. The wavelength must be shorter than the length of the pathway for re-entry to occur.[1]

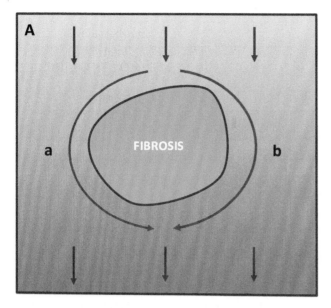
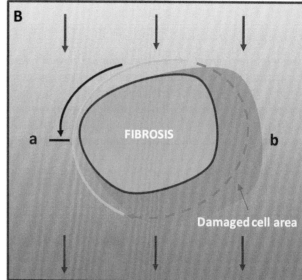

Figure 6.4 Anatomical re-entry (see text for explanation).

Macro Re-entry

Re-entry can occur within a larger circuit composed of different cardiac structures with varying conduction properties. Some examples include atrioventricular re-entry mediated by an accessory pathway (see chapter 10), atrioventricular nodal re-entry (see chapter 10) and atrial flutter (see chapter 8).

Functional Re-entry

Re-entry can also occur in contiguous fibres without any anatomical boundaries due to heterogeneous electrophysiological properties caused by local differences in transmembrane potentials. If neighbouring cells or groups of cells coexist in different states of excitability and refractoriness (dispersion of excitability and refractoriness within a tissue), re-entry may occur. Additionally, an anisotropic distribution of intercellular resistances through the gap junctions (e.g. depolarisation of adjacent cells in a transverse rather than longitudinal direction) also contributes to initiation and maintenance of re-entry. Atrial and ventricular fibrillation are examples of arrhythmias that involve functional re-entry. Several models have been proposed for functional re-entry (see Box 6.1).

Anatomical Substrates for Arrhythmogenesis within the Heart

Several cardiac structures may be involved in the genesis of arrhythmias. Atrial or ventricular myocardial remodelling secondary to either acquired or congenital heart disease may lead to atrial or ventricular tachycardia, flutter or fibrillation. Myocardial stretch, fibrosis and electrical remodelling may all play a role. Myocardial infiltration or replacement with fibrous tissue or adipocytes (e.g. arrhythmogenic right ventricular cardiomyopathy) is a common cause of ventricular arrhythmias. Fibrosis of the atrial myocardium leads to a particular rhythm disturbance called *atrial silence*, more commonly described as atrial standstill, in which atrial depolarisation simply does not occur as the myocardium is replaced by fibrous tissue. Ectopic foci are commonly present in venous structures such as the coronary sinus, vena cavae, pulmonary veins, vein of Marshall and terminal crest. Abnormal automaticity of these foci may result in atrial tachycardia and contribute to atrial fibrillation (e.g. pulmonary veins).

Specific anatomical structures are involved in other rhythm disturbances, such as accessory atrioventricular pathways in atrioventricular tachycardia or cavotricuspid isthmus in typical atrial flutter.

Arrhythmia Classification

Cardiac arrhythmias can be classified according to their site of origin, electrocardiographic criteria and clinical presentation. Most commonly, cardiac arrhythmias are divided based on the resulting heart rate into *tachyarrhythmias* (elevated heart rate), *bradyarrhythmias* (low heart rate) and *ectopic rhythms and beats* (normal heart rate). They are then further categorised based on the anatomical site of origin or re-entrant pathway.[13-15] Table 6.1 illustrates the most common rhythm disturbances in dogs and cats classified based on these criteria.

Additional classification criteria that are useful to describe rhythm disturbances include the following.

Box 6.1 Functional re-entry models

Leading circle re-entry

The re-entrant circuit propagates around a core of refractory tissue and travels through fibres with shorter refractory periods whilst being blocked in one direction in fibres with longer refractory periods. The length of the re-entry circuit is simply the shortest in which the leading wavefront is able to depolarise tissue ahead that is still relatively refractory. Changes in tissue refractoriness may lead to a change in size of the re-entry circuit, altering the rate of tachycardia. (See Figure 6.5).

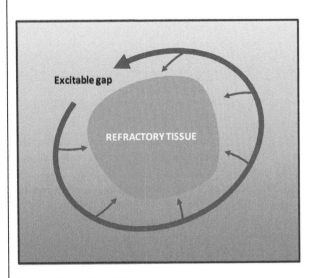

Figure 6.5 Leading circle re-entry.

Anisotropic re-entry

The conduction in cardiac fibres is anisotropic, favouring longitudinal transmission of impulses rather than transverse. This is due to a larger number of gap junctions distributed between successive cells rather than cells that are located side by side.[10] Given the right conditions, an impulse may be blocked in the longitudinal direction but still propagate slowly transversely and re-enter the area of block. This type of re-entry has been observed in atrial and myocardial muscle in the setting of myocardial infarction.[11]

Figure of eight re-entry

This type of re-entry consists of clockwise and counterclockwise wavefronts propagating around two functional or fixed arcs of block that coalesce into a central common front with slow conduction. It was first described in experimental dogs after myocardial infarction.[12] (See Figure 6.6).

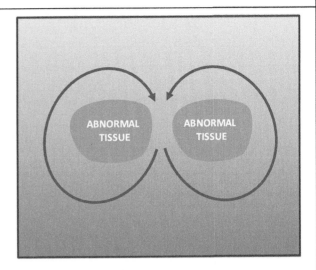

Figure 6.6 Figure of eight re-entry.

Reflection

Reflection is a special type of re-entry in which a circuit is not necessary. Instead, the impulse travels in both directions (back and forth) along the same pathway in the presence of severely impaired conduction.[11] (See Figure 6.7).

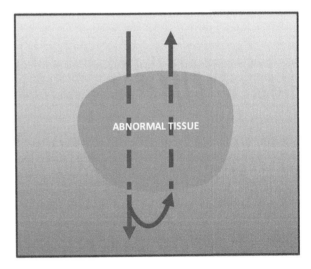

Figure 6.7 Reflection re-entry.

Spiral wave re-entry

Spiral waves represent a two-dimensional form of rotating wave propagation. When spiral wave activity occurs in three dimensions, the term *scroll waves* is used. Spiral wave activation occurs around a core of tissue that is not stimulated. The tip of the wave moves along a complex trajectory and can radiate waves into the surrounding medium. The dynamics of spiral waves may change, causing either monomorphic or polymorphic patterns (e.g. polymorphic ventricular tachycardia).[2] (See Figure 6.8).

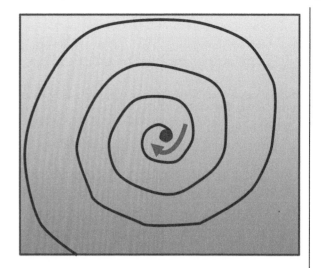

Figure 6.8 **Spiral wave re-entry.**

Electrocardiographic Criteria

- *QRS duration*
  - Narrow QRS (normal duration)
  - Wide QRS (longer duration)

  This criterion is commonly used to characterise tachyarrhythmias.
- *Narrow-QRS tachyarrhythmias* (QRS of normal duration) have a supraventricular origin as ventricular depolarisation occurs via the normal conduction system. However, ventricular arrhythmias originating high in the His–Purkinje system may also display a narrow QRS.
- *Wide-QRS tachyarrhythmias* (QRS of duration longer than normal) either have a ventricular origin or may be supraventricular with abnormal ventricular conduction (e.g. a bundle branch block).

  Chapters 13 and 14 address the approach to tachyarrhythmias with both narrow and wide presentations.
- *QRS morphology*
  - Monomorphic (all similar)
  - Polymorphic (variable)
  - Bidirectional

  This criterion is used to characterise ventricular ectopic rhythms and beats, indicating whether one (monomorphic) or more (polymorphic) ectopic sites of arrhythmia are present. Bidirectional QRS morphology is observed in ventricular tachycardia where the mean electrical axis of each beat is variable. It is a rare rhythm disturbance that is most commonly observed with severe digoxin toxicity.[16,17]
- *RR cycle length*
  - Irregular
  - Regular
  - Onset and offset

  Once again, this criterion is used to characterise tachyarrhythmias. The various arrhythmias cause either an irregular (variable RR intervals) or regular (constant RR intervals) heart rhythm, and this may be used to distinguish them (e.g. atrial fibrillation with bundle branch block versus ventricular tachycardia). The onset and offset of a tachyarrhythmia also provide a clue to the underlying arrhythmia mechanism: a sudden onset and offset (paroxysmal arrhythmia) suggest a re-entrant mechanism, whereas a progressive increase and decrease in heart rate ('warm-up' and 'cool-down') suggest abnormal automaticity.

Clinical Criteria (for tachyarrhythmias)

- *Duration*
  - Sustained (>30 s or syncope)
  - Non-sustained (<30 s)
- *Presentation*
  - Paroxysmal (sudden onset and offset)
  - Iterative (non-sustained tachycardia alternating with sinus beats/rhythm)
  - Permanent or incessant (tachycardia >12 h alternating with sinus rhythm)

Haemodynamic Consequences of Arrhythmias

The immediate effect of any rhythm disturbance is a drop in blood pressure and forward stroke volume (the amount of blood ejected from the ventricle into the arterial circulation with each beat). This change may be transient and tolerable (e.g. an isolated premature beat) or may result in significant hypotension and low cardiac output with accompanying clinical signs and

Table 6.1 Rhythm disturbances in dogs and cats

Ectopic beats and rhythms	Bradyarrhythmias	Tachyarrhythmias
Atrial	**Sinus node**	**Sinus node**
Atrial premature beat or contraction (APB or APC)	Sinus bradycardia	Sinus tachycardia
Atrial ectopic rhythm	Sinus arrest	**Atrial**
Atrial parasystole	Sinoatrial block	Focal atrial tachycardia
Atrial dissociation		Multifocal atrial tachycardia
		Atrial fibrillation
		Atrial flutter • Typical (dependent on cavotricuspid isthmus) • Typical reversed • Atypical
Junctional	**Atrial myocardium**	**Junctional**
Junctional premature beat or contraction (JPB or JPC)	Intra-atrial block	Junctional ectopic tachycardia (JET)
Junctional ectopic rhythm	Atrial silence	Junctional non-paroxysmal tachycardia
	Sino-ventricular rhythm	
Ventricular	**Atrioventricular node**	**Atrioventricular**
Ventricular premature beat or contraction (VPB or VPC)	First-degree AV block (1AVB)	Orthodromic atrioventricular reciprocating tachycardia (OAVRT)
Idioventricular rhythm	Second-degree AV block (2AVB) • Wenckebach type • Mobitz type	Antidromic atrioventricular reciprocating tachycardia (AVRT)
	Third-degree or complete AV block (3AVB)	Permanent junctional reciprocating tachycardia (PJRT) or Coumel
	Ventricular	**Ventricular**
	Bundle branch block	Accelerated idioventricular rhythm
	Ventricular asystole or arrest	Ventricular tachycardia • Monomorphic • Polymorphic • Bidirectional
		Torsades de pointes
	Pulseless electrical activity (PEA), previously known as electromechanical dissociation	
		Ventricular flutter
		Ventricular fibrillation

activation of compensatory mechanisms.[18–20] The haemodynamic effects of any particular arrhythmia depend on the nature of the rhythm disturbance (ventricular rate, rhythm and duration) and whether there is structural heart disease. Even 'benign' rhythm disturbances may have profound haemodynamic effects in patients with underlying structural disease. It is important to highlight that the haemodynamic effects of cardiac arrhythmias are not due to changes in cardiac function alone. The activation of compensatory mechanisms leads to changes in peripheral resistance, baroreceptor activity, blood volume and venous return that also play a role.

The following factors are worth considering in regard to the haemodynamic consequences of arrhythmias.

Heart Rate

Excessively high or low heart rates result in significant decreases in cardiac output (CO) and blood pressure (BP). CO represents the amount of blood leaving the heart in 1 minute (L/min) and is the product of the stroke volume (ml) and the heart rate (bpm):

$$CO = SV \times HR$$

During tachycardia, the shortened diastolic interval may impair ventricular filling, causing a decrease in stroke volume. This explains why CO is reduced despite an increase in heart rate. Coronary artery flow is also reduced during tachycardia.

During bradycardia, the decrease in heart rate is responsible for the lower CO despite an increase in SV caused by a longer diastolic interval that increases ventricular filling and contraction (Frank–Starling's law of the heart). If these changes occur abruptly, the decrease in CO and blood pressure may result in transient episodes of weakness and collapse. With more chronic rhythm disturbances, compensatory mechanisms are activated in an attempt to normalise cardiac output and blood pressure. For example, during chronic bradycardia, an increase in blood volume (via activation of the renin–angiotensin–aldosterone system) is combined with the effects of a prolonged diastolic time (as explained in this chapter) to increase the stroke volume. This, along with an increase in peripheral resistance, may be sufficient to maintain an adequate blood pressure and tissue perfusion. This explains why some of our patients with heart rates as low as 40 bpm are able to lead a normal life (e.g. chronic sinus node dysfunction or progressive atrioventricular block), whilst others display signs of collapse with a similar rate (e.g. acute atrioventricular block).

Atrioventricular Synchronisation ('atrial kick')

Another important aspect is the contribution of atrial contraction to ventricular diastolic filling and thereby stroke volume. Normally, atrial contraction contributes an additional 15–20% to the amount of blood present in the ventricles at the end of diastole. In certain cardiac diseases (e.g. degenerative valve disease), the contribution of atrial contraction may even be higher. With arrhythmias in which atrial contraction does not occur or is no longer synchronised with ventricular contraction (e.g. junctional or ventricular rhythms, atrial fibrillation, atrioventricular block, after pacemaker implantation etc.), the reduction in ventricular filling and its effect on stroke volume may have a significant impact on cardiac output.

Ventricular Activation Pattern

The pattern of ventricular activation is also important. With supraventricular arrhythmias, the ventricular activation occurs normally via the specialised conduction system. This is important as a normal sequence of ventricular activation ensures optimal contraction and ejection of blood from the ventricles. With ventricular arrhythmias, or in case of supraventricular arrhythmias that are conducted with aberrancy (e.g. bundle branch block) or via an accessory atrioventricular pathway, the loss of the normal activation of the ventricles results in a less effective contraction and adverse haemodynamic effects. The loss of 'atrial kick' and abnormal ventricular activation are the reasons why ventricular tachyarrhythmias are generally not as well tolerated as supraventricular tachyarrhythmias.

Duration of the Arrhythmias

The duration of the rhythm disturbance plays an important role in respect to the degree of haemodynamic consequences and occurrence of clinical signs. Transient arrhythmias have the potential to cause profound hypotension that may result in weakness or collapse. However, with the exception of arrhythmias that have the potential to degenerate into ventricular fibrillation, these episodes do not tend to result in the death of the patient.

More chronic arrhythmias, particularly tachyarrhythmias, have the potential to induce cardiac remodelling and congestive heart failure in addition to the immediate haemodynamic effects caused by the arrhythmia itself. A typical example is patients with incessant tachyarrhythmias who develop a form of arrhythmia-induced cardiomyopathy (AICM), also known as tachycardia-induced cardiomyopathy (TICM).[21–23] A study in dogs showed that pacing the heart at a constant rate of 180 bpm for 3 weeks resulted in left ventricular dysfunction.[24] This was regardless of whether supraventricular or ventricular pacing was used, although the degree of left ventricular enlargement and reduction in ejection fraction observed with ventricular pacing was higher. Excessive myocardial oxygen demand, chronic reduction of myocardial perfusion, abnormal cellular concentrations of calcium-ATPase and reduced production of cyclic AMP are all thought to play a role. AICM can occur with any form of tachyarrhythmia, and in humans it has been described with frequent premature beats as well, particularly those of ventricular origin.[25,26]

Clinical Signs that Commonly Accompany Cardiac Arrhythmias

Patients suffering from cardiac arrhythmias may be asymptomatic or may display signs that range from lethargy and exercise intolerance to syncope or congestive heart failure. In cases with underlying structural cardiac abnormalities, common complaints include lethargy, reduction in activity levels, poor appetite and weight loss, followed by development of signs of congestive heart failure.

Patients with transient arrhythmias tend to display signs only when experiencing the rhythm disturbance and only if the haemodynamic consequences are severe. They normally consist of periods of weakness or syncope often caused by cerebral hypoperfusion. Studies in dogs have shown a reduction in cerebral flow of approximately 7–12% with premature ectopic beats, 14% with supraventricular tachycardia, 23% with atrial fibrillation and as high as 40–75% during ventricular tachycardia.[27] Prolonged cerebral hypoxia may result in a seizure-like episode.

References

1 Gaztañaga L, Marchlinski FE, Betensky BP. Mechanisms of cardiac arrhythmias. Revista Española de Cardiología (Engl. ed.). 2012;65:174–185.

2 Issa ZF, Miller JM, Zipes DP. In Clinical arrhythmology and electrophysiology (pp. 1–26). Amsterdam: Elsevier; 2009. doi:10.1016/B978-1-4160-5998-1.00004-5

3 Dangman KH, Hoffman BF. Studies on overdrive stimulation of canine cardiac Purkinje fibers: maximal diastolic potential as a determinant of the response. J Am Coll Cardiol. 1983;2:1183–1190.

4 Yamada M, Ohta K, Niwa A, Tsujino N, Nakada T, Hirose M. Contribution of L-type Ca2+ channels to early afterdepolarizations induced by IKr and IKs channel suppression in guinea pig ventricular myocytes. J Membrane Biol. 2008;222:151–166.

5 Maruyama M, Lin S-F, Xie Y, Chua S-K, Joung B, Han S, *et al*. Genesis of phase 3 early afterdepolarizations and triggered activity in acquired long-QT syndrome. Circ Arrhythm Electrophysiol. 2011;4:103–111.

6 Kannankeril P, Roden DM, Darbar D. Drug-induced long QT syndrome. Pharmacol Rev. 2010;62:760–781.

7 Clusin WT. Calcium and cardiac arrhythmias: DADs, EADs, and alternans. Crit Rev Clin Lab Sci. 2003;40:337–375.

8 Fisch C, Miles WM. Deceleration-dependent left bundle branch block: a spectrum of bundle branch conduction delay. Circulation. 1982;65:1029–1032.

9 Kleber AG, Rudy Y. Basic mechanisms of cardiac impulse propagation and associated arrhythmias. Physiological Rev. 2004;84:431–488.

10 Barbuti A, Baruscotti M, DiFrancesco D. The pacemaker current: from basics to the clinics. J Cardiovasc Electrophysiol 18, 342–347 (2007).

11 Antzelevitch C. Basic mechanisms of reentrant arrhythmias. Curr Opin Cardio. 2001;16:1–7.

12 Gough WB, Mehra R, Restivo M, Zeiler RH, el-Sherif N. Reentrant ventricular arrhythmias in the late myocardial infarction period in the dog. 13. Correlation of activation and refractory maps. Circ Res. 1985;57:432–442.

13 Blomstrom-Lundqvist C, Scheinman MM, Aliot EM, Alpert JS, Calkins H, Camm AJ, *et al*. ACC/AHA/ESC guidelines for the management of patients with supraventricular arrhythmias – executive summary: a report of the American College of Cardiology/ American Heart Association task force on practice guidelines and the European Society of Cardiology committee for practice guidelines (writing committee to develop guidelines for the management of patients with supraventricular arrhythmias) developed in collaboration with NASPE-Heart Rhythm Society. J Am Coll Cardiol. 2003;42:1493–1531.

14 Bethge KP. Classification of arrhythmias. J Cardiovasc Pharmacol. 1991;17:S20.

15 Bethge KP. Classification of arrhythmias. J Cardiovasc Pharmacol. 1991;17(Suppl 6):S13–S19.

16 Mehta MC, Sharma VN. Experimental bidirectional ventricular tachycardia in the dog. Br Heart J. 1964;26:67–74.

17 Richter S, Brugada P. Bidirectional ventricular tachycardia. J Am Coll Cardiol. 2009;54:1189.

18 Naito M, David D, Michelson EL, Schaffenburg M, Dreifus LS. The hemodynamic consequences of cardiac arrhythmias: evaluation of the relative roles of abnormal atrioventricular sequencing, irregularity of ventricular rhythm and atrial fibrillation in a canine model. Am Heart J. 1983;106:284–291.

19 Bartel AG, McIntosh HD. Hemodynamic effects of cardiac arrhythmias. Calif Med. 1971;114:88–89.

20 Samet P. Hemodynamic sequelae of cardiac arrhythmias. Circulation. 1973;47:399–407.

21 Foster SF, Hunt GB, Thomas SP, Ross DL, Pearson M, Malik R. Tachycardia-induced cardiomyopathy in a young Boxer dog with supraventricular tachycardia due to an accessory pathway. Australian Vet J. 2006;84:326–331.

22 Schober KE, Kent AM, Aeffner F. Tachycardia-induced cardiomyopathy in a cat. Schweizer Archiv für Tierheilkunde. 2014;156:133–139.

23 Gopinathannair R, Etheridge SP, Marchlinski FE, Spinale FG, Lakkireddy D, Olshansky B. Arrhythmia-induced cardiomyopathies: mechanisms, recognition, and management. J Am Coll Cardiol. 2015;66:1714–1728.

24 Zupan I, Rakovec P, Budihna N, Brecelj A, Kozelj M. Tachycardia induced cardiomyopathy in dogs: relation between chronic supraventricular and chronic ventricular tachycardia. Int J Cardiol. 1996;56:75–81.

25 Lee GK, Klarich KW, Grogan M, Cha Y-M. Premature ventricular contraction-induced cardiomyopathy: a treatable condition. Circ Arrhythm Electrophysiol. 2012;5:229–236.

26 Park Y, Kim S, Shin J, Oh AR, Shin EJ, Lee JH, *et al.* Frequent premature ventricular complex is associated with left atrial enlargement in patients with normal left ventricular ejection fraction. Pacing Clin Electrophysiol. 2014;37:1455–1461.

27 Corday E, Irving DW. Effect of cardiac arrhythmias on the cerebral circulation. Am J Cardiol. 1960;6:803–808.

7

Bradyarrhythmias and Conduction Disturbances
Ruth Willis

Introduction

Bradycardia is defined as a heart rate that is slow. Pathological bradyarrhythmias may be due to primary disease of the cardiac conduction system or secondary to systemic illness (see chapter 23). Bradyarrhythmias are clinically relevant as they are a potential cause of cardiac syncope. Whilst some bradyarrhythmias may be haemodynamically stable, others have the potential to be life-threatening and merit medical or surgical therapy. Conduction abnormalities suggesting more localised areas of conduction block will also be discussed in this chapter.

This chapter focuses on pathological bradyarrhythmias and conduction abnormalities, such as:

1) Abnormal sinoatrial function (sinus pause, sinoatrial block SAB and sinus node arrest)
2) Abnormal atrioventricular node function (first, second and third-degree atrioventricular block)
3) Intraventricular conduction disturbances
4) Sick sinus syndrome (SSS)
5) Other conditions resulting in bradyarrhythmias.

Sinoatrial Node

Sinus Bradycardia

Sinus bradycardia is discussed in chapter 5 and is usually a physiological slowing of heart rate during periods of rest. Whilst sinus bradycardia is generally an appropriate and haemodynamically stable rhythm, inappropriate sinus bradycardia may also occur – for example, during an episode of neurally mediated syncope or secondary to systemic illness (e.g. hypothyroidism – see chapter 23)

Sinus Node Dysfunction

Under normal conditions, the sinoatrial node (SAN) has the fastest rate of spontaneous depolarisation in the heart, thereby causing overdrive suppression of other subsidiary pacemakers. Sinus node dysfunction encompasses a spectrum of changes ranging from sinus pauses to sinus node block and sinoatrial arrest.

Sinus Pause

A sinus pause is a delay in the generation of an impulse, and these pauses are followed by a sinus beat rather than an escape beat (See Figure 7.1). Sinus pauses are not an exact multiple of the preceding P-P interval, and they are frequently seen on ambulatory electrocardiograms (ECGs) during periods of sinus arrhythmia and sinus bradycardia whilst dogs are resting. Pauses of 4–6s have been documented in normal dogs during periods of rest.[1,2]

Sinus Node Block

In SAB, an impulse is generated within the SAN but is unable to exit the node and reach the working myocardium, resulting in a pause in atrial and thus ventricular activity. SAB may be intermittent or permanent.[3]

Sub-classification of Sinoatrial Block
Sinus node block is sub-classified into first, second and third-degree block:

- *First-degree sinoatrial block (1SAB)*: There is a delay between impulse generation and its transmission to the atrial myocardium, but this is not apparent on the surface ECG.
- *Second-degree sinoatrial block type I (Wenckebach) (2SAB type I)*: There is a progressive lengthening of the interval between impulse generation and transmission, eventually resulting in failure of transmission of an impulse from the SAN to the atrial myocardium. On the surface ECG, this results in:
  - A gradual shortening of the P-P interval, resulting in grouping of QRS complexes
  - At the end of each group of P-QRS complexes, there is an unconducted sinus impulse, resulting in a pause in cardiac activity.

Guide to Canine and Feline Electrocardiography, First Edition. Ruth Willis, Pedro Oliveira and Antonia Mavropoulou.
© 2018 John Wiley & Sons Ltd. Published 2018 by John Wiley & Sons Ltd.
Companion website: www.wiley.com/go/willis/electrocardiography

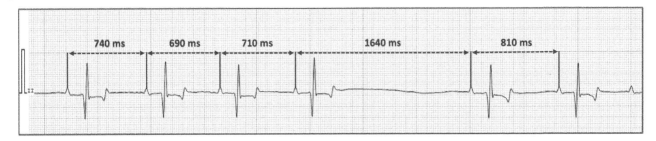

Figure 7.1 Sinus pause. A sinus pause is seen during a period of bradycardia and respiratory sinus arrhythmia in a normal dog. The duration of this pause (1640 ms) is not a multiple of the preceding P-P interval(s). [4-year-old, male neutered, Boxer dog without evidence of cardiovascular disease] (50 mm/s, 20 mm/mV)

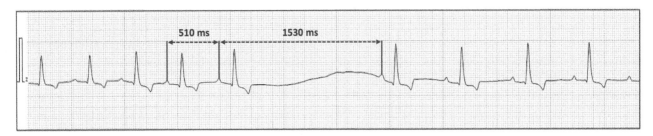

Figure 7.2 Second-degree sinoatrial block type II. A pause is seen with a duration of 1530 ms, which is three times the duration of the preceding P-P interval (510 ms × 3). This suggests that during this pause, two additional sinus depolarisations occurred but were not able to exit the sinus node and trigger a beat. This is consistent with a second-degree sinoatrial block type II. [9-year-old, male neutered, Boxer dog] (50 mm/s, 20 mm/mV)

- This pattern can be easily mistaken for sinus arrhythmia.
- *Second-degree sinoatrial block type II (2SAB type II)*: Intermittently generated impulses are not transmitted to the atrial myocardium, but, in contrast to type I, there is a constant interval between impulse generation and atrial depolarisation. On the surface ECG (Figure 7.2), this results in:
  - The underlying rhythm of the P-QRS complexes is regular (in contrast to type I, where there is clustering).
  - Intermittently, a P-QRS is absent, causing a pause.
  - The pause is an exact multiple of the preceding P-P interval.
- *Third-degree sinoatrial block (3SAB)*: None of the impulses from the SAN are transmitted to the working myocardium. On the surface ECG (Figure 7.3), this results in:
  - Complete absence of P waves
  - Long sinus pauses (sinus arrest) which may result in fatal asystole
  - These pauses may be terminated by a junctional or ventricular escape beat.
  - On the surface ECG, third-degree sinoatrial exit block is indistinguishable from sinus node arrest due to failure of impulse generation. To distinguish third-degree sinoatrial exit block from sinus arrest requires an intracardiac ECG to map activity within the SAN tissue.

Sinus Node Arrest

Sinus node arrest is more likely to be haemodynamically significant than sinus node exit block as the associated pauses are often longer (See Figure 7.4). To make the distinction between a physiological sinus pause and pathological sinus arrest, it is necessary to assess the surrounding trace. Sinus node arrest results in a marked and abrupt change in heart rhythm (See Figure 7.5), whereas physiological sinus pauses are commonly seen on ambulatory ECG recordings during periods of low heart rate in the long R-R phase of sinus arrhythmia. A definition used in human patients is that sinus arrest lasts more than three times the normal P-P interval.

Causes of sinus blocks and arrest:
• Sick sinus syndrome
• Sinus node dysfunction
• Drugs, including amiodarone, digoxin and sotalol
• Electrolyte abnormalities (see chapter 23)
• Idiopathic or vagally mediated[4]
• Atrial myocarditis.[3]

Atrioventricular Block (AVB)

Atrioventricular block is a term describing altered impulse conduction through the atrioventricular node. AVB is subdivided into first, second and third-degree

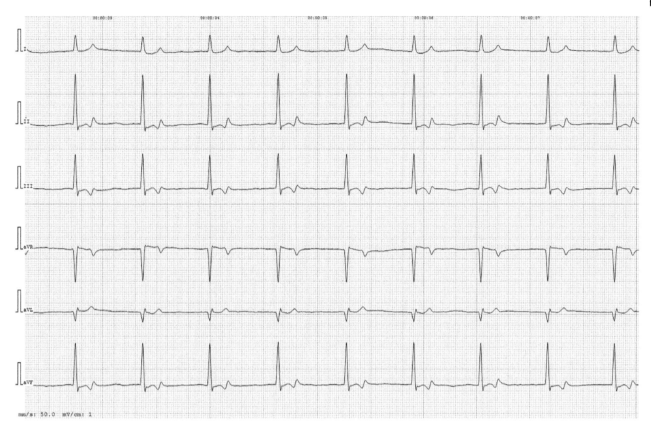

Figure 7.3 Atrial silence (atrial standstill) or third-degree sinoatrial block. A narrow-QRS rhythm is seen with a rate of 100 bpm. P waves are not seen preceding the QRS complexes that have a normal appearance (QRS duration, 60 ms; MEA, 72°). Differential diagnoses would include atrial silence or standstill in which atrial depolarisation does not occur, accounting for the lack of visible P waves; third-degree sinoatrial block, in which the sinus node depolarises but the impulse never reaches the atrial myocardium or remainder of the conduction system, and a junctional rhythm is responsible for ventricular depolarisation; a junctional rhythm with a rate higher than the sinus rate; and a sinoventricular rhythm that can be seen with hyperkalaemia in which atrial depolarisation does not occur, accounting for the lack of P waves, but sinus depolarisation and conduction through the normal conduction system still occur. In this case, atrial standstill associated with atrial myocarditis was suspected. [2-year-old, female neutered, Beagle dog with atrial myocarditis] (50 mm/s, 10 mm/mV)

atrioventricular block, as described in the remainder of this section.

First-Degree Atrioventricular Block (1 AVB)

1AVB is defined as lengthening of the PR interval to >130 ms in dogs and >90 ms in cats (Figures 7.6 and 7.7).

During the PR interval, a number of electrical and mechanical events are occurring (for further information, see chapter 3):

1) The impulse leaves the sinus node shortly before the start of the P wave and is conducted rapidly via the internodal pathways to the atrioventricular node, whilst the slower cell-to-cell depolarisation of atrial myocytes is occurring and creating the P wave on the surface ECG.
2) The impulse reaches the atrioventricular node during the early part of the P wave and continues until after the P wave has ended and the ECG trace has returned to baseline.
3) During the remainder of the PR interval, the impulse is being conducted via the His bundle, bundle branches and Purkinje system to the ventricular myocardium.
4) The Q or R wave represents depolarisation of the ventricular muscle and the conclusion of the PR interval.

An abnormal delay in conduction most commonly occurs in the atrioventricular node or the bundle of His. 1AVB is merely a delay in transmission of the impulse rather than a true block. As a result, the subsequent QRS complex is normal, providing that there is no pre-existing bundle branch block (discussed further in this chapter).

1AVB is commonly seen in cases with high resting vagal tone, especially during periods of low heart rate, and it may be seen in association with sinus arrhythmia and wandering pacemaker (see chapter 5). It is usually well tolerated without referable clinical signs but may be exacerbated by drugs or diseases likely to alter autonomic tone, for example intracranial disease.

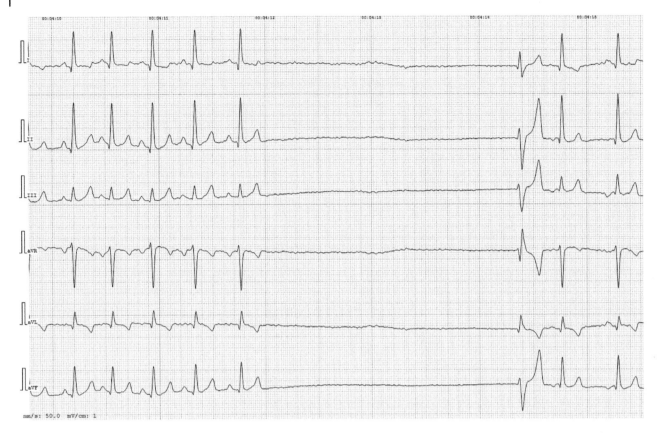

Figure 7.4 Sinus arrest in a dog. Sinus tachycardia is seen on the left of the trace with a rate of approximately 150 bpm, and it is followed by a pause lasting over 2 s, terminated by a ventricular escape beat and then a junctional rhythm. This pause occurs abruptly during sinus tachycardia, lasts for more than three times the preceding P-P interval and is interrupted by a subsidiary pacemaker, which is consistent with sinus node disease. [11-year-old, female neutered, Staffordshire Bull Terrier dog with sick sinus syndrome] (50 mm/s, 10 mm/mV)

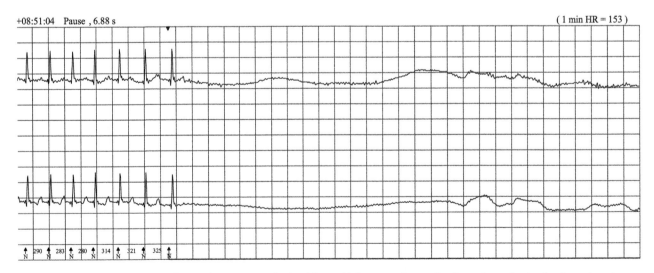

Figure 7.5 Sinus arrest causing collapse. This trace was obtained from a Holter recording at the time of an episode of collapse in a dog with sick sinus syndrome. A period of sinus tachycardia (180–200 bpm) is seen, followed by a 6.88 s period of asystole. [8-year-old, male neutered, Jack Russell terrier dog with sick sinus syndrome]

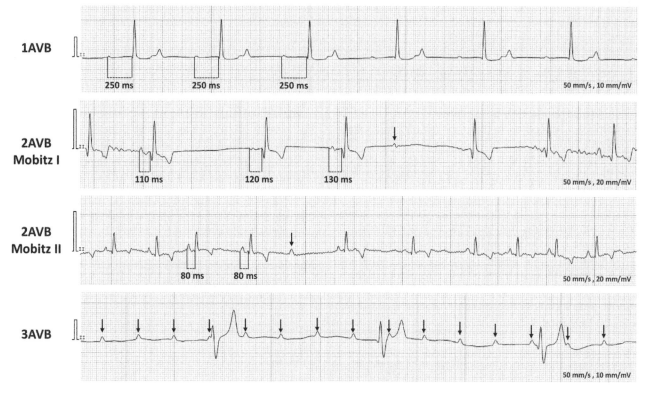

Figure 7.6 Atrioventricular block in dogs. (Top) First-degree atrioventricular block (1AVB) is characterised by a lengthening of the PR interval above >130 ms. (Middle two rows) Second-degree atrioventricular block (2AVB) Mobitz type I is characterised by a progressive lengthening of the PR interval until an impulse is blocked in the atrioventricular node and the P is not followed by a QRS (arrow). This is also often referred to as a *Wenckebach-type block*. In 2AVB Mobitz type II, one or more P waves are not followed by a QRS (arrow), but the PR interval of the conducted beats is constant. (Bottom) Third-degree atrioventricular block (3AVB) is characterised by dissociation of the atrial and ventricular rhythms. All the atrial depolarisations are blocked in the atrioventricular node, and ventricular depolarisation occurs due to a junctional (50–60 bpm) or ventricular (30–40 bpm) escape rhythm. None of the P waves (arrows) are followed by a QRS, and this becomes apparent by the fact that the interval between the P and QRS is variable.

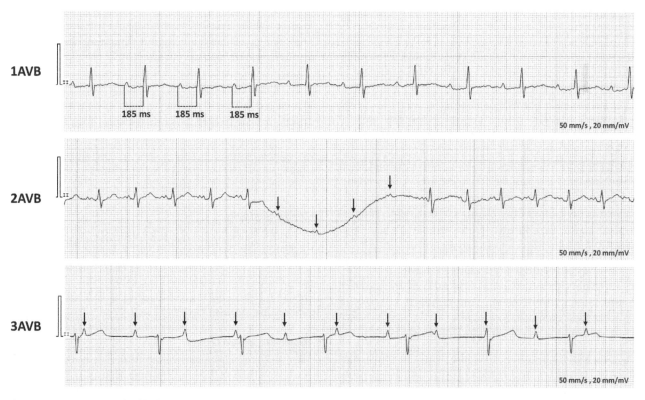

Figure 7.7 Atrioventricular block in cats. (Top) First-degree atrioventricular block (1AVB) is characterised by a lengthening of the PR interval above 90 ms. (Middle) One or more P waves are not followed by a QRS (arrows), but the PR interval of the conducted beats is usually constant. (Bottom) Third-degree atrioventricular block (3AVB) is characterised by dissociation of the atrial and ventricular rhythms, since all the atrial depolarisations are blocked in the atrioventricular node. A ventricular escape rhythm is often present with a rate between 110 and 140 bpm. None of the P waves (arrows) are followed by a QRS, and this becomes apparent by the fact that the interval between the P and QRS is variable.

> **Key features of first-degree atrioventricular block:**
>
> - Lengthening of PR interval
> - Otherwise normal P-QRS-T complex
> - Consistent coupling between P waves and QRS complexes.

Second-Degree Atrioventricular Block (2AVB)

Definition

2AVB is characterised by intermittent P waves that are not followed by a QRS complex (Figures 7.6 and 7.7). It is common to see a single unconducted P wave on ambulatory ECG (Holter) recordings from normal dogs during periods of rest, but multiple consecutive unconducted P waves occasionally occur and are more likely to be pathological.

> **Key features of second-degree atrioventricular block:**
>
> - Some P waves are not followed by a QRS complex.
> - QRS complexes are normal unless there is pre-existing bundle branch block.
> - There may be progressive lengthening of the PR interval prior to the block (Mobitz type I or Wenckebach), or the PR interval may be constant (Mobitz type II).

Sub-Classification

2AVB is sub-classified into Mobitz types I and II. In Mobitz type I (also known as Wenckebach phenomenon or Wenckebach periodicity), there is progressive lengthening of the PR interval prior to the block, whereas in Mobitz type II there is no lengthening of the PR interval prior to the block (Figures 7.6 and 7.7).

Another, arguably more clinically relevant way of describing 2AVB is to use the terms *low* and *high-grade 2AVB*. Low-grade 2AVB is the form commonly seen in resting dogs and describes 1–2 consecutive unconducted P waves during a period of low heart rate. As the resulting pause in ventricular activity is likely to be relatively brief, this rhythm may be tolerated without any referable clinical signs. In contrast, high-grade AVB has been defined as having three characteristics:

1) Several consecutive unconducted P waves
2) An atrioventricular conduction ratio of 3:1 (e.g. two unconducted P waves, then one conducted P wave for every QRS complex) or higher
3) An appropriate atrial rate (60–200 bpm).[5]

In cases with high-grade 2AVB, the pauses in ventricular activity are longer, and therefore this disorder is more likely to result in referable clinical signs. High-grade atrioventricular block (HGAVB) has also been sub-classified as follows (see Figure 7.8):

1) Class I HGAVB was defined as 2AVB with >3:1 conduction and no subsidiary pacemaker activity.
2) Class II was defined as 2AVB with subsidiary pacemaker activity.
3) Class III HGAVB was characterised by no impulses being conducted between the atria and ventricles, with complete reliance on subsidiary pacemakers to maintain ventricular activity. This is also known as 3AVB or complete heart block.

It is important to note that dogs can progress from high-grade 2AVB to 3AVB.[6]

Signalment

In a review of 124 dogs with high-grade 2AVB or 3AVB, the following breeds were reported as being predisposed: Boxer, Chow Chow, Cocker Spaniel, Golden Retriever, Labrador Retriever, Poodle and Shih Tzu.[5] In the United Kingdom, low-grade 2AVB is common in middle-aged and older Staffordshire Bull terriers.

Clinical Presentation of 2AVB

Whilst low-grade 2AVB is common in resting dogs and may be well tolerated, dogs with high-grade 2AVB are more likely to show signs such as weakness, lethargy, exercise intolerance and syncope.[5]

Investigation of Cases with Suspected High-Grade AVB

Clinical Pathology

In cases with HGAVB, it is advisable to check electrolytes as hyperkalaemia can result in delays in atrioventricular conduction (see chapter 23).[7]

ECG or Ambulatory ECG

Whilst some cases with persistent block may be diagnosed from a resting ECG, in cases with intermittent block, ambulatory ECG monitoring may be useful to document heart rate and rhythm over a longer period. It is also useful to document the simultaneous occurrence of clinical signs and bradycardia.

Echocardiography

Echocardiography is performed to screen for significant structural heart disease that could potentially damage the conduction system. For example, dogs with aortic valve endocarditis may experience extension of the infection into the septum and subsequent disruption of the conduction system.[8,9]

Atropine Response Testing

Atropine response testing (See Box 7.1) may be useful in dogs with 2AVB, and a positive response to atropine is shown by an improvement in the atrioventricular conduction ratio by at least two grades, for example from 4:1 to 2:1.[5]

Low-grade 2AVB

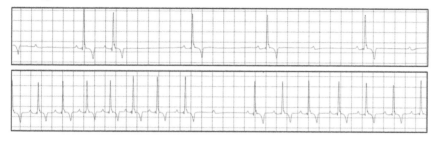

Class I high-grade AVB

Class I HGAVB is defined as 2AVB with >3:1 conduction and no subsidiary pacemaker activity.

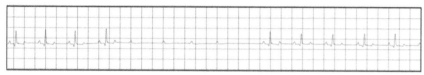

Class II high-grade AVB

Class II HGAVB is defined as 2AVB with subsidiary pacemaker activity

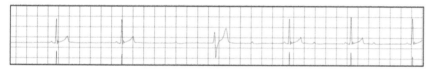

Class III high-grade AVB

Class III HGAVB is characterised by no impulses being conducted between the atria and ventricles with complete reliance on subsidiary pacemakers to maintain ventricular activity. This is also known as third degree atrioventricular block or complete heart block.

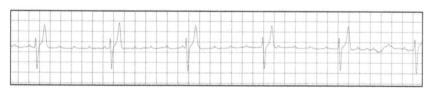

Figure 7.8 Low and high-grade atrioventricular block classification.

Box 7.1 Atropine response test

This test is sometimes performed in cases suspected of having conduction system dysfunction to assess the extent to which it is vagally mediated. Atropine is an anticholinergic drug that inhibits the parasympathetic nervous system.

Atropine response testing is performed after recording a resting ECG to document heart rate and rhythm. Atropine (0.04 mg/kg) is then injected subcutaneously or intramuscularly, and the ECG is repeated 20–30 min later. If atropine is administered intravenously, then a paradoxical bradycardia may occur prior to the onset of tachycardia. An atropine response is defined as either:

1) *Adequate*: Sinus rate increased to >150 bpm, sinus arrest abolished and improvement in the grade of 2AVB by >2 grades.

2) *Partial*: Sinus rate increased >25% from pre-atropine rate but <150 bpm and/or persistent sinus arrest; improvement in the grade of 2AVB by one grade (see Figure 7.8).

3) *Negative*: Sinus rate failed to increase >25%; persistence of sinus pauses and HGAVB.[10]

Concurrent diseases can alter autonomic tone, especially gastrointestinal, intracranial, respiratory, ocular (e.g. glaucoma) and endocrine conditions (e.g. hypothyroidism; see chapter 23 for further information).

It is important to note that, although a negative response suggests abnormal sinus node function, a positive response may still be seen in the presence of abnormal sinus node function and should not be used to rule it out.

Treatment

Cases with low-grade 2AVB during periods of rest are not likely to require any treatment. In cases with higher grade 2AVB, then sympathomimetics such as terbutaline, or methylxanthines such as theophylline, may be at least partially effective. An alternative approach would be to use vagolytics such as propantheline.

High-grade 2AVB has the potential to progress to 3AVB with a slower escape rhythm. Therefore, in dogs who do not respond to medical therapy, transvenous pacemaker implantation is a consideration.[11] The outcome for cases with HGAVB is discussed in the 'Third-degree atrioventricular block (3AVB)' section.

Third-Degree Atrioventricular Block (3AVB)

3AVB occurs when the atrioventricular node does not conduct any impulses from the atria to the ventricles. On the ECG, this results in P waves being visible but unrelated to the ventricular escape complexes (Figures 7.6 and 7.7). A junctional or ventricular escape rhythm is responsible for ventricular depolarisation (see chapters 10 and 11).

Signalment

Several studies have reported that Labradors appear to be predisposed to the development of 3AVB.[12,13] However, other breeds (including Springer spaniels and German Shepherd dogs) and crossbreed dogs have also been reported to be affected.[14]

Aetiology

The precise aetiology of 3AVB is often unknown. Whilst possible underlying pathological conditions such as cardiac conduction system fibrosis, calcification, infection (associated with endocarditis), neoplasia, amyloidosis and myocarditis have been proposed, similar changes have been documented in geriatric dogs without clinical atrioventricular nodal dysfunction.[15] Myocarditis has been reported as a cause of AVB in dogs and humans. As the associated inflammation affects the surrounding myocardium as well as the conduction system, measurement of serum levels of troponin, a marker of myocardial damage, may be useful to gauge the severity and duration of myocardial injury.[15]

A transient form of AVB, with an acute onset and fast resolution, has been reported in children with acute lymphocytic myocarditis; and a similar type of AVB has also been reported in young dogs.[16,17]

Very high serum concentrations of cardiac troponin-1 (cTn1) may suggest acute myocarditis.[15,16,18,19] However, in dogs with significant bradyarrhythmias, the reduction in cardiac output, eccentric hypertrophy secondary to volume overload and the presence of heart failure could also be at least partly responsible for the raised troponin concentrations. In acute canine experimental models of AVB, cardiac output rapidly decreases (by approximately 65–75%), resulting in diminished coronary artery perfusion and myocardial ischaemia, and these factors may also explain the subsequent increases in cTnI concentration.[20]

The reduction in cardiac output associated with 3AVB stimulates fluid retention and increased contractility in an attempt to restore cardiac output. At a microscopic level, the myocytes of dogs with AVB are longer than those of dogs in sinus rhythm. This 'stretch' happens almost immediately after the onset of AVB and may contribute to myocyte damage. Over time, the heart compensates through volume expansion and remodelling in the form of eccentric hypertrophy to optimise stroke volume, as heart rate variability is minimal.[21,22] Therefore, it is common to find cardiomegaly in these cases.

Uncommon causes of 3AVB reported in dogs include:

1) *Borrelia burgdorferi*[23]
2) *Bartonella vinsonii* (discussed further in this chapter)[15,24]
3) Endocarditis[8,25]
4) Trichinosis (*Trichinella spiralis*)[26]
5) Trypanosomiasis (Chagas disease)[27]
6) Autoimmune diseases – myasthenia gravis[28] and systemic lupus erythematosus[29]
7) Trauma, for example AVB following a road traffic accident[30]
8) Neoplasia[31–35]
9) Drug toxicity (e.g. digoxin)
10) Hypoadrenocorticism
11) Myxomatous mitral valve disease[36]
12) Phaeochromocytoma is often associated with tachyarrhythmias but occasionally may be associated with bradycardia. 3AVB and phaeochromocytoma have been reported occurring simultaneously in a small number of dogs.[30,32,37,38]

In cats, 3AVB has been seen associated with hypertrophic cardiomyopathy[39] and also hyperthyroidism.[40,41]

Clinical Findings

The presenting signs are associated with reduced cardiac output and include weakness, lethargy, exercise intolerance and syncope.[5] These signs are often acute in onset.[13] The drop in cardiac output may result in hypoperfusion of other organs, causing organ dysfunction. For example, mild azotaemia and slight increases in hepatic enzymes are common; hyperkalaemia associated with renal hypoperfusion has also been reported in one case.[42]

Diagnosis

As 3AVB is generally a persistent rhythm, the diagnosis can usually be made from a resting ECG, but in some cases the grade of block is intermittent and diagnosis is made from an ambulatory ECG.

Key ECG features of 3AVB

- No P waves are conducted through the atrioventricular node.
- Ventricular depolarisation occurs due to a junctional (QRS complex duration <70 ms with a rate of approximately 50–60 bpm) or ventricular escape rhythm (QRS complex duration >70 ms with a rate of approximately 30–40 bpm in dogs but higher in cats).
- The QRS complexes may be uniform or multiform.
- There is no coupling between the P waves and QRS complexes.

The atrial repolarisation wave (Ta) has been assessed in dogs with 3AVB (see Figure 3.14B).[43] Further studies may help to determine if the Ta wave can be used to distinguish healthy from diseased atria.

Atropine Response in 3AVB

A positive response to atropine is defined as an increase in the ventricular response rate by >20%;[5] however, many cases with 3AVB do not respond to atropine, apart from an increase in the rate of the SAN. The location of the block may be relevant as the AVN and proximal bundle of His are predominantly under parasympathetic control and hence more likely to respond to atropine than infranodal sites (i.e. more distally in the bundle of His).

Treatment of 3AVB

Some dogs with a relatively high ventricular escape rate (e.g. 60–70 bpm) and/or a high clinical suspicion of myocarditis may be treated medically with sympathomimetics (e.g. terbutaline) or methylxanthines (e.g. theophylline) to try to increase the heart rate and inodilators (e.g. pimobendan) to optimise stroke volume. Untreated and medically treated dogs with HGAVB are at high risk of sudden death, especially if the ventricular escape rate is low.[5] Dogs with 3AVB are potential candidates for transvenous pacemaker implantation. Transvenous pacemaker implantation was successful in reducing or eliminating clinical signs in over 90% of dogs with 3AVB in one large study,[12] significantly improving survival compared to dogs treated medically.[5] In another study, dogs with 3AVB treated with permanent pacemaker implantation had a median survival time of 27 months.[44] Some dogs with 3AVB and a high escape rate may appear to have minimal clinical signs but, after pacemaker implantation, show marked improvement in their demeanour and exercise tolerance.

Troponin as a Prognostic Factor?

It has been postulated that some dogs with 3AVB may have myocarditis, and therefore serum concentrations of cTnI have been studied pre- and post-pacemaker implantation. Mean cTnI concentration was significantly higher pre-pacing versus post-pacing, but in the majority of dogs post-pacing levels remained above the reference range.[15] The median time between these cTnI assays was 51 days (range, 11–162 days). In this small study, it was observed that the dogs with the highest pre-pacing cTnI concentrations (ranging from 0.36 to 10.66 ng/ml) were found to have progressive left ventricular enlargement and myocardial failure when compared to their pre-pacing examination.[15]

Outcome/Natural Progression of Disease

The vast majority of dogs with HGAVB have been shown to have persistence or progression of their bradyarrhythmia; in one study, improvement was seen in only 13% (of 92 dogs).[11] However, transient AVB associated with acute myocarditis and myocardial interstitial oedema has been reported in humans.[45]

Studies in humans suggest that patients with infranodal block (within the bundle branches) have a shorter survival time than those with nodal AVB (within the AVN). Nodal AVB would likely result in a narrower escape rhythm QRS complex, generated in the proximal junctional tissues such as the proximal bundle of His, whereas infranodal AVB would likely result in a wider escape rhythm complex originating in the Purkinje fibres. Therefore, in human patients, a wider QRS complex escape rhythm suggests an infranodal block and a shorter survival time. However, dogs appear to behave differently; dogs with wide-QRS complex escape rhythms had a longer survival than those with narrow-QRS complex escape rhythms in one study.[5] This suggests either that the QRS width of escape rhythms is not an accurate method of assessing site of AV block in dogs or that dogs with escape rhythms generated in more proximal junctional tissue had a poorer prognosis.[5]

Future Potential Treatments

Sub-epicardial injection of modified canine mesenchymal stem cells into dogs with experimentally produced AVB has been described, and these cells appeared to fulfil a stable biological pacing function during the relatively short 6-week follow-up period.[46,47] Further studies are required to determine whether this technique could be used in a clinical setting.

Intraventricular Conduction Disturbances

To understand conduction blocks, it is important first to review the anatomy of the conduction system in chapter 1 and cardiac vectors in chapter 3. The principal underlying conduction block is that if one (or more) sections of the conduction system is damaged and cannot conduct the impulse, then an area of the ventricular myocardium will depolarise more slowly as the wave of depolarisation travels from adjacent, normally depolarised myocardium by cell-to-cell conduction, rather than using the specialised fast conduction tissue. This results in a wider QRS complex with a different morphology from beats of supraventricular origin conducted normally.

Key point

The wide-QRS complexes associated with some intraventricular conduction abnormalities may be mistaken for a ventricular rhythm, potentially resulting in inappropriate treatment. To differentiate supraventricular beats with aberrant conduction from a ventricular rhythm, look for consistent P-QRS coupling.

Intraventricular conduction blocks are sub-classified on the basis of the anatomical region of the block into monofascicular, bifascicular and trifascicular blocks, as shown in Table 7.1. As described in human literature, the anterior (cranial) and posterior (caudal) bundle branches pass through the corresponding papillary muscles of the left ventricle. If the path to one of these papillary muscles is blocked, then ventricular activation will originate from the other papillary muscle, and, as a result, the net vector of ventricular depolarisation will shift towards the blocked fascicle.

Key point

Although the presence of conduction blocks is undisputed, it is controversial whether the origin of the block can be reliably determined from the resting ECG in dogs and cats. This is due to differences in anatomy between humans and small animal patients and inaccuracies of Einthoven's triangle to predict axis changes.[48]

The ECG traces described in the following section follow descriptions in other texts, but readers are encouraged to exercise a degree of caution when trying to determine the origin of a conduction deficit from a resting ECG, similar to that exercised when evaluating the mean electrical axis.

The intraventricular conduction disturbances discussed in this section include:

- Right bundle branch block
- Bifascicular left bundle branch block (block of both the anterior and posterior fascicles)
- Left anterior (cranial) fascicular block
- Bifascicular block affecting the left anterior (cranial) fascicle and right bundle branch
- Bifascicular block affecting the left posterior (caudal) fascicle and right bundle branch
- Trifascicular block.

The splintered QRS complex with a delta wave in the upstroke of the R wave suggestive of ventricular preexcitation via antegrade conduction through an accessory pathway is described in chapter 10.

It is logical to assume that a conduction disturbance is more likely to occur in a long thin fascicle than in a shorter, thicker fascicle. This may explain why the right bundle branch is most vulnerable to block, followed by the left anterior (cranial) fascicle and the left bundle branch, with the left posterior (caudal) fascicle being the least vulnerable.[49] Bundle branch blocks result in asynchronous ventricular depolarisation, and therefore myocardial function should be carefully evaluated in cases with bundle branch block.[50,51]

Right Bundle Branch Block (RBBB)

RBBB is an uncommon finding in healthy dogs and cats.[4] The precise site of the block is variable, and this can result in variation in the resulting QRS morphology; the more proximal the area of the block, the more marked the change in the surface ECG. The initial part of ventricular depolarisation via the bundle of His and then conduction down the left bundle branch is unaffected, so the initial portion of the QRS complex appears normal. However, the right ventricle depolarises by cell-to-cell transmission, which is slower and results in a vector of depolarisation spreading towards the right, resulting in increased prominence of the S wave.

Table 7.1 Anatomical classification of conduction disturbances in humans[49]

Monofascicular blocks	Bifascicular blocks	Trifascicular blocks
Right bundle branch	Right bundle branch and either left anterior *OR* left posterior fascicle	Both right and left bundle branch conduction is interrupted by infranodal disease
Left anterior (cranial) hemi-block	Left bundle branch block (includes both anterior and posterior fascicles)	Bifascicular block with atrioventricular nodal block
Left posterior (caudal) hemi-block		

<table>
<tr><td>

Key features of RBBB (see Figures 7.9 and 7.10)[52]

- QRS duration of >80 ms in dogs and >60 ms in cats
- Right axis deviation (up to −110°)
- Large wide S waves in leads II, III and aVF
- R wave in lead aVR
- An r' or R' wave is usually present in V1.
- No echocardiographic evidence of right ventricular enlargement
- The block can be intermittent and related to the heart rate (especially after sudden shortening of the preceding R-R interval[53]).

</td></tr>
</table>

Causes of right bundle branch block include:[54]

- Occasionally found in healthy dogs and cats
- A rate-dependent phenomenon (also known as Ashman's phenomenon) – see Figure 7.11[53,55]
- With sinus tachycardia[56]
- In association with severe structural heart disease, for example cardiac neoplasia, cardiomyopathy or heartworm
- In conjunction with a ventricular septal defect
- Post–cardiac arrest rhythm.

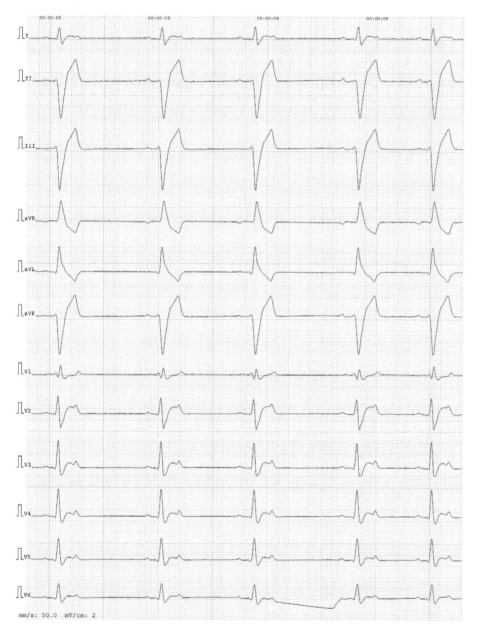

Figure 7.9 Right bundle branch block in a dog. A sinus rhythm is present with a rate of approximately 60 bpm. The QRS is wide (≈120 ms; >80ms) with large S waves in leads II, III, aVF; and R waves in leads aVR and aVL. A concomitant left anterior fascicular block may also be present given an R wave in lead I and a MEA ≈−80° (−60 to −90°). [10-year-old, male neutered, Cairn Terrier dog without echocardiographic evidence of structural heart disease] (50 mm/s, 5 mm/mV)

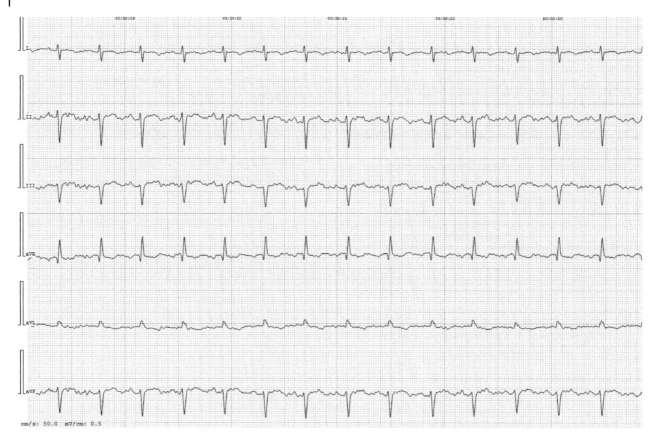

Figure 7.10 Right bundle branch block in a cat. A sinus rhythm is present with a rate of approximately 160 bpm. A normal P wave (20 ms; MEA, ≈70°) is present, preceding each QRS with a fixed PR interval within normal limits (80 ms). The QRS is wide (60 ms) with a right deviation of the MEA (≈−95°). [11-month-old, female neutered, Domestic Shorthair cat without evidence of structural heart disease] (50 mm/s, 20 mm/mV)

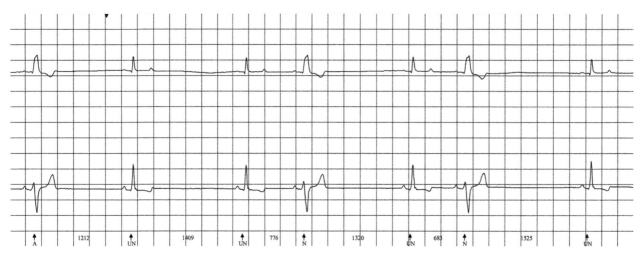

Figure 7.11 Example of Ashman's phenomenon from an ambulatory ECG. Beats 1, 4 and 6 are conducted with a bundle branch block following a long R-R interval (beats 2 to 3 and 4 to 5), followed by a short RR interval (beats 3 to 4 and 5 to 6) suggestive of Ashman's phenomenon. All beats are sinus with a consistent PR interval. It is postulated that the right bundle branch has a longer refractory period than the left bundle branch, and therefore during the shorter cycle it has not had time to fully repolarise, hence the block.[55] Ashman's phenomenon may also be observed at or near the onset of re-entrant narrow-QRS complex tachycardias due to the sudden shortening of the R-R interval. [9-year-old, male Boxer dog]

Incomplete Right Bundle Branch Block (IRBBB)

In dogs, incomplete right bundle branch block has been described.[57]

Key features of IRBBB[52]

- QRS duration of <80 ms in dogs (not described in cats)
- Right axis deviation (up to −80°)
- Large S waves in leads II, III and aVF
- R wave in lead aVR
- An r′ or R′ wave is normally present in lead V1.
- An S wave or W pattern is usually present in V10.
- No echocardiographic evidence of right ventricular enlargement.

Left Bundle Branch Block (LBBB)

LBBB results from conduction delay or block in both the anterior and posterior fascicles of the left bundle branch, and it is rare in healthy dogs and cats.[4] Initially, the impulse is transmitted normally via the His bundle and right bundle branch, but then, due to block of conduction through the left bundle branch, the left ventricle is depolarised more slowly by cell-to-cell transmission through the left ventricular myocardium.

Key features of LBBB (see Figure 7.12)

- Prolonged QRS complex – canine >80 ms, feline >60 ms
- There is an R wave in leads I, II, III and aVF.
- Absence of Q wave in lead I
- No echocardiographic evidence of LV enlargement
- May be rate dependent
- Prominent J point deviation and/or ST segment deviation due to altered left ventricular depolarisation and repolarisation.[58]

Causes of LBBB include:

- Significant underlying cardiac disease (e.g. dilated cardiomyopathy)[59]
- In association with sinus tachycardia[58,60]
- Congenital aortic stenosis[61]
- Drug toxicities (e.g. doxorubicin)[62]
- Severe ischaemia.[63]

Left Anterior Fascicle Block (LAFB)

The position of the left anterior fascicle is shown in Figure 1.3. It is worthwhile noting that different degrees of conduction disturbance can be observed and also that conduction disturbances can be intermittent.[49,64]

Key features of LAFB (Figure 7.13)[49,54,65]

- Left axis deviation (usually between −45 and −90°)
- Small Q waves with tall R waves (qR complexes) in leads I and aVL
- Small R waves with deep S waves (rS complexes) in leads II, III and aVF
- QRS duration normal or slightly prolonged (by up to 20 ms).

Causes of LAFB include:

- LAFB is seen most commonly in cats with marked LV hypertrophy.[66]
- A ventricular septal defect in the cranial (anterior) septum.

Clinical Significance

In cats, LAFB is generally well tolerated, and no specific therapy is required. In human patients without underlying cardiac disease, LAFB is regarded as an incidental finding.[49]

Bifascicular Block – Left Anterior Fascicle Block with Right Bundle Branch Block

This is a rare conduction disturbance in dogs. See Figure 7.9 for possible example.

Key features of LAFB and RBBB[67]

- Prolonged QRS duration (>80 ms)
- Small or absent S wave in lead I
- qR in lead aVL and r′ or R′ in lead V1
- Mean electrical axis shift to left (−60 to −90°).

Bifascicular Block – Left Posterior Fascicle Block with Right Bundle Branch Block

This conduction abnormality has been reported in experimental conditions but not in clinical practice. The left posterior fascicle is short, wide and located close to the left ventricular inflow tract (which is subject to less turbulent flow than the outflow tract) and also has a double blood supply. These factors may at least partly explain why it is less susceptible to damage than other parts of the intraventricular conduction system.[49]

Experimental studies in dogs have shown that with left posterior fascicle block, the mean electrical axis is deviated to the right and the QRS duration shows no significant prolongation. If RBBB is created in addition to an existing left posterior fascicle block, then the mean electrical axis is rotated to the right and the QRS duration shows significant prolongation.[67]

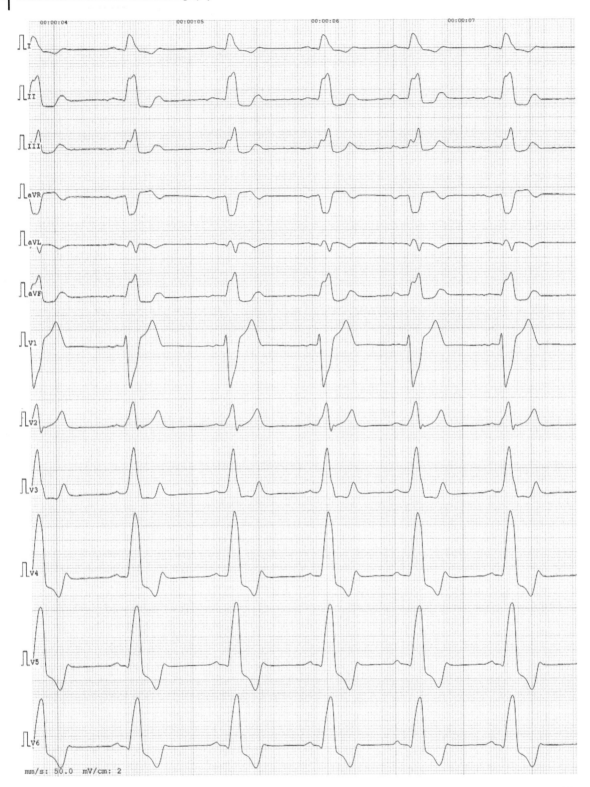

Figure 7.12 Left bundle branch block in a dog. A sinus rhythm is present with a rate of approximately 80 bpm. A normal P wave (40 ms; MEA, 60°) is present, preceding each QRS with a fixed PR interval within normal limits (120 ms). The QRS is wide (≈120 ms; >80 ms) with a normal MEA (68°). The QRS is predominantly positive in leads I, II, III, aVF and V2 to V6. [8-year-old, male, Gordon Setter dog with preclinical dilated cardiomyopathy] (50 mm/s, 5 mm/mV)

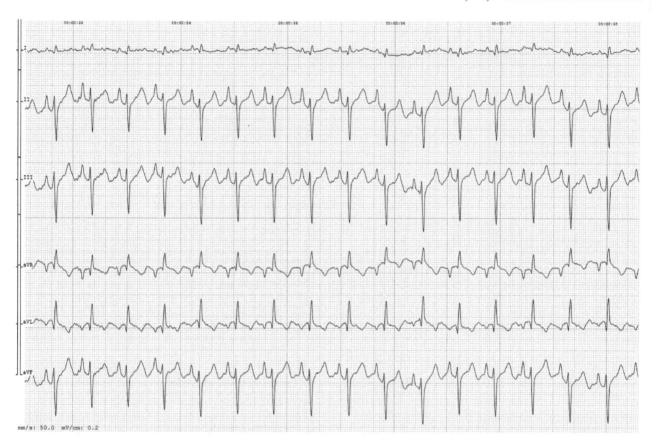

Figure 7.13 Left anterior fascicle block (LAFB) in a cat. A sinus rhythm is present with a rate of approximately 150 bpm. A normal P wave (30 ms; MEA, 82°) is present, preceding each QRS with a fixed PR interval within normal limits (60 ms). The QRS duration is slightly longer than normal (≈45–50 ms; <40 ms), with a left MEA deviation (−80°; −45 to −90°). Deep S waves (rS complexes) may be seen in leads II, III, and aVF, with qr and qR complexes in leads I and aVL, respectively. [16-year-old, male neutered, Bengal cat with equivocal hypertrophic cardiomyopathy] (50 mm/s, 50 mm/mV)

Trifascicular Block

Multiple forms of trifascicular block have been described in dogs but are rarely encountered in clinical practice. The subtypes described include:

- Both right and left bundle branch interruption by infranodal disease[68]
- 2AVB with concurrent LBBB.[69]

Key features of trifascicular block with 2AVB and concurrent LBBB are:

- 2AVB
- Prolongation of the QRS complexes (≥80 ms)
- Tall, slurred, delayed R waves in leads II, III, aVF and left precordial leads
- May be mild prolongation of the QT interval
- Mean electrical axis within the reference range
- V1 precordial lead has an rS type configuration (see chapter 4).
- If Q waves are present in lead I, then this suggests normal depolarisation of the proximal interventricular

---

septum and implies that the block of conduction is situated more distally – termed *post-divisional block*. In contrast, if Q waves are absent in lead I, this suggests that the area of block is located proximally – termed *truncular* or *divisional bundle branch block*.

Causes of trifascicular block include:

- Hereditary stenosis of the bundle of His[68]
- Cardiomyopathy[70]
- Myocardial infarction[63,71]
- Severe complex congenital disease
- Myocarditis.[16]

Given the potential for trifascicular block to be haemodynamically significant, permanent pacemaker implantation is advised.[69]

Intermittent Left or Right Bundle Branch Block

Intermittent right or left bundle branch block is diagnosed when QRS complexes with LBBB or RBBB

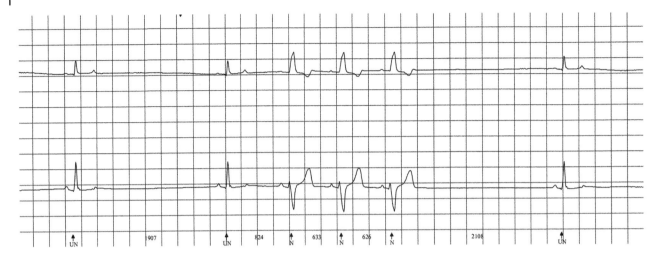

Figure 7.14 Intermittent bundle branch block in a dog. This ambulatory ECG trace shows a sinus rhythm with varying QRS complex morphologies. The coupling between the P waves and QRS complexes is consistent in all beats, suggesting sinus rhythm (or sinus arrhythmia) with an intermittent intraventricular conduction disturbance resulting in the wide-QRS complexes (complexes 3, 4 and 5). The bundle branch block occurs when the heart rate increases, suggesting a phase 3 or acceleration-dependent block. [9-year-old, male neutered, Boxer dog]

morphology are interspersed between the sinus beats, and this may be a heart rate–dependent phenomenon (see Figure 7.14).[56,58] There are multiple possible mechanisms for heart rate–dependent bundle branch block:

1) Tachycardia-dependent (also called phase 3) block, when the refractory period of the bundle branch is greater than the sinus cycle length. This is generally considered to be a physiological form of block.[72]

2) Acceleration-dependent aberrant conduction – the sinus cycle length is shorter than the action potential duration of damaged bundle branch tissue which, as a result of pathological injury, has a longer refractory period. This is also known as tachycardia-dependent alternans.

3) Bradycardia-dependent or pause-dependent aberrant conduction (also called phase 4 block). In this condition, the aberrant conduction is preceded by a pause. The pause may be a compensatory pause, spontaneous slowing of the sinus rate or overdrive suppression of the sinus rate after a fast atrial rhythm. Several causes have been proposed, including concealed conduction, hypoxia, vagal effects and supernormality of the affected bundle.[73]

Supernormal Conduction

Supernormal conduction is defined as conduction that occurs faster than expected or that occurs when block is expected,[74] for example a normal-duration QRS in a patient with persistent left or right bundle branch block (see Figure 7.15). It does not mean that conduction is faster than normal, just less altered or closer to normal in a patient with abnormal conduction. The underlying mechanism is conduction during a period of supernormal excitability and altered membrane potential. Imagine a case with an abnormal left bundle branch and a normal right bundle. When an impulse reaches the bundle branches, it finds the right bundle in an excitable state and the left in a period of refractoriness. This results in a beat conducted with an LBBB. However, during the repolarisation phase at the end of stage 3, the cells experience a period of 'supernormal excitability' where a weaker stimulus that would not normally trigger cell depolarisation may be able to do so (see chapter 2). If a premature impulse happens to reach the bundle branches when the left bundle is experiencing this stage of repolarisation, conduction may be normal or less aberrant. Supernormal conduction may be seen during sinus rhythm, supraventricular tachycardia (SVT) or atrial fibrillation.

Sick Sinus Syndrome

Introduction

The distinction between sinus node dysfunction (SND) and sick sinus syndrome (SSS) depends on whether there are referable clinical signs – dogs with SSS will show both abnormal sinus node activity on the ECG and also referable clinical signs such as syncope, ataxia and weakness. The ECG abnormalities seen are due to failure of impulse generation, failure of exit of the impulse from the SAN or failure of entrance to the adjacent atrial tissue. The ECG abnormalities seen include sinus bradycardia, sinus arrest, low mean heart rate and sometimes pathological SVT.[10] In some papers, slow atrial fibrillation is described as a manifestation of SAN dysfunction.[75–78]

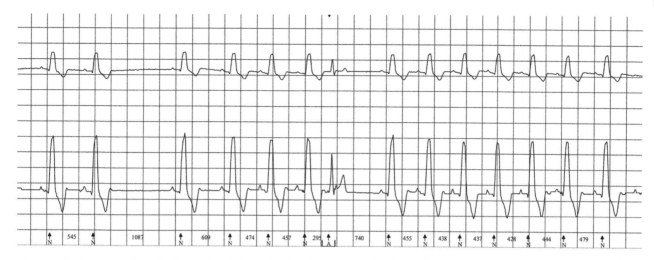

Figure 7.15 Supernormal conduction. This ambulatory ECG tracing was recorded from a dog with persistent left bundle branch block. A sinus rhythm is seen with a wide QRS (≈80 ms) in all beats except for the seventh beat, which presents a shorter duration (≈60 ms) which was unexpected. This beat was premature and is likely to have occurred during the supernormal excitability period, accounting for its normal or less aberrant conformation. [6-year-old, male, crossbreed dog]

Signalment

In a retrospective review of 93 dogs with this disorder or SAN dysfunction, Miniature Schnauzers, West Highland White terriers (WHWTs), Cocker Spaniels and females were overrepresented. The mean age at diagnosis was 11 ± 3 years.[10] In a previous publication, Cocker Spaniels, WHWTs, Pugs and Dachshunds were reported as being predisposed.[79] A European study reported that the condition was more common in Miniature Schnauzers and American Cocker Spaniels.[13] In this report, the mean age at presentation was similar at 10 ± 3.5 years, and female dogs slightly outnumbered males (57 vs. 43%).[13] There are sporadic reports of SSS in other breeds, such as a 2-year-old Boxer dog[80] and a Bull Terrier.[81]

Aetiology

Research in humans suggests that multiple aetiologies produce a similar syndrome. In human patients, the most common cause of SSS is an idiopathic degenerative fibrosis of the nodal tissue. However, the pathogenesis may be multifactorial as degeneration of the sinus node artery, alterations in the innervation regulating the SAN, autoantibodies to proteins within the SAN and ion channel alterations within the SAN have also been described.[82–84]

A postmortem histological study of SAN tissue and the transitional region (between the node and atrial tissue – see chapter 1) from seven dogs with naturally occurring SSS consistently revealed severe depletion of SAN cells, with a corresponding increase in fibrous or fibro-fatty tissue that interrupted contiguity between the SAN and the surrounding atrial myocardium. It is logical that these changes would disrupt conduction of the

electrical impulse. Sclerotic changes in the intramural coronary arteries supplying the SAN (SAN arteries) with thickening of the vessel walls and a slight to moderate decrease in luminal size were observed in all cases, but only one case showed severe narrowing of the lumen.[85] Physiological studies on a canine model using optical mapping have demonstrated that at a cellular level, there is dysfunction of both calcium and voltage clocks in SSS.[86]

SSS is not simply a disease of the SAN. The atrial myocardium in dogs with naturally occurring SSS was reported to show increased fibrous tissue and disruption of the muscle bundle architecture (interstitial myocardial fibrosis) in both the left and right atrial walls to varying degrees.[85] This is supported by experimental studies showing that if the SAN is excised from healthy dogs, subsidiary pacemakers (usually located in the atrioventricular junctional region) take over the role of dominant pacemaker within 10 days postoperatively.[87] However, dogs with SSS do not reliably have these escape rhythms, resulting in periods of asystole.

In cases with SSS, altered autonomic tone is likely to contribute to disease development. For example, older Miniature Schnauzers are predisposed to the development of diabetic cataracts, and it has been postulated that these ocular changes may influence autonomic tone.[88]

Presenting Signs

Dogs with *sinus node dysfunction* may have no clinical signs, but bradycardia or bradyarrhythmias may be identified as an incidental finding at routine clinical evaluation or may be an unexpected finding during general anaesthesia.[10] In contrast, dogs with SSS may be presented with syncope, lethargy, exercise intolerance or left-sided congestive heart failure if there is concomitant valvular heart disease.[10] Sudden death is reported to be rare, however.[10] Although the pathological changes may have a chronic course, the signs often seem to appear acutely.[13]

Clinical Findings

- Bradyarrhythmia which may be sinus bradycardia
- Arrhythmia – for example, short pauses during sinus rhythm or profound sinus arrhythmia that seems inappropriate
- Usually normal cardiac output signs unless there is significant concurrent structural heart disease
- Heart murmur if there is concomitant atrioventricular valve disease
- Comorbidities in older populations.

Diagnosis

Whilst the predominant rhythm in dogs with SSS may be sinus rhythm or sinus arrhythmia, ECG abnormalities documented in SSS include:

- Intermittent sinus arrest – whilst pauses of 4–6s can be seen in normal dogs during periods of rest, longer pauses may be seen in dogs with SSS.
- Low 24h mean heart rate (<60bpm)
- Prolonged periods of sinus bradycardia
- Intermittent 1AVB and 2AVB
- Intermittent pathological narrow-QRS complex tachycardia
- Junctional escape beats
- Intermittent SAN dysfunction progressing to a more permanent state
- Periods of tachycardia may cause overdrive suppression of the SAN and be followed by sinus pauses and/ or periods of bradycardia (see chapter 2 for an explanation on overdrive suppression).

See Figure 7.16 for an example of arrhythmias associated with SSS.

Poincaré Plots in Sick Sinus Syndrome

Poincaré plots have been studied in a dog with SSS and may be useful in the assessment of global autonomic influence and also illustrate the short-term beat-to-beat impact on rhythm (see chapter 16 for further information on heart rate variability). Poincaré plots are generated by plotting one R-R interval against the following R-R interval (R-R + 1). Distinctive patterns of bradycardia and 1:1, 2:1, 3:1, 4:1 and 5:1 AV block were evident in the tachogram and Poincaré plots in a dog with SSS.[77]

The patterning of beats in this patient seemed to be independent of the forces of sympathetic and parasympathetic tone, as there was clustering of the R-R intervals caused by episodes of SVT and also AV block.[89] Studies in human patients suggest that the chronobiology of cardiac rhythm can provide greater understanding than routine short ECGs.[90]

Atropine Response Test

Some dogs with SND or SSS may respond to atropine administration. Dogs with frequent syncope are less likely to be atropine responsive.[10] The length of the periods of sinus arrest and the presence of a disease likely to alter vagal tone were not helpful in predicting response to atropine.[10] Whilst some reports suggest that response to atropine predicts response to medical therapy,[10] another study, looking at SSS in WHWTs, stated that responses to parenteral atropine were variable and were not necessarily predictive of the subsequent response to oral anticholinergic agents.[91] The test is performed as described in this chapter, and dogs are considered to show a positive response if the atrial rate increases by 20% above the resting sinus rate.[5] Higher doses of atropine have also been recommended.[92]

Echocardiography in dogs with SSS may be unremarkable or may show signs typical of AV valve disease that is a common comorbidity in this patient group.

Clinical pathology in cases with SSS is generally unremarkable or shows evidence of concomitant conditions commonly encountered in older dogs, for example azotaemia. Thyroid function testing may merit consideration if there are clinical signs of hypothyroidism. If there is clinical suspicion of hypoadrenocorticism, then measuring electrolytes and basal cortisol may be indicated.

Treatment

Medical

Many positive chronotropic drugs have been used to treat SSS, including theophylline, propantheline, hyoscyamine and terbutaline. Generally, patients are started on monotherapy before consideration of whether to use multiple chronotropes. Side effects reported with positive chronotropic drugs include hyperactivity, panting and diarrhoea.

Dogs that respond appropriately to parenteral atropine can be treated orally with anticholinergic drugs such as hyoscyamine sulphate. Hyoscyamine sulphate elixir is easily dispensed in amounts appropriate for administration to small-breed dogs, and the dose can be accurately titrated. Adverse effects of anticholinergic drugs include dryness of the mouth, mydriasis, lethargy, anorexia,

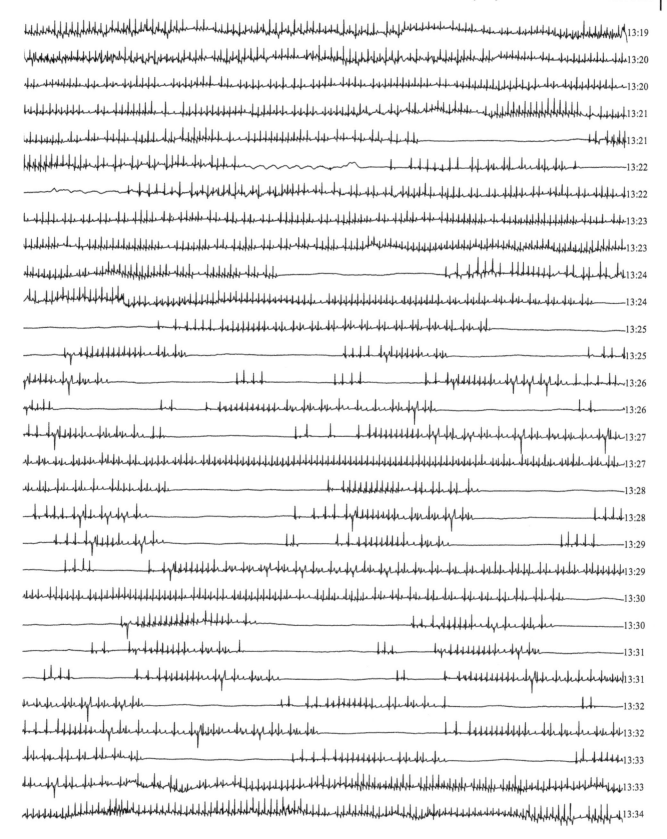

Figure 7.16 Sick sinus syndrome. Example of an ambulatory ECG recorded from a dog with sick sinus syndrome. Periods of sinus rhythm and short paroxysms of narrow-QRS tachycardia are abruptly interrupted by frequent long pauses. [12-year-old, female neutered, West Highland White Terrier with SSS]

gastric distension, ileus and other gastrointestinal tract problems. Urine retention may also occur, but with proper dosing and monitoring adverse effects are usually minimal.[93]

In an experimental model of heart failure, there was up-regulation of adenosine receptors, thereby supporting use of the adenosine receptor antagonist theophylline.[94] However, whilst theophylline is occasionally of benefit, it is generally less effective than anticholinergic treatment.[93] The combination of an anticholinergic agent and theophylline can be administered to dogs that respond inadequately to the former as monotherapy. If medical treatment fails to control clinical signs, then pacemaker implantation is the treatment of choice.[93]

Surgical Pacemaker Implantation

Pacemaker implantation is used in this condition to prevent the prolonged sinus pauses that may cause pre-syncope, syncope or hypoxic seizures (see chapter 18 for further information on pacemakers). In one study, survival did not vary between dogs with SND and SSS whether they were treated medically or surgically, but the reduction in frequency of clinical signs likely improved the quality of life for both dogs and their owners.[10]

Although transvenous pacemaker implantation is associated with complications, these were rarely life-threatening, and good survival was documented in the majority of cases in one large retrospective study.[12] Encouraging survival times have been reported after pacemaker implantation, especially considering that SSS tends to affect older dogs. In another retrospective study, the mean survival time for the 60 dogs that died during the study period was 2.2 years (range, 0.1–5.8 years).[13] Another study reported that most dogs succumbed to disease unrelated to their arrhythmia or the pacemaker.[95]

Transthoracic external pacing has been described as a temporary bridge to permanent pacemaker implantation, but delivery of the current across the chest wall is painful, and therefore general anaesthesia is required.[96] Dual-chamber and atrial pacing for treatment of SSS have also been reported.[80,97]

Treatment of Tachyarrhythmias in Sick Sinus Syndrome

Dogs with concurrent SVT are more likely to be candidates for pacemaker implantation than medical therapy, as sympathomimetics may exacerbate the episodes of SVT. If SVT persists after pacemaker implantation, then medical therapy (e.g. with diltiazem) may be indicated depending on clinical findings and the results of other tests. Progression to congestive heart failure was reported to be more likely in cases with concurrent tachycardias.[10]

Outcome

Many dogs with SSS can experience good quality life, and sudden death is reported to be a rare outcome for these dogs.[10] Some dogs with SSS and valvular heart disease may develop congestive heart failure secondary to the valvular heart disease.

One study identified 93 dogs with SSS or SND, and during the 12-year study period the outcomes were:

- 63 (68%) dogs had died at the time of writing.
  - 43 were euthanised for non-cardiac disease.
  - 13 were euthanised due to congestive heart failure.
  - 3 due to complications associated with pacemaker placement.
  - 2 because of frequent syncope, despite medical therapy where pacemaker implantation was declined.
  - 1 died from atrial thromboembolism.
  - 1 dog died suddenly.
- 16 dogs (17%) were still alive at the time of writing, with a median follow-up time of 653 days.
- 14 dogs (15%) were lost to follow-up.

Of the 63 dogs that died, in this study there was no significant difference in survival between dogs with SSS and SND; however, these groups were managed differently. In this study, median survival time for all dogs after diagnosis was 538 days (interquartile range, 195–990 days), and did not differ between SSS (480 days) and SND (754 days) dogs.[10]

Sick Sinus Syndrome in Cats

This disorder is rarely diagnosed in cats, but we should perhaps be mindful that many cats have a sedentary lifestyle and also cats have a high inherent escape rhythm rate, so they may therefore better tolerate bradyarrhythmias. There is one case report of 3AVB with suspected concurrent SSS in a cat.[98] Figure 7.17 shows an example of SND in a cat.

Selected Conditions Resulting in Bradyarrhythmias

Neurally Mediated Syncope

Neurally mediated syncope is the most common form of syncope in human patients without structural cardiac disease,[99] and this condition is also recognised in dogs. Reflex or neurally mediated syncope is a heterogeneous group of conditions characterised by an inappropriate autonomic response to a stimulus, resulting in bradycardia and hypotension. In human patients, the autonomic response can be sub-classified as cardio-inhibitory or vasodepressor. Cardio-inhibitory syncope results from

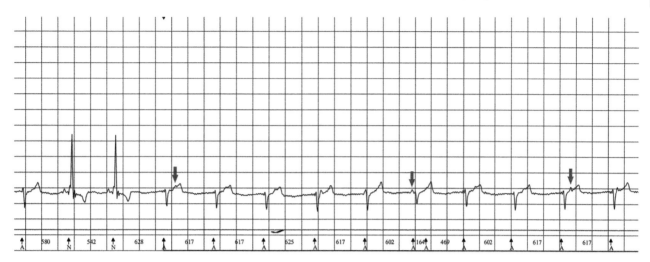

Figure 7.17 Sinus node dysfunction in a cat with bradycardia detected as an incidental finding. Ambulatory ECG recording from a cat showing two sinus beats followed by a ventricular escape rhythm with a rate of 100 bpm. P waves are seen intermittently and highlighted by arrows. [4-year-old, neutered, male Domestic Shorthair cat]

an inappropriate increase in vagal tone producing bradycardia and asystole. Vasodepressor syncope is characterised by a sudden withdrawal of sympathetic tone resulting in profound hypotension. Regardless of mechanism, the consequent hypotension and cerebral hypoperfusion may result in syncope. As ambulatory blood pressure measurements are difficult in dogs, ambulatory ECGs help us to identify dogs with the cardio-inhibitory form. Cardio-inhibition is likely to be the predominant mechanism if there are long sinus pause(s); shorter sinus pauses suggest a vasodepressor component with vasodilation.[100]

Pathophysiology of Cardio-Inhibitory Syncope

Syncope may arise via a combination of reflexes resulting in a surge in vagal activity. The effects of vagal stimulation on the heart include:

- Inhibition of impulse generation in the SAN, resulting in bradycardia or sinus arrest
- Slowed conduction through the AV node resulting in AVB.[101]

Other changes that may occur after vagal stimulation and favour the onset of atrial fibrillation after a long sinus pause are:[100]

- Changes in the electrophysiological properties of atrial cells. The surge in parasympathetic activity shortens the effective refractory period and action potential duration in atrial tissue. This dispersion of repolarisation favours the formation of re-entrant circuits and can form a substrate for paroxysmal or sustained atrial fibrillation.[102]
- In pulmonary vein cells, the shortened action potential duration enhances the transient calcium current and

sodium–calcium exchange, which can set up favourable conditions for early afterdepolarisations, thereby enabling the formation of ectopic foci.[103]

Dogs with outflow tract obstruction may be more susceptible to the Bezold Jarisch reflex (BJR). This reflex is initiated by the activation of pressure sensors in the left ventricle that detect stretch and activate C fibre afferent nerves, causing a vagally mediated reflex arc, increased parasympathetic activity and withdrawal of sympathetic tone. This autonomic change leads to bradycardia, vasodilation and hypotension.[104] The reason for this seemingly paradoxical response may be to reduce myocardial work and oxygen consumption, thus providing myocardial protection during periods of compromised myocardial oxygen supply.[105]

The BJR is not the only reflex causing bradycardia and hypotension; other reflexes, such as the *reverse-Bainbridge reflex* (which originates from atrial rather than ventricular stretch receptors), have also been reported.[106] However, it is difficult to differentiate the exact origins of such reflexes in a clinical setting.[104,107]

Signalment

Neurally mediated syncope is common in young, otherwise healthy brachycephalic dogs and has also been reported in other breeds, including Dobermanns.[108]

History

A detailed history is very important in these cases, as diagnosis may rely on history and exclusion of concurrent disease. Typically, neurally mediated syncope affects young, active dogs, and the episode occurs after a sudden change in activity such as a transition from rest to excitement or a surge of activity during exercise. The owner may describe the dog gradually slowing over a few seconds, sometimes followed by ataxia, prior to becoming recumbent. There may or may not be loss of consciousness, and mucous membranes are pale during the episode; if there is significant cerebral hypoxia, then extension of the forelimbs and neck may be seen and occasionally urination. Recovery is gradual over several minutes, but after this time dogs will usually stand and are able to continue exercise.

Neurally mediated syncope is more common in brachycephalics due to high resting vagal tone secondary to upper airway obstruction. In humans, the triggers may be:

1) Vasovagal (emotional, orthostatic)
2) Situational (vomiting, coughing, after exercise)
3) Mechanical (e.g. carotid sinus pressure).

In dogs, emotional triggers are unlikely. Dogs are sometimes described as having events after a change in body position, especially if accompanied by a surge in activity – for example, a fast transition from sleep to rushing to the door – which may have some elements of an orthostatic response.

Syncope associated with vomiting, with coughing or after surges in activity is recognised in dogs. Intracranial disease and gastrointestinal disease may also lower the threshold for vasovagal events.

Clinical Examination

Dogs are generally normal at the time of examination. A systolic murmur at the heart base may raise suspicion of outflow tract obstruction that may predispose dogs to developing a BJR.

Further Investigation

- Clinical pathology – usually unremarkable
- Resting ECG – usually unremarkable
- Echocardiography
- Ambulatory ECG Holter findings.

If an event is documented during the recording, then, prior to the event, the trace typically shows sinus rhythm or sinus tachycardia, which is followed by a rapid decrease in heart rate (see Figure 7.18). The bradycardia may be absolute (<60 bpm) or relative with a >30% reduction in heart rate over a short period. Sinus pauses, 2AVB, ventricular asystole followed by escape beat(s) and sinus bradycardia may be seen prior to the resumption of sinus rhythm.[109] If an episode does not occur during the recording, then there may be other findings suggesting high resting vagal tone, such as a low mean heart rate (<65 bpm), and unexpected changes in heart rate and rhythm without an associated diary entry.

In occasional cases, atrial fibrillation may be seen after the episode (see Figure 9.15).[100]

Treatment

Neurally mediated syncope is generally regarded as a benign disorder and therefore unlikely to be life-threatening, but the possibility of further episodes of collapse can have an impact on the owner and dog's quality of life. If the events are highly situational (i.e. always associated with a particular activity), then avoiding that activity may be sufficient to prevent the events occurring. Sympathomimetics have been used and are especially effective in cases with tussive syncope, as they may alleviate underlying airway disease.

Whilst the use of β-blockers seems logical to dampen the effect of surges of catecholamines in excitable dogs, the response to treatment seems to be variable, with some dogs having more frequent episodes after β-blocker administration. Fludrocortisone, midodrine and serotonin reuptake inhibitors have also been used in human patients, with varying reports regarding efficacy, and use of these medications is under review in human patients.[110]

Transvenous pacemaker implantation was successful in reducing or eliminating clinical signs in dogs with vasovagal syncope in one study.[12] Six of eight dogs had greatly reduced frequency of collapse, and two became asymptomatic. Although the procedure was associated with complications, these were rarely life-threatening, and good survival was documented in the majority of cases.[12]

Other Causes of Bradyarrhythmia

Bartonella Myocarditis

Myocyte injury is suspected to play a role in some symptomatic bradyarrhythmias, and infection with *Bartonella*, a gram-negative bacterium, has been implicated as one possible cause.[15,24,111] The myocardium of infected dogs showed multifocal areas of neutrophils and macrophage infiltration histologically. However, it is important to note that, in some human cases of *Bartonella henselae*–induced myocarditis, the organism may not be apparent in the myocardium.[112] A possible explanation for this is that some infectious agents may have surface proteins similar to host cells, thereby inducing a cross-reactive autoimmune response to host proteins. In some susceptible individuals, this may tip the balance of immunological response versus tolerance towards response and subsequently lead to autoimmune disease.[113] The importance of *Bartonella* exposure or infection in dogs with signs of inflammatory cardiomyopathy or

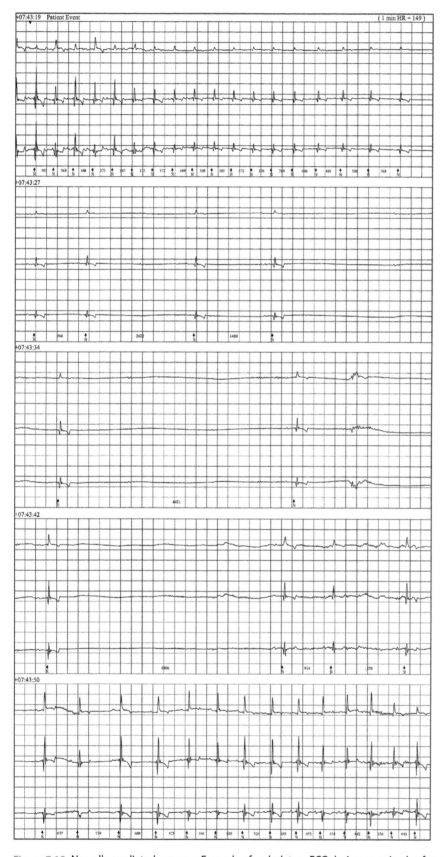

Figure 7.18 Neurally mediated syncope. Example of ambulatory ECG during an episode of syncope in a Boxer. Prior to the event, the trace shows sinus rhythm with a rate of approximately 140 bpm, and this is followed by an abrupt transition to sinus bradycardia with a minimum instantaneous rate of 14 bpm, followed by a gradual return to sinus rhythm.

symptomatic bradyarrhythmias, in particular 3AVB, merits further study.[15,111]

Stenosis of the Bundle of His in Pugs

This defect was reported in a colony of purebred dogs but does not appear to be commonly seen in clinical practice. In the 21 dogs identified as being affected by this disorder, the AV node and bundle branches appeared normal at postmortem examination, but in all cases there was significant stenosis of the mid-portion of the bundle of His. Sinus pauses and 2AVB were identified on the resting ECG of affected dogs.[68]

Trypanosomiasis (Chagas myocarditis)

Chagas disease is caused by the protozoan organism *Trypanosoma cruzi*, which is a recognised cause of myocarditis in dogs in the southern United States and Latin American countries. Transmission is commonly via a bite from or ingestion of an infected insect vector and, less commonly, via blood transfusions or transplacental or transmammary infection. Trypomastigotes enter cardiac myocytes and develop into amastigotes in about 14 days. The amastigotes multiply, causing myocyte destruction, parasite release into the circulation and an inflammatory response that results in lethargy, enlargement of the liver or spleen, lymphadenopathy and arrhythmias. Chronic myocarditis can result in conduction abnormalities, arrhythmias, ventricular myocardial dysfunction, heart failure and sudden death.[27]

Persistent Atrial Standstill

This condition is also known as *parchment atrium* on account of the marked thinning of the atrial walls that can result in them becoming almost translucent when seen at postmortem examination. It is a rare condition recognised in English Springer Spaniels and also sporadically in other pure or mixed-breed dogs.[3,19] Dogs affected by this condition may show signs of sudden-onset severe bradyarrhythmias, with the ECG trace persistently showing no P waves and with cardiac output maintained by a ventricular escape rhythm. Some dogs show upper forelimb muscle atrophy, suggesting a more widespread muscular dystrophy.

Clinical pathology in affected cases reveals normal or high basal cortisol concentrations, and electrolytes within their respective reference ranges. Echocardiographic findings include marked right atrial or biatrial enlargement, often with progression to ventricular systolic failure. Cardiac histopathological findings include lymphocytic inflammation, fibrosis, fibroelastosis and steatosis of one or both atria and associated conduction tissue; these may also spread to affect the ventricle(s).[3,114]

Four dogs treated with pacemaker implantation showed a good outcome.[115]

Bradycardia in Cats

Cats have a higher ventricular escape rate than dogs that, in conjunction with a sometimes sedentary lifestyle, can result in some bradyarrhythmias being well tolerated. As a result, reports of cats with symptomatic bradyarrhythmias are rare. Bradyarrhythmias in conjunction with cardiomyopathy[40] and systemic disease[41] are recognised, and this is discussed in chapters 21 and 23.

In cats, bradycardia is often defined as a heart rate of 100–120 bpm or less.[116] Cats with bradyarrhythmias may have seizure-like episodes, as was described in three cats with HGAVB.[117] In this case series, one cat improved with terbutaline administration, and another cat had a pacemaker fitted.

Syncope associated with intermittent AVB and ventricular asystole has been reported in a cat. This cat was treated by transvenous pacemaker implantation but developed chylothorax postoperatively. The chylothorax may have been due to either partial obstruction of thoracic duct flow or progression of the arrhythmia from intermittent to permanent AVB, resulting in worsening heart failure.[118] Another case report describes successful transvenous pacemaker implantation in a cat for treatment of complete AVB and asystole. During the 18-month follow-up period after pacemaker implantation, there was no recurrence of syncope.[119] The outcomes of 21 cats with 3AVB has been described,[40] and further information is shown in chapter 21.

Bradycardia Secondary to Drug Administration and Toxicity

Drug administration can potentially result in bradyarrhythmias, especially if agents from different drug classes (e.g. diltiazem and amiodarone) are used concurrently. Numerous toxicities can also result in bradycardia, and therefore obtaining a thorough patient history is essential in cases with unexplained bradyarrhythmias. See chapter 23 for further information.

Conclusion

Bradyarrhythmias are clinically significant as a potential cause of intermittent syncope and exercise intolerance in dogs. Whilst some bradyarrhythmias may be life-threatening and require urgent intervention, others may be tolerated and may reflect physiological change. As ever, it is important to assess the patient as well as the ECG trace.

References

1 Ulloa HM, Houston BJ, Altrogge DM. Arrhythmia prevalence during ambulatory electrocardiographic monitoring of beagles. Am J Vet Res. 1995;56:275–281.

2 Hall LW, Dunn JK, Delaney M, Shapiro LM. Ambulatory electrocardiography in dogs. Vet Rec. 1991;129:213–216.

3 Robinson WF, Thompson RR, Clark WT. Sinoatrial arrest associated with primary atrial myocarditis in a dog. J Small Anim Pract. 1981;22:99–107.

4 Buchanan JW. Spontaneous arrhythmias and conduction disturbances in domestic animals. Ann N Y Acad Sci. 1965;127:224–238.

5 Schrope DP, Kelch WJ. Signalment, clinical signs, and prognostic indicators associated with high-grade second- or third-degree atrioventricular block in dogs: 124 cases (January 1, 1997–December 31, 1997). J Am Vet Med Assoc. 2006;228:1710–1717.

6 Winter RL, Bright JM. ECG of the month: AV block in a dog. J Am Vet Med Assoc. 2011;239:1060–1062.

7 Schrope DP, Fox PR, Hahn AW, Bond B, Rosenthal S. Effects of electrocardiograph frequency filters on P-QRS-T amplitudes of the feline electrocardiogram. Am J Vet Res. 1995;56:1534–1540.

8 Robertson BT, Giles HD. Complete heart block associated with vegetative endocarditis in a dog. J Am Vet Med Assoc. 1972;161:180–184.

9 Peddle GD, Boger L, Van Winkle TJ, Oyama MA. Gerbode type defect and third degree atrioventricular block in association with bacterial endocarditis in a dog. J Vet Cardiol. 2008;10:133–139.

10 Ward JL, DeFrancesco TC, Tou SP, Atkins CE, Griffith EH, Keene BW. Outcome and survival in canine sick sinus syndrome and sinus node dysfunction: 93 cases (2002–2014). J Vet Cardiol. 2016;18:199–212.

11 Santilli RA, Porteiro Vázquez DM, Vezzosi T, Perego M. Long-term intrinsic rhythm evaluation in dogs with atrioventricular block. J Vet Intern Med. 2016;30:58–62.

12 Johnson MS, Martin MWS, Henley W. Results of pacemaker implantation in 104 dogs. J Small Anim Pract. 2007;48:4–11.

13 Wess G, Thomas WP, Berger DM, Kittleson MD. Applications, complications, and outcomes of transvenous pacemaker implantation in 105 dogs (1997–2002). J Vet Intern Med. 2006;20:877–884.

14 Oyama MA, Sisson DD, Lehmkuhl LB. Practices and outcome of artificial cardiac pacing in 154 dogs. J Vet Intern Med. 2001;15:229–239.

15 Trafny DJ, Oyama MA, Wormser C, Reynolds CA, Singletary GE, Peddle GD. Cardiac troponin-I concentrations in dogs with bradyarrhythmias before and after artificial pacing. J Vet Cardiol. 2010;12:183–190.

16 Church WM, Sisson DD, Oyama MA, Zachary JF. Third degree atrioventricular block and sudden death secondary to acute myocarditis in a dog. J Vet Cardiol. 2007;9:53–57.

17 Atwell RB, Sutton RH. Focal lymphocytic non-suppurative myocarditis and 3 degrees heart block in a 2-year-old dog. Aust Vet J. 1990;67:265.

18 Fonfara S, Loureiro J, Swift S, James R, Cripps P, Dukes McEwan J. Cardiac troponin I as a marker for severity and prognosis of cardiac disease in dogs. Vet J. 2010;184:334–339.

19 Fonfara S, Loureiro JF, Swift S, James RA, Pereira YM, Lopez-Alvarez J, Summerfield N, Dukes McEwan J. English springer spaniels with significant bradyarrhythmias – presentation, troponin I and follow-up after pacemaker implantation. J Small Anim Pract. 2010;51:155–161.

20 de Groot SH, Schoenmakers M, Molenschot MM, Leunissen JD, Wellens HJ, Vos MA. Contractile adaptations preserving cardiac output predispose the hypertrophied canine heart to delayed afterdepolarization-dependent ventricular arrhythmias. Circulation. 2000;102:2145–2151.

21 Verduyn SC, Ramakers C, Snoep G, Leunissen JD, Wellens HJ, Vos MA. Time course of structural adaptations in chronic AV block dogs: evidence for differential ventricular remodeling. Am J Physiol Heart Circ Physiol. 2001;280:H2882–H2890.

22 Volders PGA, Sipido KR, Vos MA, Kulcsár A, Verduyn SC, Wellens HJJ. Cellular basis of biventricular hypertrophy and arrhythmogenesis in dogs with chronic complete atrioventricular block and acquired torsade de pointes. Circulation. 1998;98:1136–1147.

23 Levy SA, Duray PH. Complete heart block in a dog seropositive for *Borrelia burgdorferi*: similarity to human Lyme carditis. J Vet Intern Med. 1988;2:138–144.

24 Breitschwerdt EB, Atkins CE, Brown TT, Kordick DL, Snyder PS. *Bartonella vinsonii* subsp. berkhoffii and related members of the alpha subdivision of the Proteobacteria in dogs with cardiac arrhythmias, endocarditis, or myocarditis. J Clin Microbiol. 1999;37:3618–3626.

25 Sykes JE, Kittleson MD, Chomel BB, MacDonald KA, Pesavento PA. Clinicopathologic findings and outcome in dogs with infective endocarditis: 71 cases (1992–2005). J Am Vet Med Assoc. 2006;228:1735–1747.

26 Sleeper MM, Bissett S, Craig L. Canine trichinosis presenting with syncope and AV conduction disturbance. J Vet Intern Med. 2006;20:1228–1231.

27 Saunders AB, Gordon SG, Rector MH, DeMaster A, Jackson N, Clubb FJ, *et al.* Bradyarrhythmias and

pacemaker therapy in dogs with Chagas disease. J Vet Intern Med. 2013;27:890–894.

28 Hackett TB, Van Pelt DR, Willard MD, Martin LG, Shelton GD, Wingfield WE. Third degree atrioventricular block and acquired myasthenia gravis in four dogs. J Am Vet Med Assoc. 1995;206:1173–1176.

29 Malik R, Zunino P, Hunt GB. Complete heart block associated with lupus in a dog. Aust Vet J. 2003;81:398–401.

30 Nicholls PK, Watson PJ. Cardiac trauma and third degree AV block in a dog following a road accident. J Small Anim Pract. 1995;36:411–415.

31 Stern JA, Tobias JR, Keene BW. Complete atrioventricular block secondary to cardiac lymphoma in a dog. J Vet Cardiol. 2012;14:537–539.

32 Mak G, Allen J. Simultaneous pheochromocytoma and third-degree atrioventricular block in 2 dogs. J Vet Emerg Crit Care. 23, 610–614 (2013).

33 Gallay J, Belanger M-C, Helie P, Cote E, Johnson TO, Peters ME. Cardiac leiomyoma associated with advanced atrioventricular block in a young dog. J Vet Cardiol. 2011;13:71–77.

34 Dupuy-Mateos A, Wotton PR, Blunden AS, White RN. Primary cardiac chondrosarcoma in a paced dog. Vet Rec. 2008;163:272–273.

35 Schuller S, Van Israel N, Else RW. Third degree atrioventricular block and accelerated idioventricular rhythm associated with a heart base chemodectoma in a syncopal Rottweiler. J Vet Med A Physiol Pathol Clin Med. 2007;54:618–623.

36 Kaneshige T, Machida N, Yamamoto S, Nakao S, Yamane Y. A histological study of the cardiac conduction system in canine cases of mitral valve endocardiosis with complete atrioventricular block. J Comp Pathol. 2007;136:120–126.

37 Gilson SD, Withrow SJ, Wheeler SL, Twedt DC. Pheochromocytoma in 50 dogs. J Vet Intern Med. 1994;8:228–232.

38 Zelinka T, Petrak O, Turkova H, Holaj R, Strauch B, Krsek M, *et al.* High incidence of cardiovascular complications in pheochromocytoma. Horm Metab Res. 2012;44:379–384.

39 Kaneshige T, Machida N, Itoh H, Yamane Y. The anatomical basis of complete atrioventricular block in cats with hypertrophic cardiomyopathy. J Comp Pathol. 2006;135:25–31.

40 Kellum HB, Stepien RL. Third-degree atrioventricular block in 21 cats (1997–2004). J Vet Intern Med. 2006;20:97–103.

41 Fox PR, Peterson ME, Broussard JD. Electrocardiographic and radiographic changes in cats with hyperthyroidism: comparison of populations evaluated during 1992–1993 vs. 1979–1982. J Am Anim Hosp Assoc. 1999;35:27–31.

42 Jung S, Jandrey KE. Hyperkalemia secondary to renal hypoperfusion in a dog with third-degree atrioventricular block. J Vet Emerg Crit Care. 2012;22:483–487.

43 Perego M, Skert S, Santilli RA. Analysis of the atrial repolarization wave in dogs with third-degree atrioventricular block. Am J Vet Res. 2014;75:54–58.

44 Ward JL, DeFrancesco TC, Tou SP, Atkins CE, Griffith EH, Keene BW. Complication rates associated with transvenous pacemaker implantation in dogs with high-grade atrioventricular block performed during versus after normal business hours. J Vet Intern Med. 2015;29:157–163.

45 Morimoto S-I, Kato S, Hiramitsu S, Uemura A, Ohtsuki M, Kato Y, *et al.* Role of myocardial interstitial edema in conduction disturbances in acute myocarditis. Heart Vessels. 2006;21:356–360.

46 Lu W, Yaoming N, Boli R, Jun C, Changhai Z, Yang Z, *et al.* mHCN4 genetically modified canine mesenchymal stem cells provide biological pacemaking function in complete dogs with atrioventricular block. Pacing Clin Electrophysiol. 36, 1138–1149 (2013).

47 Hou Y-B, Zou C-W, Wang Y, Li D-C, Li Q-B, Li H-X, *et al.* Establishing a new electrical conduction pathway by anastomosis of the right auricle and right ventricle assisted by mesenchymal stem cells in a canine model. Transplant Proc. 2011;43:3980–3986.

48 Spodick DH. Fascicular blocks: not interpretable from the electrocardiogram. Am J Cardiol. 1992;70:809–810.

49 Elizari MV, Acunzo RS, Ferreiro M. Hemiblocks revisited. Circulation. 2007;115:1154–1163.

50 Littmann L, Goldberg JR. Apparent bigeminy and pulsus alternans in intermittent left bundle-branch block. Clin Cardiol. 1999;22:490.

51 Littmann L, Symanski JD. Hemodynamic implications of left bundle branch block. J Electrocardiol. 2000;33(Suppl):115–121.

52 Watt TBJ, Pruitt RD. Cocaine-induced incomplete bundle branch block in dogs. Circ Res. 1964;15:234–239.

53 Watt TBJ, Freud GE, Durrer D, Pruitt RD. Left anterior arborization block combined with right bundle branch block in canine and primate hearts. An electrocardiographic study. Circ Res. 1968;22:57–63.

54 Tilley LP. Essentials of canine and feline electrocardiography. St. Louis: Mosby; 1995.

55 Bailey JC, Lathrop DA, Pippenger DL. Differences between proximal left and right bundle branch block action potential durations and refractoriness in the dog heart. Circ Res. 1977;40:464–468.

56 Moise S. Right bundle branch block in a dog with sinus tachycardia. J Am Vet Med Assoc. 1984;184:1458–1459.

57 Moore EN, Boineau JP, Patterson DF. Incomplete right bundle-branch block. An electrocardiographic enigma and possible misnomer. Circulation. 1971;44:678–687.

58 Tou SE, DeFrancesco TC, Keene BW. ECG of the month. Intermittent tachycardia-dependent left bundle branch block in a dog during anesthesia. J Am Vet Med Assoc. 2011;239:55–57.

59 Brownlie SE, Cobb MA. Observations on the development of congestive heart failure in Irish wolfhounds with dilated cardiomyopathy. J Small Anim Pract. 1999;40:371–377.

60 Rausch WP, Keene BW. ECG of the month: sinus tachycardia with left bundle branch block. J Am Vet Med Assoc. 2002;220:980–981.

61 Patterson DF. Congenital defects of the cardiovascular system of dogs: studies in comparative cardiology. Adv Vet Sci Comp Med. 1976;20:1–37.

62 Mauldin GE, Fox PR, Patnaik AK, Bond BR, Mooney SC, Matus RE. Doxorubicin-induced cardiotoxicosis: clinical features in 32 dogs. J Vet Intern Med. 1992;6:82–88.

63 el-Sherif N, Scherlag BJ, Lazzara R. Conduction disorders in the canine proximal His-Purkinje system following acute myocardial ischemia. II. The pathophysiology of bilateral bundle branch block. Circulation. 1974;49:848–857.

64 Liu SK, Tilley LP, Tashjian RJ. Lesions of the conduction system in the cat with cardiomyopathy. Recent Adv Stud Cardiac Struct Metab. 1975;10:681–693.

65 Tilley LP, Liu SK, Gilbertson SR, Wagner BM, Lord PF. Primary myocardial disease in the cat: a model for human cardiomyopathy. Am J Pathol. 1977;86:493–522.

66 Ferasin L, Sturgess CP, Cannon MJ, Caney SMA, Gruffydd-Jones TJ, Wotton PR. Feline idiopathic cardiomyopathy: a retrospective study of 106 cats (1994–2001). J Feline Med Surg. 2003;5:151–159.

67 Okuma K. ECG and VCG changes in experimental hemiblock and bifascicular block. Am Heart J. 1976;92:473–480.

68 James TN, Robertson BT, Waldo AL, Branch CE. De subitaneis mortibus. XV. Hereditary stenosis of the His bundle in Pug dogs. Circulation. 1975;52:1152–1160.

69 Toaldo MB, Critelli M, Santilli RA. ECG of the month. J Am Vet Med Assoc. 2011;239:438–440.

70 Billen F, Van Israel N. Syncope secondary to transient atrioventricular block in a German shepherd dog with dilated cardiomyopathy and atrial fibrillation. J Vet Cardiol. 2006;8:63–68.

71 el-Sherif N, Scherlag BJ, Lazzara R. Conduction disorders in the canine proximal His-Purkinje system following acute myocardial ischemia. I. The pathophysiology of intra-His bundle block. Circulation. 1974;49:837–847.

72 Chilson DA, Zipes DP, Heger JJ, Browne KF, Prystowsky EN. Functional bundle branch block: discordant response of right and left bundle branches to changes in heart rate. Am J Cardiol. 1984;54:313–316.

73 Shenasa M, Josephson ME, Wit AL. Paroxysmal atrioventricular block: electrophysiological mechanism of phase 4 conduction block in the His-Purkinje system: a comparison with phase 3 block. Pacing Clin Electrophysiol. 2017;40:1234–1241. doi:10.1111/pace.13187

74 Moore EN, Spear JF, Fisch C. 'Supernormal' conduction and excitability. J Cardiovasc Electrophysiol. 1993;4:320–337.

75 Ferrer MI. The sick sinus syndrome. Circulation. 1973;47:635–641.

76 Duhme N, Schweizer PA, Thomas D, Becker R, Schroter J, Barends TRM, et al. Altered HCN4 channel C-linker interaction is associated with familial tachycardia-bradycardia syndrome and atrial fibrillation. Eur Heart J. 2013;34:2768–2775.

77 Ki C-S, Jung CL, Kim H-J, Baek K-H, Park SJ, On YK, et al. A KCNQ1 mutation causes age-dependant bradycardia and persistent atrial fibrillation. Pflugers Arch. 2014;466:529–540.

78 Ishikawa T, Ohno S, Murakami T, Yoshida K, Mishima H, Fukuoka T, et al. Sick sinus syndrome with HCN4 mutations shows early onset and frequent association with atrial fibrillation and left ventricular noncompaction. Heart Rhythm. 2017;14:717–724.

79 Saunders AB. ECG of the month: sick sinus syndrome. J Am Vet Med Assoc. 2005;227:51–52.

80 Burrage H. Sick sinus syndrome in a dog: treatment with dual-chambered pacemaker implantation. Can Vet J. 2012;53:565–568.

81 Kavanagh K. Sick sinus syndrome in a bull terrier. Can Vet J. 2002;43:46–48.

82 Adan V, Crown LA. Diagnosis and treatment of sick sinus syndrome. Am Fam Physician. 2003;67:1725–1732.

83 Mangrum JM, DiMarco JP. The evaluation and management of bradycardia. N Engl J Med. 2000;342:703–709.

84 Monfredi O, Dobrzynski H, Mondal T, Boyett MR, Morris GM. The anatomy and physiology of the sinoatrial node: a contemporary review. Pacing Clin Electrophysiol. 2010;33:1392–1406.

85 Nakao S, Hirakawa A, Fukushima R, Kobayashi M, Machida N. The anatomical basis of bradycardia-tachycardia syndrome in elderly dogs with chronic degenerative valvular disease. J Comp Pathol. 2012;146:175–182.

86 Joung B, Chen P-S, Lin S-F. The role of the calcium and the voltage clocks in sinoatrial node dysfunction. Yonsei Med J. 2011;52:211–219.

87 Fabry-Delaigue R, Duchene-Marullaz P, Lemaire P, Chambon M. Long-term observation of cardiac rhythm and automaticity in the dog after excision of the sinoatrial node. J Electrocardiol. 1982;15:209–220.

88 Hamlin RL, Smetzer DL, Breznock EM. Sinoatrial syncope in Miniature Schnauzers. J Am Vet Med Assoc. 1972;161:1022–1028.

89 Gladuli A, Moïse NS, Hemsley SA, Otani NF. Poincaré plots and tachograms reveal beat patterning in sick sinus syndrome with supraventricular tachycardia and varying AV nodal block. J Vet Cardiol. 2011;13:63–70.

90 Li Y-C, Ge L-S, Guang X-Q, Chen P, Wu L-P, Yang P-L, *et al.* Establishment of a canine model of cardiac memory using endocardial pacing via internal jugular vein. BMC Cardiovasc Disord. 2010;10:30.

91 Moneva-Jordan A, Corcoran BM, French A, Dukes McEwan J, Martin MW, Luis-Fuentes V, *et al.* Sick sinus syndrome in nine West Highland white terriers. Vet Rec. 2001;148:142–147.

92 Rishniw M, Kittleson MD, Jaffe RS, Kass PH. Characterization of parasympatholytic chronotropic responses following intravenous administration of atropine to clinically normal dogs. Am J Vet Res. 1999;60:1000–1003.

93 Thomason JD, Fallaw TL, Calvert CA. ECG of the month: pacemaker implantation for sick sinus syndrome. J Am Vet Med Assoc. 2008;233:1406–1408.

94 Lou Q, Hansen BJ, Fedorenko O, Csepe TA, Kalyanasundaram A, Li N, *et al.* Upregulation of adenosine A1 receptors facilitates sinoatrial node dysfunction in chronic canine heart failure by exacerbating nodal conduction abnormalities revealed by novel dual-sided intramural optical mapping. Circulation. 2014;130:315–324.

95 Sisson D, Thomas WP, Woodfield J, Pion PD, Luethy M, DeLellis LA. Permanent transvenous pacemaker implantation in forty dogs. J Vet Intern Med. 1991;5:322–331.

96 DeFrancesco TC, Hansen BD, Atkins CE, Sidley JA, Keene BW. Noninvasive transthoracic temporary cardiac pacing in dogs. J Vet Intern Med. 2003;17:663–667.

97 Estrada AH, Pariaut R, Hemsley S, Gatson BH, Moise NS. Atrial-based pacing for sinus node dysfunction in dogs: initial results. J Vet Intern Med. 2012;26:558–564.

98 Hogan KM, Quinn RL. ECG of the month: third-degree AV block with sick sinus syndrome. J Am Vet Med Assoc. 2015;246:843–845.

99 Fu Q, Levine BD. Pathophysiology of neurally mediated syncope: role of cardiac output and total peripheral resistance. Auton Neurosci. 2014;184:24–26.

100 Porteiro Vázquez DM, Perego M, Santos L, Gerou-Ferriani M, Martin MWS, Santilli RA. Paroxysmal atrial fibrillation in seven dogs with presumed neurally-mediated syncope. J Vet Cardiol. 2016;18:1–9.

101 Hamlin RL, Smith CR. Effects of vagal stimulation on S-A and A-V nodes. Am J Physiol. 1968;215:560–568.

102 Liu L, Nattel S. Differing sympathetic and vagal effects on atrial fibrillation in dogs: role of refractoriness heterogeneity. Am J Physiol. 1997;273:H805–H816.

103 Patterson E, Lazzara R, Szabo B, Liu H, Tang D, Li Y-H, *et al.* Sodium-calcium exchange initiated by the Ca2+ transient: an arrhythmia trigger within pulmonary veins. J Am Coll Cardiol. 2006;47:1196–1206.

104 McMillan MW, Aprea F, Leece EA. Potential Bezold-Jarisch reflex secondary to a 180 degrees postural change in an anaesthetized dog. Vet Anaesth Analg. 2012;39:561–562.

105 Salo LM, Woods RL, Anderson CR, McAllen RM. Nonuniformity in the von Bezold-Jarisch reflex. Am J Physiol Regul Integr Comp Physiol. 2007;293:R714–R720.

106 Crystal GJ, Salem MR. The Bainbridge and the 'reverse' Bainbridge reflexes: history, physiology, and clinical relevance. Anesth Analg. 2012;114:520–532.

107 Kinsella SM, Tuckey JP. Perioperative bradycardia and asystole: relationship to vasovagal syncope and the Bezold-Jarisch reflex. Br J Anaesth. 2001;86:859–868.

108 Calvert CA, Jacobs GJ, Pickus CW. Bradycardia-associated episodic weakness, syncope, and aborted sudden death in cardiomyopathic Doberman Pinschers. J Vet Intern Med. 1996;10:88–93.

109 Moya A, Sutton R, Ammirati F, Blanc J-J, Brignole M, Dahm JB, *et al.* Guidelines for the diagnosis and management of syncope (version 2009). Eur Heart J. 2009;30:2631–2671.

110 McLeod KA. Dysautonomia and neurocardiogenic syncope. Curr Opin Cardiol. 2001;16:92–96.

111 Santilli RA, Battaia S, Perego M, Tursi M, Grego E, Marzufero C, *et al.* Bartonella-associated inflammatory cardiomyopathy in a dog. J Vet Cardiol. 2017;19:74–81.

112 Meininger GR, Nadasdy T, Hruban RH, Bollinger RC, Baughman KL, Hare JM. Chronic active myocarditis following acute Bartonella henselae infection (cat scratch disease). Am J Surg Pathol. 2001;25:1211–1214.

113 Davies JM. Molecular mimicry: can epitope mimicry induce autoimmune disease? Immunol Cell Biol. 1997;75:113–126.

114 Jeraj K, Ogburn PN, Edwards WD, Edwards JE. Atrial standstill, myocarditis and destruction of cardiac conduction system: clinicopathologic correlation in a dog. Am Heart J. 1980;99:185–192.

115 Thomason JD, Kraus MS, Fallaw TL, Calvert CA. Survival of 4 dogs with persistent atrial standstill treated by pacemaker implantation. Can Vet J. 2016;57:297–298.

116 Sicken J, Neiger R. Addisonian crisis and severe acidosis in a cat: a case of feline hypoadrenocorticism. J Feline Med Surg. 2013;15:941–944.

117 Penning VA, Connolly DJ, Gajanayake I, McMahon LA, Luis-Fuentes V, Chandler KE, *et al*. Seizure-like episodes in 3 cats with intermittent high-grade atrioventricular dysfunction. J Vet Intern Med. 2009;23:200–205.

118 Ferasin L, van de Stad M, Rudorf H, Langford K, Hotston MA. Syncope associated with paroxysmal atrioventricular block an ventricular standstill in a cat. J Small Anim Pract. 2002;43:124–128.

119 Forterre S, Nurnberg JH, Forterre F, Skrodzki M, Lange PE. Transvenous demand pacemaker treatment for intermittent complete heart block in a cat. J Vet Cardiol. 2001;3:21–26.

8

Atrial Rhythms
Pedro Oliveira

Introduction

In this chapter, we will discuss abnormal rhythms originating from atrial structures other than the sinus node and without involvement of the junctional area or ventricular structures. These include ectopic atrial beats and rhythms, atrial flutter and atrial fibrillation, although the latter is discussed in a dedicated chapter (chapter 9). Rhythms involving the junctional area are discussed in chapter 10.

Atrial Ectopic Beats (AEBs)

AEBs arise from atrial structures outside the sinus node. These may include the working atrial myocardium, the coronary sinus, the pulmonary veins, the venae cavae and the ligament (or vein) of Marshall.[1]

Depending on the origin of the ectopic focus, the direction of the atrial depolarisation wave will vary, and therefore the ectopic P' waves will be different from the normal P waves on the electrocardiogram (ECG). This helps distinguish ectopic beats from sinus beats, and determining the electrical axis of the ectopic P' waves provides a clue as to their likely origin in the atria (Box 8.1). It can be very useful when trying to distinguish between the different narrow-complex tachycardias as discussed in chapter 13.

Classification

An ectopic beat that occurs before the next expected sinus depolarisation is said to be *premature*.[2] The coupling interval between the premature beat and the preceding sinus beat (P-P' interval) is shorter than the interval between sinus beats (P-P interval) (Box 8.2). The terms *atrial premature complex* (APC), *atrial premature beat* (APB) and *atrial premature contraction* (APC) are often used to describe a premature ectopic atrial beat. Less commonly, *premature atrial contraction* (PAC) may also be used. The terms that are commonly mentioned in veterinary literature include *atrial premature contraction* or *complex* (APC), and this will be used throughout this book.

A premature beat may be followed by a pause that is characterized as non-compensatory or compensatory depending on whether the depolarisation resets the sinus node (Figures 8.2 and 8.3). If a pause is not present after the premature beat, it is described as an *interpolated beat* (Figure 8.4).

An ectopic beat that occurs after a sinus pause is described as an *escape beat*. The P-P' interval is longer than the sinus P-P. In this case, the ectopic focus 'fires' after the sinus node fails to do so, preventing cardiac arrest and effectively 'escaping' death. Most commonly, the ectopic beat originates from a subsidiary pacemaker in the junctional area (Figure 10.4) or the ventricles (Figure 11.7).

Ectopic beats can occur in an isolated fashion or may appear in more organized forms. Examples include *bigeminy*, in which a sequence of a normal beat followed by an ectopic beat is seen (Figure 8.5); a sequence of two normal beats followed by an ectopic beat is called *trigeminy* (see Figure 11.9), and a sequence of three normal beats followed by an ectopic beat is called *quadrigeminy*. A sequence of two consecutive ectopic beats is a *couplet* and of three consecutive beats is a *triplet* (Figures 8.6 and 8.7).

Atrial Ectopic Beats, Ventricular Activation and the PR Interval

When an ectopic beat fails to result in ventricular activation, it is described as *blocked* or *non-transmitted*. Depending on how premature an ectopic beat is, it may encounter the atrioventricular node (AVN) tissues in a

Guide to Canine and Feline Electrocardiography, First Edition. Ruth Willis, Pedro Oliveira and Antonia Mavropoulou.
© 2018 John Wiley & Sons Ltd. Published 2018 by John Wiley & Sons Ltd.
Companion website: www.wiley.com/go/willis/electrocardiography

Box 8.1 How to determine the origin of atrial ectopic beats

To estimate the origin of ectopic beats in the atria, one must examine the axis of the P' wave. See Figure 8.1.

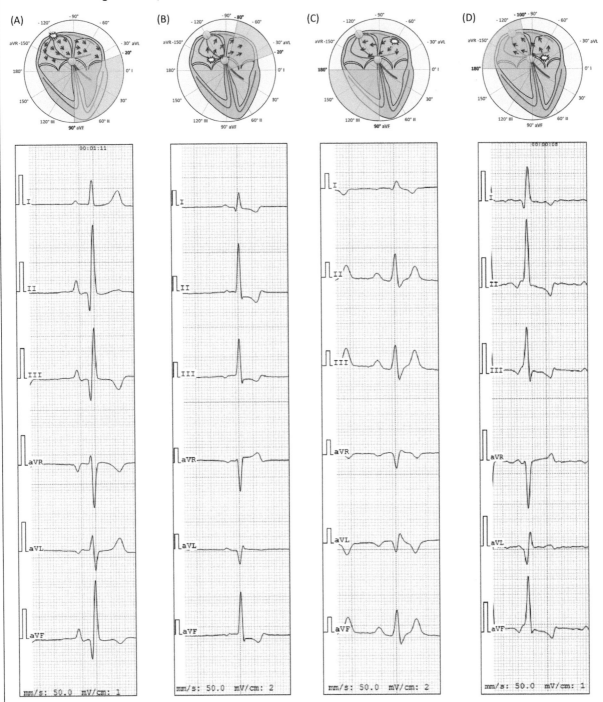

Figure 8.1 Different P' wave morphologies depending on the ectopic site location.

A) *Roof of right atrium*: P' electrical axis between −20 and +90° (in this example, +78°). The P' wave is positive in leads I, II, III and aVF, and negative in leads aVR and aVF as sinus P waves.

B) *Floor of right atrium*: P' electrical axis between −20 and −80° (in this example, −30°). The P' wave is positive in leads I, II and aVL, and negative in leads III, aVR and aVF.

C) *Roof of left atrium*: P' electrical axis between +90 and +180° (in this example, +109°). The P' wave is positive in leads II, III and aVF, and negative in leads I, aVR and aVL.

D) *Floor of left atrium*: P' electrical axis between −100 and +180° (in this case, −106°). The P' wave is negative in leads I, II, III and aVF, and positive in leads aVL and aVR.

Box 8.2 Interpolated beats, and compensatory and non-compensatory post-extrasystolic pauses

Atrial premature complex followed by a compensatory pause:

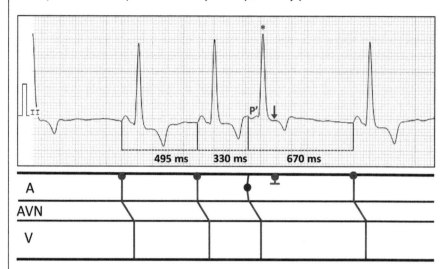

Figure 8.2 Atrial premature complex (*) followed by a compensatory pause. (50 mm/s; 5 mm/mV)

In Figure 8.2, the underlying rhythm was sinus with a cycle length (P-P) of 495 ms. In other words, the sinus node "fired" every 495 ms. Given that an ectopic beat (*) occurred, the atrial myocardium was still refractory when the next sinus beat was supposed to happen (arrow), and a pause is seen instead. The P-P' interval was 330 ms, and the pause lasted for 670 ms (P'-P). The sum of P-P' and P'-P is 1000 ms, which is approximately the same as twice the sinus cycle length (P-P). This suggests that after the premature beat, the sinus node still "fired" but was unable to result in atrial depolarisation as the myocardium was still refractory from the ectopic beat. Another cycle had to occur before the next sinus beat appeared on the electrocardiogram.

Atrial premature complex followed by a non-compensatory pause:

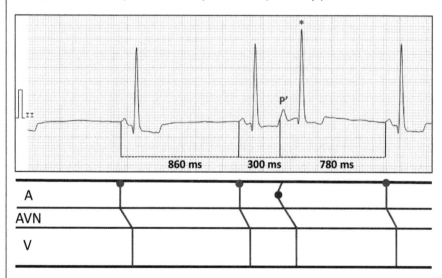

Figure 8.3 Atrial premature complex (*) followed by a non-compensatory pause. (50 mm/s; 5 mm/mV)

In Figure 8.3, the underlying rhythm was sinus with a cycle length (P-P) of 860 ms. The P-P' interval was 300 ms, and the pause lasted for 780 ms (P'-P). The sum of P-P' and P'-P was now less than a multiple of the cycle length P-P at 1080 ms. This suggests that the depolarisation wave created by the ectopic beat was able to depolarise the sinus node, thereby resetting it. As a result, the next sinus beat occurred sooner than in Figure 8.2.

Interpolated atrial premature complex:

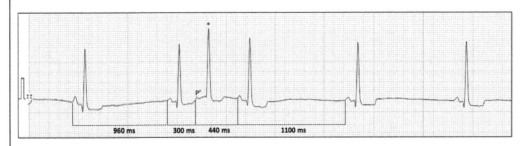

Figure 8.4 Interpolated atrial premature complex (*). (50 mm/s; 5 mm/mV)

In Figure 8.4, the underlying rhythm was sinus with a variable cycle length (P-P) due to respiratory sinus arrhythmia. The third beat was an ectopic atrial beat but was not followed by a pause, which implies that it did not interfere with either the AVN and or sinus node activities. This was an interpolated beat.

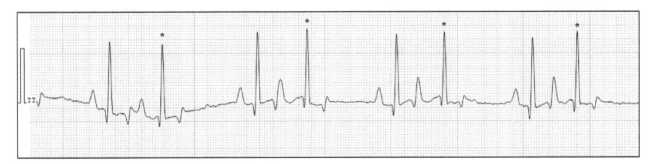

Figure 8.5 Atrial bigeminy. The * highlights the premature beats which alternate with the sinus beats. [6-year-old, female neutered, crossbreed dog without obvious structural heart disease] (50 mm/s; 10 mm/mV)

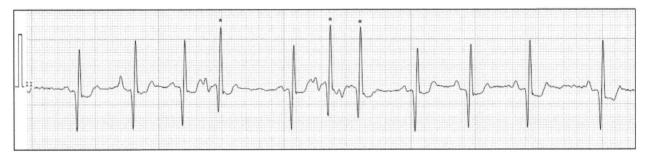

Figure 8.6 Atrial couplet – two consecutive atrial ectopic beats (*). [10-year-old, male Giant Schnauzer with lymphoma and no obvious structural heart disease]

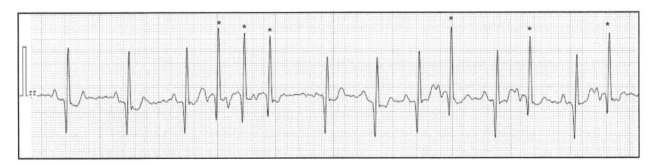

Figure 8.7 Atrial triplet – three consecutive atrial ectopic beats (*). [10-year-old, male Giant Schnauzer with lymphoma and no obvious structural heart disease] (50 mm/s; 10 mm/mV)

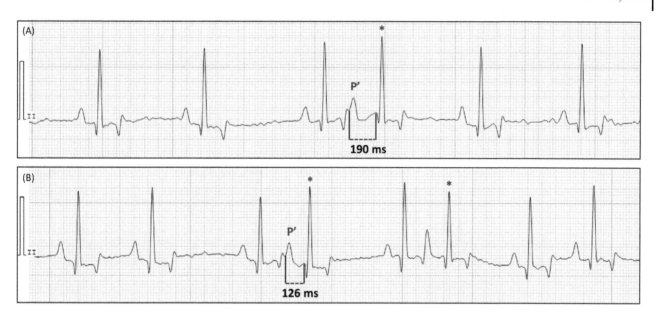

Figure 8.8 Blocked atrial premature contraction. (A) Ectopic atrial beat (*) with a prolonged P'Q attributed to slower conduction through the atrioventricular node. (B) Example of an ectopic atrial beat from the same patient without prolonged P'R. [6-year-old, female neutered, crossbreed dog without obvious structural heart disease] (50 mm/s; 10 mm/mV)

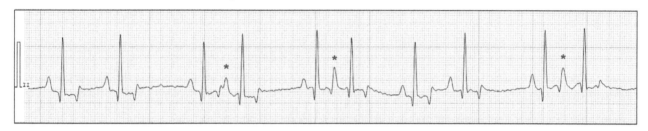

Figure 8.9 Example of a 'hidden' P' wave (6-lead trace available online). The fourth, sixth and tenth beats are ectopic, originating from the roof of the right atrium. The P' wave of the sixth and tenth beats is superimposed on the T wave, resulting in an increase in amplitude in comparison to the T wave conformation of the normal beats. [6-year-old, female neutered, crossbreed dog without obvious structural heart disease] (50 mm/s; 10 mm/mV)

state of refractoriness that prevents them from being conducted to the ventricles. Alternatively, conduction may be slower than normal (Wenckebach periodicity) in cases of AVN relative refractoriness resulting in a prolonged P'R (Figure 8.8).

'Hidden' Atrial Ectopic Beats

The diagnosis of an AEB relies on the identification of a P' wave on the ECG. However, the P' wave may overlap another wave or complex, commonly the T wave of the preceding beat. This is particularly common when the ectopic focus is located in the pulmonary veins on the roof of the left atrium.[3,4] Close analysis of the T wave conformation of the beat preceding a premature beat is essential when trying to identify differences, such as an increase in amplitude or different morphology (e.g. double hump or biphasic), that might suggest the presence of an ectopic P' (Figure 8.9).

Ectopic Atrial Rhythms

If more than three consecutive ectopic beats occur, this is described as an atrial rhythm or tachycardia depending on the heart rate (Figures 8.10 and 8.13). In humans, an ectopic atrial rhythm is considered tachycardia if the rate is above 100 bpm.[2] In our patients, this has not been well described, but most would consider a rate above 140–160 bpm as tachycardia.

Distinguishing an ectopic atrial rhythm from a sinus rhythm can be quite challenging, particularly if it originates from the roof of the right atrium. Variations of the P' wave morphology and electrical axis in comparison to the sinus P as well as variations of the PR interval are valuable clues. The PR interval may be within the normal range or slightly longer or shorter than normal, depending on the location of the ectopic focus. The further away it is from the AVN, the longer the PR interval and vice versa.

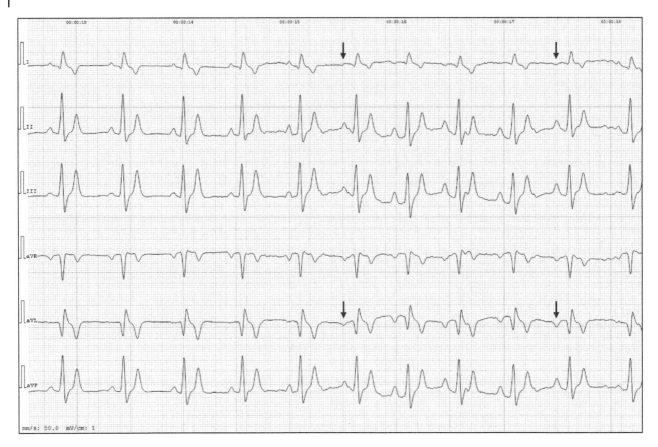

Figure 8.10 Ectopic atrial rhythm. The first five beats are sinus in origin (P axis of +64°) with a heart rate of approximately 100 bpm and a regular rhythm. From beat 6 to beat 10, there is an ectopic atrial rhythm originating from the roof of the left atrium (P′ axis of +127°) with a heart rate of approximately 120 bpm and a regular rhythm. The change in P wave morphology is most obvious in leads I and aVL (arrows). [8-year-old, female neutered, Great Dane with dilated cardiomyopathy] (50 mm/s; 10 mm/mV)

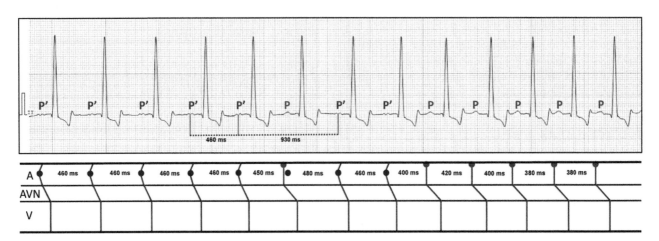

Figure 8.11 Atrial parasystole. A concomitant ectopic atrial rhythm (P′ and red dot on laddergram) and sinus rhythm (P and black dot on laddergram) can be seen. As illustrated on the laddergram, the cycle length of the ectopic rhythm (P′-P′) is approximately 460 ms; when it is interrupted by a sinus beat (beat 6), the following ectopic beat occurs at an interval of 930 ms which is approximately double 460 ms. This suggests that the sinus depolarisation did not reset the ectopic focus (entrance block) and that it continued to discharge at the same rate. This is a feature of atrial parasystole in which the P′-P′ interval is a multiple of a common denominator that is the discharge rate of the ectopic focus. [11-year-old, male Gordon Setter with suspicion of inflammatory myocardial disease] (50 mm/s; 10 mm/mV)

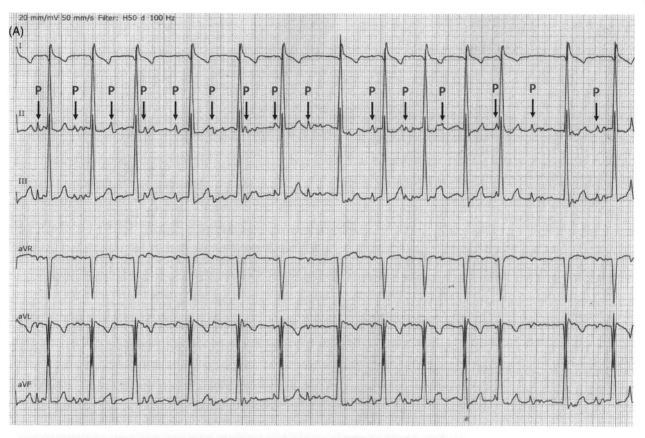

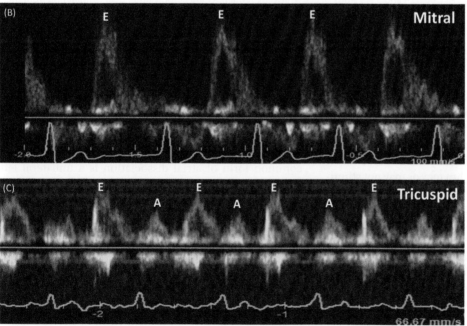

Figure 8.12 Atrial dissociation. (A) Electrocardiographic trace showing a narrow-QRS tachycardia with an irregular rhythm and a ventricular rate of approximately 140–160 bpm. Waves consistent with P waves may be seen (P) and appear dissociated from the QRS complexes. The atrial depolarisation rate is approximately 200 bpm. Additional small undulations of the baseline may be seen. (B) Echocardiographic pulsed-wave Doppler image showing the mitral inflow pattern in the same patient. Passive early diastolic flow (E waves) from the left atrium to the left ventricle may be seen, but flow resulting from atrial contraction (A waves) is not present in contrast to the tricuspid flow pattern from the same patient shown in (C), where both early diastolic filling (E waves) and flow resulting from organised atrial contraction (A waves) may be seen. These findings suggest the presence of a disorganized atrial rhythm (atrial fibrillation) at the level of the left atrium, whilst an organized rhythm (sinus or ectopic rhythm) is present on the right atrium as a result of atrial dissociation. [7-year-old, male neutered, Newfoundland dog referred for investigation of cardiac arrhythmia without evidence of structural heart disease] *Source*: Courtesy of Julia Sargent, Royal Veterinary College, London.

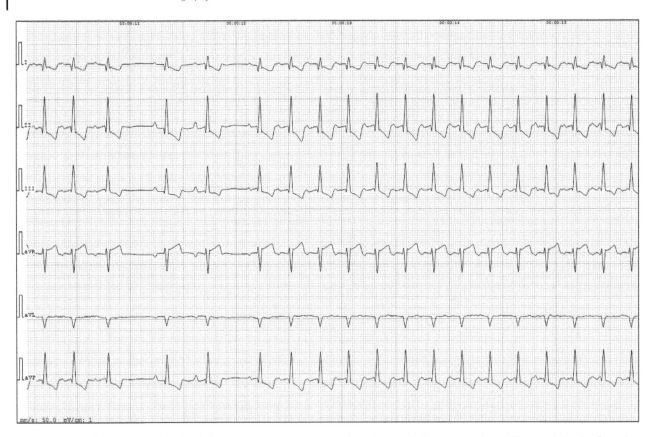

Figure 8.13 Focal atrial tachycardia (FAT). Beats 4 and 5 are sinus beats, whilst the remainder are ectopic atrial beats originating from the floor of the right atrium (P' axis of +30° and PR of 100–120 ms). From the sixth beat, an episode of FAT starts with a rate of 220 bpm. From beats 8 to 14, the P wave appears superimposed on the T wave. [10-year-old, male Border Terrier without obvious structural heart disease]. (50 mm/s; 10 mm/mV)

Atrial Parasystole

An ectopic atrial rhythm may coexist with the sinus rhythm if the sinus depolarisation wave is unable to depolarise the myocardium around the ectopic focus and effectively suppress it. This phenomenon is described as *entrance block*, and the resulting rhythm is called *atrial parasystole*.[5–8] The ectopic rhythm may or may not stimulate the surrounding area of myocardium, depending on whether it happens to be in an excitable or refractory state. On the ECG, ectopic P' waves are seen amidst normal P waves with a P'-P' interval that is a multiple of a common denominator (the ectopic discharge rate) (Figure 8.11). Additionally, the entrance block may be complete or incomplete. With complete entrance block, the ectopic focus is never influenced by the sinus depolarisation wave and discharges at a fixed rate – *fixed parasystole*. With incomplete entrance block, the sinus depolarisation wave may interfere transiently with the ectopic focus, altering its discharge rate – *modulated parasystole*.[9–11]

Atrial Dissociation

Rarely, an ectopic focus and surrounding myocardium may be completely isolated due to concomitant *entrance and exit block* resulting in *atrial dissociation* (Figure 8.12).[12–14] In this instance, the ectopic atrial rhythm does not result in ventricular depolarisation, nor does it interfere with the sinus rhythm. The ectopic P' waves are seen in the background amidst the underlying rhythm without influencing the P-P and R-R. The most common form of atrial dissociation is a unilateral left atrial rhythm with an underlying sinus rhythm. However, unilateral tachycardia, flutter and fibrillation have also been described.[15]

Atrial Tachycardia

Atrial tachycardia refers to an ectopic atrial rhythm that has an elevated heart rate (usually >200 bpm). It is caused by rapid depolarisation of an ectopic focus in the atrial myocardium or venous structures (e.g. vena cavae, pulmonary veins and coronary sinus).[16,17] The terms *focal atrial tachycardia* (FAT) or *multifocal atrial tachycardias* are used depending on whether one or multiple foci are present. These foci are normally located at or near well-defined anatomical areas such as the terminal crest, the interatrial septum, the triangle of

Koch, the coronary sinus, the right or left auricular appendages, the ligament of Marshall and pulmonary veins.[16,18] In both people and dogs, the ectopic focus seems to be more commonly located in the right atrium (63%) in contrast to the left atrium (37%).[18,19] The terminal crest, tricuspid annulus, coronary sinus on the right atrium, and ostia of the pulmonary veins on the left atrium are the most common sites for ectopic foci in both humans and dogs.[18,20] Possible arrhythmia mechanisms include abnormal automaticity, triggered activity or micro re-entry. In a group of dogs, abnormal automaticity was identified as the underlying mechanism for the majority of cases.[18] Atrial tachycardia may occur in the absence of cardiac structural abnormalities, or it may be secondary to acquired or congenital defects, myocarditis, neoplastic infiltration, cardiac surgery, anti-arrhythmic drugs (e.g. digitalis intoxication), hyperthyroidism, general anaesthesia and electrolyte imbalances (e.g. hypokalaemia).[1]

Electrocardiographic features

Atrial tachycardia has the same features as an ectopic atrial rhythm but with a higher heart rate which in dogs often may range from 210 to 340 bpm (Figure 8.13).[21] In cats it has not been well described, but an ectopic atrial rhythm with a rate above 200 bpm could reasonably be termed atrial tachycardia. A ventricular rate above 300–400 bpm has been reported in cats with paroxysmal supraventricular tachycardia.[22,23] However, without endocardial mapping, the exact underlying mechanism could not be confirmed, and other supraventricular tachyarrhythmias (e.g. AVRT and atrial flutter) could be present in these cases.

Rhythm

Rhythm is generally regular; however, a gradual increase (warm-up) and decrease (cool-down) in heart rate may be seen during onset and offset of tachycardia, respectively.[1,24] This is due to a progressive increase and decrease of the discharge rate of the ectopic focus and suggests that the underlying mechanism is abnormal automaticity or triggered activity. Similarly, a variation of the cycle length (R-R interval) of over 20 ms may be caused by oscillations of the discharge rate of the ectopic focus and changes in AVN conduction velocity (block and conduction via the fast and slow pathways). With micro re-entry, a constant discharge rate and sudden onset and offset are expected.

Ectopic P'

The ectopic P' wave is different from the sinus P as discussed in this chapter, and its morphology will depend on the location of the ectopic focus. In the majority of

cases reported in dogs, the P' wave had a dorsoventral (supero-inferior) axis, suggesting a location in the roof of the left or right atrium (positive in leads II, III and aVF).[18,19] If the ectopic focus is located in the crista terminalis, the ectopic P' will be similar to the sinus P and therefore difficult to distinguish from inappropriate sinus tachycardia (see chapter 5). Unfortunately, the identification of P' waves during tachycardia may be challenging, as at higher heart rates they are often superimposed on the T wave of the previous complex. A comparison of the electrocardiographic waves and segments in sinus rhythm and tachycardia is essential for this purpose. If an electrocardiographic recording during sinus rhythm is not available due to sustained tachycardia, a precordial thump may be attempted to temporarily interrupt the tachycardia, allowing documentation of one or two sinus beats (see chapter 13).[21]

P'R

The P'R interval is normal or prolonged, and the P' wave is normally seen closer to the following QRS complex than the preceding QRS (RP' is longer than P'R; RP'/P'R > 0.7).[18,25] At higher rates, the P' may overlap the T wave of the preceding complex (Figure 8.13). Atrioventricular conduction is normal (1:1) or with second-degree atrioventricular block Wenckebach type.

QRS

Given that this is an atrial rhythm, the QRS complex is expected to be similar to the QRS of the sinus beats. Normally, it is normal in both appearance and duration (<70 ms in dogs and <40 ms in cats) unless aberrancy or bundle branch block is present. QRS alternans has been reported in approximately 33% of dogs with this arrhythmia.[21]

Clinical Presentations

The clinical presentation depends on the duration and rate of tachycardia. Brief episodes of tachycardia may not result in referable clinical signs and may be well tolerated. Sustained or incessant tachycardia may result in tachycardia-induced cardiomyopathy and congestive heart failure, or episodes of weakness and syncope. A retrospective study in 65 dogs with supraventricular tachycardia reported that the most common complaint was syncope (30%), followed by laboured breathing (23%), cough (21%), exercise intolerance (14%), vomiting (14%), ascites (12%) and weakness (11%).[26] Fifteen (23%) dogs were asymptomatic. In the author's experience, subtle signs such as panting and lethargy are commonly observed in patients with sustained or incessant tachycardias before syncope or congestive heart failure occurs. Unfortunately, these signs are often missed by the carer/owner.

Ectopic atrial tachycardia	
Rate	Dog: 210–340 bpm
	Cat: unknown; likely >200 bpm
Regularity	Regular. Up to 20% RR variability.
Onset and offset	Sudden or gradual increase (warm-up) and decrease (cool-down) in heart rate
P' wave	Ectopic P' with variable morphology
P':QRS ratio	1:1, AV block can occur
P'R and R'P	P'R normal or prolonged
	R'P/P'R > 0.7
QRS	Normal

Treatment

The ideal treatment strategy for ectopic atrial tachycardia would be suppression (or destruction) of the ectopic focus, effectively preventing it from occurring. However, this often proves difficult, and heart rate control may be a more realistic goal for most patients.

Medical Treatment

Emergency Treatment

For unstable patients presented in cardiogenic shock due to marked tachycardia, heart rate control should be the priority. Fast-acting drugs that delay atrioventricular conduction are preferred such as calcium channel blockers (e.g. intravenous diltiazem or verapamil) or less commonly β-blockers (e.g. intravenous esmolol). Systolic function should be assessed before using these drugs, particularly β-blockers, as hypotension and congestive heart failure are possible complications. If the patient is relatively stable or intravenous drugs are not available, oral medication may also be used with the disadvantage that the effects are not immediate. Intravenous procainamide may also be successful for conversion to a sinus rhythm. In the author's experience, oral sotalol or diltiazem act relatively quickly (30 min–3 h) in these cases and may be used safely, providing that there is no underlying structural cardiac disease.

Long-term Treatment

Maintenance of sinus rhythm may be achieved with class III anti-arrhythmics (sotalol or amiodarone), but recurrence seems to be common in many patients. Combination therapy may be necessary to ensure effective rate control. The following is an example of treatment options that may be used in these cases:

1) Sotalol (1–3 mg/kg q12h) *or* diltiazem (1–3 mg/kg q8–12h)
2) Sotalol combined with mexiletine (especially if a response to lidocaine is seen)
3) Sotalol combined with diltiazem (care with bradycardia and risk of death)

4) Amiodarone (side effects with long-term treatment)
5) Flecainide (risk of ventricular arrhythmias).

Electrical Cardioversion

Electrical cardioversion is effective in resetting the ectopic focus and restoring sinus rhythm. However, recurrence is very common, making this option undesirable. It is normally reserved for unstable patients that do not respond to medical treatment as a temporary measure before a more definitive option can be achieved (e.g. radiocatheter ablation).

Radiocatheter Ablation

Radiocatheter ablation provides a definitive solution for ectopic atrial tachycardia without the need for further treatment. It is the preferred treatment method in humans with ectopic atrial tachycardia. After the location of the ectopic focus is known from an electrophysiology study and mapping, it is destroyed with catheter ablation. More information on radiocatheter ablation of ectopic atrial tachycardia can be found in chapter 19.

Monitoring

Effective monitoring in these patients requires periodic Holter recordings, ideally every 6 months. The aim of medical therapy is to achieve acceptable control of ventricular rate (e.g. 24h mean heart rate of <110 bpm/24h; <140 bpm/24h for some cardiologists) or ideally complete suppression of the arrhythmia, although this is often not possible. It is particularly important that a 24h Holter recording be obtained 10–20 days after any treatment change as this is the only reliable way to assess its efficacy. Echocardiography should also be used as necessary to assess for structural changes and underlying disease if present.

Multifocal Atrial Tachycardia

Multifocal atrial tachycardia is caused by the presence of multiple ectopic atrial foci causing irregular atrial activation. This is an uncommon rhythm disturbance normally associated with significant atrial structural disease secondary to cardiac or chronic pulmonary disease and, less commonly, digoxin intoxication, acid–base and electrolytic abnormalities.[27–29] In fact, some authors argue that a distinction should be made between multifocal atrial tachycardia and multiple focal atrial tachycardias.[20] The latter refers to the presence of more than one ectopic focus of atrial tachycardia in the same patient, whereas multifocal atrial tachycardia represents a continuously changing site of focal triggering most usually seen in human patients with severe lung disease and reportedly caused by delayed afterdepolarisations potentiated by

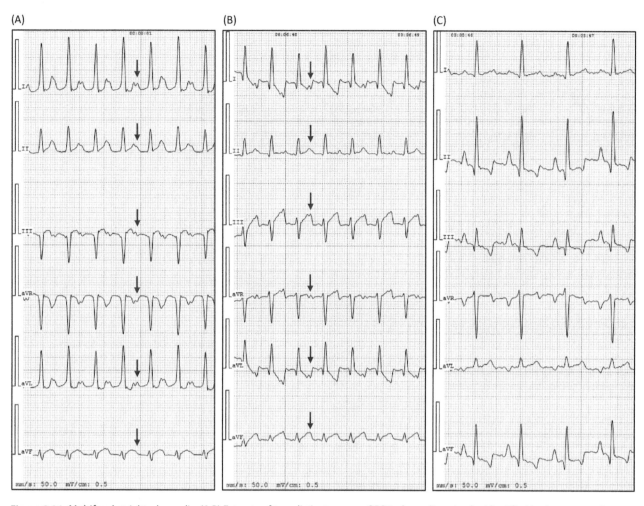

Figure 8.14 Multifocal atrial tachycardia. (A,B) Extracts of two distinct narrow-QRS tachycardia episodes identified in the same patient. The P′ wave (arrows) conformations are different, as is the cycle length of tachycardia: 220–240 ms in (A) and 200–220 ms in (B). (C) An extract of sinus rhythm of the same patient for comparison. An electrophysiology study confirmed the presence of three distinct ectopic foci along the terminal crest. [6-year-old, male Hamilton Hound without obvious structural heart disease] (50 mm/s; 20 mm/mV)

adrenergic stimulation.[20,28] According to this classification, the electrocardiographic findings with multiple focal atrial tachycardias are similar to those with focal atrial tachycardia but with at least two distinct atrial foci of sustained tachycardia (different P′) (Figure 8.14). With multifocal atrial tachycardia, at least three morphologically distinct P waves should be identified, with irregular P-P intervals and an isoelectric baseline between them.[27,29] In veterinary medicine, information is lacking in regard to these rhythm disturbances, particularly since diagnosis based on electrocardiographic findings alone is challenging.

Atrial Flutter

Atrial flutter refers to a very rapid atrial tachycardia caused by the presence of a macro re-entrant circuit in the atrial wall (Figure 8.15).[30] Its first description dates

back to 1886, when John McWilliam observed very rapid atrial activation during experiments in hearts of several animals, including dogs and cats.[31] Subsequently, the electrocardiographic findings of this arrhythmia were documented, featuring characteristic 'sawtooth' waves in the surface ECG (Figure 8.16).[32,33]

Some Considerations on Classification

For a long time, the term *atrial flutter* was used to describe any regular atrial tachycardia with a heart rate above 240 bpm and the absence of an isoelectric baseline in at least one lead.[34] The possible underlying mechanism was not taken into account, even though it had already been shown that this specific arrhythmia was caused by atrial macro re-entry from experiments in dogs since 1921.[35] More recently, with the widespread use of electrophysiology studies in human medicine, the

Typical flutter

Reverse typical flutter

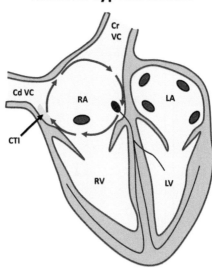

Figure 8.15 Cavotricuspid isthmus–dependent atrial flutter. The depolarisation wave travels in a loop around the atrial septum, the lateral wall of the right atrium and the tricuspid annulus. It traverses an area of slower conduction between the ostium of the caudal vena cava, the Eustachian ridge and the tricuspid annulus termed the *cavotricuspid isthmus* (CTI). Most commonly, the direction of travel is counterclockwise – *typical flutter* – although it may also occur in a clockwise fashion – *reverse typical flutter*. RA, Right atrium; LA, left atrium; RV, right ventricle; LV, left ventricle; Cd VC, caudal vena cava; Cr VC, cranial vena cava; CTI, cavotricuspid isthmus.

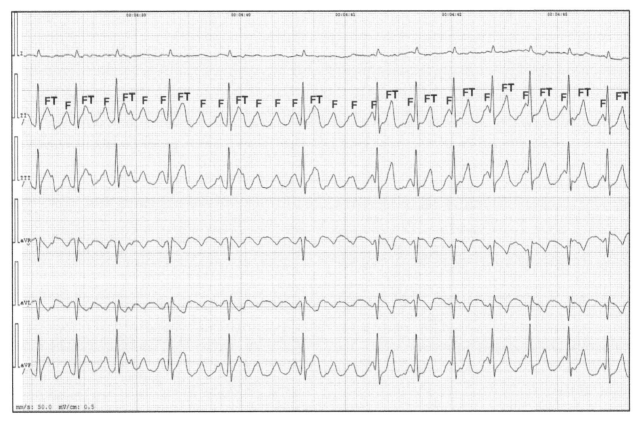

Figure 8.16 Typical atrial flutter. Flutter waves (F) can be seen in a characteristic sawtooth pattern. After each QRS, an F wave is superimposed with a T wave (T), causing small variations in its appearance. [9-year-old, female Bernese Mountain dog without obvious structural heart disease] (50 mm/s; 20 mm/mV)

classification of atrial tachycardias evolved to include their corresponding mechanisms. The current recommendations suggest a distinction between *macro re-entrant atrial tachycardias* (atrial flutter and other recognized atrial macro re-entrant circuits) and *focal atrial tachycardia* for arrhythmias caused by micro re-entry, abnormal automaticity or triggered activity.[1,17] The obvious disadvantage of this classification is that an electrophysiology study is necessary to confirm the arrhythmia mechanism, and this is not readily available to our patients. In 1979, Wells and colleagues distinguished two types of flutter: type I (typical) and type II (atypical) atrial flutter.[36] This was based on the baseline heart rate (>350 bpm in type II), stable intracardiac ECG rate and baseline, and whether it could be transiently entrained with pacing (type I) or not (type II) during an electrophysiology study. This classification was widely accepted, and some still refer to atrial flutter as Wells type I or II. However, most macro re-entrant atrial tachycardias and atrial flutters fit the description of Wells type I flutter, and therefore this classification is not useful to specify the exact location of the macro re-entry circuit.[17] Current recommendations suggest a division into *typical* or *atypical flutter*.

Typical Atrial Flutter

This is the most common type of atrial flutter with the re-entrant circuit being located in the right atrium. The depolarisation wave travels in a loop, most commonly in a counterclockwise direction, up the atrial septum and down the lateral wall of the right atrium between the terminal crest caudally and the tricuspid annulus cranially to enter an area of slower conduction between the ostium of the caudal vena cava, the Eustachian ridge and the tricuspid annulus termed the *cavotricuspid isthmus* (CTI) (Figure 8.15).[17,37] For this reason, it is also called *cavotricuspid isthmus–dependent atrial flutter*. The CTI has been identified as the slow conduction area of the circuit accounting for approximately 30% of the cycle length.[38] The depolarisation wave may also travel in a clockwise manner, in which case the term *reverse typical atrial flutter* is used.

Atypical Atrial Flutter

In atypical atrial flutter, the re-entrant circuit may be present in the right or left atrium but differs from the typical circuit described in the 'Typical atrial flutter' subsection. In humans, it most commonly occurs following cardiac surgery that leads to formation of areas of myocardial fibrosis around which re-entry can occur.[39] In dogs, atypical atrial flutter was reported in five dogs with two distinct isthmic areas in the right atrium: one at the level of the right septal wall, and another in the right atrial free wall.[40] To the best of our knowledge, this type of atrial flutter has not been described in cats.

Other Atrial Macro Re-entrant Tachycardias

In humans, other macro re-entrant atrial tachycardias have been described in both the right and left atria that do not involve the CTI and that are not due to scarring of the myocardium.[17,38,41] Additionally, other circuits that involve the CTI have also been described which could be considered as unusual forms of typical atrial flutter: (1) a 'lower loop' with a counterclockwise circuit around the inferior vena cava, and (2) and a 'double wave' in which two wavefronts briefly circulate in the same re-entrant circuit of flutter.[17,42–44] To the best of our knowledge, these have not been identified in our patients to date.

Atrial Fibrillo-flutter (fibrillatory conduction)

Occasionally, atrial depolarisation waves suggestive of atypical flutter are seen on electrocardiographic recordings that, when examined closely, display irregularities in frequency and morphology more consistent with atrial fibrillation (Figure 8.18). The terms *atrial fibrillo-flutter* and *fibrillatory conduction* have been used to describe these findings.[17,38] Multiple endocardial recordings have shown localized areas of relatively organized activation sequences with simultaneous irregular activation patterns in other areas of the atrial myocardium.[17,45] These findings also prompted the use of the term *focal atrial fibrillation*.[17] Progression to atrial fibrillation seems to be common in these cases, although reorganization back to atrial flutter is also observed.

Electrocardiographic Features of Atrial Flutter

Atrial flutter is characterized by an atrial rate between 300 and 600 bpm and a ventricular rate between 180 and 350 bpm in dogs.[46–50] P waves are replaced by flutter (F) waves that represent the cyclic atrial activation loop, and normal-looking QRS complexes are normally seen.

Flutter (F) Waves

In typical atrial flutter, an inverted sawtooth F-wave pattern is seen in leads II, III and aVF, with low-amplitude F waves in leads I and aVL (Figure 8.16).[37] This is characteristic of typical atrial flutter, and a unique feature of this pattern is that there is never a return to baseline.[17] In contrast, the F wave pattern observed in typical reversed atrial flutter is less specific and variable with a positive deflection in leads II, III and aVF and a return to baseline (Figure 8.17).[37,51] The determinants of the F wave pattern are largely determined by the activation of the left atrium as a result of re-entry in the right atrium. In typical atrial flutter, the left atrial activation occurs initially via the inferior interatrial pathway (coronary sinus musculature), whilst in reversed typical atrial flutter it occurs via Bachman's bundle. Given that the re-entry mechanism is the same in both forms of atrial flutter, the cycle length and resulting heart rates are normally similar.

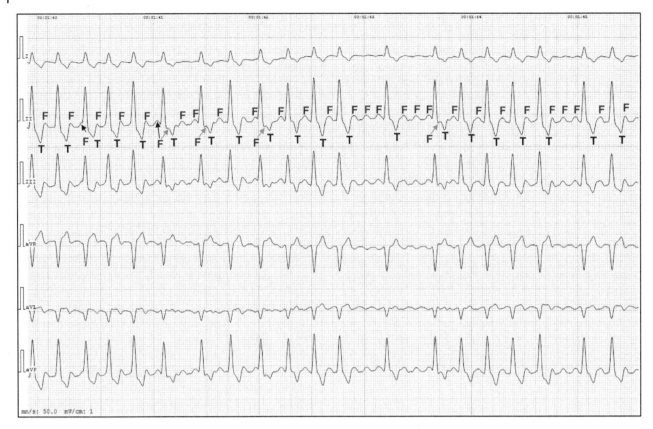

Figure 8.17 Reverse typical atrial flutter. Flutter waves (F) can be seen with the appearance of a sine wave and a return to baseline. After each QRS, an F wave occurs superimposed with a T wave (T) appearing as a small positive deflection in lead II, although in some areas the real appearance of the T wave is disclosed by separation of the two waves. [10-year-old, male neutered, Bull Terrier with mitral valve dysplasia] (50 mm/s; 10 mm/mV)

It is important to note that the typical F wave pattern depends on the sequence of activation of the left atrium and function of the interatrial pathways.[52,53] Neither the rate nor absence of isoelectric baseline should be considered specific to typical atrial flutter, as it can occur with other tachycardias.[17]

Rhythm

Since atrial flutter is due to re-entry via a fixed circuit, the rate of atrial depolarisation is constant. In other words, the atrial rate is fixed and regular. The ventricular rhythm, on the contrary, may be either regular or irregular depending on whether the atrioventricular conduction remains constant.[38] Commonly, a 2:1 conduction ratio is seen, although it may vary from 1:1 to 6:1 and variations of the atrioventricular conduction ratio may be seen in the same patient (Figures 8.17 and 8.19). This is influenced by concealed conduction in the AVN in which a 'blocked' atrial impulse delays conduction of the following beat. On the ECG, this can be seen as variation in the distance between the F waves

and the resulting QRS (Figure 8.16). Conduction ratios that are even (2:1, 4:1, 6:1) are more common than odd ratios (3:1, 5:1), and a 1:1 conduction is uncommon. It may occur with lower atrial rates, a short AVN refractory period or the presence of an accessory pathway (Figure 8.19).

The atrioventricular conduction ratio will determine the ventricular rate, which in dogs is often between 180 and 350 bpm.

QRS

Given that this is an atrial rhythm, the QRS complex is expected to be normal in both appearance and duration (<70 ms in dogs and <40 ms in cats). Exceptions include pre-existing aberrancy, bundle branch block or ventricular pre-excitation. Tachycardia-dependent aberrancy (see chapter 7) may occur during elevated heart rates in cases with 1:1 AV conduction. Isolated aberrancy may also occur during atrioventricular conduction ratio changes (e.g. 4:1 to 2:1) that result in a long RR–short RR change (Ashman phenomenon).

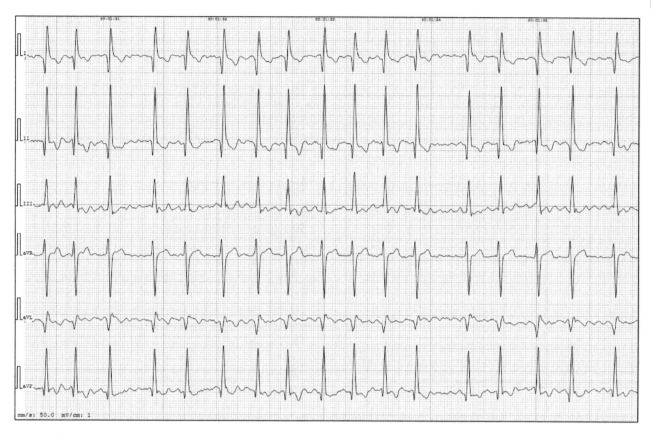

Figure 8.18 Atrial fibrillo-flutter or fibrillatory conduction. A narrow-QRS tachycardia can be seen with an irregular rhythm and a rate of approximately 200 bpm. P waves are not discernible, and instead undulations of the baseline can be seen suggestive of atrial depolarisation waves; in leads III and aVL, these waves seem relatively organised and have an appearance suggestive of flutter waves, but closer analyses reveal that their cycle length is not constant and that this is indeed atrial fibrillation. [13-year-old, male neutered, Cocker Spaniel with chronic valvular degenerative disease] (50 mm/s; 10 mm/mV)

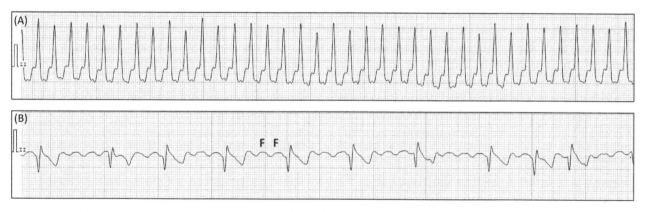

Figure 8.19 (A) Atrial flutter with 1:1 conduction. Narrow-QRS complex tachycardia with a heart rate of 425 bpm. (B) After treatment with intravenous verapamil, flutter waves (F) are now visible with a change in atrioventricular conduction ratio to 3:1 and 4:1, resulting in a heart rate of 120–130 bpm. The flutter rate (F-F interval) remains at 425 bpm [12-year-old, male neutered, Irish Setter without obvious structural heart disease]. (50 mm/s; 5 mm/mV)

Clinical Presentation

In the author's experience, Holter monitoring in patients with atrial flutter often reveals paroxysms of sustained (>30 s) or incessant (>12 h) atrial flutter alternating with periods of sinus rhythm. Periods of change between atrial flutter and atrial fibrillation may also be seen. Depending on the ventricular rate and duration of tachycardia, the clinical signs may range from lethargy, weakness or syncope to signs of congestive heart failure due to tachycardia-induced cardiomyopathy or underlying structural disease.

Atrial flutter	
Rate	Dog: 180 to >300 bpm Cat: unknown
Regularity	Regular or irregular
Onset/offset	Sudden
F wave	Sawtooth pattern in typical atrial flutter without return to baseline Sine-wave pattern in reverse typical atrial flutter with return to baseline
F:QRS ratio	1:1 to 6:1
QRS	Normal

Treatment

Treatment strategies for atrial flutter are aimed at controlling the ventricular response during flutter or restoring and maintaining sinus rhythm.

Medical Treatment

Heart rate control may be achieved with drugs that delay atrioventricular conduction such as calcium channel blockers (e.g. diltiazem), β-blockers (e.g. propranolol, atenolol and metoprolol) or class III anti-arrhythmic drugs (amiodarone and sotalol). The latter may also result in a return to sinus rhythm, as they influence atrial myocardial conduction velocity by effectively interfering with the re-entry circuit.[54,55] This can also occur with class I anti-arrhythmics (e.g. procainamide, flecainide and propafenone) through an increase in atrial refractoriness.[55,56] In the author's experience, sotalol provides good results in most patients at dosages of up to 3 mg/kg every 12 h. In patients with systolic dysfunction, lower doses may be used (1 mg/kg), but if ineffective or not well tolerated, amiodarone may be used instead. Alternatively, diltiazem at 2–3 mg/kg every 12 h often provides a good alternative with the disadvantage of only providing rate control.

Electrical Cardioversion

Electrical cardioversion is effective in interrupting re-entry and restoring sinus rhythm. However, since the re-entrant circuit remains, recurrence is very common, making this option undesirable. It is normally reserved for unstable patients that do not respond to medical treatment as a temporary measure before a more definitive option can be achieved (e.g. radiocatheter ablation).

Radiocatheter Ablation

Radiocatheter ablation provides a definitive solution for atrial flutter without the need for further treatment. In typical atrial flutter, the CTI is the target for ablation, resulting in permanent interruption of the re-entrant circuit.[37,57] In atypical atrial flutter, the ablation site varies depending on the re-entrant circuit location and structures involved. In human medicine, this is considered the best treatment option for atrial flutter with a reported success rate of 90–100%.[57] In veterinary medicine, these procedures are currently only available in a few specialist centres worldwide, but in the future they will become more widespread and available to our patients. More information on radiocatheter ablation of atrial flutter can be found in chapter 19.

Monitoring

Effective monitoring in these patients requires periodic Holter recordings, ideally every 6 months. The aim of medical therapy is to achieve acceptable control of the ventricular rate or, ideally, complete suppression of the arrhythmia. In the author's opinion, a 24 h average heart rate of <110 bpm/24 h would be ideal, although some veterinary cardiologists aim for <140 bpm/24 h. It is particularly important that a 24 h Holter recording be obtained after any treatment change, as this is the only reliable way to assess its efficacy. This is usually done 10–20 days after the change has occurred. Echocardiography should also be used as necessary to assess for structural changes and underlying disease if present.

References

1 Blomstrom-Lundqvist C, Scheinman MM, Aliot EM, Alpert JS, Calkins H, Camm AJ, *et al*. ACC/AHA/ESC guidelines for the management of patients with supraventricular arrhythmias – executive summary: a report of the American College of Cardiology/American Heart Association task force on practice guidelines and the European Society of Cardiology committee for practice guidelines (writing committee to develop guidelines for the management of patients with supraventricular arrhythmias) developed in collaboration with NASPE-Heart Rhythm Society. J Am Coll Cardiol. 2003;42:1493–1531.

2 Robles de Medina EO, Bernard R, Coumel P, Damato AN, Fisch C, Krikler D, *et al*. Definition of terms related to cardiac rhythm. WHO/ISFC Task Force. Eur J Cardiol. 1978;8:127–144.

3 Shah D, Yamane T, Choi K-J, Haissaguerre M. QRS subtraction and the ECG analysis of atrial ectopics. Ann Noninvasive Electrocardiol. 2004;9:389–398.

4 Rajawat YS, Gerstenfeld EP, Patel VV, Dixit S, Callans DJ, Marchlinski FE. ECG criteria for localizing the pulmonary vein origin of spontaneous atrial premature complexes: validation using intracardiac recordings. Pacing Clin Electrophysiol. 2004;27:182–188.

5 Schamroth L. The definition of parasystole. Cardiology. 1965;44:37–45.

6 Friedberg HD, Schamroth L. Atrial parasystole. Br Heart J. 1970;32:172–180.

7 Mekhamer YE, Kittleson MD. ECG of the month: generalized cardiomegaly and an enlarged left atrium in a dog. J Am Vet Med Assoc. 1989;194:1198–1199.

8 Waner T, Ohad DG. Apparent atrial parasystole associated with *Ehrlichia canis* infection in a dog: a clinical case report. Israel J Vet Med. 2008;63(4):116–121.

9 Satullo G, Donato A, Luzza F, Saporito F, Oreto G. Atrial parasystole and tachycardia: modulation and automodulation of a parasystolic focus. Chest. 1992;102:622–625.

10 Oreto G, Luzza F, Satullo G, Coglitore S, Schamroth L. Sinus modulation of atrial parasystole. Am J Cardiol. 1986;58:1097–1099.

11 Satullo G, Oreto G, Luzza F, Consolo A, Donato A. Sinus parasystole. Am Heart J. 1991;121:1507–1512.

12 Kovacevic A, Sastravaha A. Clinically silent atrial dissociation in a dog. J Vet Cardiol. 2007;9:135–137.

13 Scollan K, Bulmer BJ, Heaney AM. Electrocardiographic and echocardiographic evidence of atrial dissociation. J Vet Cardiol. 2008;10:53–55.

14 Chung KY, Walsh TJ, Massie E. A review of atrial dissociation, with illustrative cases and critical discussion. Am J Med Sci. 1965;250:72–78.

15 Chung EK. In Principles of cardiac arrhythmia (ed. Chung EK, pp. 462–469). Philadelphia: Williams & Wilkins; 1989.

16 Fenelon G, Shepard RK, Stambler BS. Focal origin of atrial tachycardia in dogs with rapid ventricular pacing-induced heart failure. J Cardiol Electrophysiol. 2003;14:1093–1102.

17 Saoudi N, Cosio F, Waldo A, Chen SA, Iesaka Y, Lesh M, *et al*. Classification of atrial flutter and regular atrial tachycardia according to electrophysiologic mechanism and anatomic bases: a statement from a joint expert group from the Working Group of Arrhythmias of the European Society of Cardiology and the North American Society of Pacing and Electrophysiology. J Cardiovasc Electrophysiol. 2001;12:852–866.

18 Santilli RA, Perego, M, Perini, A, Moretti, P, Spadacini, G. Electrophysiologic characteristics and topographic distribution of focal atrial tachycardias in dogs. J Vet Intern Med. 2010;24:539–545.

19 Kistler PM, Haqqani H, Singarayar S, Roberts-Thomson KC, Spence SJ, Morton JB, *et al*. P wave morphology in focal atrial tachycardia. Heart Rhythm. 2005;2:50–51.

20 Schubart AF, Marriott HJL, Gorten RJ. Isorhythmic dissociation. Am J Med. 1958;24:209–214.

21 Santilli RA, Perego M, Crosara S, Gardini F, Bellino C, Moretti P, *et al*. Utility of 12-lead electrocardiogram for differentiating paroxysmal supraventricular tachycardias in dogs. J Vet Intern Med. 2008;22:915–923.

22 Schober KE, Kent AM, Aeffner F. Tachycardia-induced cardiomyopathy in a cat. Schweizer Archiv für Tierheilkunde. 2014;156:133–139.

23 Ferasin L. Recurrent syncope associated with paroxysmal supraventricular tachycardia in a Devon Rex cat diagnosed by implantable loop recorder. J Feline Med Surg. 2009;11:149–152.

24 Goldreyer BN, Gallagher JJ, Damato AN. The electrophysiologic demonstration of atrial ectopic tachycardia in man. Am Heart J. 1973;85:205–215.

25 Santilli RA, Perego M, Crosara S, Gardini F, Bellino C, Moretti P, *et al*. Utility of 12-lead electrocardiogram for differentiating paroxysmal supraventricular tachycardias in dogs. J Vet Intern Med. 2008;22:915–923.

26 Finster ST, DeFrancesco TC, Atkins CE. Supraventricular tachycardia in dogs: 65 cases (1990–2007). J Vet Emerg Crit Care. 2008;18:503–510.

27 Shine KI, Kastor JA, Yurchak PM. Multifocal atrial tachycardia: clinical and electrocardiographic features in 32 patients. New Engl J Med. 1968;279:344–349.

28 McCord J, Borzak S. Multifocal atrial tachycardia. Chest. 1998;113:203–209.

29 Hebbar AK, Hueston WJ. Management of common arrhythmias: part I. Supraventricular arrhythmias. Am Fam Physician. 2002;65:2479–2486.

30 Boyden PA. Animal models of atrial flutter. J Interv Cardiol. 1995;8:687–696.

31 McWilliam JA. Fibrillar contraction of the heart. J Physiol (Lond.). 1887;8:296–310.

32 Lewis T. Observations upon a curious and not uncommon form of extreme acceleration of the auricle: atrial flutter. Heart. 1913;4:171.

33 Jolly WA, Ritchie WT. Auricular flutter and fibrillation. Ann Noninvasive Electrocardiol. 2003;8:92–96.

34 Puech P. L'Activité électrique auriculaire normale et pathologique. Paris: Masson & Cie; 1956.

35 Lewis ST, Drury AN, Iliescu CC. A demonstration of circus movement in clinical flutter of the auricles. Heart. 1921;341.

36 Wells JL, MacLean WA, James TN, Waldo AL. Characterization of atrial flutter: studies in man after open heart surgery using fixed atrial electrodes. Circulation. 1979;60:665–673.

37 Santilli RA, Perego M, Perini A, Carli A, Moretti P, Spadacini G. Radiofrequency catheter ablation of cavo-tricuspid isthmus as treatment of atrial flutter in two dogs. J Vet Cardiol. 2010;12:59–66.

38 García Cosío F, Pastor A, Núñez A, Magalhaes AP, Awamleh P. [Atrial flutter: an update]. Rev Esp Cardiol. 2006;59:816–831.

39 Ricard P, Imianitoff M, Yaici K, Coutelour JM, Bergonzi M, Rinaldi JP, *et al.* Atypical atrial flutters. Europace. 2002;4:229–239.

40 Santilli RA, Ramera L, Perego M, Moretti P, Spadacini G. Radiofrequency catheter ablation of atypical atrial flutter in dogs. J Vet Cardiol. 2014;16:9–17.

41 Bochoeyer A, Yang Y, Cheng J, Lee RJ, Keung EC, Marrouche NF, *et al.* Surface electrocardiographic characteristics of right and left atrial flutter. Circulation. 2003;108:60–66.

42 Zhang S, Younis G, Hariharan R, Ho J, Yang Y, Ip J, *et al.* Lower loop reentry as a mechanism of clockwise right atrial flutter. Circulation. 2004;109:1630–1635.

43 Cheng J, Cabeen WR, Scheinman MM. Right atrial flutter due to lower loop reentry: mechanism and anatomic substrates. Circulation. 1999;99:1700–1705.

44 Cheng J, Scheinman MM. Acceleration of typical atrial flutter due to double-wave reentry induced by programmed electrical stimulation. Circulation. 1998;97:1589–1596.

45 Zipes DP, Dejoseph RL. Dissimilar atrial rhythms in man and dog. Am J Cardiol. 1973;32:618–628.

46 Frame LH, Page RL, Boyden PA, Fenoglio JJJ. Circus movement in the canine atrium around the tricuspid ring during experimental atrial flutter and during reentry in vitro. Circulation. 1987;76:1155–1175.

47 Schoels W, Restivo M, Caref EB, Gough WB, el-Sherif N. Circus movement atrial flutter in canine sterile pericarditis model: activation patterns during entrainment and termination of single-loop reentry in vivo. Circulation. 1991;83:1716–1730.

48 Boyden PA, Frame LH, Hoffman BF. Activation mapping of reentry around an anatomic barrier in the canine atrium: observations during entrainment and termination. Circulation. 1989;79:406–416.

49 Uno K, Kumagai K, Khrestian CM, Waldo AL. New insights regarding the atrial flutter reentrant circuit: studies in the canine sterile pericarditis model. Circulation. 1999;100:1354–1360.

50 Pariaut R, Santilli R, Moise SN. In Kirks Current veterinary therapy XV (eds. Bonagura JD, Twedt DC, pp. 737–748). Amsterdam: ElsSevier Saunders; 2009.

51 Yang Y, Cheng J, Bochoeyer A, Hamdan MH, Kowal RC, Page R, *et al.* Atypical right atrial flutter patterns. Circulation. 2001;103:3092–3098.

52 Irie T, Kaneko Y, Nakajima T, Saito A, Ota M, Kato T, *et al.* Typical atrial flutter with atypical flutter wave morphology due to abnormal interatrial conduction. Cardiol J. 2011;18:450–453.

53 Yan S-H, Cheng W-J, Wang L-X, Chen M-Y, Hu H-S, Xue M. Mechanisms of atypical flutter wave morphology in patients with isthmus-dependent atrial flutter. Heart Vessels. 2009;24:211–218.

54 Boyden PA, Graziano JN. Activation mapping of reentry around an anatomical barrier in the canine atrium: observations during the action of the class III agent, d-sotalol. J Cardiovasc Electrophysiol. 1993;4:266–279.

55 Spinelli W, Hoffman BF. Mechanisms of termination of reentrant atrial arrhythmias by class I and class III antiarrhythmic agents. Circ Res. 1989;65:1565–1579.

56 Boyden PA. Effects of pharmacologic agents on induced atrial flutter in dogs with right atrial enlargement. J Cardiovasc Pharmacol. 1986;8:170.

57 Chen SA, Chiang CE, Wu TJ, Tai CT, Lee SH, Cheng CC, *et al.* Radiofrequency catheter ablation of common atrial flutter: comparison of electrophysiologically guided focal ablation technique and linear ablation technique. J Am Coll Cardiol. 1996;27:860–868.

9

Atrial Fibrillation

Ruth Willis

Introduction

Atrial fibrillation (AF) is the commonest pathological supraventricular tachyarrhythmia in dogs[1,2] and has also been reported in cats.[3] The key features are rapid, disorganized atrial electrical activity resulting in loss of the atrial contribution to ventricular filling, and an irregular, typically rapid ventricular rate resulting in a reduction in cardiac output.[4] The majority of dogs and cats with AF have concurrent cardiac disease and atrial enlargement.[5] Occasionally, AF is diagnosed in the absence of underlying overt structural heart disease, and this occurs most often in large and giant-breed dogs.[5,6] Haemodynamic status, chronicity of the arrhythmia and the presence of concurrent cardiac disease influence treatment decisions and prognosis.[7,8]

Mechanisms of Atrial Fibrillation

Multiple electrical and structural derangements occur during the formation and maintenance of atrial fibrillation. Initiation of atrial fibrillation is attributed to abnormal automaticity or re-entry (see chapter 6). Historically, multiple atrial ectopic foci were believed to be the underlying cause, although currently other mechanisms are known to be involved. Two major models – the multiple-wavelet model and also the focal model – have been proposed and shown to be sustainable in animals.[9–12]

1. Multiple-wavelet Model

In this model, multiple wavelets of electrical activity propagate within the atria due to functional re-entry circuits. For re-entry to be possible, an electrical impulse must leave a starting point and then return to the same point after a sufficient time that the refractory period is over and the tissue is excitable again. Therefore, re-entry is favoured by conditions that:

- Shorten the refractory period.
- Slow conduction velocity.
- Provide a larger atrial mass.

A minimum number of wavelets (usually six or more) must coexist at all times for AF to be maintained.[13] These wavelets travel in different directions, depolarising small areas of atrial tissue, colliding with each other and then dividing or extinguishing one another in a random fashion (Figure 9.1).[14] The term *critical mass* is used to describe atria of sufficient mass that these wavelets can propagate rather than extinguishing each other.[13] Re-entry is favoured by heterogeneous atrial electrophysiology that can be created or enhanced by pathological change, resulting in atrial fibrosis, inflammation and wall stretch.[15]

2. Focal Model

One or multiple ectopic atrial foci or re-entry circuits are present, and they discharge so rapidly that conduction through the atria cannot occur uniformly and the wavefronts break into irregular wavelets (fibrillatory conduction) (Figure 9.2). The existence of both ectopic foci and micro re-entrant circuits (rotors) has been proved in both human and animal studies, and most are located in the pulmonary veins at their junction with the left atrium.[12,16]

Guide to Canine and Feline Electrocardiography, First Edition. Ruth Willis, Pedro Oliveira and Antonia Mavropoulou.
© 2018 John Wiley & Sons Ltd. Published 2018 by John Wiley & Sons Ltd.
Companion website: www.wiley.com/go/willis/electrocardiography

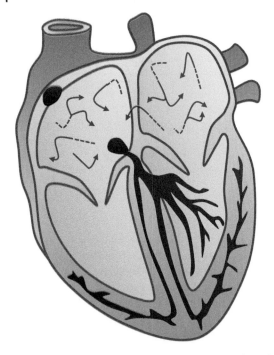

Figure 9.1 Multiple wavelet model. Multiple wavelets of electrical activity propagate within the atria due to functional re-entry circuits (red arrows). A minimum number of wavelets (usually six or more) must coexist for AF to be maintained. These wavelets travel in different directions, depolarising small areas of atrial tissue, colliding with each other and then dividing or extinguishing one another in a random fashion.

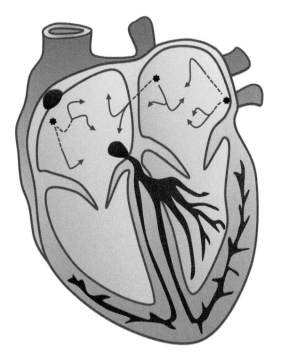

Figure 9.2 Focal activation model. One or multiple ectopic atrial foci or micro re-entry circuits are present (dark blue stars), and they discharge so rapidly that conduction through the atria cannot occur uniformly and the wavefronts break into irregular wavelets (red arrows).

Factors Predisposing to Initiation and Maintenance of Atrial Fibrillation

Multiple factors need to occur simultaneously to create conditions favourable for the existence of AF. To establish a re-entrant rhythm, areas of myocardium with different conduction velocities and refractory periods are necessary – hence, phrases such as *heterogeneous electrophysiological state* and *dispersion of refractoriness* are used to describe the atrial substrate.[9] These changes facilitate some tissue being repolarised and therefore ready to transmit an impulse whilst other adjacent areas remain refractory, thereby allowing an impulse loop to be propagated.

Cardiac Anatomy – Myocyte Fibre Orientation and Critical Mass

In normal animals, the myocytes around the pulmonary veins show numerous and abrupt changes in fibre orientation, resulting in slow and complex conduction patterns, thereby creating conditions that favour the initiation and maintenance of atrial fibrillation.[17] A large mass of atrial tissue is more likely to have this dispersion of refractoriness, which is why atrial fibrillation is more common in larger patients,[5,9] and giant-breed dogs can attain this critical mass in the apparent absence of cardiac disease.[18]

Atrial Pathology and Stretch

Atrial stretch is a common consequence of heart failure in dogs. Atrial stretch results in electrophysiological changes that promote dispersion of refractoriness.[11,19] Moreover, the association of AF with heart failure in dogs has been attributed to local fibrosis interfering with impulse conduction.[15] Shortly after the onset of AF, cellular changes can be seen in the atria – infiltration of leukocytes supports the presence of tissue inflammation, and this is followed by cell death. Inflammation and cell death result in the production of cytokines that promote the production of fibrous tissue,[20] and local angiotensin II production is thought to be one of the key signalling molecules in this process.[20] The atrial fibrosis seen in congestive heart failure occurs between the muscle bundles, especially around the pulmonary veins, thereby creating zones of slowed conduction within the atria; and the resulting dispersion of conduction velocities becomes more apparent at higher heart rates.[15,17]

Electrical Remodelling

Electrical remodelling before and also during atrial fibrillation has been described in detail.[16] Changes include:

- A decrease in the outward Ca^{2+} current and increased inward K+ current (I_{k1}) shorten the action potential duration, thereby favouring re-rentry.[12]
- Increased expression in the $3Na^+/1Ca^{2+}$ exchanger results in increased movement of Na^+ into cardiomyocytes during phase 4 that may permit afterdepolarisations.[21]
- Impaired Ca^{2+} handling and reduced Ca^{2+} transients in atrial myocytes during AF may contribute to a reduction in contractility.[22]
- A decrease in the Na^+ current slows conduction velocity.

Rate-dependent electrical remodelling also occurs, and once AF is established it often becomes persistent – hence the phrase 'Atrial fibrillation begets atrial fibrillation.'[23]

Atrial Myocyte Ultrastructural Changes

AF alters cell ultrastructural properties in several ways, including:

- Loss of myofibrils
- Glycogen accumulation
- Dispersion of nuclear chromatin
- Changes in mitochondrial properties
- Loss of sarcoplasmic reticulum and transverse tubules
- Alterations in the expression and organization of structural proteins, such as smooth muscle actin, titin, myosin heavy chain, troponin and desmin.[24]

These ultrastructural changes help to explain why AF often becomes a persistent arrhythmia.

Autonomic Nervous System Influence

Autonomic nervous system influence changes in sympathetic and, more importantly, parasympathetic tone can create the dispersion of refractoriness vital for the creation of re-entrant circuits. Perhaps counterintuitively, both the sympathetic and parasympathetic nervous systems have the same shortening effect on the refractory period of atrial myocytes, thereby promoting the formation of more circulating wavelets.[25–29] Experimental studies have also shown that vagal stimulation increases the spatial dispersion in atrial refractoriness and shortening of the action potential.[26–28] Additionally, vagal stimulation may enhance ectopic firing from pulmonary vein cardiomyocytes, which may contribute to triggering AF.

Wavelength

The wavelength of a circuit is defined as the distance travelled by the depolarisation wave during the functional refractory period. The wavelength is calculated by multiplying conduction velocity by refractory period. The number of wavelets that can occur simultaneously is determined by the atrial tissue mass and also wavelength. The wavelength will be shortened by vagal stimulation (which decreases the refractory period) and intra-atrial conduction defects. Drugs that increase wavelength by increasing conduction velocity or prolonging the refractory period will favour termination of AF by reducing the number of wavelets that can be sustained to below the critical threshold.[23]

Ventricular Response

The atrial rate in AF is somewhere between 400 and 700 bpm. Fortunately, the atrioventricular (AV) node is not able to respond in a 1:1 conduction, and many depolarisation waves are blocked in this structure and do not reach the ventricles (Figure 9.3).

The ventricular response will depend on how many impulses are able to travel through the AV node and depolarise the ventricles. The ventricular response is irregular, as varying penetration of the blocked atrial impulses into the AV node (concealed conduction) affects the propagation of subsequent impulses.[30] Typically, the ventricular response in dogs is 120–260 bpm[6] and in cats is 200–280 bpm.[3] Several factors can influence the ventricular response in the course of AF by affecting conduction through the AV node:[30]

1) *Autonomic nervous system*: The autonomic nervous system greatly influences conduction through the AV node. Sympathetic stimulation increases conduction and therefore increases the ventricular response rate, whilst parasympathetic stimulation has the opposite effect.[31]
2) *AV node disease*: Intrinsic disease of the AV node or the conduction system may exist in many patients with AF, as most have some form of structural heart disease.[32,33]
3) *Drugs*: Several drugs influence conduction through the AV node, and this constitutes the mainstay for medical treatment of AF (see the 'Treatment' section).

Electrocardiographic Findings

The diagnosis of AF can be made from a resting electrocardiogram (ECG). Atrial fibrillation is characterized on the surface ECG by irregular RR intervals and the absence of discernible P waves. *Fibrillatory* (f) *waves* may be

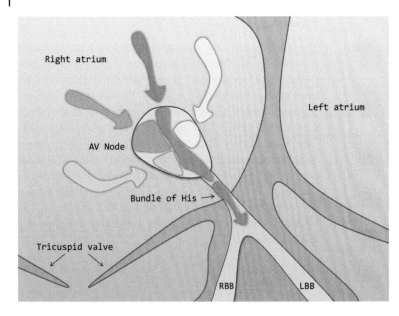

Figure 9.3 The atrioventricular node and atrial fibrillation. Diagram illustrating four concomitant depolarisation waves (coloured arrows) reaching the atrioventricular node (AVN) at the same time. Each of these waves causes depolarisation of an area of the AVN tissue depending on their point of entry (coloured areas). The yellow, green and purple waves are cancelled out as they reach areas of refractory tissue. The red wave is able to traverse the AVN and goes on to depolarise the ventricles via the His–Purkinje system. The AVN acts as a filter, allowing only a few of the depolarisation waves to actually reach the ventricles and preventing the ventricular rate from being so high that it would be incompatible with life. The depolarisation waves that reach the ventricles do so in a random way that accounts for the irregularity of the ventricular response seen in atrial fibrillation. LBB, Left bundle branch; RBB, right bundle branch.

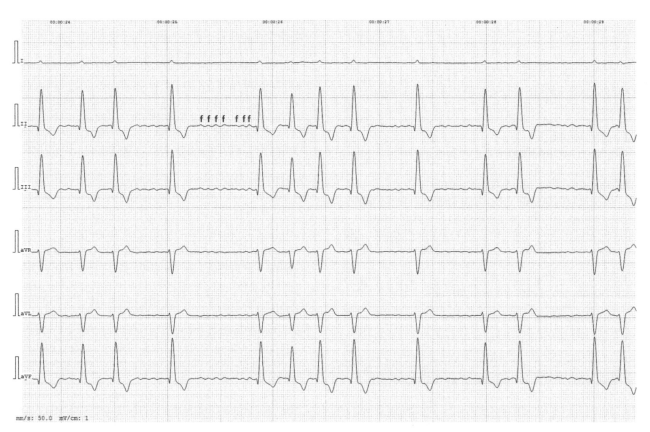

Figure 9.4 Atrial fibrillation. Narrow-QRS complex tachycardia with irregular R-R intervals, no discernible P waves and visible f waves (f) typical of atrial fibrillation. [7-year-old, male German Shepherd dog] (Lead II, 50 mm/s, 10 mm/mV)

visible as a series of continuous and randomly occurring oscillations of the baseline (Figure 9.4). Table 9.1 shows a summary of the characteristics of AF.

Depending on the amount of atrial tissue involved in each depolarisation wavelet, the resulting f waves will be different. Fewer ectopic foci are able to depolarise a larger area of atrial tissue (larger vectors) and will result in larger f waves – *coarse atrial fibrillation* (Figure 9.5). These waves should not be confused with flutter waves (F) (see chapter 8). If many ectopic foci exist concomitantly, the resulting vectors and amount of tissue involved will be small, resulting in smaller f waves – *fine atrial*

Table 9.1 Characteristics of atrial fibrillation

	Dog	Cat
Heart rate	Atrial: 400–700 bpm (f waves) Ventricular: 120–260 bpm	Atrial: 400–700 bpm (f waves) Ventricular: 200–280 bpm
Rhythm (RR intervals)	Irregular	
P wave	Absent. Fibrillatory (f) waves may be visible as a series of continuous and randomly occurring oscillations of the baseline	
AV conduction	Variable; occult AV conduction	
QRS width	Normal (<70 ms), except if abnormal intraventricular conduction is present or significant cardiac enlargement	Normal (<40 ms), except if abnormal intraventricular conduction is present or significant cardiac enlargement
VA conduction	Absent	
Dropped beats	Not applicable	
Onset/offset	Usually incessant	Paroxysmal or incessant

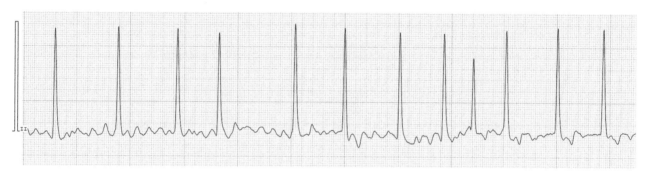

Figure 9.5 Coarse atrial fibrillation. The f waves have higher amplitude with more of a sine wave appearance. [18-year-old, male neutered, crossbreed dog with chronic valvular degenerative disease] (Lead II, 50 mm/s, 50 mm/mV)

fibrillation. The f waves may in fact be so small that they are barely visible on the surface ECG (Figure 9.6).

QRS Morphology

The QRS complex usually has a normal appearance and duration in patients with AF, as the impulses travel through the AV node and the normal ventricular electrical conduction system. In the next section, the reasons for wide-QRS complexes during AF are discussed.

Wide-QRS Complexes During Atrial Fibrillation

In patients with marked ventricular enlargement or hypertrophy, the duration of the QRS may be longer than normal (see chapter 4).

Wide-QRS complexes may occur in cases with AF for several reasons:[57]

- Ventricular enlargement (Figure 9.7)
- Bundle branch block (Figure 9.8)
- Ashman's phenomenon (see Figure 7.11 and chapter 7 for more details)[58,59]
- AF and ventricular ectopy (Figure 9.9)
- Pre-excitation and AF (Figure 9.10)[60,61]
- AF and third-degree atrioventricular block (AVB) (Figure 9.11).

ST Segments and T Wave Morphology

The characteristics of the ST segments and T waves are usually normal in patients with AF, although they may appear abnormal due to the presence of overlying f waves. This is particularly true in cases of coarse AF, in which the ST segments and T waves may be completely obscured (Figure 9.5).

Ambulatory ECGs in Atrial Fibrillation

The ventricular response rate to AF, and also the frequency and complexity of ventricular ectopy, will determine whether anti-arrhythmic treatment is required. Holter analysis software generates a tachogram that plots ventricular rate against time for the duration of the recording and also calculates the mean 24 h heart rate

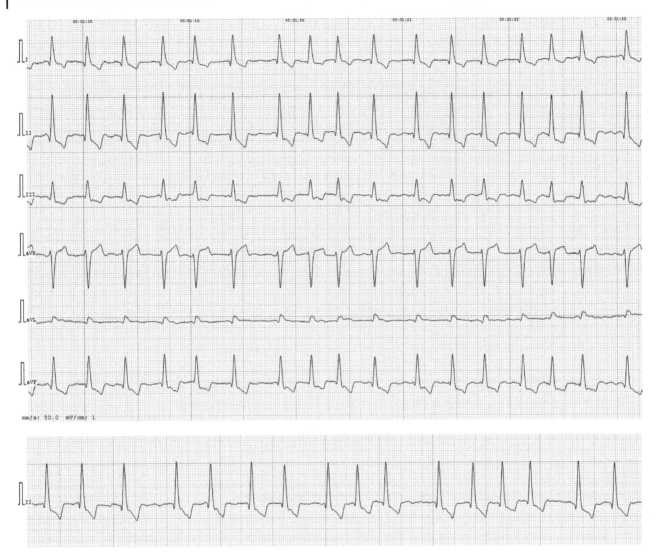

Figure 9.6 Fine atrial fibrillation. The f waves are not readily visible, although the irregularity of the rhythm and absence of visible P waves signal the presence of atrial fibrillation. [11-year-old, male neutered, Norfolk Terrier dog with chronic valvular degenerative disease] (Lead II, 50 mm/s, 10 mm/mV)

(Figure 9.12). Time is represented on the x-axis using the 24 h clock, and instantaneous heart rate is represented on the left-hand y-axis. An additional y-axis on the right-hand side of the graph represents the frequency of ventricular ectopy over the 24 h period. Analysis of the tachogram allows assessment of the need for treatment or the effectiveness of rate control during treatment.

Whilst a resting ECG will document heart rate, it has been shown that the resting ECG tends to overestimate the ventricular rate of dogs with AF.[62] This has been attributed to the stress associated with visiting the veterinary centre and being restrained for a resting ECG, resulting in adrenergic stimulation which raises heart rate.[63] Therefore, Holter monitoring is frequently performed in cases with AF to assess the ventricular rate over a longer period (typically 24 h) with the dog at home. Whilst shorter recordings of perhaps 1 h with the dog close to the clinic have been suggested as being superior for evaluation of rate control compared to a resting ECG, and may be tempting in view of convenience, the ventricular rate during this first hour was similar to that seen in the clinic, presumably as a result of stress associated with the clinic visit and also the presence of the recording equipment (see Figure 9.12).[62]

The ventricular rate response to AF is very variable – some dogs may have a relatively slow rate, referred to as *lone atrial fibrillation*,[6,41] whereas other dogs may have a fast ventricular response that may require treatment to optimise cardiac output and also ameliorate the risk of tachycardia-induced cardiomyopathy. Additionally, some breeds (e.g. Great Danes) with AF may have concurrent malignant ventricular dysrhythmias which may

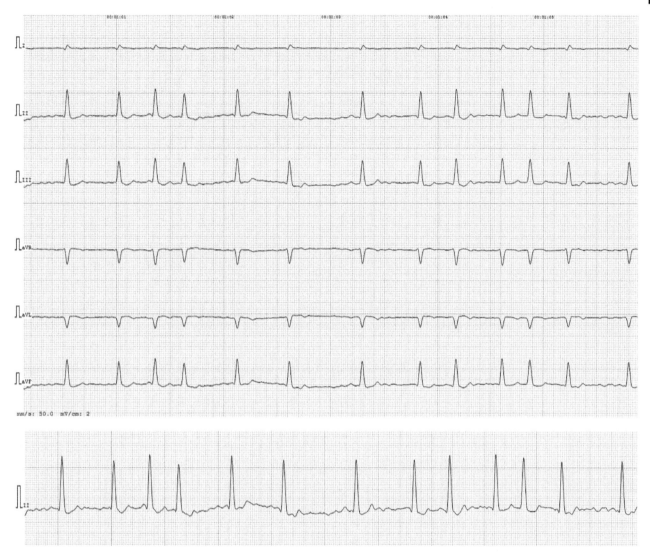

Figure 9.7 Wide QRS in atrial fibrillation secondary to ventricular enlargement or hypertrophy. Atrial fibrillation in a dog with dilated cardiomyopathy. The QRS complexes are wide (75 ms) due to left ventricular enlargement. [9-year-old, male neutered, Saint Bernard dog with dilated cardiomyopathy] (Lead II, 50 mm/s, 5 mm/mV)

not be detected on a 1–5 min rhythm strip, and the presence of ventricular arrhythmias in dogs with AF may influence treatment decisions.[64]

Ambulatory ECG monitoring over 24 h can help to stratify cases with AF into three groups:

1) 'Lone' atrial fibrillation
   - Holter-derived mean 24 h ventricular rate <110 bpm (Figure 9.13)
   - Minimal ventricular ectopy
   - No complex ventricular ectopy
   - No echocardiographic evidence of structural heart disease
   - Further monitoring advisable given the potential to progress to a dilated cardiomyopathy phenotype.[6]

2) Rapid atrial fibrillation
   - Holter-derived mean 24 h ventricular rate >110 bpm (Figure 9.12)
   - Likely to require treatment to slow the ventricular response.

3) Rapid atrial fibrillation with complex ventricular ectopy
   - Holter-derived mean 24 h ventricular rate >110 bpm
   - Frequent ventricular ectopy
   - Complex ventricular ectopy (e.g. couplets, triplets and ventricular tachycardia)
   - Possible echocardiographic evidence of structural heart disease
   - Likely to require treatment to slow the ventricular response ± reduce risk of sudden death.

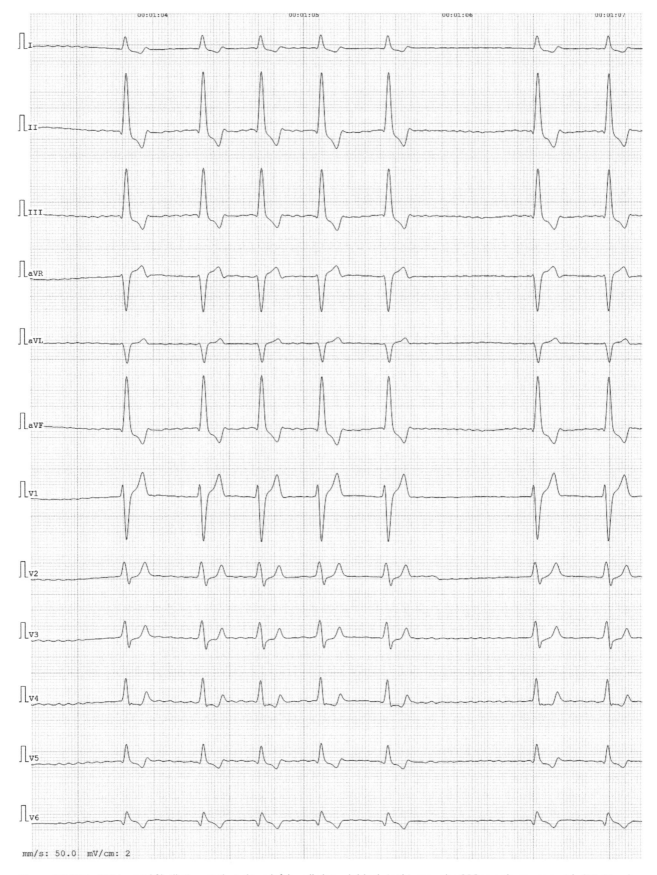

Figure 9.8 Wide QRS in atrial fibrillation attributed to a left bundle branch block. In this case, the QRS complexes were wide (80–85 ms), with an absence of precordial concordance suggesting a left bundle branch block. Concordance exists when all the QRS complexes in the chest leads are either predominantly positive or predominantly negative (see chapters 7 and 14). The QRS duration was thought to be excessive due to left ventricular enlargement. [7-year-old, female crossbreed dog with a patent ductus arteriosus] (50 mm/s, 5 mm/mV)

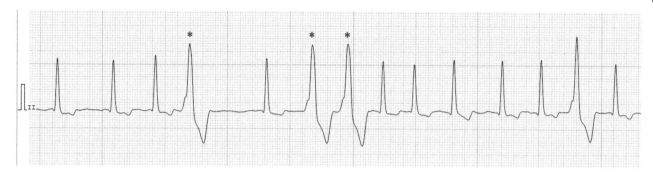

Figure 9.9 Atrial fibrillation accompanied by ventricular ectopic beats. Ventricular ectopic beats (*) occur randomly and do not follow the long RR–short RR sequence observed in Ashman's phenomenon. A post-extrasystolic pause may also be observed due to occult retro-conduction of the ventricular impulse through the atrioventricular node as shown in the example above (fourth beat from left). A tendency to organization into couplets, triplets, bigeminy, trigeminy and runs of tachycardia is also observed with ventricular arrhythmias.[57] [8-year-old, male Golden Retriever dog] (50 mm/s; 10 mm/mV)

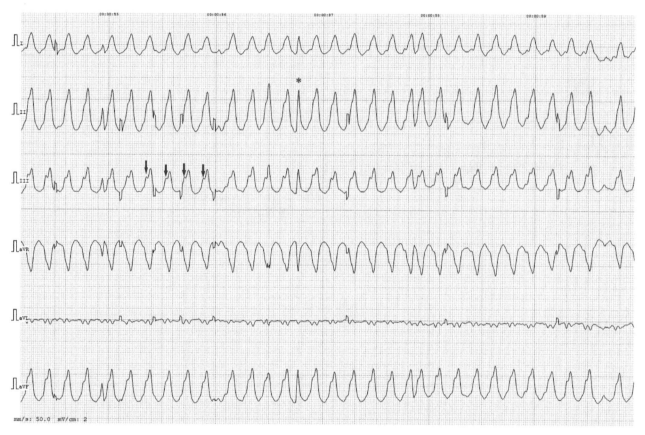

Figure 9.10 Atrial fibrillation with pre-excitation. The QRS complexes are wide (85–90 ms) except for the 15th beat (*), which presents a normal duration (60 ms). A positive deflection may be seen in the initial portion of the R wave consistent with a delta wave (δ, highlighted by arrow), particularly in lead III (arrows). The RR intervals are irregular, as would be expected in AF and allowing differentiation with ventricular tachycardia.[60,61] This dog also presented periods of atrial fibrillation without pre-excitation. [9-year-old, male neutered, Boxer dog] (50 mm/s; 5 mm/mV)

Pathophysiology of Atrial Fibrillation

Reduction in Cardiac Output

The atria normally function as reservoirs for blood returning from the pulmonary and systemic circulation, and atrial contraction augments passive ventricular filling, contributing approximately 20% of end diastolic volume at rest.[34] Therefore, the loss of organised atrial contraction results in reduced ventricular filling and impaired ventricular diastolic function.[10] This reduction in cardiac output is likely to be more noticeable during periods of

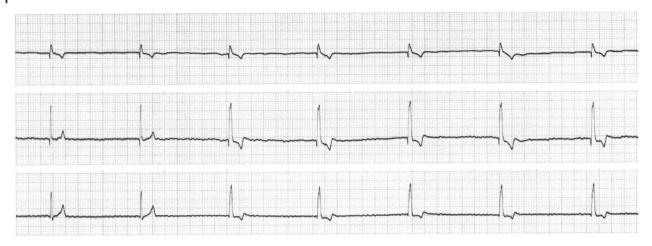

Figure 9.11 Atrial fibrillation and complete atrioventricular block. The baseline shows fine undulations typical of f waves. The QRS complexes exhibit variable width and morphology, likely reflecting change in the site of the ventricular escape focus. Despite the presence of atrial fibrillation, the ventricular rhythm is regular as none of the impulses are conducted from the atria to the ventricles. [7-year-old, male Labrador Retriever dog] (Leads I-III; 25 mm/s; 10 mm/mV) *Source*: Courtesy of Paul Wotton.

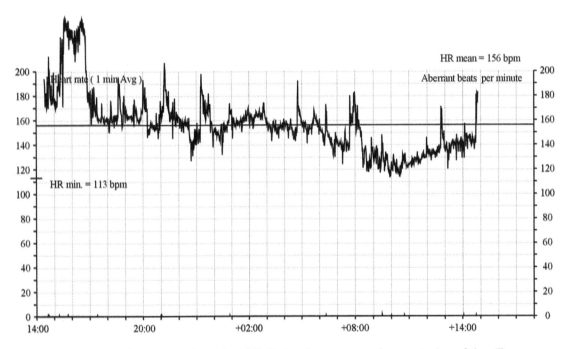

Figure 9.12 Tachogram from a dog with rapid atrial fibrillation after treatment of congestive heart failure. The average ventricular rate over 24 h is 156 bpm, suggesting that this patient could benefit from anti-arrhythmic treatment to lower the ventricular rate. Frequent peaks of elevated heart rate are also seen – for example, around 16:00. [7-year-old, male neutered, Labrador Retriever dog]

high demand, such as during exercise, and, in some dogs, the development of AF may result in collapse.

Tachycardia

The drop in cardiac output is compounded by tachycardia that:

- Reduces the diastolic interval available for ventricular filling

- Increases myocardial oxygen demand
- Reduces myocardial perfusion during diastole
- Persistent tachycardia impairs systolic function both directly and also indirectly through alterations in cellular and neurohormonal systems.[35]

Sustained tachycardia results in left ventricular systolic dysfunction. This is subclassified into *arrhythmia-induced*, where the arrhythmia is the sole cause of the ventricular dysfunction, and *arrhythmia-mediated*,

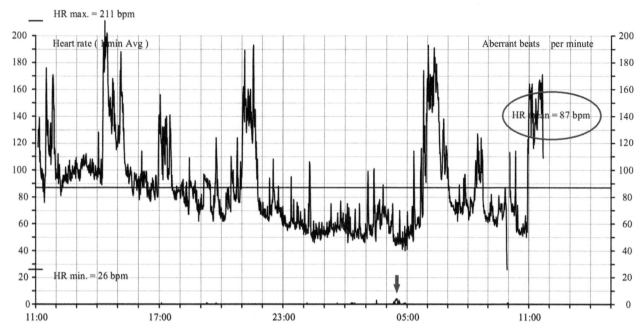

Figure 9.13 Tachogram from dog with lone atrial fibrillation The average 24 h ventricular rate is 87 bpm (blue circle). The right-hand *y*-axis shows the frequency of ventricular ectopy plotted against time on the *x*-axis. Over the 24 h recording, there was minimal ventricular ectopy that occurred singly as escape beats during periods of low heart rate, and these beats occurred most frequently between 04:00 and 05:00 (red arrow). [5-year-old, male German Shepherd dog]

where the arrhythmia worsens left ventricular dysfunction or heart failure in a patient with underlying heart disease.[35]

Cardiac Asynchrony

AF results in ventricular asynchrony as the ventricle contracts in a disorganised manner.[36] Ventricular asynchrony is highlighted by echocardiographic M-mode images of the left ventricle in short axis, showing the asynchronous movement of the left ventricular free wall and interventricular septum. This asynchrony compromises cardiac output and the efficiency of the contraction.

Thromboembolic Disease

Thromboembolic disease is a recognised complication of AF in human patients and may occur in cats due to their concurrent structural heart disease.[3] Thromboembolic complications are less common in dogs, although they have been reported occasionally.[37,38]

Situations When Atrial Fibrillation May Occur

1. Secondary to Structural Heart Disease

This is the most common setting for the development of AF, particularly with diseases that lead to marked

enlargement of one or both atria.[39] In dogs, AF is commonly associated with dilated cardiomyopathy (DCM).[39,40] In studies of Wolfhounds with congestive heart failure, almost all have AF at the time of onset of clinical signs.[41,42] DCM tends to affect middle-aged and older large and giant-breed dogs, and the prevalence of AF increases with age.[40] Less commonly, AF can occur with other forms of heart disease, such as secondary to advanced mitral valve disease or severe congenital heart disease and heart failure.[6,39] In Dobermans with DCM, the development of AF is a poor prognostic indicator.[43] In cats, AF tends to accompany severe cardiac disease with marked atrial enlargement and congestive heart failure.[3]

2. Atrial Fibrillation Without Structural Heart Disease – *Lone AF*

AF in the absence of significant structural heart disease is usually referred to as *lone atrial fibrillation*. This condition has been documented in a number of large and giant breeds, including Irish Wolfhounds,[41,44] Great Danes[45,46] Mastiffs, Newfoundlands, Rottweilers[6] and a Pointer.[47]

In a study involving 500 Irish Wolfhounds, rhythm disturbances without evidence of DCM were detected in 48 dogs.[41] In another study of Irish Wolfhounds with AF who eventually progressed to show signs of congestive heart failure and a DCM phenotype, the mean age at which AF was first detected was 45 months in males and

24 months in female dogs.[42] The time from detection of AF to the onset of congestive heart failure signs in this small study was 27 months in males and 24 months in females.[42] Reports of idiopathic lone AF in cats are rare.[48]

3. Paroxysmal Atrial Fibrillation

In humans, it is recognised that initial episodes of AF may be paroxysmal, but, with time, the paroxysms may lengthen and the arrhythmia may become permanent; the same may be true for dogs. Dogs with paroxysmal AF are likely to have underlying structural heart disease resulting in atrial stretch, as this may create the mechanical and electrical changes required for AF to be initiated and then perpetuated, even if only for short periods. Familial AF has been documented in humans,[49–51] but further work is likely to be required in view of likely genetic heterogenicity. No such information is available for dogs to date.

The presenting sign with paroxysmal AF seems to be variable, with some dogs showing no referable clinical signs; but, in occasional cases, collapse at the onset of AF has been documented. Figures 9.14 and 9.15 illustrate examples of paroxysmal AF.

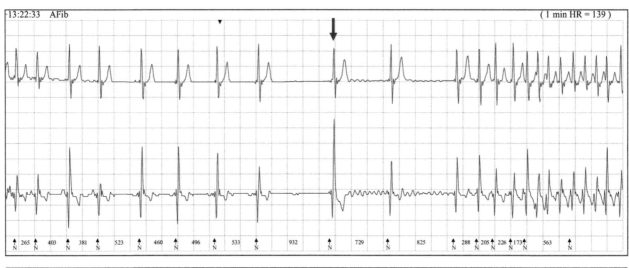

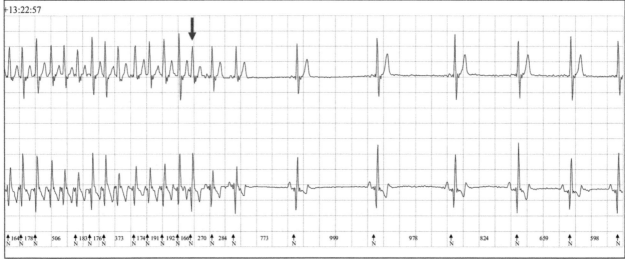

Figure 9.14 Paroxysmal atrial fibrillation. The blue arrow highlights the onset of atrial fibrillation, and the red arrow shows offset approximately 24 s later. Prior to the onset of atrial fibrillation (trace to left of blue arrow), the P morphology is variable, suggesting an ectopic focus or foci. There is a short pause prior to onset, and the morphology of the first beat in the paroxysm of atrial fibrillation is subtly different from the sinus beat in lead II, suggesting that it may originate from an ectopic focus and/or that it has been conducted aberrantly. There are reports of ectopic atrial foci resulting in paroxysmal atrial fibrillation in dogs, and this remains a possibility in this case, but an electrophysiological study would be required to investigate this further.[52] Note the increase in the ventricular rate during the paroxysm of atrial fibrillation. [3-year-old, female English Cocker Spaniel dog with signs consistent with congestive heart failure]

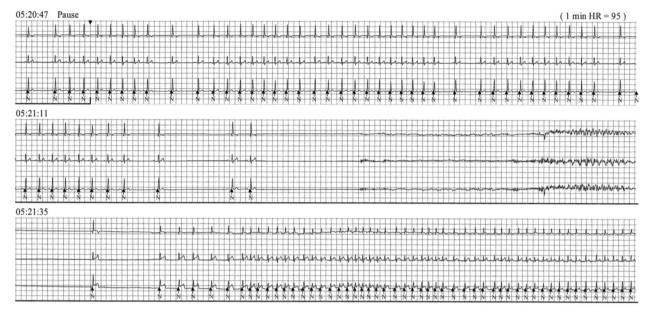

Figure 9.15 Atrial fibrillation after a long sinus pause. An ambulatory ECG trace from a Cavalier King Charles Spaniel (CKCS) with a long history of atrioventricular valve disease and, more recently, multiple episodes of collapse. Whilst no episodes of collapse were noted by the owner during the recording, during a period of presumed rest at 05:20 a.m., the dog had a 17 s period of sinus node arrest with ventricular asystole followed by atrial fibrillation which persisted for the remainder of the recording (7 h). The trace shows some baseline artefact around 05:21:30, and this raises suspicion that the dog may have experienced a hypoxic seizure given the likely hypotension associated with such a long period of ventricular asystole. The reason for the long period of sinus node and/or autonomic dysfunction seen in this case is unclear. CKCS are recognised as being predisposed to upper airway obstruction and also intracranial disease,[55] and both these conditions could potentially alter autonomic tone, but neither condition readily explains the abrupt change seen in this case. Heart rate variability has been studied in dogs with naturally occurring myxomatous mitral valve disease, and whilst in early disease there may be hypervagal autonomic imbalance, later in the disease process parasympathetic tone appears to be reduced.[56] Alternatively, we can speculate that this trace may show a form of sick sinus syndrome or an abortive sudden death.[33] Pacemaker implantation was discussed but declined by the owner due to the severe pre-existing atrioventricular valve disease. [12-year-old, female Cavalier King Charles Spaniel]

4. Vagally Induced Atrial Fibrillation

Vagally induced AF has been demonstrated in canine experimental models and also occurs, albeit uncommonly, in certain disease states which involve a sudden change in autonomic tone (e.g. gastrointestinal surgery) or cardiac stretch (e.g. after drainage of pericardial effusion). Vagal AF tends to be paroxysmal (Figure 9.15).[53]

In German Shepherd dogs with experimentally induced vagal AF, administration of lidocaine during the first hour after onset of AF has been shown to convert the rhythm back to sinus.[54] Lidocaine blocks the fast sodium channels preferentially in the atria and increases post-depolarisation refractoriness. Ranolazine, a piperazine derivate with antianginal activity, also affects fast sodium channels and could also have a role in the treatment of vagally mediated AF.

Clinical Features of Atrial Fibrillation

Although dogs with lone AF may tolerate their condition without any referable signs, the majority of dogs will have a history of signs potentially referable to cardiac disease, such as lethargy, exercise intolerance, change in respiratory rate or pattern, coughing, syncope, reduced appetite, weight loss and/or ascites.[4]

In addition to a tachyarrhythmia, physical examination findings in cases with AF may include signs of reduced cardiac output such as mucous membrane pallor, cold extremities, prolonged capillary refill time, jugular distension, reduced precordial impulse strength, systolic heart murmur, absence of respiratory sounds and/or adventitious lung sounds.[4]

Cats with AF are likely to have signs of severe heart failure and atrial enlargement; they may also present with signs suggestive of thromboembolic disease, such as hindlimb paralysis.[3]

Key Clinical Features

- Irregularly irregular heart rhythm
- Heart rate can vary from 70 to 300 bpm.
- Variable femoral pulse quality, with pulse deficits depending on the time available for diastolic filling
- Pulse rate is usually approximately half of the heart rate.

Treatment

Rate or Rhythm Control

There are two possible treatment strategies in AF: restore and then maintain sinus rhythm, or control the ventricular rate in response to AF. Whilst rhythm control is appealing to improve cardiac function, lower the risk of tachycardia-induced cardiomyopathy and reduce any associated clinical signs, dogs and cats with AF often have severe underlying structural heart disease, making this goal challenging. Dogs with AF have molecular and structural changes within the atria,[9,10] making it more challenging to restore and then maintain sinus rhythm. Therefore, in the majority of cases, therapy is aimed at controlling the ventricular rate in response to AF.

The benefits of rate versus rhythm control in dogs are yet to be firmly established.[65] Indeed, some cases with lone AF and an acceptable mean heart rate may not require treatment at all. Human patients showed no significant benefit to rhythm versus rate control when mortality was used as the end point; however, rhythm control improves the ability to exercise and also the possibility of preventing atrial remodelling.[66]

Rhythm Control

Converting AF or another abnormal heart rhythm back into a sinus rhythm is called *cardioversion*. This may be performed via the use of drugs – *pharmacological cardioversion* – or by applying an electrical shock to the heart that resets the myocardial cells and allows resumption of normal sinus activity – *electrical cardioversion* (Figure 9.16). In humans, electrophysiological or surgical interventions are also routinely used to restore sinus rhythm in patients with AF.[67] If cardioversion is to be attempted, then this is likely to have the best results in cases with recent-onset AF and no evidence of underlying structural heart disease.[8,68,69] Pharmacological cardioversion has been attempted in dogs with several drugs, including propafenone, flecainide, dofetilide, ibutilide, lidocaine, sotalol and amiodarone.[8,70–73] Successful cardioversion of AF has been reported in six dogs treated with amiodarone, despite the presence of underlying structural cardiac disease.[74] Cardioversion was also possible with lidocaine in dogs with vagally mediated AF.[54,75]

Electrical Cardioversion

Electrical cardioversion is performed under general anaesthesia and consists in delivering an electrical shock to the heart synchronized with the R wave on the ECG (see Figure 9.16). This electrical current may be delivered either transthoracically[68] or transvenously.[76–78] The principle is that depolarisation of a large area of atrial myocardium will disrupt the multiple re-entrant circuits and produce a more electrically homogeneous environment promoting the resumption of sinus rhythm. Synchronization with the R wave (QRS) is very important and distinguishes electrical cardioversion from defibrillation that is unsynchronized. R wave synchronisation prevents shock delivery during ventricular repolarisation, when a shock could trigger ventricular fibrillation. The most vulnerable period for ventricular fibrillation occurs at the peak of the T wave. It is important to note that most defibrillators automatically switch back to asynchronous mode by default after a synchronized discharge. This is to allow immediate defibrillation in case ventricular fibrillation occurs. **Therefore, it is vital that the synchronization mode be switched on before each individual cardioversion attempt.**

Rate Control

Rate control involves the use of pharmacological treatment or electrophysiological/surgical interventions to reduce ventricular response in atrial fibrillation and effectively maintain the heart rate at acceptable levels.

Overview of Drugs and Strategies used to Treat Atrial Fibrillation

Diltiazem (monotherapy)

Diltiazem is a non-dihydropyridine calcium channel blocker that decreases the ventricular response by reducing the AV node conduction. It has a fast onset of action and is normally well tolerated with few side effects in both dogs and cats. It should be used with care in patients with systolic dysfunction and/or congestive heart failure due to its negative inotropic effects.

- *Oral dose – dog*: 1–4 mg/kg q8h or up to 3–5 mg/kg q12h for sustained or extended-release preparations
- *Oral dose – cat*: 1–2.5 mg/kg q8h
- *Adverse reactions*: Bradycardia in dogs and vomiting in cats.

Digoxin (monotherapy)

Digoxin causes an increase in parasympathetic tone and a reduction in sympathetic tone. This inhibits AV nodal conduction and results in a decrease in heart rate. Additionally, digoxin also has a mild positive inotropic effect. Digoxin has a narrow therapeutic range and a slow onset of action. Serum levels should be checked 5–7 days after starting treatment, and the sample should be taken at least 8 h post pill. The ideal serum concentration is between 0.9 and 1.2 ng/mL.

- *Oral dose – dog*: 2.5–3 μg/kg q12h or 0.22 mg/m^2 in dogs >20 kg
- *Oral dose – cat*: 10 μg/kg q24–48 h

• *Adverse reactions*: Anorexia, vomiting, diarrhoea, depression and arrhythmias (e.g. ventricular arrhythmias). Cats are more sensitive to the toxic effects of digoxin. Hypokalaemia predisposes to toxicity.

Digoxin + Diltiazem

Heart rate control with digoxin monotherapy is not always appropriate as increases in sympathetic tone with excitement, exercise or other causes can override the

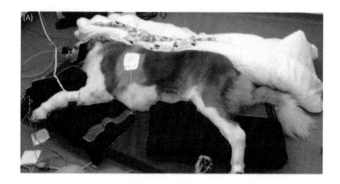

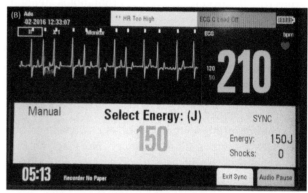

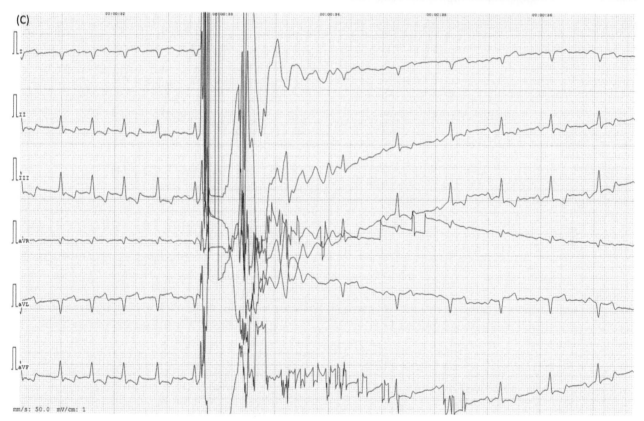

Figure 9.16 Electrical cardioversion. (A) Electrical cardioversion is performed with the patient under general anaesthesia as it is painful. The patient is placed in right or left lateral recumbency on a soft mattress and protected by padding or blankets to avoid physical damage caused by involuntary limb movement. Adhesive electrodes are placed on both sides of the chest dorsally where the atria are located (not ventrally as for ventricular pacing). Continuous electrocardiographic monitoring and additional anaesthesia monitoring should be available (e.g. pulse oximetry, blood pressure etc.). (B) The quality of the electrocardiogram should be checked on the defibrillator monitor, and the synchronization option should be selected (SYNC on the monitor). It is important to ensure that the R waves are being correctly detected (white markers on top of the R waves on the electrocardiogram) to make sure that electrical discharge is delivered synchronized with the R wave and not the T wave, as this could lead to ventricular fibrillation. The energy of the impulse may then be selected. (C) Six-lead electrocardiographic recording during successful electrical cardioversion. Atrial fibrillation may be seen on the left of the trace (first five beats). This is followed by a baseline artefact caused by patient movement during the electrical discharge. A return to a regular sinus rhythm may then be seen. [2-year-old, male Saint Bernard dog that developed AF during anaesthesia and without structural heart disease] (50 mm/s; 10 mm/mV)

vagal effects of this drug. The combination of digoxin and diltiazem has been reported to be more effective for rate control in dogs than monotherapy with either of these drugs.[79]

β-blockers

Drugs with β-blocking effects (e.g. propranolol, atenolol, sotalol etc.) cause inhibition of AV nodal conduction and may be used for rate control in cases of AF. Care must be taken as the accompanying negative inotropic effects may result in hypotension or even precipitate congestive heart failure.

Amiodarone (monotherapy)

Amiodarone primarily blocks potassium channels but also has potent sodium channel blocking effects. Additionally, it also has some α/β-adrenergic blocking effects and calcium channel blocking effects that result in inhibition of AV nodal conduction. It has a slow onset of action and has a less negative inotropic effect in comparison to the drugs discussed in this chapter. One report described a >20% decrease in heart rate in 76% of dogs and conversion to sinus rhythm in 35%. Due to its potential for toxicity, this drug is usually used when other anti-arrhythmic drugs have failed or are not well tolerated.[74] Hepatic enzyme activities and thyroid hormone levels should be determined prior to the start of treatment and every 3 months thereafter.

- *Oral dose – dog*: 10–15 mg/kg q12h for 7 days, followed by 5–7.5 mg/kg q12h for 14 days and then 5–7.5 mg/kg q24h
- *Adverse reactions*: Anorexia, gastrointestinal disturbances, hepatotoxicity, reduced thyroid hormone levels, bradycardia, QT interval prolongation and hypotension.

Lidocaine

Lidocaine may result in conversion to sinus rhythm in cases of acute vagally mediated AF, especially if given within 1 h after onset.[75]

Note: All doses shown above were obtained from BSAVA Small Animal Formulary, 8th edition.

More information on anti-arrhythmic therapy may be found in chapter 17 and appendix 4.

Targets for Ventricular Rate Control

The ideal target range for dogs and cats with AF is not known.[65] Typically, a ventricular response rate lower than 150–160 bpm (as determined by an ECG at the clinic) in a dog would be considered by many as acceptable. However, the heart rate that is determined in such conditions is highly influenced by stress, and, when compared to the heart rate obtained from dogs at home, it was consistently overestimated at the clinic.[62] The average 24 h heart rate determined from a Holter recording with the patient in its normal environment and performing normal activities is the best way to assess rate control. Ideally, this should be performed before treatment is started, 10–20 days after starting or changing medication, and also if disease status changes to assess the mean ventricular rate and also the frequency and complexity of ventricular ectopy.

There is little information in veterinary literature regarding when treatment should be started and the ideal mean 24 h ventricular rate in these cases. In normal dogs in sinus rhythm, the accepted 24 h mean heart rate is 65–90 bpm and, for cases with persistent AF, a 24 h mean ventricular rate of over 140–150 bpm has been suggested as a threshold for starting treatment.[8,79] Whilst the ideal target heart rate for dogs with persistent AF is not known, many clinicians are comfortable using a similar target range for ventricular rate to that used in human patients with persistent AF of 80–110 bpm, with the caveat that this relatively tight control may not be achievable in cases with severe systolic dysfunction.[62,80,81]

Treating Atrial Fibrillation in Patients with Congestive Heart Failure

In patients with structural heart disease, congestive heart failure and AF, priority should always be given to management of congestive heart failure before considering anti-arrhythmic treatment. Elevated sympathetic tone during congestive heart failure will invariably lead to an increase in heart rate, making it impossible to assess the need for rate control until after stabilisation. Additionally, most of the drugs used to lower the ventricular rate are negative inotropes and therefore should be used with caution in cases with congestive heart failure. Similarly, other conditions that may contribute to an increase in sympathetic tone (especially potentially painful conditions) should also be addressed in any case with atrial fibrillation. However, in some cases, extreme tachycardia compromises cardiac function, and, in this situation, control of congestive heart failure cannot be obtained until the ventricular rate is reduced.

Treating Atrial Fibrillation in Cats

AF in cats is rare and tends to be associated with severe underlying structural heart disease. Treatment should aim for management of the underlying disease, and if necessary β-blockers (e.g. atenolol) or calcium channel blockers (e.g. diltiazem) may be used to slow the ventricular response rate to AF.

Other Treatment Strategies

Radiocatheter Ablation

Radiocatheter ablation is increasingly becoming a first-line therapy for the treatment of AF in humans.[82] As mentioned in this chapter, the pulmonary veins are the source of ectopic foci and/or micro re-entrant circuits that play an important role in triggering and maintaining AF. For this reason, radiocatheter ablation is used to electrically isolate the pulmonary veins from the rest of the atrium in an attempt to attain a long-lasting cure. With the aid of three-dimensional electrophysiology mapping techniques, the pulmonary veins are located and the adjoining tissue between the veins and the atrium is ablated to effectively stop electrical continuity through these structures.[82] Other sites are also investigated during the procedure and ablated if necessary (e.g. vena cava, crista terminalis, ligament of Marshall and atrial wall). The reported rates of success are variable but around 54% after a first procedure and 80% after multiple procedures (average of 1.5 procedures).[83] The complication rate is low.

The use of radiocatheter ablation for treatment of AF has not been reported in veterinary medicine, although it may become available in the future.

Pacemaker Therapy

A number of applications for pacemaker therapy have been described for human patients with AF.[84] The most common indication is to prevent bradycardia in patients with concomitant conduction system abnormalities such as AVB (see Figure 9.11). AVB can also be caused purposely via radiocatheter ablation of the AV node, and this is followed by artificial ventricular pacing. This option provides effective ventricular rate control in patients who are refractory to medical treatment and are not eligible for other treatment options. However, it has the disadvantage of the need for permanent artificial pacing.

Other strategies include atrial or ventricular pacing. Pacing the ventricles at a rate that is near the mean heart rate of intrinsically conducted AF has been shown to contribute to a reduction in cycle length variability, leading to a more regular and better tolerated rhythm.[36] Atrial pacing is used in patients with paroxysmal AF in an attempt to prevent its onset. This is based on the fact that initiation of AF may occur with atrial premature complexes (APCs) and episodes of bradycardia or tachycardia. Atrial pacing algorithms are aimed at suppressing the APCs and reducing the dispersion of atrial refractoriness caused by bradycardia.

The use of these strategies for the treatment of AF has not been described in veterinary patients.

References

1 Patterson DF, Detweiler DK, Hubben K, Botts RP. Spontaneous abnormal cardiac arrhythmias and conduction disturbances in the dog: a clinical and pathologic study of 3,000 dogs. Am J Vet Res. 1961;22:355–369.

2 Buchanan JW. Spontaneous arrhythmias and conduction disturbances in domestic animals. Ann NY Acad Sci. 1965;127:224–238.

3 Cote E, Harpster NK, Laste NJ, MacDonald KA, Kittleson MD, Bond BR, *et al*. Atrial fibrillation in cats: 50 cases (1979–2002). J Am Vet Med Assoc. 2004;225:256–260.

4 Saunders A, Gordon S, Miller M. Canine atrial fibrillation. Compend Contin Educ Vet. 2009;31:E1–E9; quiz, E10.

5 Guglielmini C, Chetboul V, Pietra M, Pouchelon JL, Capucci A, Cipone M. Influence of left atrial enlargement and body weight on the development of atrial fibrillation: retrospective study on 205 dogs. Vet J. 2000;160:235–241.

6 Menaut P, Belanger MC, Beauchamp G, Ponzio NM, Moïse NS. Atrial fibrillation in dogs with and without structural or functional cardiac disease: a retrospective study of 109 cases. J Vet Cardiol. 2005;7:75–83.

7 Jung SW, Sun W, Griffiths LG, Kittleson MD. Atrial fibrillation as a prognostic indicator in medium to large-sized dogs with myxomatous mitral valvular degeneration and congestive heart failure. J Vet Intern Med. 2015;30:51–57.

8 Gelzer ARM, Kraus MS. Management of atrial fibrillation. Vet Clin North Am Small Anim Pract. 2004;34:1127–1144–vi.

9 Schotten U, Verheule S, Kirchhof P, Goette A. Pathophysiological mechanisms of atrial fibrillation: a translational appraisal. Physiol Rev. 2011;91:265–325.

10 Iwasaki Y-K, Nishida K, Kato T, Nattel S. Atrial fibrillation pathophysiology: implications for management. Circulation. 2011;124:2264–2274.

11 Brundel BJJM, Melnyk P, Rivard L, Nattel S. The pathology of atrial fibrillation in dogs. J Vet Cardiol. 2005;7:121–129.

12 Nattel S. New ideas about atrial fibrillation 50 years on. Nature. 2002;415:219–226.

13 Moore EN, Spear JF. Electrophysiological studies on atrial fibrillation. Heart Vessels. 1987;(Suppl 2):32–39.

14 Moe GK, Rheinboldt WC, Abildskov JA. A computer model of atrial fibrillation. Am Heart J. 1964;67:200–220.

15 Li D, Fareh S, Leung TK, Nattel S. Promotion of atrial fibrillation by heart failure in dogs: atrial remodeling of a different sort. Circulation. 1999;100:87–95.

16 Nattel S, Burstein B, Dobrev D. Atrial remodeling and atrial fibrillation: mechanisms and implications. Circ Arrhythm Electrophysiol. 2008;1:62–73.

17 Hocini M, Ho SY, Kawara T, Linnenbank AC, Potse M, Shah D, *et al*. Electrical conduction in canine pulmonary veins: electrophysiological and anatomic correlation. Circulation. 2002;105:2442–2448.

18 Vollmar C, Keene B, Kohn B, Vollmar A. Long term outcome of Irish Wolfhounds with lone atrial fibrillation. J Vet Int Med. 2015;29:C19.

19 De Jong AM, Maass AH, Oberdorf-Maass SU, Van Veldhuisen DJ, Van Gilst WH, Van Gelder IC. Mechanisms of atrial structural changes caused by stretch occurring before and during early atrial fibrillation. Cardiovasc Res. 2011;89:754–765.

20 Cardin S, Li D, Thorin-Trescases N, Leung T-K, Thorin E, Nattel S. Evolution of the atrial fibrillation substrate in experimental congestive heart failure: angiotensin-dependent and -independent pathways. Cardiovasc Res. 2003;60:315–325.

21 Li D, Melnyk P, Feng J, Wang Z, Petrecca K, Shrier A, *et al*. Effects of experimental heart failure on atrial cellular and ionic electrophysiology. Circulation. 2000;101:2631–2638.

22 Sun H, Gaspo R, Leblanc N, Nattel S. Cellular mechanisms of atrial contractile dysfunction caused by sustained atrial tachycardia. Circulation. 1998;98:719–727.

23 Wijffels MC, Kirchhof CJ, Dorland R, Allessie MA. Atrial fibrillation begets atrial fibrillation: a study in awake chronically instrumented goats. Circulation. 1995;92:1954–1968.

24 Ausma J, Litjens N, Lenders MH, Duimel H, Mast F, Wouters L, *et al*. Time course of atrial fibrillation-induced cellular structural remodeling in atria of the goat. J Mol Cell Cardiol. 2001;33:2083–2094.

25 Sharifov OF, Fedorov VV, Beloshapko GG, Glukhov AV, Yushmanova AV, Rosenshtraukh LV. Roles of adrenergic and cholinergic stimulation in spontaneous atrial fibrillation in dogs. J Am Coll Cardiol. 2004;43:483–490.

26 Ninomiya I. Direct evidence of nonuniform distribution of vagal effects on dog atria. Circ Res. 1966;19:576–583.

27 Alessi R, Nusynowitz M, Abildskov JA, Moe GK. Nonuniform distribution of vagal effects on the atrial refractory period. Am J Physiol. 1958;194:406–410.

28 Liu L, Nattel S. Differing sympathetic and vagal effects on atrial fibrillation in dogs: role of refractoriness heterogeneity. Am J Physiol. 1997;273:H805–H816.

29 Chen J, Wasmund SL, Hamdan MH. Back to the future: the role of the autonomic nervous system in atrial fibrillation. Pacing Clin Electrophysiol. 2006;29:413–421.

30 Langendorf R, Pick A. Ventricular response in atrial fibrillation: role of concealed conduction in the AV junction. Circulation. 1965;32:69–75.

31 Nagayoshi H, Janota T, Hnatkova K, Camm AJ, Malik M. Autonomic modulation of ventricular rate in atrial fibrillation. Am J Physiol. 1997;272:H1643–H1649.

32 Reid DS, Jachuck SJ, Henderson CB. Cardiac pacing in incomplete atrioventricular block with atrial fibrillation. Br Heart J. 1973;35:1154–1160.

33 van den Berg MP, van Gelder IC. Atrial fibrillation and sinus node dysfunction. J Am Coll Cardiol. 2001;38:1585–1586.

34 Ishida Y, Meisner JS, Tsujioka K, Gallo JI, Yoran C, Frater RW, *et al*. Left ventricular filling dynamics: influence of left ventricular relaxation and left atrial pressure. Circulation. 1986;74:187–196.

35 Gopinathannair R, Etheridge SP, Marchlinski FE, Spinale FG, Lakkireddy D, Olshansky B. Arrhythmia-induced cardiomyopathies: mechanisms, recognition, and management. J Am Coll Cardiol. 2015;66:1714–1728.

36 Barold SS. What is cardiac resynchronization therapy? Am J Med. 2001;111:224–232.

37 Usechak PJ, Bright JM, Day TK. Thrombotic complications associated with atrial fibrillation in three dogs. J Vet Cardiol. 2012;14:453–458.

38 Nishida K, Chiba K, Iwasaki Y-K, Katsouras G, Shi Y-F, Blostein MD, *et al*. Atrial fibrillation-associated remodeling does not promote atrial thrombus formation in canine models. Circ Arrhythm Electrophysiol. 2012;5:1168–1175.

39 Westling J, Westling W, Pyle RL. Epidemiology of atrial fibrillation in the dog. Intl J Appl Res Vet Med. 2008;6:151–154.

40 Tidholm A, Häggström J, Borgarelli M, Tarducci A. Canine idiopathic dilated cardiomyopathy. Part I: Aetiology, clinical characteristics, epidemiology and pathology. Vet J. 2001;162:92–107.

41 Vollmar AC. The prevalence of cardiomyopathy in the Irish wolfhound: a clinical study of 500 dogs. J Am Anim Hosp Assoc. 2000;36:125–132.

42 Brownlie SE, Cobb MA. Observations on the development of congestive heart failure in Irish

wolfhounds with dilated cardiomyopathy. J Small Anim Pract. 1999;40:371–377.

43 Calvert CA, Pickus CW, Jacobs GJ, Brown J. Signalment, survival, and prognostic factors in Doberman pinschers with end-stage cardiomyopathy. J Vet Intern Med. 1997;11:323–326.

44 Brownlie SE. An electrocardiographic survey of cardiac rhythm in Irish wolfhounds. Vet Rec. 1991;129:470–471.

45 Meurs KM, Miller MW, Wright NA. Clinical features of dilated cardiomyopathy in Great Danes and results of a pedigree analysis: 17 cases (1990–2000). J Am Vet Med Assoc. 2001;218:729–732.

46 Tarducci A, Borgarelli M, Zanatta R, Cagnasso A. Asymptomatic dilated cardiomyopathy in Great Danes: clinical, electrocardiographic, echocardiographic and echo-Doppler features. Vet Res Commun. 2003;27(Suppl 1):799–802.

47 Takemura N, Nakagawa K, Hirose H. Lone atrial fibrillation in a dog. J Vet Med Sci. 2002;64:1057–1059.

48 Connolly DJ. A case of sustained atrial fibrillation in a cat with a normal sized left atrium at the time of diagnosis. J Vet Cardiol. 2005;7:137–142.

49 Volders PGA, Zhu Q, Timmermans C, Eurlings PMH, Su X, Arens YH, *et al.* Mapping a novel locus for familial atrial fibrillation on chromosome 10p11-q21. Heart Rhythm. 2007;4:469–475.

50 Ishikawa T, Ohno S, Murakami T, Yoshida K, Mishima H, Fukuoka T, *et al.* Sick sinus syndrome with HCN4 mutations shows early onset and frequent association with atrial fibrillation and left ventricular noncompaction. Heart Rhythm. 2017;14:717–724.

51 Duhme N, Schweizer PA, Thomas D, Becker R, Schroter J, Barends TRM, *et al.* Altered HCN4 channel C-linker interaction is associated with familial tachycardia-bradycardia syndrome and atrial fibrillation. Eur Heart J. 2013;34:2768–2775.

52 Santilli RA, Perego M, Perini A, Moretti P, Spadacini G. Electrophysiologic characteristics and topographic distribution of focal atrial tachycardias in dogs. J Vet Intern Med. 2010;24:539–545.

53 Porteiro Vázquez DM, Perego M, Santos L, Gerou-Ferriani M, Martin MWS, Santilli RA. Paroxysmal atrial fibrillation in seven dogs with presumed neurally-mediated syncope. J Vet Cardiol. 2016;18:1–9.

54 Pariaut R, Moïse NS, Koetje BD, Flanders JA, Hemsley SA, Farver TB, *et al.* Evaluation of atrial fibrillation induced during anesthesia with fentanyl and pentobarbital in German Shepherd dogs with inherited arrhythmias. Am J Vet Res. 2008;69:1434–1445.

55 Penderis J. Chiari-like malformation: a substantive health and welfare problem in the Cavalier King Charles spaniel. Vet J. 2013;195:133–134.

56 Rasmussen CE, Falk T, Zois NE, Moesgaard SG, Häggström J, Pedersen HD, *et al.* Heart rate, heart rate variability, and arrhythmias in dogs with myxomatous mitral valve disease. J Vet Intern Med. 2012;26:76–84.

57 Brady WJ, Skiles J. Wide QRS complex tachycardia: ECG differential diagnosis. Am J Emerg Med. 1999;17:376–381.

58 Chenevert M, Lewis RJ. Ashman's phenomenon – a source of nonsustained wide-complex tachycardia: case report and discussion. J Emerg Med. 1992;10:179–183.

59 Harrigan RA, Garg M. An interesting cause of wide complex tachycardia: Ashman's phenomenon in atrial fibrillation. J Emerg Med. 2013;45:835–841.

60 Gatzoulis K, Carlson MD, Johnson NJ, Biblo LA, Waldo AL. Regular wide QRS complex tachycardia during atrial fibrillation in a patient with preexcitation syndrome: a case report. J Cardiovasc Electrophysiol. 1995;6:493–497.

61 Obeyesekere MN, Leong-Sit P, Massel D, Manlucu J, Krahn AD, Skanes AC, *et al.* Incidence of atrial fibrillation and prevalence of intermittent pre-excitation in asymptomatic Wolff-Parkinson-White patients: a meta-analysis. Int J Cardiol. 2012;160:75–77.

62 Gelzer AR, Kraus MS, Rishniw M. Evaluation of in-hospital electrocardiography versus 24-hour Holter for rate control in dogs with atrial fibrillation. J Small Anim Pract. 2015;56:456–462.

63 Miller RH, Lehmkuhl LB, Bonagura JD, Beall MJ. Retrospective analysis of the clinical utility of ambulatory electrocardiographic (Holter) recordings in syncopal dogs: 44 cases (1991–1995). J Vet Intern Med. 1999;13:111–122.

64 Wess G, Schulze A, Geraghty N, Hartmann K. Ability of a 5-minute electrocardiography (ECG) for predicting arrhythmias in Doberman Pinschers with cardiomyopathy in comparison with a 24-hour ambulatory ECG. J Vet Intern Med. 2010;24:367–371.

65 Pariaut R. Atrial fibrillation: current therapies. Vet Clin North Am Small Anim Pract. 2017;47:977–988.

66 Wyse DG, Waldo AL, DiMarco JP, Domanski MJ, Rosenberg Y, Schron EB, *et al.* A comparison of rate control and rhythm control in patients with atrial fibrillation. N Engl J Med. 2002;347:1825–1833.

67 van Gelder IC, Tuinenburg AE, Schoonderwoerd BS, Tieleman RG, Crijns HJ. Pharmacologic versus direct-current electrical cardioversion of atrial flutter and fibrillation. Am J Cardiol. 1999;84:147R–151R.

68 Bright JM, Martin JM, Mama KA retrospective evaluation of transthoracic biphasic electrical cardioversion for atrial fibrillation in dogs. J Vet Cardiol. 2005;7:85–96.

69 Bright JM, zumBrunnen J. Chronicity of atrial fibrillation affects duration of sinus rhythm after transthoracic cardioversion of dogs with naturally occurring atrial fibrillation. J Vet Intern Med. 2008;22:114–119.

70 Feld GK, Cha Y. Electrophysiologic effects of the new class III antiarrhythmic drug dofetilide in an experimental canine model of pacing-induced atrial fibrillation. J Cardiovasc Pharmacol Ther. 1997;2:195–203.

71 Madan BR, Pendse VK. Interaction of quinidine and propranolol in experimental cardiac arrhythmias in the dog. Arch Int Pharmacodyn Ther. 1977;225:287–293.

72 Pyle RL. Conversion of atrial fibrillation with quinidine sulfate in a dog. J Am Vet Med Assoc. 1967;151:582–589.

73 Oyama MA, Prosek R. Acute conversion of atrial fibrillation in two dogs by intravenous amiodarone administration. J Vet Intern Med. 2006;20:1224–1227.

74 Saunders AB, Miller MW, Gordon SG, Van De Wiele CM. Oral amiodarone therapy in dogs with atrial fibrillation. J Vet Intern Med. 2006;20:921–926.

75 Moïse NS, Pariaut R, Gelzer ARM, Kraus MS, Jung SW. Cardioversion with lidocaine of vagally associated atrial fibrillation in two dogs. J Vet Cardiol. 2005;7:143–148.

76 Kumagai K, Yamanouchi Y, Tashiro N, Hiroki T, Arakawa K. Low energy synchronous transcatheter cardioversion of atrial flutter/fibrillation in the dog. J Am Coll Cardiol. 1990;16:497–501.

77 Dunbar DN, Tobler HG, Fetter J, Gornick CC, Benson DWJ, Benditt DG. Intracavitary electrode catheter cardioversion of atrial tachyarrhythmias in the dog. J Am Coll Cardiol. 1986;7:1015–1027.

78 Sanders RA, Ralph AG, Olivier NB. Cardioversion of atrial fibrillation in a dog with structural heart disease using an esophageal-right atrial lead configuration. J Vet Cardiol. 2014;16:277–281.

79 Gelzer ARM, Kraus MS, Rishniw M, Moise NS, Pariaut R, Jesty SA, et al. Combination therapy with digoxin and diltiazem controls ventricular rate in chronic atrial fibrillation in dogs better than digoxin or diltiazem monotherapy: a randomized crossover study in 18 dogs. J Vet Intern Med. 2009;23:499–508.

80 Van Gelder IC, Van Veldhuisen DJ, Crijns HJGM, Tuininga YS, Tijssen JGP, Alings AM, et al. Rate control efficacy in permanent atrial fibrillation: a comparison between lenient versus strict rate control in patients with and without heart failure. Background, aims, and design of RACE II. Am Heart J. 2006;152:420–426.

81 Kotecha D, Piccini JP. Atrial fibrillation in heart failure: what should we do? Eur Heart J. 2015;36:3250–3257.

82 Verma A, Natale A. Should atrial fibrillation ablation be considered first-line therapy for some patients? Why atrial fibrillation ablation should be considered first-line therapy for some patients. Circulation. 2005;112:1214–1222, disc. 1231.

83 Ganesan AN, Shipp NJ, Brooks AG, Kuklik P, Lau DH, Lim HS, et al. Long-term outcomes of catheter ablation of atrial fibrillation: a systematic review and meta-analysis. J Am Heart Assoc. 2013;2:e004549.

84 Knight BP, Gersh BJ, Carlson MD, Friedman PA, McNamara RL, Strickberger SA, et al. Role of permanent pacing to prevent atrial fibrillation: science advisory from the American Heart Association Council on Clinical Cardiology (Subcommittee on Electrocardiography and Arrhythmias) and the Quality of Care and Outcomes Research Interdisciplinary Working Group, in collaboration with the Heart Rhythm Society. Circulation. 2005;111:240–243.

10

Junctional Rhythms
Pedro Oliveira

Introduction

In this chapter, we will discuss abnormal rhythms arising from the atrioventricular (AV) junction or atrioventricular node (AVN), as it is commonly known. This area is composed of the atrionodal bundles converging into the proximal AV bundle, the compact node and the distal AV bundle which includes the Bundle of His (see chapter 1). Ectopic junctional beats and rhythms, junctional tachycardia and rhythm disturbances caused by macro reentry circuits that involve the AVN and accessory pathways (APs; e.g. AV re-entrant tachycardia) will be discussed.

Junctional Ectopic Beats

As the name suggests, junctional ectopic beats arise from the junctional area. All three areas of the AVN possess cells that are capable of spontaneous depolarisation similar to the P cells in the sinus node.[1-3] Ectopic beats may arise from any of these areas, and the appearance of the electrocardiogram (ECG) will differ with respect to the position of the P' wave in relation to the QRS (Figure 10.1). If the ectopic beat originates in the atrionodal bundles or proximal AV bundle, the depolarisation wave will still need to travel through the compact node to reach the ventricles and will suffer the normal physiologic delay across this area. In the meantime, the atria will be depolarised retrogradely before the impulse reaches the ventricles. As a result, the P' wave will appear before the QRS with either a normal or a short P'R interval (Figure 10.1A). If the ectopic beat originates in the compact node itself, atrial and ventricular depolarisation will occur roughly at the same time, and the P' wave will be buried in the QRS (Figure 10.1B). This is a common presentation of junctional ectopic beats or rhythms.

Lastly, if the ectopic beat arises from the distal AV bundle, the depolarisation wave will have to travel up the compact node before it reaches the atrial side, suffering delay. The atrial depolarisation will occur after ventricular depolarisation, and a P' wave will be seen after the QRS, commonly in the descending R or ST segment (Figure 10.1C).

The appearance of the P' wave is the other important clue pointing to the origin of ectopic beats in the junctional area. Given its location in the central fibrous body (see chapter 1), atrial activation will occur in a retrograde fashion with a P' electrical axis between −80 to −100° (Figure 10.2). On the ECG, it will appear as a negative wave in leads II, III and aVF and positive in leads aVL and aVR (Figure 10.2).

Classification

As described for atrial ectopic beats, junctional ectopic beats may be *premature* (P-P' < P-P) (Figure 10.3) or *escape beats* if they occur after a sinus pause (P-P' > P-P)[4] (Figure 10.4). Junctional premature beats are often referred to as *junctional premature complexes* or *contractions* (JPCs). The term JPC will be used throughout this chapter.

Non-compensatory or *compensatory pauses* may be seen after a JPC, as described for atrial premature beats (see Box 8.2), depending on whether the atrial depolarisation wave is able to reset the sinus node or not, respectively (Figure 10.3). If a pause is not present after the premature beat, it is described as an *interpolated beat* (Figure 10.3).

Ectopic beats can occur in an isolated fashion or may appear in more organized forms such as *bigeminy*, *trigeminy* or *quadrigeminy*. A sequence of two consecutive ectopic beats is a *couplet* and of three consecutive beats is a *triplet*.

Guide to Canine and Feline Electrocardiography, First Edition. Ruth Willis, Pedro Oliveira and Antonia Mavropoulou.
© 2018 John Wiley & Sons Ltd. Published 2018 by John Wiley & Sons Ltd.
Companion website: www.wiley.com/go/willis/electrocardiography

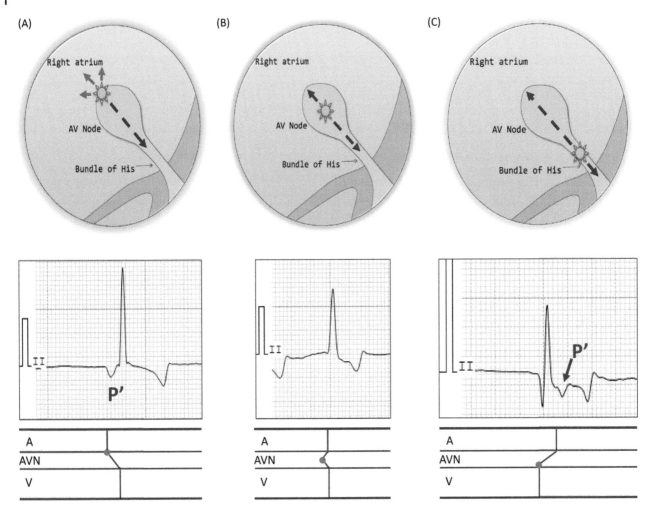

Figure 10.1 Position of the P' wave in relation to the QRS in junctional ectopic beats originating from different areas of the junctional region. (A) The impulse originates from the atrionodal bundles or proximal AVB activating the atria before the ventricles, as the impulse still needs to travel through the AVN suffering delay. As a result, an ectopic P' is seen with a concentric retrograde activation pattern just before the QRS and with a short P'R. (B) The impulse originates from within the AVN itself, causing atrial and ventricular activation to occur simultaneously. An ectopic P' is not seen, as it is buried within the QRS. (C) The impulse originates from the distal AVB, and since it needs to travel through the AVN retrogradely, the impulse reaches the ventricles first and then the atria. As a result, an ectopic P' is seen at the end of the QRS or ST segment. The P' axis is also consistent with concentric retrograde atrial activation.

Junctional Rhythms

If more than three consecutive junctional ectopic beats occur, this is described as a *junctional rhythm* or *tachycardia* depending on the heart rate (Figures 10.5 and 10.6). Additionally, if this occurs due to activity of a subsidiary pacemaker during bradycardia (e.g. abnormal sinus node function or AV block), the term *junctional escape rhythm* is used.[4] In dogs with an experimentally induced junctional rhythm, a spontaneous depolarisation rate of approximately 54–112 bpm has been described.[5] This is consistent with the clinical findings in dogs with junctional escape rhythm that typically present a heart rate of approximately 40–60 bpm[6] (Figure 10.7). A junctional rhythm with a depolarisation rate above 100 bpm would normally be considered

tachycardia in this species. In cats, a junctional escape rhythm (narrow QRS) with a heart rate of 110 to 140 bpm is commonly seen. This is consistent with the results of a retrospective study in cats with AV block that found escape rates of 100–140 bpm with both narrow and wide-QRS complexes, but frequently above 120 bpm if the QRS was narrow.[7]

Junctional Tachycardia

Junctional tachycardia is a unique type of supraventricular arrhythmia defined by a narrow-QRS complex and atrioventricular (AV) dissociation or retrograde atrial conduction in a 1:1 pattern. In human medicine, several terms have been used to describe this rhythm disturbance, such as junctional ectopic tachycardia (JET)

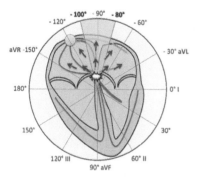

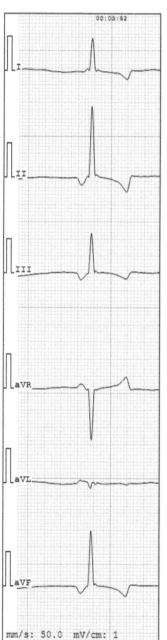

Figure 10.2 Appearance of the P' wave of junctional ectopic beats. The P' is negative in leads II, III and aVF, and positive in leads aVR and aVF. The P' axis is approximately −90°. In this example, the PR is also short at 60 ms.

and automatic junctional tachycardia (AJT), the latter implying that the dominant mechanism is abnormal automaticity.[8] However, other arrhythmia mechanisms are also possible, and therefore the term *focal junctional tachycardia* (FJT) is preferred.[8] FJT is driven by an ectopic focus within or immediately adjacent to the AV junction of the cardiac conduction system. It may occur in the setting of a structurally normal heart (idiopathic) or as a consequence of cardiac surgery to repair congenital defects. This rhythm disturbance has been reported in dogs, particularly in young Labrador Retrievers.[9,10] A non-paroxysmal form of junctional tachycardia may also occur and is briefly discussed in this chapter.

Focal Junctional Tachycardia
Electrocardiographic Features

This arrhythmia is characterized by a narrow-QRS complex tachycardia with a heart rate in dogs of 100–180 bpm or higher (Table 10.1).[11] Isorhythmic AV dissociation (discussed here) is often present, although occasional 1:1 retrograde ventriculo-atrial conduction may be observed.[8,12] Incessant forms of FJT can lead to tachycardia-induced cardiomyopathy.

Isorhythmic Atrioventricular Dissociation

The term *isorhythmic atrioventricular dissociation* (IAVD) indicates the presence of two rhythms (a sinus and an ectopic rhythm) that coexist and show some degree of synchronization (have similar discharge rates). On the ECG, this is seen as normal P waves that are not associated with the QRS; the P-P and R-R intervals are similar, but the PR interval varies. When the two rhythms synchronize for only brief periods of time and then resume their original discharge rates, the term *accrochage* is used.[13,14] If the two rhythms maintain similar discharge rates for longer periods, the term *synchronization* is used instead.[13–15]

Two types of synchronization may occur:

Type 1: A rhythmic variation of the sinus P wave position is seen in relation to the QRS. It is often seen moving closer to and then away from the QRS. Occasionally, the P wave might move into and get buried within the QRS complex, only to move back out again in front of the QRS in the subsequent beats (Figure 10.8). The explanation for type 1 synchronization is based on cyclical variations of the parasympathetic and sympathetic tone influenced by the baroreceptor reflex.[16–20] When the P wave is closer to or buried within the QRS, the contribution of atrial contraction to ventricular filling is lost, causing a slight drop in stroke volume and blood pressure. This will cause a reflex increase in sympathetic stimulation of the sinus node, increasing its discharge rate. As a

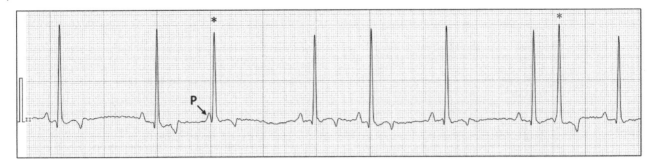

Figure 10.3 Junctional premature complex. The underlying rhythm is respiratory sinus arrhythmia. A junctional premature complex (red *) is seen, followed by a post-extrasystolic pause; the sinus P wave may be seen almost buried within the QRS of the premature beat, supporting the fact that this is indeed a junctional ectopic beat rather than an atrial ectopic one. Another junctional premature complex (blue *) may be seen at the end of the trace without a post-extrasystolic pause; this was an interpolated ectopic beat. [4-year-old, female neutered, Labrador Retriever without obvious structural disease] (50 mm/s; 20 mm/mV)

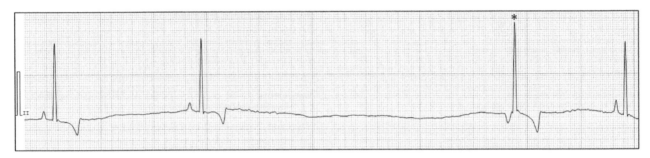

Figure 10.4 Junctional escape beat. The underlying rhythm is sinus bradycardia. A junctional escape beat (*) is seen after a sinus pause, characterized by a narrow QRS, a negative P' and a short P'R. [11-year-old, female neutered, West Highland White Terrier with sinus node dysfunction] (50 mm/s; 20 mm/mV)

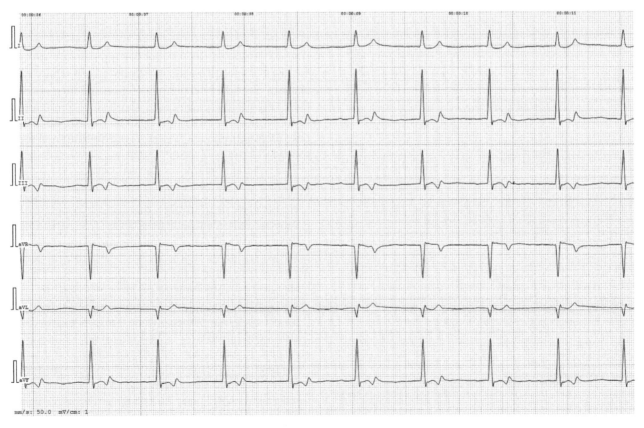

Figure 10.5 Junctional rhythm. A narrow-QRS rhythm is seen with a rate ≈ 96 bpm. A P wave is not seen preceding the QRS, suggesting a junctional ectopic rhythm. [1-year-old, male Beagle dog with myocarditis] (50 mm/s; 10 mm/mV)

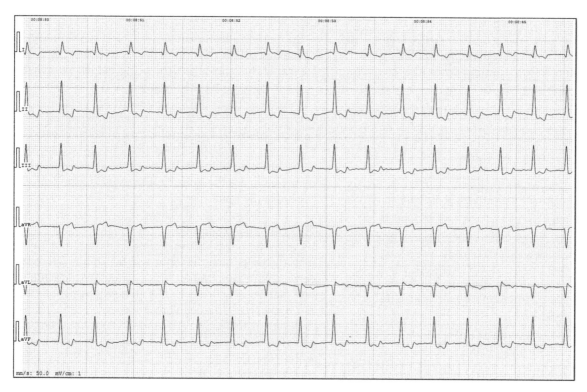

Figure 10.6 Junctional tachycardia. A narrow-QRS rhythm is seen with a rate ≈ 180 bpm. A P wave is not seen preceding the QRS, suggesting a junctional ectopic rhythm that at this rate is considered tachycardia (>100 bpm). Alternatively, a ventricular rhythm originating high in the His–Purkinje could also be possible, with ventricular activation still occurring via the normal conduction system. [10-year-old, female neutered, Labrador Retriever with suspicion of arrhythmia-induced cardiomyopathy] (50 mm/s; 10 mm/mV)

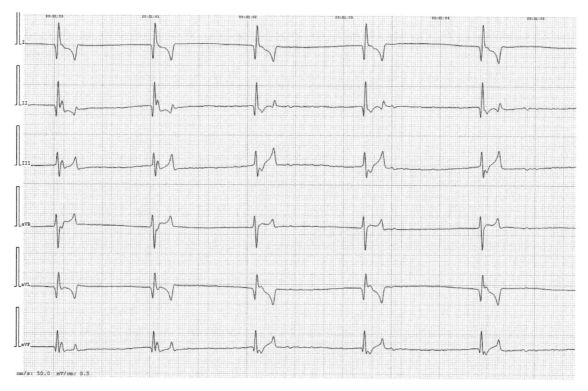

Figure 10.7 Junctional escape rhythm. This electrocardiogram was recorded from a dog with sick sinus syndrome and a junctional escape rhythm during periods of sinus bradycardia or arrest. A narrow-QRS rhythm is seen with a rate ≈ 60 bpm, consistent with a junctional escape rhythm. On the third to fifth beats, a P wave is not seen preceding the QRS, and instead, a small wave is seen buried in the ST segment consistent with concentric retrograde atrial activation (P'). On the first two beats, a sinus P wave is seen on the descending limb of the R wave, suggesting two competing rhythms: sinus and junctional. [9-year-old, female neutered, West Highland White Terrier with sick sinus syndrome] (50 mm/s; 20 mm/mV)

consequence, the P wave will move out of the QRS. Once this occurs, an increase in stroke volume and blood pressure will have the opposite effect via the baroreceptor reflex, slowing down the sinus rate again, and the cycle will start over.

Table 10.1 Focal junctional tachycardia

Rate	Dog: often <180 bpm Cat: not reported, likely above 140 bpm
Regularity	Regular
Onset/offset	Gradual increase (warm-up) and decrease (cool-down) in heart rate
P or P' wave	Sinus P wave present with IAVD *or* retrograde concentric P' (−80° to −100° axis) in ST segment during ventriculo-atrial conduction 1:1
P':QRS ratio	Absent
PR and RP	Variable in type 1 IAVD Fixed in type 2 IAVD
QRS	Normal

Type 2: The relationship between P and QRS is fixed, and the rhythmic fluctuation seen in type 1 synchronization does not occur. The P wave may precede the QRS complex, may coincide with it being hidden or may be superimposed on the ST segment or the first half of the T wave[19] (Figure 10.9). The underlying mechanism for type 2 synchronization is unclear. A hypothesis supports the existence of an electrical interaction between the two pacemakers.[21] Another hypothesis suggests that the mechanical pulsation of the sinus node artery may influence the sinus P cells to synchronize with the ectopic rhythm.[22]

Ventriculo-atrial Conduction
If the discharge rate of the ectopic focus becomes higher than the sinus rate, the latter will be suppressed (over-drive suppression), and a 1:1 ventriculo-atrial conduction pattern may be seen. The atria will be depolarised retrogradely by the depolarisation wave originating in the junctional area. A retrograde P' (axis between −80° to −100°, as discussed in this chapter) may be buried within the QRS or may be seen in the ST segment (Figure 10.10).

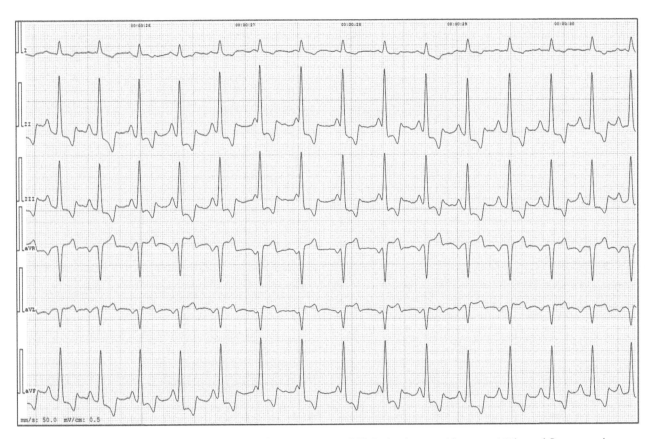

Figure 10.8 Isorhythmic atrioventricular dissociation of type 1. A narrow-QRS rhythm is seen with a rate ≈ 160 bpm. A P wave can be seen before each QRS with a PR interval that is progressively shorter until the P is slightly buried in the QRS and then longer again. This suggests that the atria and ventricles are dissociated (P does not cause QRS) but are synchronized with similar rates. The atrial depolarisation is caused by the normal sinus rhythm, and the ventricular activation is the result of an ectopic junctional rhythm with a rate that is similar to the sinus rhythm. [12-year-old, male Labrador Retriever with suspicion of myocarditis] (50 mm/s; 20 mm/mV)

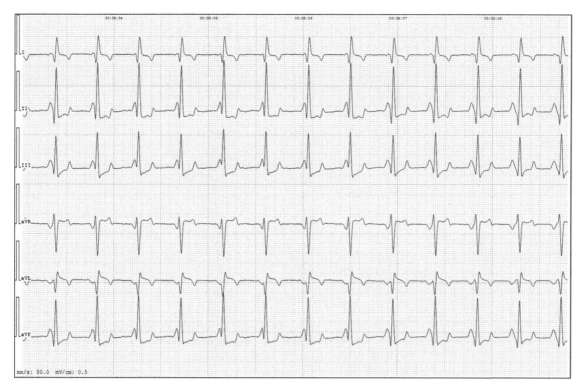

Figure 10.9 Isorhythmic atrioventricular dissociation of type 2. A narrow-QRS rhythm is seen with a rate ≈ 140 bpm. A P wave can be seen before each QRS with a very short and slightly variable PR interval. This suggests that the atria and ventricles are dissociated (P does not cause QRS) but are synchronized with very similar rates. The P wave appears at a relatively fixed position in relation to the QRS, in contrast with the example in Figure 10.8. [13-year-old, male neutered, Labrador Retriever with suspicion of dilated cardiomyopathy] (50 mm/s; 20 mm/mV)

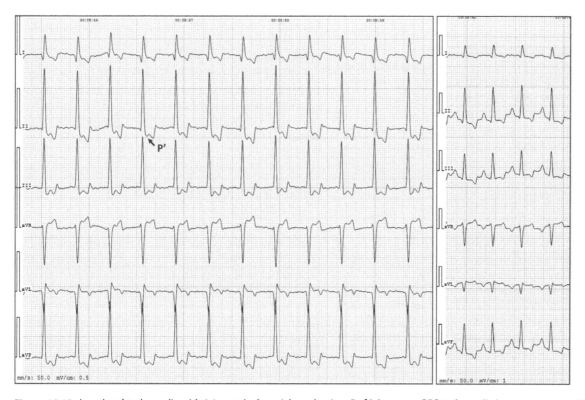

Figure 10.10 Junctional tachycardia with 1:1 ventriculo-atrial conduction. (Left) A narrow-QRS tachycardia is seen at a rate ≈ 160 bpm. (50 mm/s; 20 mm/mV) P waves are not visible before each QRS, suggesting a junctional tachycardia originating from the AVN or distal AV bundle. Instead, small waves can be seen buried in the ST segment (arrow), consistent with a concentric retrograde atrial activation pattern (P'). These can be seen after each beat, indicating a 1:1 ventriculo-atrial conduction. (Right) Appearance of the ST segment of this dog during sinus rhythm can be seen for comparison. (50 mm/s; 10 mm/mV) These findings suggest a junctional tachycardia originating from the distal AV bundle. [12-year-old, female neutered, Labrador Retriever with suspicion of myocardial disease/myocarditis]

QRS

Given that ventricular activation occurs via the normal conduction pathways (bundle branches), the QRS complex is expected to be similar to the QRS of the sinus beats. Normally, it is normal in both appearance and duration (<70 ms in dogs and <40 ms in cats) unless aberrancy or bundle branch block is present.

Onset and Offset

Onset and offset of FJT are normally gradual, with a warm-up and cool-down period.

Non-paroxysmal Junctional Tachycardia

This arrhythmia usually begins as an accelerated junctional rhythm, and the heart rate gradually increases to above 100 bpm. A typical 'warm-up' and 'cool-down' pattern is seen on the ECG. The underlying mechanism is thought to be enhanced automaticity of a junctional focus or triggered activity.[8,23] In humans, it is considered a benign arrhythmia, although it can also signal the presence of serious underlying disease such as digitalis toxicity, severe systemic disease and myocardial ischemia.[8] In our patients, non-paroxysmal junctional tachycardia is occasionally seen, although it is not well described. In the author's experience, this may be seen in young Labrador Retrievers, and, as in humans, it tends to be benign in most cases.

Treatment

Anti-arrhythmic therapy is used with the aim of controlling the ventricular rate. The decision to treat will depend on the presence of associated clinical signs or an elevated average heart rate over 24 h (Holter) and the perceived risk of arrhythmia-induced cardiomyopathy. Ideally, suppression of the ectopic focus would be achieved, but this may prove difficult. In cases of extracardiac disease, appropriate management should be prioritized, including the correction of any underlying abnormalities (e.g. electrolyte imbalances).

Medical Treatment

Class I, II and III anti-arrhythmics may be effective in these cases, although drug therapy is not always successful. In humans, β-blockers are often used as first-line treatment but are seldomly effective in achieving appropriate rate control.[24,25] Varying degrees of success were reported with digoxin, magnesium, intravenous procainamide, amiodarone, amiodarone combined with ivabradine, flecainide, propafenone and sotalol.[24,26–28]

In dogs, long-term administration of amiodarone, particularly to a young dog, is not desirable due to the risk of adverse side effects. Sotalol can be used instead with relatively good results in the author's experience. Propranolol, atenolol or metoprolol may also be effective.

Class IV anti-arrhythmics (calcium channel blockers) may be effective if the underlying arrhythmia mechanism is enhanced automaticity or if the ectopic focus is located above the compact node.[23]

Radiocatheter Ablation

Radiocatheter ablation is used in human patients when medical treatment fails.[24,29] This includes two different approaches: (1) ablation of the ectopic focus, preserving AV function; and (2) as a last resort, ablation of the AV node and placement of a pacemaker. Unfortunately, mapping the ectopic focus is challenging, as arrhythmias due to abnormal automaticity are not amenable to entraining with pacing techniques. Modern navigation systems are used to plot the entire His bundle and mark the spot of earliest retrograde conduction during tachycardia, which is later empirically ablated during sinus rhythm. The risk of AV block and subsequent need for a pacemaker associated with this approach has been reported at 5–10%.[24] In veterinary medicine, these techniques are not widely available, although this may change in the future. Ablation of the AV node followed by artificial pacing has been used to successfully manage atrial and junctional tachycardias in dogs.

Monitoring

Effective monitoring in these patients requires periodic Holter recordings, ideally every 6 months. It is particularly important that a 24 h Holter recording be obtained after any treatment change, as this is the only reliable way to assess its efficacy. This is usually done 10–20 days later. Echocardiography should also be used as necessary to assess for structural changes and underlying disease if present.

Atrioventricular Reciprocating Tachycardia

Atrioventricular reciprocating tachycardia (AVRT) is caused by a macro re-entrant circuit involving the AVN, the atrial and ventricular myocardium, and an AP. Normally, the AVN is the only point of electrical communication between the atria and the ventricles, but in some patients one or more points of communication may exist via APs. These are the result of a congenital malformation in which one or more strands of muscle fail to regress during the formation of the fibrous skeleton of the heart and connect the atrial and ventricular myocardium directly. They were first described by Albert Kent in 1893,[30] which is why some authors still use the term *bundles of Kent* when referring to APs. One or more APs may be present in the same patient.

Accessory Pathways

Anatomical Properties

As mentioned in this chapter, APs are aberrant muscle bundles that connect the atrium to the ventricle outside the regular AV conduction system.[31] They are found most often in the AV junctional areas, breaching the insulation provided by the fibrofatty tissues of the AV groove and the fibrous annulus of the AV valves. Histologically, most pathways are composed of working myocardium, although APs containing specialized cells have been described in humans.[32] Regardless of the type of myocyte present, normal gap junctions were identified, arranged in a pattern suggestive of working ventricular myocardium.[33]

Location

Depending on their location around the tricuspid and mitral annulus, APs are divided into right (cranial, lateral and caudal), septal (cranial, mid- and caudal) and left (cranial, lateral and caudal) pathways (Figure 10.11).

In dogs, APs have been described more commonly around the tricuspid annulus, with most patients having only a single pathway.[34–37]

Conduction Properties

Conduction through an AP may be anterograde (from atrium to ventricle) or retrograde (from ventricle to atrium). In humans, most APs are capable of bidirectional conduction.[38,39] In dogs, one report suggested that most APs (11/15) were only capable of retrograde conduction, with the remaining (4/15) being capable of bidirectional conduction.[40]

The conduction properties of APs differ from the normal electrical conduction system (e.g. AVN–His–Purkinje),

and this is important when considering how the macro re-entrant circuit is formed in AVRT. Most APs exhibit fast and non-decremental conduction properties (no decrease in conduction velocity along the pathway in response to repetitive stimuli), in contrast to the AVN.[41] Additionally, the velocity of conduction does not change with the heart rate as it does in the normal conduction system, which means that impulses will travel at the same velocity through an AP regardless of autonomic tone and heart rate variations. Exceptions have been described in humans with APs that exhibit slow and decremental conduction properties (progressive decrease in conduction velocity along the pathway in response to increasing prematurity of repetitive stimuli).[41,42] These are uncommon and, to the best of the author's knowledge, have not been described in dogs or cats to date. Another important aspect is that the refractory period of an AP is normally longer than the AVN, making it possible for a premature impulse to induce AVRT (see discussion in this chapter on AVRT re-entry circuits).

Pre-excitation

With an AP capable of anterograde conduction, a phenomenon called *ventricular pre-excitation* may occur (Figures 10.12 and 10.13 and Table 10.2).[43,44] Under normal circumstances, an atrial impulse reaches the AP and AVN almost simultaneously. Whilst the impulse traveling through the AVN is subjected to the normal conduction delay, the impulse moving though the AP is not and reaches the ventricular side sooner, causing early ventricular depolarisation – *pre-excitation*. Conduction through the pre-excited ventricular myocardium is slow, as it occurs via cell-to-cell transmission in contrast to the AVN–His–Purkinje system. For this reason, once the impulse travelling through the AVN reaches the ventricular side

Figure 10.11 Anatomical location of accessory pathways in dogs. The designation used in human medicine is also included, as it has been used in several veterinary publications. AV, Aortic valve; AVN, atrioventricular node; PV, pulmonic valve.

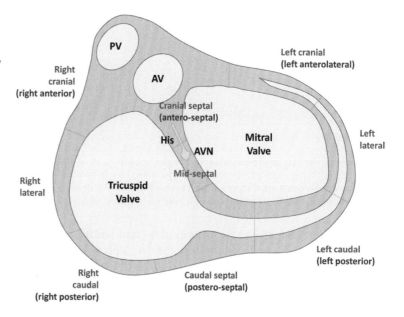

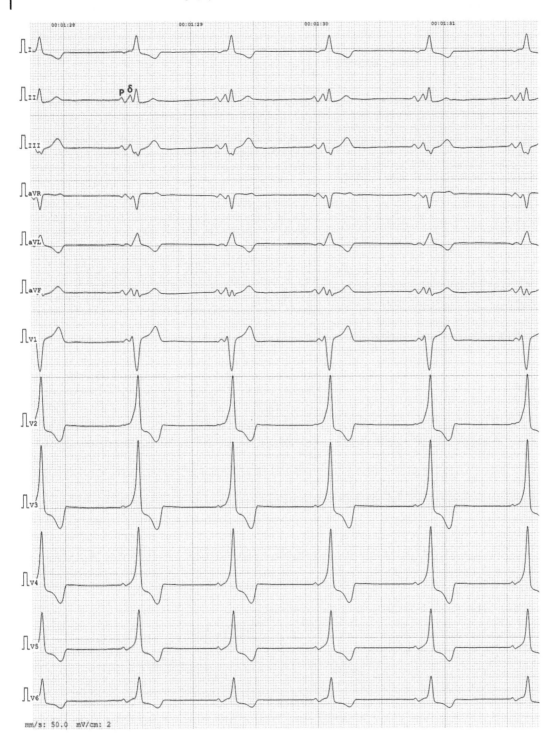

Figure 10.12 Ventricular pre-excitation on the electrocardiogram. A wide-QRS rhythm is seen with a rate of 80 bpm. A P wave is visible before each QRS with a short PR interval and is followed by a delta wave (δ) that is most visible in leads II, III, aVR, avL and aVF in this case. The PR interval is constant, distinguishing it from idioventricular rhythm with atrioventricular dissociation (see chapter 11). [8-year-old, female neutered, Labrador Retriever; OAVRT confirmed with EP study] (50 mm/s; 5 mm/mV)

and is quickly transmitted to the majority of the ventricular myocardium via the conduction system, the two depolarisation waves collide and merge. On the ECG, this is seen as a shorter PQ interval with an initial wave – *delta* (δ) *wave* – that gives the QRS a wide and bizarre appearance (Figure 10.13). The δ wave is the result of early depolarisation

of ventricular myocardium via the AP, and its amplitude and duration are proportional to the extent of myocardium depolarised before the rapid depolarisation wave front from the AVN–His–Purkinje collides with it (Figure 10.13). Since ventricular depolarisation does not occur in a normal fashion with pre-excitation, repolarisation is also affected. On the ECG, this is seen as either ST segment depression or elevation and asymmetric T waves with an opposite polarity to that of the δ wave (Figure 10.12).

The occurrence of pre-excitation depends on the velocity of conduction of the electrical impulse and refractoriness of the atrial tissue and AP relative to the AVN.[44] This may change in response to autonomic tone or drugs; for this reason, pre-excitation may be intermittent, or various degrees of pre-excitation may be seen in the same patient. It is particularly common for pre-excitation to become apparent only after drugs such as sotalol are used to treat tachycardia. The location of the

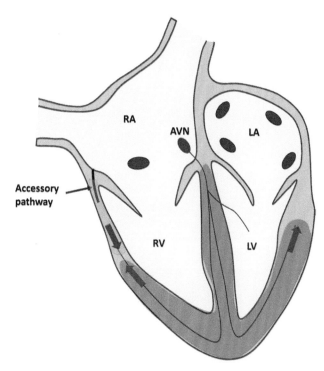

Figure 10.13 Ventricular activation during pre-excitation. The green arrow/area represents antegrade ventricular depolarisation via the accessory pathway, and the red arrows/area represent ventricular depolarisation via the normal conduction system. The two depolarisation waves eventually collide and merge. Depending on the proportion of ventricle activated anterogradely via the AP, the resulting QRS will be wider or narrower, similar to what happens with fusion beats caused by ventricular ectopic depolarisations (see chapter 11).

AP is also important for pre-excitation.[38,45] For example, left-sided APs are more distant from the sinus node than right-sided APs, and as it takes longer for the atrial impulse to reach the AP, the degree of pre-excitation may be very low or non-existent. The refractory period of APs located in the left free wall has also been shown to be lower in comparison to APs in the septal or right free wall.[38]

Identification of pre-excitation strongly suggests the presence of an AP. If the pathway is only capable of retrograde conduction, it is said to be *concealed*.

Lown–Ganong–Levine Syndrome

In 1952, Lown, Ganong and Levine described a clinical syndrome (LGL) characterized by paroxysms of tachycardia and electrocardiographic findings of a short PR interval and a normal QRS duration that had already been identified 15 years earlier by Clerc and colleagues.[46,47] The presence of pathways connecting the atrial tissue to the bundle of His, bypassing the AVN, were proposed to explain these findings.[48–52] Alternatively, enhanced AVN conduction (faster than normal) was also suggested as a possible explanation.[53] Subsequent findings based on electrophysiology and histopathologic studies revealed that several mechanisms could account for the presence of a short PR interval and a normal QRS duration, including enhanced conduction through the AVN, several types of fibres that bypass all or part of the AVN, and an anatomically small AVN. The accompanying episodes of tachycardia documented in these cases have been identified as concomitant supraventricular (e.g. atrioventricular nodal reciprocating tachycardia [AVNRT], AVRT, atrial fibrillation and atrial flutter) or ventricular tachycardias. For these reasons, LGL is no longer considered a clinical syndrome but rather the presence of concomitant abnormalities in the same patient causing tachycardia episodes, a short PR interval and normal QRS. To the best of the author's knowledge, LGL has not been described in dogs or cats. However, in Figure 10.14, an example of a case presenting all the diagnostic criteria for LGL may be seen, suggesting that it may occur in our patients.

Table 10.2 Pre-excitation

Pre-excitation		Differential diagnoses
Short PR	Dogs <60 ms Cats <50 ms	1) Atrial or junctional rhythm with a short P'R and bundle branch block
δ wave	Deflection in the beginning of QRS	2) Ventricular rhythm with sinus P waves that happen to fall before the QRS with an apparent short P'R
Wide QRS	Dogs >70 ms Cats >40 ms	3) Junctional rhythm with isorhythmic AV dissociation (type II)
		4) Splintered QRS (wide-QRS complex – see chapter 4)
ST and T wave	ST elevation or depression T wave polarity opposite the δ wave	

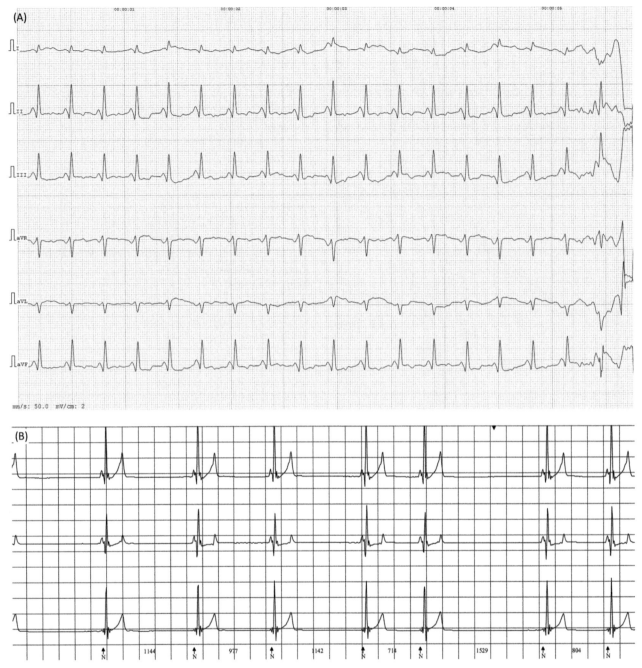

Figure 10.14 Suspicion of Lown–Ganong–Levine in a dog. (A) A narrow-QRS rhythm is seen with a rate of ≈ 200 bpm. The QRS is normal in duration and appearance (50–60 ms; MEA, 85°), as is the P wave (40 ms; P axis, 76°), but the PR interval is non-existent. The most likely differential diagnoses for this finding would be a junctional tachycardia with isorhythmic atrioventricular dissociation of type 2, or a pre-excited sinus/atrial rhythm, although some degree of QRS prolongation would be expected with the latter. Alternatively, it is possible that conduction through the atrioventricular node is abnormally fast or that an accessory pathway exists connecting the atrial tissues directly to the conduction system beneath the atrioventricular node (e.g. His bundle), allowing the impulse to bypass this structure completely. In this case, the latter was suspected as the PR duration was always constant during tachycardia and bradycardia, as shown during a 24 h Holter monitor suggesting a sinus rhythm without conduction delay through the atrioventricular node. This dog was asymptomatic, and this was an incidental finding during a pre-anaesthetic assessment. Although an electrophysiological study was offered to the client, it was not performed as the dog was not showing any referable clinical signs; as a result, a definitive rhythm diagnosis has not been obtained in this case. (B) Example of the rhythm in the same dog during bradycardia (59 bpm) whilst wearing the Holter monitor. [9-year-old, male neutered, Cocker Spaniel]

Prevalence and Clinical Significance

In dogs, APs have been described more commonly in the Labrador Retriever and Boxer and may be associated with other congenital defects such as tricuspid dysplasia, atrial septal defect and pulmonic stenosis.[54–57] In cats, a higher prevalence has been reported in the American shorthair with a concomitant primary cardiomyopathy.[57]

Clinical signs vary depending on the presence, rate and duration of tachycardia. Episodes of lethargy often accompanied by panting, weakness and collapse are the most common complaints in cases experiencing acute episodes of tachycardia. More prolonged tachycardia may result in tachycardia-induced cardiomyopathy with myocardial dysfunction and congestive heart failure.[35,36,58]

The clinical significance of APs extends beyond AVRT. The presence of an AP capable of anterograde conduction may lead to excessively elevated heart rates in patients with other supraventricular tachycardias, such as atrial tachycardia and atrial fibrillation, by allowing atrial impulses to reach the ventricles without being filtered by the AVN.

Macro Re-entry Circuits in AVRT

The re-entry circuit in AVRT is formed from the atrial myocardium, the AVN, the ventricular myocardium and the AP. Depending on the direction of the electrical impulse, it may be divided into *orthodromic AVRT* or *antidromic AVRT* (Figure 10.15).

Orthodromic AVRT (OAVRT)

This is the most common type of AVRT. The impulse travels down the AVN–His–Purkinje to the ventricles and retrogradely back to the atria via the AP. The direction of the impulse within the re-entry circuit is clockwise. On the ECG, a narrow-QRS tachycardia is seen (Figure 10.16). A P wave resulting from retrograde conduction to the atria may be seen on the descending segment of the R wave or the ST segment, although this often proves difficult, particularly at higher rates.

Initiation and Cessation

OAVRT may be initiated by either a premature atrial or ventricular beat. A premature atrial beat may reach the AP while it is still refractory and unable to conduct anterogradely; therefore, it is effectively blocked. However, it is conducted to the ventricles via the AVN–His–Purkinje, and, by the time it reaches the ventricular side of the AP, retrograde conduction may now be possible, triggering OAVRT. Less commonly, a premature ventricular beat may be conducted retrogradely via the AP whilst being blocked via the Purkinje–His–AVN; by the time the depolarisation wave reaches the AVN via the atrial side, anterograde conduction may be possible, initiating OAVRT (Figure 10.17).

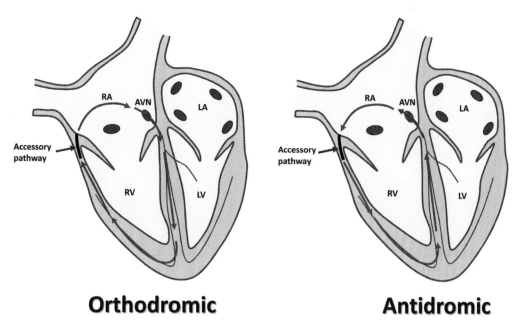

Orthodromic   **Antidromic**

Figure 10.15 Macro re-entry circuit in atrioventricular reciprocating tachycardia (AVRT). In orthodromic AVRT, the impulse travels down the AVN and normal conduction system, activating the ventricles in a normal fashion, and then travels back to the atria retrogradely via the accessory pathway, causing eccentric retrograde atrial activation and reaching the AVN again for another cycle. In antidromic AVRT, the impulse travels down the accessory pathway anterogradely, activates the ventricles slowly via the working myocardium and then travels back up the conduction system to reach the atria retrogradely via the AVN, causing concentric retrograde atrial activation before it reaches the AP again.

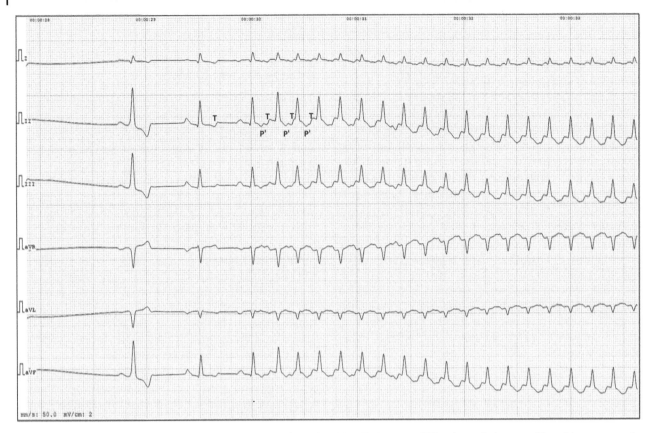

Figure 10.16 Orthodromic atrioventricular reciprocating tachycardia (OAVRT). A narrow-QRS tachycardia is seen with sudden onset and a rate of ≈ 280 bpm. A P' wave caused by retrograde atrial activation may be seen in the ST segment during tachycardia and after the last sinus beat before tachycardia initiation. It is useful to compare the ST segment during tachycardia with sinus beats (the first three beats) to identify the P' wave. In this example, we can see that this wave is not present in the first two beats. Additionally, the first beat is pre-excited (shorter PR and wide QRS), adding more evidence to the presence of an AP. [10-month-old, male Labrador Retriever; OAVRT confirmed with EP study] (50 mm/s; 5 mm/mV)

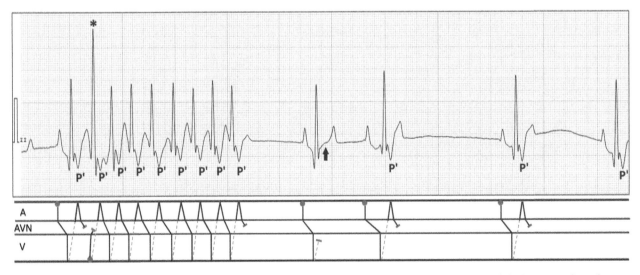

Figure 10.17 Initiation of OAVRT. A premature ventricular ectopic depolarisation (*) is blocked at the AVN whilst being conducted retrogradely via the AP (dotted line); by the time the retrograde atrial depolarisation wave reaches the AVN, it has had time to recover and is able to allow anterograde conduction again; the impulse is allowed to proceed to the ventricles and back to the atria again retrogradely via the AP, effectively initiating OAVRT. Retroconducted P' waves are also seen after beats 1, 11, 12 and 13 without initiation of OAVRT, as the retrograde atrial depolarisation wave is blocked at the AVN anterogradely. A retrograde P' is not seen in beat 10 (arrow). [10-month-old, male Staffordshire Terrier; OAVRT confirmed with EP study]

Cessation may occur spontaneously due to block at either the AVN (anterograde) or the AP (retrograde), or it may occur with premature atrial or ventricular depolarisations that are able to reset the re-entrant circuit. A precordial thump may achieve the same result by inducing a ventricular ectopic depolarisation (Figure 10.18).

Initiation and cessation of OAVRT are always sudden.

Electrocardiographic Features of OAVRT

Narrow-QRS tachycardia: The QRS complexes are of normal duration since the ventricular activation occurs via the normal conduction pathways. Exceptions may exist due to intraventricular conduction delays that are often rate-dependent (see chapter 7). Heart rate is commonly between 190 and 300 bpm in dogs.[35,36,58–60]

Regular RR intervals: Since this is a re-entrant arrhythmia, its cycle length is constant. Some degree of variation may be seen in cases in which more than one AP is present, or due to alternating conduction through the fast and slow AVN pathways.[59]

Retrograde atrial depolarisation: The atria are depolarised retrogradely with a 1:1 ventricular conduction (one P' for each QRS); otherwise, OAVRT would stop. The atrial activation is almost always eccentric, with the exception of pathways located close to the junctional area. The P' wave conformation may vary but always with a ventrodorsal (infero-superior) orientation (see Box 8.1).[59]

The RP' interval is short (<50% of RR interval), since it is due to ventriculo-atrial conduction via the AP which is normally fast. The RP' is thus shorter than the P'R interval, with an RP'/P'R ratio of less than 0.7 in contrast to atrial tachycardia (see chapter 8).[59]

QRS alternans: QRS electrical alternans is a beat-to-beat variation of the QRS amplitude larger than 0.1 mV and visible in at least one lead (Figure 10.18B). It has been identified as an independent predictor for AVRT in both humans and dogs.[59,61,62] However, it should not be used as the only electrocardiographic feature suggestive of AVRT, as it may also occur in dogs with focal atrial tachycardia.[59]

Antidromic AVRT (AAVRT)

In AAVRT, the impulse travels via the AP from the atrium to the ventricle and up the Purkinje–His–AVN retrogradely back to the atria (Figures 10.13 and 10.19). The direction of the impulse is said to be counterclockwise within the re-entry circuit, and an AP capable of anterograde conduction must be present. On the ECG, a wide-QRS tachycardia is seen with a regular RR interval that must be distinguished from ventricular tachycardia or other supraventricular tachycardias with aberrant

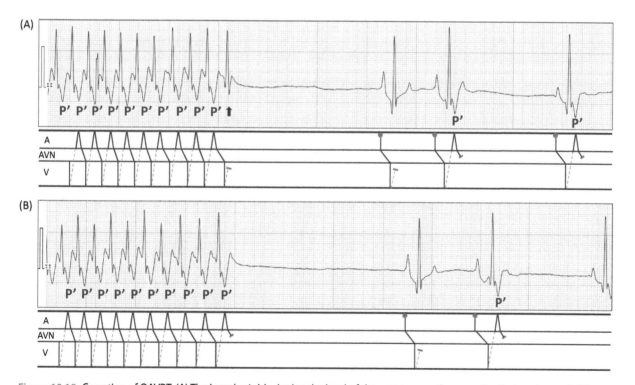

Figure 10.18 Cessation of OAVRT. (A) The impulse is blocked at the level of the accessory pathway; notice that a retrograde P' is not present in the last beat of tachycardia (arrow), as the depolarisation wave never reaches the atria retrogradely via the AP (blocked dotted line on laddergram). (B) A retrograde P' is seen in the last beat of tachycardia but is not followed by a QRS, meaning that it was blocked at the level of AVN. [10-month-old, male Staffordshire Terrier; OAVRT confirmed with EP study]

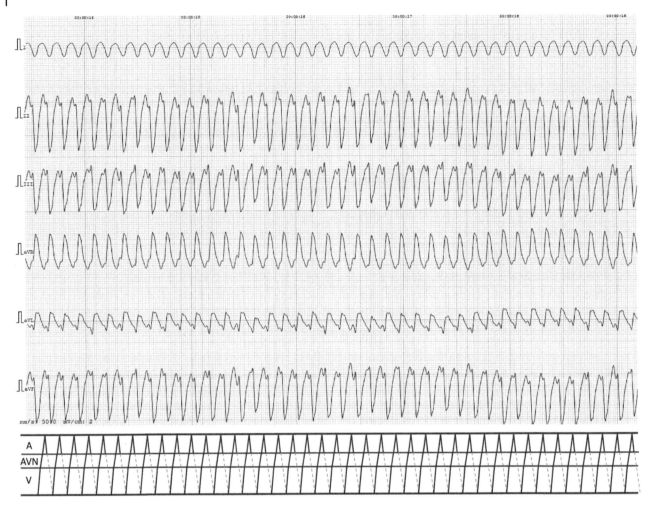

Figure 10.19 Antidromic atrioventricular reciprocating tachycardia (AAVRT). A wide-QRS (≈100 ms) tachycardia is seen with a rate of approximately 480 bpm. Differential diagnoses include ventricular tachycardia and supraventricular tachycardia conducted with bundle branch block or pre-excited. In cases of AAVRT, ventricular depolarisation occurs via an accessory pathway, and the ventricles are depolarised slowly via the working myocardium, explaining the wide QRS; ventriculo-atrial conduction occurs retrogradely via the bundle branches–His–AVN, causing concentric retrograde atrial activation, although the retrograde P' waves are not visible on the ECG as they occur at the same time as the QRS. This example is from a dog with very high suspicion of AAVRT that presented with both narrow- and wide-complex tachycardia with features of OAVRT and AAVRT, respectively. Additionally, pre-excitation was also documented, increasing the level of suspicion. Unfortunately, the dog died suddenly only a few days before an electrophysiology study was due to be performed. [10-month-old, female Labrador Retriever with tachycardia-induced cardiomyopathy] (50 mm/s; 5 mm/mV) *Source:* Courtesy of Paul Motskula from Anderson Moores Veterinary Specialists, UK.

conduction. Retrograde P' waves resulting from concentric retrograde activation are superimposed on the QRS.

To the best of the author's knowledge, this type of AVRT has not been described in dogs or cats, although it likely exists considering the example in Figure 10.19. Unfortunately, these patients are at risk of ventricular fibrillation and sudden death.

Permanent Junctional Reciprocating Tachycardia (PJRT)

PJRT, or tachycardia of Coumel, is a type of OAVRT mediated by an AP that exhibits slow and decremental conduction. One case has been described in a dog

(Figure 10.20).[63] The anterograde limb of the circuit is the AVN–His–Purkinje, and the retrograde limb is a concealed, slowly conducting AP with decremental properties.[64–66] Since conduction is slow through the AP, the RP' interval is long rather than short, and whilst this makes it easier to identify the retrograde P' after the QRS, it can be easily mistaken for an atrial tachycardia. Permanent junctional reciprocating tachycardia is often incessant, with a long RP' interval and narrow QRS complex, and inverted P waves in the inferior leads (leads II, III and aVF) of the surface ECG[67] (Figure 10.20). As mentioned in this chapter, differential diagnoses include focal atrial tachycardia, but also OAVRT with a prolonged ventriculo-atrial conduction (e.g. induced by amiodarone) and atypical forms of AVNRT (discussed further here). An electrophysiology study is required for a definitive diagnosis.[66]

Treatment

Anti-arrhythmic therapy is used with the aim of controlling the ventricular rate which in this case means preventing re-entry from occurring. Since the atrial and ventricular myocardium, the AVN–His–Purkinje and the AP are all part of the re-entrant circuit, this provides several possible targets to stop re-entry. Typically with medical treatment, the aim is to slow conduction through the AVN, and to a lesser extent the myocardium.[68] For a more definitive treatment, radiocatheter ablation is used to destroy the AP.

Medical Treatment

Class IV (e.g. diltiazem) and class II (β-blockers) are often the first choice in human patients who do not undergo ablation.[69] The aim is to slow AVN conduction. Similarly, most veterinary cardiologists prefer diltiazem as the first-line treatment, and in most cases this provides good results, at least initially. β-blockers are not used as frequently since by the time of diagnosis, there is often evidence of systolic dysfunction in our patients. Otherwise, atenolol or metoprolol may also be used with success.[69–71]

Class III anti-arrhythmics (amiodarone and sotalol) are a good alternative and are commonly the next choice after diltiazem.[72,73] Sotalol is usually preferred due to the

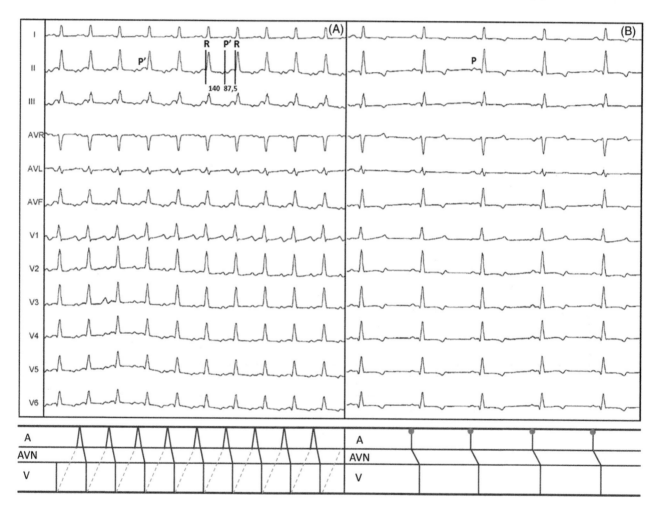

Figure 10.20 Permanent junctional reciprocating tachycardia (PJRT) in a dog. (A) Twelve-lead surface electrocardiogram during permanent junctional reciprocating tachycardia. A narrow-QRS rhythm is seen with a ventricular of approximately 230 bpm. A P' wave is seen with a P'R of 87.5 ms and RP' of 140 ms, suggesting that this would likely be a case of focal atrial tachycardia with a likely origin in the atrial floor (negative in leads II, III and aVF). Instead, this was PJRT confirmed via an electrophysiology study. The anterograde limb of the re-entrant circuit is the AVN–His–Purkinje, and the retrograde limb is a concealed, slowly conducting, accessory pathway with decremental properties (dashed blue line on laddergram). Since conduction is slow through the AP, the RP' interval is long rather than short; and whilst this makes it easier to identify the retrograde P' after the QRS, it can be easily mistaken for an atrial tachycardia. The laddergram on the bottom of the picture illustrates the re-entrant circuit. (B) Twelve-lead surface electrocardiogram of the same dog during sinus rhythm showing a normal QRS complex and a PR interval of 75 ms. [5-year-old, male English Bulldog with PJRT] (50 mm/s; 1 mV/cm) *Source*: With permission from Santilli RA *et al.* Permanent junctional reciprocating tachycardia in a dog. J Vet Cardiol. 2013;15(3):225–230.[63]

undesirable possible side effects with long-term administration of amiodarone, although the latter may be more effective.[68,74]

Other drugs used in humans with AVRT that are not commonly used in veterinary medicine include propafenone and flecainide (class Ic anti-arrhythmics).[68,73,75] These drugs slow conduction through the AVN–His–Purkinje and also through the AP.[72] Conversion to sinus rhythm may be obtained with lidocaine (class Ib) or procainamide (class Ia).

In refractory cases, the combination of more than one antiarrhythmic drug is often necessary. An example is the combination of mexiletine (class Ib) with sotalol. In the author's experience, this is not very effective, possibly because class Ib drugs do not significantly alter conduction through the AVN or AP, but there is some evidence to support the use of mexiletine in these cases.[76] Another combination used is sotalol and diltiazem, although it is not universally accepted due to the risk of bradycardia and, in some cases, even death; therefore, it should be used with care. Other combinations are used in humans and may also prove useful in our patients. An example is the combination of a β-blocker with amiodarone and flecainide.[77]

In the author's experience, it is common for acceptable rate control to be achieved initially with medical treatment, only to be followed by episodes of relapse and progressive treatment failure over a period ranging from months to a few years.

Electrical Cardioversion

Electrical cardioversion is effective in restoring sinus rhythm. It may be very useful in the unstable patient with poor response to medical treatment, until a more definitive treatment option is achieved.

Radiocatheter Ablation

Radiocatheter ablation has become the first-line treatment for AVRT in human patients, as it provides a definitive resolution without the need for further treatment.[73] It is a very safe procedure with a success rate of 89–97%.[78] This is also available for our patients and hopefully will become commonplace for the treatment of AVRT. It should be strongly considered as early as possible, especially in case of inappropriate results with medical treatment and the need to combine anti-arrhythmic drugs.

Monitoring

Patients on medical treatment should have periodic Holter recordings ideally at least every 6 months. It is particularly important that a 24 h Holter recording be obtained after any treatment change, as this is the only reliable way to assess treatment efficacy. This is usually done 10–20 days later. Echocardiography should also be used as necessary to assess cardiac dimensions and function given the risk of tachycardia-induced cardiomyopathy.

Monitoring is no longer required after successful radiocatheter ablation confirmed with a Holter recording post procedure (e.g. 1–3 months later) and with appropriate remodelling in case of tachycardia-induced structural changes or other structural abnormalities.

Atrioventricular Nodal Reciprocating Tachycardia

AVNRT is caused by a re-entry circuit within the AVN itself or perinodal tissue.[79,80] It is the most common regular supraventricular tachycardia in humans, but to the best of our knowledge has never been described in dogs or cats. The electrocardiographic features of typical (slow-fast) AVNRT include a narrow-QRS complex tachycardia (unless aberrant conduction is present) with often indiscernible retrograde P' waves that occur just before, at the onset of, or immediately after the QRS complex. Atypical forms of AVNRT (fast-slow and slow-slow) also exist where retrograde atrial activation occurs after ventricular activation with a retrograde P' appearing after the QRS.[79] Distinction between AVNRT, AVRT and even junctional tachycardia if P' waves are not visible can be very challenging based on only the 12-lead ECG, and an electrophysiology study is required for a definitive diagnosis.

References

1 Laske TG, Shrivastav M, Iaizzo PA. In Handbook of cardiac anatomy, physiology, and devices (ed. Iaizzo PA, pp. 159–175). New York: Springer; 2009. doi:10.1007/978-1-60327-372-5_11

2 Dobrzynski H, Boyett MR, Anderson RH. New insights into pacemaker activity: promoting understanding of sick sinus syndrome. Circulation. 2007;115:1921–1932.

3 James TN, Sherf L. Ultrastructure of the human atrioventricular node. Circulation. 1968;37:1049–1070.

4 Robles de Medina EO, Bernard R, Coumel P, Damato AN, Fisch C, Krikler D, *et al.* Definition of terms related to cardiac rhythm. WHO/ISFC Task Force. Eur J Cardiol. 1978;8:127–144.

5 Tanahashi Y. An experimental study on canine A-V junctional pacemaker: evaluation of the automaticity by overdrive suppression and autonomic blockade by practolol and atropine. Japan Circ J. 41, 1043–1049 (1977).

6 Detweiler DK. In Comprehensive electrocardiology 1861–1908. Springer: London; 2010. doi:10.1007/978-1-84882-046-3_41

7 Kellum HB, Stepien RL. Third-degree atrioventricular block in 21 cats (1997–2004). J Vet Intern Med. 2006;20:97–103.

8 Blomstrom-Lundqvist C, Scheinman MM, Aliot EM, Alpert JS, Calkins H, Camm AJ, *et al.* ACC/AHA/ESC guidelines for the management of patients with supraventricular arrhythmias – executive summary: a report of the American College of Cardiology/ American Heart Association task force on practice guidelines and the European Society of Cardiology committee for practice guidelines (writing committee to develop guidelines for the management of patients with supraventricular arrhythmias) developed in collaboration with NASPE-Heart Rhythm Society. J Am Coll Cardiol. 2003;42:1493–1531.

9 Perego M, Ramera L, Santilli RA. Isorhythmic atrioventricular dissociation in Labrador Retrievers. J Vet Intern Med. 2012;26:320–325.

10 Bright JM, Lombard CW. ECG of the month: atrioventricular junctional tachycardia producing atrioventricular dissociation. J Am Vet Med Assoc. 1983;182:580–581.

11 Pariaut R, Santilli R, Moise SN. In Kirks current veterinary therapy XV (eds. Bonagura JD, Twedt DC, pp. 737–748). Amsterdam: Elsevier Saunders; 2009.

12 Perego M, Ramera L, Santilli RA. Isorhythmic atrioventricular dissociation in Labrador Retrievers. J Vet Intern Med. 2012;26:320–325.

13 Fletcher E, Morton P, Murtagh JG, Bekheit S. Atrioventricular dissociation with accrochage. Br Heart J. 1971;33:572–577.

14 Marriott HJ. Atrioventricular synchronization and accrochage. Circulation. 1956;14:38–43.

15 Segers M, Lequime J, Denolin H. Synchronization of auricular and ventricular beats during complete heart block. Am Heart J. 1947;33:685–691.

16 Levy MN, Zieske H. Mechanism of synchronization in isorhythmic A-V dissociation. 3. Computer model. Circ Res. 1971;28:23–33.

17 Levy MN, Zieske H. Mechanism of synchronization in isorhythmic dissociation. I. Experiments on dogs. Circ Res. 1970;27:429–443.

18 Schubart AF, Marriott HJ, Gorten RJ. Isorhythmic dissociation; atrioventricular dissociation with synchronization. Am J Med. 1958;24:209–214.

19 Levy MN, Edelstein J. The mechanism of synchronization in isorhythmic A-V dissociation. II. Clinical studies. Circulation. 1970;42:689–699.

20 Paulay KL, Damato AN, Bobb GA. Atrioventricular interaction in isorhythmic dissociation. Am Heart J. 1972;82:647–653.

21 Segers M. Les phénomènes de synchronisation au niveau du coeur. Arch Int Physiol. 1946;54:87–106.

22 James TN. Pulse and impulse in the sinus node. Henry Ford Hosp Med J. 1967;275–282.

23 Lee KL, Chun HM, Liem LB, Sung RJ. Effect of adenosine and verapamil in catecholamine-induced accelerated atrioventricular junctional rhythm: insights into the underlying mechanism. Pacing Clin Electrophysiol. 1999;22:866–870.

24 Hamdan MH, Badhwar N, Scheinman MM. Role of invasive electrophysiologic testing in the evaluation and management of adult patients with focal junctional tachycardia. Card Electrophysiol Rev. 2002;6:431–435.

25 Ruder MA, Davis JC, Eldar M, Abbott JA, Griffin JC, Seger JJ, *et al.* Clinical and electrophysiologic characterization of automatic junctional tachycardia in adults. Circulation. 1986;73:930–937.

26 Amrousy DE, Elshehaby W, Feky WE, Elshmaa NS. Safety and efficacy of prophylactic amiodarone in preventing early junctional ectopic tachycardia (JET) in children after cardiac surgery and determination of its risk factor. Pediatr Cardiol. 2016;37:734–739.

27 Dieks J-K, Klehs S, Müller MJ, Paul T, Krause U. Adjunctive ivabradine in combination with amiodarone: a novel therapy for pediatric congenital junctional ectopic tachycardia. Heart Rhythm. 2016;13:1297–1302.

28 Paul T, Reimer A, Janousek J, Kallfelz HC. Efficacy and safety of propafenone in congenital junctional ectopic tachycardia. J Am Coll Cardiol. 1992;20:911–914.

29 Hamdan MH, Scheinman MM. Role of invasive EP testing in the evaluation and management of junctional tachycardia. Card Electrophysiol Rev. 2000;4:50–53.

30 Kent AF. Researches on the structure and function of the mammalian heart. J Physiol (Lond). 1893;14:i2–254.

31 Ho SY. Accessory atrioventricular pathways: getting to the origins. Circulation. 2008;117:1502–1504.

32 Becker AE, Anderson RH, Durrer D, Wellens HJ. The anatomical substrates of Wolff-Parkinson-White syndrome: a clinicopathologic correlation in seven patients. Circulation. 1978;57:870–879.

33 Peters NS, Rowland E, Bennett JG, Green CR, Anderson RH, Severs NJ. The Wolff-Parkinson-White syndrome: the cellular substrate for conduction in the accessory atrioventricular pathway. Eur Heart J. 1994;15:981–987.

34 Santilli RA, Spadacini G, Moretti P, Perego M, Perini A, Crosara S, *et al.* Anatomic distribution and electrophysiologic properties of accessory atrioventricular pathways in dogs. J Am Vet Med Assoc. 2007;231:393–398.

35 Atkins CE, Kanter R, Wright K, Saba Z, Baty C, Swanson C, *et al.* Orthodromic reciprocating tachycardia and heart failure in a dog with a concealed

posterosptal accessory pathway. J Vet Intern Med. 1995;9:43–49.

36 Wright KN, Mehdirad AA, Giacobbe P, Grubb T, Maxson T. Radiofrequency catheter ablation of atrioventricular accessory pathways in 3 dogs with subsequent resolution of tachycardia-induced cardiomyopathy. J Vet Intern Med. 1999;13:361–371.

37 Scherlag BJ, Wang X, Nakagawa H, Hirao K, Santoro I, Dugger D, *et al*. Radiofrequency ablation of a concealed accessory pathway as treatment for incessant supraventricular tachycardia in a dog. J Am Vet Med Assoc. 1993;203:1147–1152.

38 DeChillou C, Rodriguez LM, Schläpfer J, Kappos KG, Katsivas A, Baiyan X, *et al*. Clinical characteristics and electrophysiologic properties of atrioventricular accessory pathways: importance of the accessory pathway location. J Am Coll Cardiol. 1992;20:666–671.

39 Haissaguerre M, Gaïta F, Marcus FI, Clementy J. Radiofrequency catheter ablation of accessory pathways: a contemporary review. J Cardiovasc Electrophysiol. 1994;5:532–552.

40 Santilli RA, Spadacini G, Moretti P, Perego M, Perini A, Crosara S, *et al*. Anatomic distribution and electrophysiologic properties of accessory atrioventricular pathways in dogs. J Am Vet Med Assoc. 2007;231:393–398.

41 Hluchy J, Schickel S, Schlegelmilch P, Jörger U, Brägelmann F, Sabin GV. Decremental conduction properties in overt and concealed atrioventricular accessory pathways. Europace. 2000;2:42–53.

42 Zipes DP, Dejoseph RL, Rothbaum DA. Unusual properties of accessory pathways. Circulation. 1974;49:1200–1211.

43 Ohnell RF. Pre excitation: a cardiac abnormality. Acta Med Scan. 1944;1952:77.

44 Bhatia A, Sra J, Akhtar M. Preexcitation syndromes. Curr Prob Cardiol. 2016;41:99–137.

45 Svenson RH, Miller HC, Gallagher JJ, Wallace AG. Electrophysiological evaluation of the Wolff-Parkinson-White syndrome: problems in assessing antegrade and retrograde conduction over the accessory pathway. Circulation. 1975;52:552–562.

46 Lown B, Ganong WF, Levine SA. The syndrome of short P-R interval, normal QRS complex and paroxysmal rapid heart action. Circulation. 1952;5:693–706.

47 Clerc A, Levy R, Cristesco C. A propos du raccourcissement permanent de l'espace PR de l'electrocardiogramme sans deformation du complex ventriculaire. Arch Mal Coeur. 1938;569.

48 Burch GE, Kimball JL. Notes on the similarity of QRS complex configurations in the Wolff-Parkinson-White syndrome. Am Heart J. 1946;32:560–570.

49 James TN. Morphology of the human atrioventricular node, with remarks pertinent to its electrophysiology. Am Heart J. 1961;62:756–771.

50 Brechenmacher C, Laham J, Iris L, Gerbaux A, Lenègre J. Histological study of abnormal conduction pathways in the Wolff-Parkinson-White syndrome and Lown-Ganong-Levine syndrome. Arch Mal Coeur Vaiss. 1974;67:507–519.

51 Ward DE, Camm AJ. Dual AH pathways in patients with and without the Lown-Ganong-Levine syndrome. Brit Heart J. 1981;356.

52 Mahaim I. Kent's fibers and the A-V paraspecific conduction through the upper connections of the bundle of His-Tawara. Am Heart J. 1947;33:651–653.

53 Wiener I. Syndromes of Lown-Ganong-Levine and enhanced atrioventricular nodal conduction. Am J Cardiol. 1983;52:637–639.

54 Santilli RA, Spadacini G, Moretti P, Perego M, Perini A, Crosara S, *et al*. Anatomic distribution and electrophysiologic properties of accessory atrioventricular pathways in dogs. J Am Vet Med Assoc. 2007;231:393–398.

55 Finster ST, DeFrancesco TC, Atkins CE. Supraventricular tachycardia in dogs: 65 cases (1990–2007). J Vet Emerg Crit Care. 2008;18:503–510.

56 Wright KN, Atkins CE, Kanter R. Supraventricular tachycardia in four young dogs. J Am Vet Med Assoc. 1996;208:75–80.

57 Hill BL, Tilley LP. Ventricular preexcitation in seven dogs and nine cats. J Am Vet Med Assoc. 1985;187:1026–1031.

58 Santilli RA, Spadacini G, Moretti P, Perego M, Perini A, Tarducci A, *et al*. Radiofrequency catheter ablation of concealed accessory pathways in two dogs with symptomatic atrioventricular reciprocating tachycardia. J Vet Cardiol. 2006;8:157–165.

59 Santilli RA, Perego M, Crosara S, Gardini F, Bellino C, Moretti P, *et al*. Utility of 12-lead electrocardiogram for differentiating paroxysmal supraventricular tachycardias in dogs. J Vet Intern Med. 2008;22:915–923.

60 Wang X, Nakagawa H, Hirao K, Santoro I, Dugger D, Gwin RM, *et al*. Radiofrequency ablation of a concealed accessory pathway as treatment for incessant supraventricular tachycardia in a dog. J Am Vet Med Assoc. 1993;203:1147–1152.

61 Kalbfleisch SJ, El-Atassi R, Calkins H, Langberg JJ, Morady F. Differentiation of paroxysmal narrow QRS complex tachycardias using the 12-lead electrocardiogram. J Am Coll Cardiol. 1993;21:85–89.

62 Erdinler I, Okmen E, Oguz E, Akyol A, Gurkan K, Ulufer T. Differentiation of narrow QRS complex tachycardia types using the 12-lead electrocardiogram. Ann Noninvasive Electrocardiol. 2002;7:120–126.

63 Santilli RA, Santos LFN, Perego M. Permanent junctional reciprocating tachycardia in a dog. J Vet Cardiol. 2013;15:225–230.

64 Coumel PH, Cabrol C, Fabiato A, Gourgon R, Slama R. Tachycardie permanente par rythme reciproque. Arch Mal Coeur. 1967;60:1850.

65 Coumel P. Junctional reciprocating tachycardias: the permanent and paroxysmal forms of A-V nodal reciprocating tachycardias. J Electrocardiol. 1975;8:79–90.

66 Farré J, Ross D, Wiener I, Bär FW, Vanagt EJ, Wellens HJ. Reciprocal tachycardias using accessory pathways with long conduction times. Am J Cardiol. 1979;44:1099–1109.

67 Gaïta F, Haissaguerre M, Giustetto C, Fischer B, Riccardi R, Richiardi E, *et al.* Catheter ablation of permanent junctional reciprocating tachycardia with radiofrequency current. J Am Coll Cardiol. 1995;25:648–654.

68 Lévy, S, Ricard, P. Using the right drug: a treatment algorithm for regular supraventricular tachycardias. Eur Heart J. 1997;18(Suppl. C):C27–C32.

69 Ko JK, Ban JE, Kim YH, Park IS. Long-term efficacy of atenolol for atrioventricular reciprocating tachycardia in children less than 5 years old. Pediatr Cardiol. 2004;25:97–101.

70 Gaïta F, Giustetto C, Riccardi R, Brusca A. Wolff-Parkinson-White syndrome. Identification and management. Drugs. 1992;43:185–200 (1992).

71 Gmeiner R, Ng CK. Metoprolol in the treatment and prophylaxis of paroxysmal reentrant supraventricular tachycardia. J Cardiovasc Pharmacol. 1982;4:5–13.

72 Honerjäger P, Schmidt G. Pharmacology of modern anti-arrhythmia drugs in therapy of supraventricular tachycardia. Z Gesamte Inn Med. 1993;48:425–429.

73 Page RL, Joglar JA, Caldwell MA, Calkins H, Conti JB, Deal BJ, *et al.* 2015 ACC/AHA/HRS guideline for the management of adult patients with supraventricular tachycardia. Heart Rhythm. 2016;13:e136–e221.

74 Kuga K, Yamaguchi I, Sugishita Y. Effect of intravenous amiodarone on electrophysiologic variables and on the modes of termination of atrioventricular reciprocating tachycardia in Wolff-Parkinson-White syndrome. Japan Circ J. 1999;63:189–195.

75 Kohli V. Oral flecainide is effective in management of refractory tachycardia in infants. Indian Heart J. 2013;65:168–171.

76 Touboul P, Gressard A, Kirkorian G, Atallah G. Effects of mexiletine in the Wolff-Parkinson-White syndrome. Arch Mal Coeur Vaiss. 1981;74:1315–1323.

77 Ergül Y, Özyılmaz İ, Saygı M, Tola HT, Akdeniz C, Tuzcu V. The use of flecainide in critical neonates and infants with incessant supraventricular tachycardias. Turk Kardiyol Dern Ars. 2015;43:607–612.

78 Petrelis B, Skanes AC, Klein GJ, Krahn AD, Yee R. In Catheter ablation of cardiac arrhythmias (eds. Huang SKS, Miller JM, pp. 496–517). Amsterdam: Elsevier Saunders; 2015.

79 Katritsis DG, Camm AJ. Atrioventricular nodal reentrant tachycardia. Circulation. 2010;122:831–840.

80 Blomstrom-Lundqvist C, Scheinman MM, Alpert JS. ACC/AHA/ESC guidelines for the management of patients with supraventricular arrhythmias – executive committee. JACC. 2003;42:1493–1531.

11

Ventricular Rhythms
Antonia Mavropoulou

Introduction

Ventricular rhythms are abnormal rhythms arising from the ventricles. They are among the most clinically relevant arrhythmias for their potential to cause significant haemodynamic compromise and even death.

A rhythm is considered ventricular in origin when the ectopic pacemaker is located distally to the atrioventricular junction. This includes the remainder of the specialised conduction system (bundle branches and Purkinje system) and the ventricular myocardium. Some authors choose to also include the bundle of His in this classification as it traverses the fibrous skeleton to appear on the ventricular side; however, others believe that only rhythms originating beneath the His bundle ramifications should be deemed ventricular as the bundle of His is still part of the atrioventricular junction.

Ventricular rhythms are commonly associated with either structural heart disease or systemic disease, although in a minority of cases they may also occur as a primary or idiopathic arrhythmia.[1,2] They may be the result of abnormal automaticity, triggered activity or re-entry depending on the underlying cause.[3] Throughout this chapter, several examples of ventricular rhythms caused by different aetiologies will be discussed (see also chapters 20, 21, 23 and 24).

Ventricular Ectopic Beats

Ventricular ectopic beats (VEBs) are caused by spontaneous depolarisation of an ectopic pacemaker located anywhere in the ventricular specialised conduction system or working myocardium. If the beat originates from the working myocardium, impulse conduction will occur via cell-to-cell depolarisation which is a slow process and will depolarise the ventricles asynchronously. For this reason, the resulting QRS complex is wide (QRS >70 ms

in dogs and >40 ms in cats) and bizarre, which constitutes one of the main characteristics of ventricular rhythms. If the beat originates from within or close to the specialised conduction tissue, then at least part of the impulse conduction may occur via the specialised system. In some instances, if the origin is high in the conduction system (e.g. close to the bundle of His), the QRS may even appear normal, making it very difficult to distinguish it from a supraventricular beat.[4-7]

Origin of Ventricular Ectopic Beats

The appearance of the QRS complex will vary depending on the location of the ectopic focus and the route of ventricular depolarisation as the impulse propagates through the ventricles. Typically, an ectopic beat is suspected to originate from the left ventricle if the QRS displays a right bundle branch block morphology (negative in leads II, III and aVF) and from the right ventricle if it displays a left bundle branch block morphology (positive in leads II, III and aVF) (see Figure 11.1).[8] In human medicine, the origin of ectopic ventricular beats can be determined more precisely, and several algorithms have been developed for their localisation.[9-12] Unfortunately, this cannot be applied to our patients due to differences in chest conformation and the position of the heart inside the chest, resulting in limitations in our electrocardiogram (ECG) lead systems.[8] Studies that describe the electrocardiographic characteristics of ectopic beats originating from various areas of the ventricles supported by electrophysiological evidence in dogs and cats are lacking, although some information may be found in the veterinary literature (see Table 11.1).[13]

Unifocal or Multifocal Ventricular Ectopy

Beats that originate in the same ectopic focus and that always depolarise the ventricles via the same route are called *unifocal*, *uniform* or *monomorphic beats*

Guide to Canine and Feline Electrocardiography, First Edition. Ruth Willis, Pedro Oliveira and Antonia Mavropoulou.
© 2018 John Wiley & Sons Ltd. Published 2018 by John Wiley & Sons Ltd.
Companion website: www.wiley.com/go/willis/electrocardiography

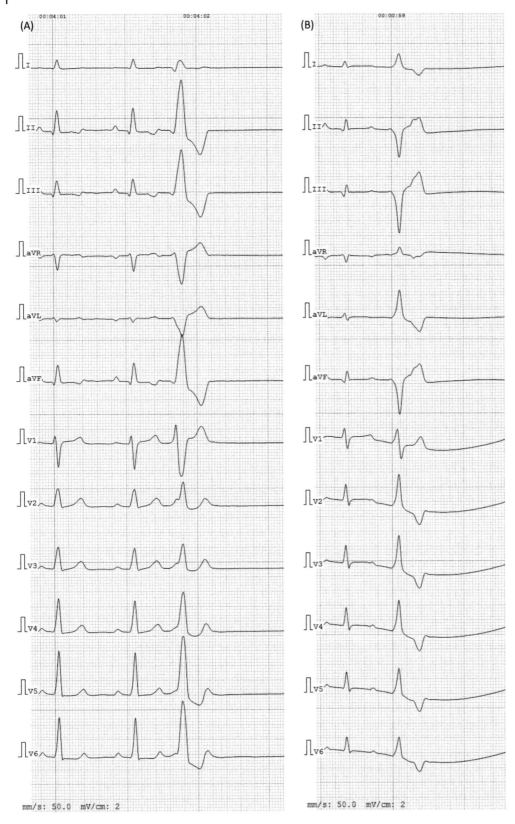

Figure 11.1 Ventricular ectopic beats. (A) The third beat is a ventricular beat with likely origin in the right ventricle as the QRS complex displays a left bundle branch block morphology (positive in leads II, III and aVF). [9-year-old, male neutered, Boxer with suspicion of arrhythmogenic right ventricular cardiomyopathy (ARVC)] (50 mm/s, 5 mm/mV) (B) The second beat is a ventricular beat with likely origin in the left ventricle as the QRS complex displays a right bundle branch block morphology (negative in leads II, III and aVF). [8-year-old, female neutered, Boxer with suspicion of ARVC] (50 mm/s, 5 mm/mV)

Table 11.1 Characteristics of ventricular ectopic beats based on their origin[13]

Ectopic beat origin	QRS characteristics
Right ventricle	
Apex	>70 ms; largest deflection positive in leads II, III and aVF; positive in lead I; negative in V1 and V2; positive in V3 to V6
Septum	>70 ms; largest deflection positive in leads II, III and aVF; usually positive in lead I; variable in V1; positive in V2 to V6
Outflow tract	>70 ms; largest deflection positive in leads II, III and aVF; negative in lead I if cranial origin; negative, diphasic or isodiphasic if caudal origin; negative in aVL if origin is beneath pulmonic valve, or positive if further away; notches in leads II, III and aVF suggest an origin between the pulmonic and aortic trunk; variable in V1; positive in V2 to V6.
His region	<70 ms; aberrant morphology; MEA between +60° and +80°
Left ventricle	
Apex	>70 ms; largest deflection negative in leads II, III and aVF; MEA with a ventro-dorsal orientation (infero-superior); negative in V1 to V6
Inflow and septum	>70 ms; largest deflection negative in leads II, III and aVF; MEA with a ventro-dorsal orientation (infero-superior)
Outflow tract	>70 ms; largest deflection negative in leads II, III and aVF; MEA is variable

(Figure 11.2). The ectopic beats are all similar in appearance on the same ECG lead and may present with a regular timing or randomly. Unifocal beats commonly display a constant coupling interval (R-R'). *Multifocal* or *polymorphic beats* originate from multiple ectopic pacemakers (foci) located in different areas of the ventricles, or alternatively may originate from the same ectopic focus but with different routes taken to depolarise the ventricles. Their appearance on the ECG varies with each beat, and the coupling intervals are also different in contrast to unifocal beats (Figure 11.3).

Premature or Escape Beats

As described for atrial and junctional ectopic beats, VEBs may be *premature* if they occur prematurely when compared to the underlying rhythm (R-R' < R-R) (Figures 11.4, 11.5 and 11.6), and they are commonly referred to as *ventricular premature complexes* or *contractions* (VPCs). If an ectopic beat occurs after a pause, it is described as an *escape beat* (R-R' > R-R)[14] (Figure 11.7).

When a VEB occurs very prematurely, it may exhibit the so-called *R on T phenomenon*. This term refers to the superimposition of the ventricular depolarisation (R wave) to the T wave of the preceding beat.[15] Superimposition can happen on the ascending limb, on top of the T wave or on the descending limb. The T wave represents a period of ventricular vulnerability due to the dispersion of repolarisation, and stimulation may induce re-entrant life-threatening arrhythmias, including ventricular fibrillation (VF).[16–18]

Compensatory Versus Non-compensatory Pauses

A pause is often seen after a VPC (as was described for atrial and junctional ectopic beats), and the duration of this pause will depend on whether the sinus node is reset or not by the ectopic depolarisation wave. The depolarisation wave triggered by the VPC may reach the atria retrogradely, and occasionally a retrograde P' wave may be seen after the QRS.

If left undisturbed, the sinus node will continue to 'fire' at the same rate as the underlying rhythm (R-R); therefore, it will discharge normally after the ectopic beat, but it may be unable to depolarise the ventricles. On the ECG, this will be seen as a pause after the VPC in which the sum of the R-R' and the R'-R will be twice as long as the R-R (Figure 11.4). This will be a *compensatory pause*. Alternatively, if the depolarisation wave propagating through the atria invades and resets the sinus node, the next sinus beat will happen sooner, and the pause that follows the VPC is a *non-compensatory pause* (Figure 11.5). The interval given by the sum of R-R' and R'-R will be less than twice that of the R-R interval of the underlying rhythm. If a VPC is not followed by a pause and happens between two sinus beats without altering the normal R-R cycle, it is called an *interpolated beat* (Figure 11.6).

Single or Organised Forms of Ventricular Ectopy

As already discussed in this chapter for the atrial ectopic beats, ventricular premature beats can occur in an isolated fashion or may appear in more organised forms. The latter include *bigeminy* in which there is a

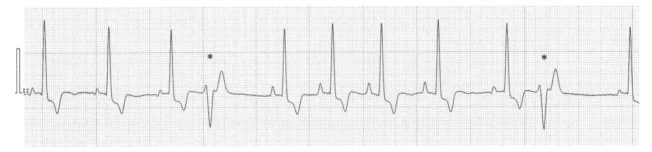

Figure 11.2 Monomorphic ventricular ectopic beats. This trace shows a sinus rhythm interrupted by two examples of single ventricular premature beats (*). The QRS of the ventricular beats has the same morphology, is wider than the normal complexes (100 ms) and has a right bundle branch block conformation. [8-year-old, male Siberian Husky with a patent ductus arteriosus] (50 mm/s, 10 mm/mV)

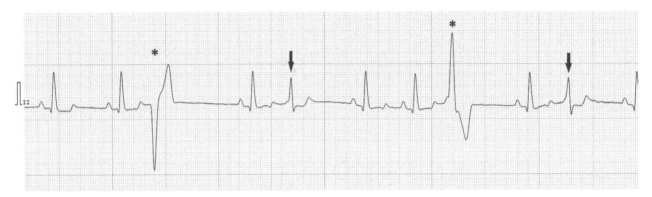

Figure 11.3 Polymorphic ventricular ectopic beats. The trace shows a sinus rhythm interspersed with single ventricular ectopic beats (*) that display varying QRS morphologies suggesting different origins in the ventricular myocardium. The arrows highlight fusion beats that represent a merging of depolarisation waves originating from the sinus node and the ventricular ectopic focus (see the 'Fusion and capture beats' section). [7-year-old, male neutered, Rhodesian Ridgeback with a splenic mass] (50 mm/s, 5 mm/mV)

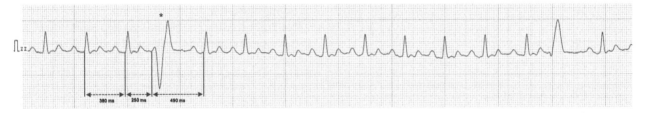

Figure 11.4 Ventricular premature beat with a compensatory pause. The fourth beat is a ventricular premature beat (*) with a coupling interval (R-R') of 250 ms and is followed by a 490 ms pause. The R-R of the sinus beats is 380 ms, which is half of the sum of R-R' and R'R (250 + 490 = 740 ms), indicating that the pause was compensatory. In other words, the VPC did not reset the sinus node, although it prevented a normal QRS from happening as the ventricular myocardium was not ready to depolarise. The sinus node still depolarised every 380 ms with the following visible sinus depolarisation occurring 740 ms after the one before the VPC. [8-year-old, female neutered, Great Dane dog with dilated cardiomyopathy] (50 mm/s, 5 mm/mV)

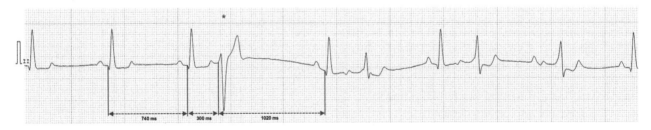

Figure 11.5 Ventricular premature beat with a non-compensatory pause. The fourth beat is a ventricular premature beat (*) with a coupling interval (R-R') of 300 ms and is followed by a 1020 ms pause. The R-R of the sinus beats is 740 ms. If the depolarisation wave resulting from the ventricular premature beat had left the sinus node undisturbed, the next sinus beat would have been expected 1480 ms later (2 x 740 ms); however, it occurred only 1320 ms later (300 + 1020 ms). This suggests that the sinus node was depolarised and reset by the ectopic depolarisation wave and that this pause was a non-compensatory pause. [8-year-old, female neutered, Great Dane dog with dilated cardiomyopathy] (50 mm/s, 10 mm/mV)

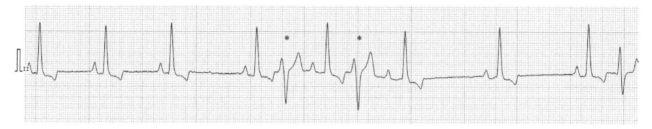

Figure 11.6 Interpolated ventricular premature complex. Between the fourth and fifth and the fifth and sixth sinus beats, there are two premature ventricular beats (*) that do not influence the sinus rhythm and are not followed by a pause. The R-R interval of the sinus beats remains unchanged despite the premature beats. In this case, the R-R is even shorter than the previous due to respiratory sinus arrhythmia. Premature beats that do not alter the underlying sinus rhythm are called *interpolated beats*. [13-year-old, male Border Collie dog with chronic valvular degenerative disease] (50 mm/s, 10 mm/mV)

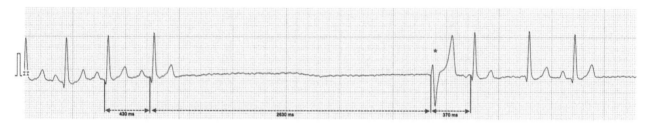

Figure 11.7 Ventricular escape beat. The trace shows three sinus beats followed by a 2630 ms sinus pause that is concluded with a ventricular escape beat (*) and then resumption of sinus rhythm. Escape beats occur after the next expected sinus beat (R-R' > R-R) in contrast to premature beats. [9-year-old, female neutered, Staffordshire Bull Terrier dog with sinus node dysfunction] (50 mm/s, 10 mm/mV)

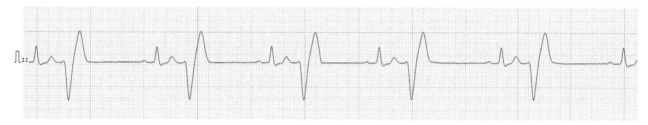

Figure 11.8 Ventricular bigeminy. Sinus beats alternate with ventricular premature beats in a 1:1 sequence. [8-year-old, female neutered, Great Dane dog with dilated cardiomyopathy] (50 mm/s, 5 mm/mV)

repetitive sequence of a normal beat followed by an ectopic beat (Figure 11.8), *trigeminy* in which two normal beats are followed by an ectopic beat (see Figure 11.9) and *quadrigeminy* in which three normal beats are followed by an ectopic beat. Furthermore, *couplets* (a sequence of two consecutive ectopic beats) and *triplets* (three consecutive ectopic beats) (Figure 11.10) can also occur.

Fusion and Capture Beats

Ventricular fusion beats occur when two different pacemakers compete for control of the ventricles. Most commonly, the sinus node and the ventricular ectopic focus are the two pacemakers competing with each other, although an atrial, junctional or even second ventricular ectopic focus can produce ventricular fusion. The two depolarisation waves collide, producing a QRS complex with intermediate morphology between the two complexes (e.g. when a sinus and a ventricular beat collide, a P wave will precede a QRS complex that has intermediate features between a sinus and a ventricular complex) (Figures 11.3 and 11.11). Fusion beats are particularly useful in the diagnosis of more complex arrhythmias when there is doubt about whether they are supraventricular with aberrant conduction or ventricular in origin.[19,20]

Capture beats occur when an impulse originating from the sinus node 'captures' transiently the ventricles during atrioventricular dissociation (e.g. during a ventricular arrhythmia) and produces a QRS complex of normal morphology and duration.[19,21]

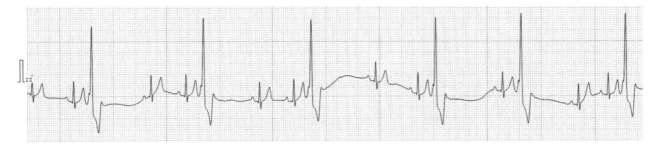

Figure 11.9 Ventricular trigeminy. Two sinus beats are followed by a ventricular premature beat for four cycles. [4-year-old, male Great Dane dog with dilated cardiomyopathy] (50 mm/s, 10 mm/mV)

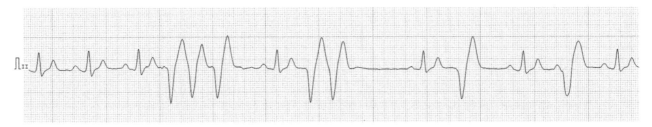

Figure 11.10 Ventricular triplet, couplet and bigeminy. Three sinus beats are followed by a triplet of ventricular beats followed by a sinus beat, and then a couplet of ventricular beats followed by ventricular bigeminy until the end of the trace. [8-year-old, female neutered, Great Dane dog with dilated cardiomyopathy] (50 mm/s, 5 mm/mV)

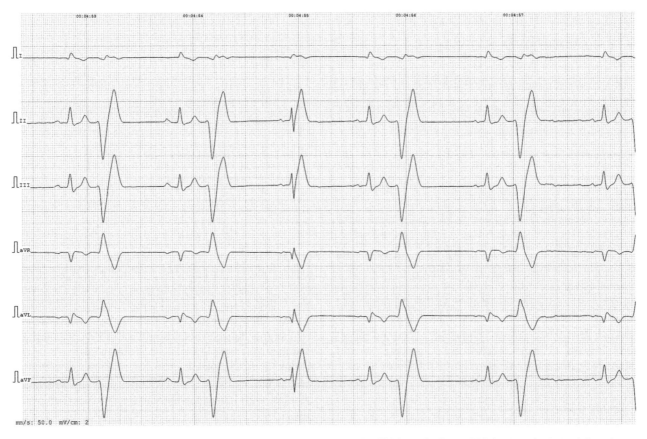

Figure 11.11 Fusion beat. The predominant rhythm is ventricular bigeminy. The fifth beat displays a QRS that is wider (80 ms) than the QRS of the sinus beats (70 ms) but less aberrant than the other ventricular beats (100 ms). This is a fusion beat caused by simultaneous sinus and ventricular depolarisations with the QRS assuming a morphology that is a mixture between a sinus and ventricular ectopic beat. A sinus P wave may be seen before the QRS with a normal PR interval supporting this fact. [8-year-old, female neutered, Great Dane dog with dilated cardiomyopathy] (50 mm/s, 5 mm/mV)

Clinical Significance and Treatment

Isolated VEBs normally do not cause significant haemodynamic disturbances and do not warrant anti-arrhythmic treatment. However, in humans a link has been established between frequent VEBs and arrhythmia-induced systolic dysfunction.[22–24] For this reason, in patients with frequent VEBs and unexplained systolic dysfunction, it would be prudent to consider anti-arrhythmic treatment (see 'Treatment' section in this chapter).

Efforts should always be made to identify and address their underlying cause. This may be a primary cardiac disease (e.g. acquired or congenital structural disease, congestive heart failure, myocardial infarction, myocarditis or neoplasia),[25–36] a systemic disease (e.g. inflammatory or infectious diseases, increased sympathetic tone due to excitement, hypoxia or pain, electrolyte imbalances, etc.)[37–41] or the effect of drugs (e.g. sympathomimetics, digoxin, anaesthetic agents etc.) (see also chapters 23 and 24).[42–44]

In 1971, Lown and Wolf[17] proposed a grading system to categorise VEBs in humans based on their severity (see Table 11.2). According to this system, there are seven different grades of arrhythmias (0, 1, 2, 3, 4A, 4B and 5), where in grade 0 the patient presents no VEBs, while in grade 5 there are R on T phenomena. Grades 1, 2 and 3 are considered benign, and they do not require treatment if the patient is asymptomatic and haemodynamically stable. On the contrary, human patients with grades 4A, 4B and 5 are advised to have anti-arrhythmic treatment due to the risk of dangerous life-threatening arrhythmias. Although this system is popular in human medicine, it has not been studied in veterinary medicine, and it is uncertain whether the same criteria for treatment should be applied in dogs and cats. For more information, please consult chapters 20, 21, 22 and 23.

Table 11.2 Grading system proposed by Lown and Wolf to categorise the severity of ventricular arrhythmias

Ventricular arrhythmia categorisation	
Grade 0	No ventricular ectopic beats (VEBs)
Grade 1	Infrequent unifocal/monomorphic single VEBs (<30 VPCs/h)
Grade 2	Frequent unifocal/monomorphic single VEBs (>30 VPCs/h)
Grade 3	Multifocal/polymorphic VEBs
Grade 4A	Presence of couplets
Grade 4B	Presence of triplets or more than 3 VPCs (ventricular tachycardia)
Grade 5	VEBs with R-on-T phenomena

Ventricular Rhythms

More than three consecutive VEBs are described as a ventricular rhythm. A sequence of 4–6 consecutive ventricular beats is also occasionally described as a 'salvo' of ventricular beats. A ventricular rhythm that becomes apparent during bradycardia (e.g. abnormal sinus node function or atrioventricular block) is termed an *idioventricular rhythm* or a *ventricular escape rhythm* (see also chapter 7). The rate of the inherent ventricular escape rhythm is determined by the subsidiary pacemakers. A ventricular rhythm with a rate above the inherent ventricular escape rate is considered an *accelerated idioventricular rhythm* (AIVR), while the term *ventricular tachycardia* (VT) is used for rhythms with faster rates. Although a clear demarcation between these rhythms exists in human patients, the distinction in veterinary medicine is arbitrary, and different heart rate ranges for each rhythm exist in the literature. The clinical significance of this differentiation is that AIVR is considered to be a relatively 'benign' self limiting rhythm that does not require treatment, whereas VT often has the potential for significant haemodynamic consequences and even death.

Idioventricular or Ventricular Escape Rhythm

An idioventricular rhythm is a ventricular rhythm (>3 consecutive VEBs) with a heart rate that has ranges in literature of 20–65 bpm in dogs and 60–140 bpm in cats (see Figures 11.12 and 11.13).[45–48] It is due to the activity of subsidiary pacemakers present in the ventricles that are normally inhibited by the higher sinus rate (overdrive suppression) but, during periods of bradycardia, become apparent. They effectively ensure that cardiac arrest does not occur in the event of sinus node failure and simultaneous absence of subsidiary pacemaker activity higher up in the conduction system (e.g. a junctional escape rhythm).

Accelerated Idioventricular Rhythm

An AIVR is a ventricular rhythm (>3 consecutive VEBs) at a rate faster than the intrinsic ventricular escape rate but slower than the rate of VT. It usually occurs when the ectopic ventricular focus depolarises faster than the sinus node due to either slowing of the sinus rate or acceleration of the ventricular ectopic focus.[49–51]

Generally, an AIVR occurs at heart rates similar to the physiological sinus rate. In humans, a clear demarcation between AIVR and VT exists, and a ventricular rhythm with a rate above 100–120 beats/min is considered VT based on the upper limit of the physiological sinus rate.[49,52] A cut-off rate value is not universally accepted in dogs or cats due to the wide range of physiological

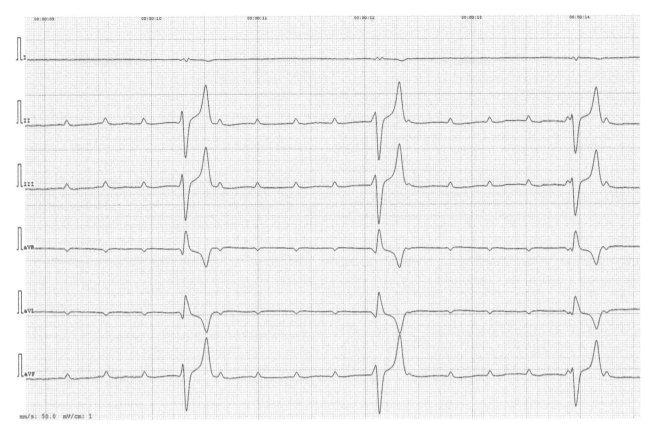

Figure 11.12 Idioventricular or escape rhythm in a dog. The underlying rhythm is sinus with third-degree (complete) atrioventricular block and a ventricular escape rhythm. P waves with characteristics consistent with a sinus rhythm are seen with a rate of approximately 160 bpm and a regular rhythm, but they are not coupled with the QRS complexes. The QRS complexes are wide (120 ms) and bizarre with a rate of approximately 40 bpm and a regular rhythm indicating a ventricular escape rhythm. [11-year-old, male Jack Russell Terrier dog with third-degree atrioventricular block] (50 mm/s, 10 mm/mV)

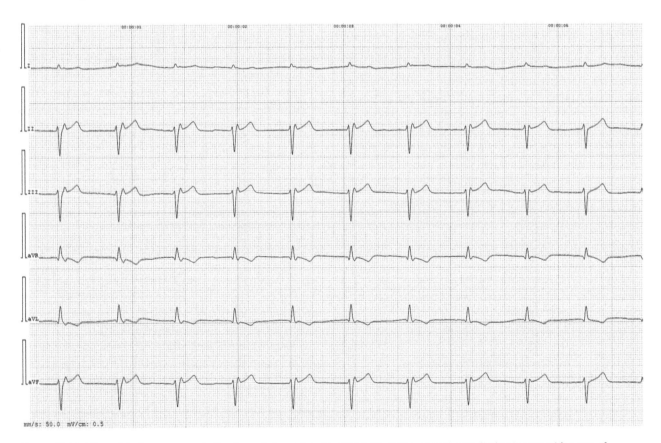

Figure 11.13 Idioventricular or escape rhythm in a cat. A regular wide-QRS (≈75–80 ms, normal <40) rhythm is seen with a rate of approximately 110 bpm and without visible P waves in a cat with hyperkalaemia (7 mmol/L, normal 3.5–5.5). The heart rate and QRS complex characteristics are suggestive of an idioventricular rhythm. [4-year-old, female neutered, Domestic Shorthair cat with urethral obstruction] (50 mm/s, 5 mm/mV)

heart rates in these species, and different ranges for AIVR exist in veterinary literature.[19,45,47,50,53–57] Depending on the source, the lower limit of an AIVR in dogs ranges between 50 and 70 beats/min, while the upper limit ranges between 100 and 180 beats/min. Similarly, no general consensus exists in cats, and AIVR heart rate ranges between 100–140 beats/min and 180–240 beats/min (Figure 11.14).

AIVR is considered a benign and self-limiting rhythm that is thought to be caused by enhanced normal automaticity of subsidiary pacemakers present in the ventricles (e.g. Purkinje fibres);[55] it may be more apparent in instances where vagal tone predominates over sympathetic tone, such as during anaesthesia (see chapter 24).[42,43] It may also be seen in cases with structural heart disease (e.g. myocardial disease, including myocarditis and acute infarction),[53,58–60] extracardiac disease (e.g. pancreatitis, sepsis, splenic neoplasia, hypoxia, trauma etc.)[45,61,62] or the administration of certain drugs (e.g. digoxin and isoprenaline).[44,63] In these instances, triggered activity or re-entry may also be present.[54,55] It usually presents as a monomorphic ventricular arrhythmia, although irregular and multiform AIVR has been described in humans.[58,64]

Monomorphic Ventricular Tachycardia (monomorphic VT)

This rhythm consists of more than three consecutive VEBs with a rate above 180 bpm in which every beat has the same morphology in all leads (Figures 11.15, 11.16 and 11.17). Some degree of variation in morphology may be seen due to fusion or due to changes in exit sites from a re-entrant circuit (pleomorphism),[65] but all beats share the same origin and ventricular depolarisation route. Additionally, the R-R intervals of the ectopic beats tend to be constant. It may occur as paroxysms of non-sustained (<30 s) or sustained (>30 s) tachycardia, or less commonly may be incessant (>12 h). The two most likely underlying arrhythmia mechanisms are re-entry and triggered activity.[66] In dogs with arrhythmogenic right ventricular cardiomyopathy (see chapter 20), repetitive paroxysms of non-sustained or sustained monomorphic VT alternating with sinus beats or sinus rhythm are frequently seen (Figure 11.17).[25,27,67–70] In this case, due to its repetitive nature, it is also called *iterative monomorphic ventricular tachycardia*. Increases in sympathetic tone may accentuate this arrhythmia by reducing the action potential duration, increasing the intracellular calcium and favouring phase 4 afterdepolarisations.[71,72]

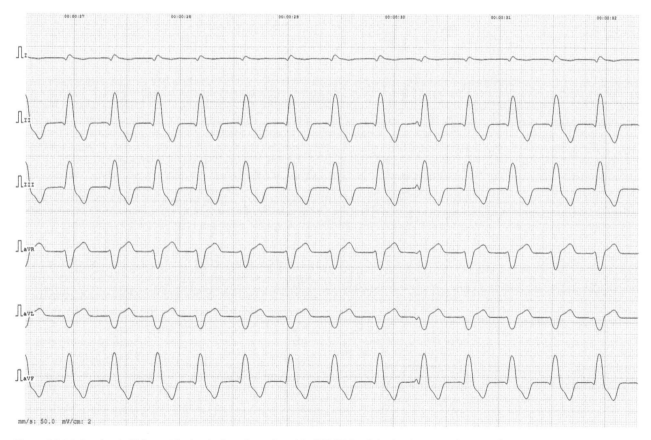

Figure 11.14 Accelerated idioventricular rhythm. A regular wide-QRS (120 ms) rhythm is seen with a rate of approximately 140 bpm and no consistently obvious P waves, consistent with an accelerated idioventricular rhythm. [9-year-old, male Borzoi dog with a splenic mass] (50 mm/s, 5 mm/mV)

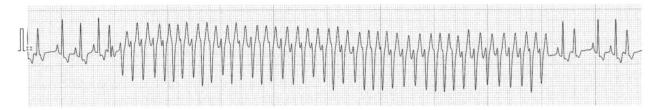

Figure 11.15 Non-sustained monomorphic ventricular tachycardia. Several sinus beats are followed by a paroxysm of rapid (320 bpm) monomorphic ventricular tachycardia. Onset and offset are sudden, and offset is followed by sinus beats interspersed with two single VPCs. The QRS morphology is the same for all ventricular beats (monomorphic), and the episode lasts less than 30 s (non-sustained). [8-year-old, male neutered, Siberian Husky with myocardial disease] (25 mm/s, 10 mm/mV)

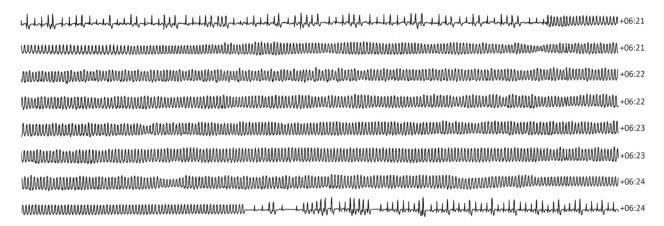

Figure 11.16 Sustained monomorphic ventricular tachycardia. Ambulatory ECG trace from a Boxer suspected to have arrhythmogenic right ventricular cardiomyopathy (ARVC) showing an episode of rapid monomorphic ventricular tachycardia lasting for a little longer than 3 min (sustained >30 s). [5-year-old, female Boxer dog with suspicion of ARVC]

Figure 11.17 Iterative monomorphic ventricular tachycardia. Ambulatory ECG trace from a Boxer suspected to have arrhythmogenic right ventricular cardiomyopathy (ARVC) showing short paroxysms of monomorphic ventricular tachycardia alternating with sinus beats. Due to its repetitive nature, the term *iterative* is used to describe this arrhythmia. [8-year-old, male Boxer dog with suspicion of ARVC]

Ventricular Flutter

Ventricular flutter is a form of very rapid monomorphic VT in which the rate is so high that the QRS and T waves are no longer possible to distinguish. This creates a sine wave–like appearance on the ECG (Figure 11.18). The heart rate during ventricular flutter is often above 300 bpm, causing serious haemodynamic compromise and often degenerating into VF.[18,73,74] Urgent treatment is necessary (see section on 'Treatment' further in this chapter).

Polymorphic Ventricular Tachycardia (PVT)

PVT also consists in more than three consecutive VEBs with a rate above 180 bpm; however, the QRS morphology

is variable, suggesting the presence of more than one ectopic focus (Figures 11.19 and 11.20). The R-R intervals of the ectopic beats are also frequently variable as they originate from various ectopic pacemakers with different intrinsic depolarisation rates.

PVT may occur in patients with structural heart disease (e.g. cardiomyopathies, chronic valvular disease and congenital disease) as a result of myocardial cell damage leading to re-entry or triggered activity. It is also described in human patients with cardiac channelopathies,[75] and although these disorders have been extensively studied and described in humans, they are not well documented in dogs and cats. A particular type of PVT occasionally seen in our patients is known as *torsades de*

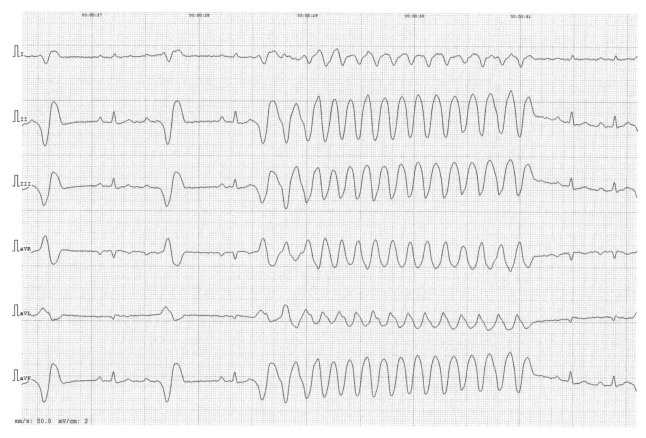

Figure 11.18 Ventricular flutter. Electrocardiographic trace showing a brief episode of very rapid monomorphic ventricular tachycardia, where the QRS and T waves are no longer distinguishable, causing a sine wave–like appearance. The rate during tachycardia is approximately 380–400 bpm. [8-year-old, female neutered, Great Dane dog with dilated cardiomyopathy] (50 mm/s, 5 mm/mV)

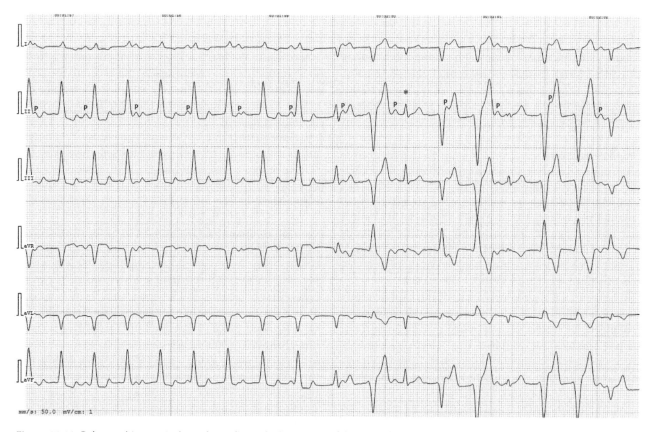

Figure 11.19 Polymorphic ventricular tachycardia. In the beginning of this trace (first nine beats), a wide-QRS rhythm is seen with a regular rhythm and rate of approximately 180–185 bpm. The QRS is wide (80 ms) with a left bundle branch block morphology; P waves are visible (P) but are not coupled with the QRS. These findings are consistent with ventricular tachycardia. For the remainder of the trace, a ventricular rhythm is seen with varying QRS morphologies with a right bundle branch block conformation. The 12th beat (*) presents a normal QRS duration (60 ms) and is preceded by a P wave with PR interval within normal limits (100 ms). This was a sinus beat. [9-year-old, female neutered, Labrador Retriever dog with suspicion of myocarditis] (50 mm/s, 10 mm/mV)

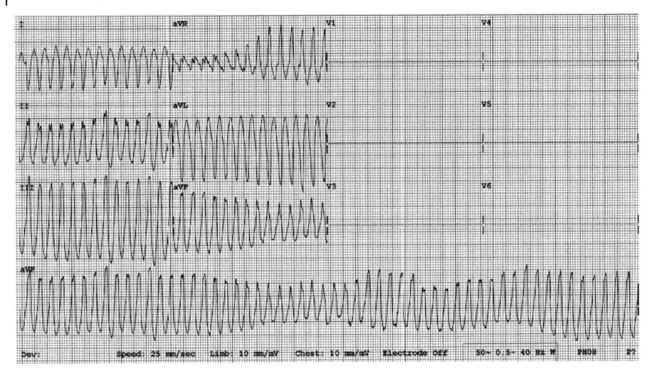

Figure 11.20 Torsades de pointes. A very rapid wide-QRS tachycardia is seen with a rate of approximately 340 bpm. The QRS complex amplitudes continuously change, appearing to twist around the baseline. This trace was recorded from a Boxer dog with arrhythmogenic right ventricular cardiomyopathy (ARVC) on treatment with sotalol, suggesting a pharmacologic QT interval prolongation as the presumed cause for torsades de pointes. (25 mm/s, 10 mm/mV) *Source*: Courtesy of Joel Silva, North Downs Specialist Referrals, UK.

pointes (TP) and may occur in the presence of either structural heart disease or systemic disease. Finally, when PVT is identified in the absence of known structural cardiac disease, channelopathy or systemic disease, it may be termed as *idiopathic*.

Torsades de Pointes

This rhythm disturbance is characterised by a rapid PVT with a distinctive appearance of the QRS complexes that continuously change in amplitude and appear to twist around the baseline (Figure 11.20), although this feature may not be apparent in every lead. It usually results in very pronounced haemodynamic effects, and although TP may terminate spontaneously, it commonly recurs and may degenerate into VF.

In humans, TP is closely associated with cardiac repolarisation abnormalities seen on the ECG such as a prolonged QT interval. A number of congenital (e.g. channelopathies) or acquired (e.g. electrolyte imbalances or drugs) abnormalities may contribute to abnormal repolarisation by interfering with potassium (reduced I_{Ks}, I_{Kr} or I_{K1}), calcium (increased I_{Ca}) or sodium currents (increased late I_{Na}) during stages 1–3 of the action potential[76] (see chapters 2 and 6). The increase in repolarisation time favours the development of early afterdepolarisation-induced triggered activity

(see chapter 6), and multiple foci of triggered activity may result in TP.[76] Additionally, heterogeneous repolarisation of cells in adjacent areas of myocardium can create a substrate for re-entry that may also be involved in maintenance of TP.[76,77]

An adequate trigger is necessary to induce TP, consisting of a short RR–long RR–short RR sequence. This is a sequence of a premature ectopic beat (most commonly ventricular) followed by a sinus beat and then another ectopic beat before TP starts.[78–80]

Long QT Syndrome (LQTS) and Short QT Syndrome (SQTS)

LQTS is a disorder recognised in human patients and characterised by repolarisation abnormalities with a propensity to cause life-threatening arrhythmias. It can be congenital or acquired. The congenital form is associated with gene mutations encoding for ion channels and/or associated proteins (generally potassium or sodium ion channels), whereas the acquired LQTS is usually associated with drugs and electrolyte imbalances (hypokalaemia, hypocalcaemia and hypomagnesaemia). In humans, three major congenital LQTS subtypes with 'benign' and 'malignant' variants within each subgroup have been described.[81,82] Recently, sudden death and LQTS were reported together in a family of Springer Spaniels and were associated with a KCNQ1 mutation (a gene encoding for the α-subunit of the slow component of the delayed rectifier [I_{Ks}] channel).[83]

SQTS is another example of abnormal cardiac ion channel function recognised in human patients that leads to a shorter action potential duration and faster repolarisation, and may cause atrial fibrillation and VF.[84–88] To the best of the authors' knowledge, it has not been described in dogs or cats.

Catecholaminergic Polymorphic Ventricular Tachycardia (CPVT)

This is a rare rhythm disturbance described in children and young adults in which stress- or emotion-induced syncope occurs due to PVT, with high risk of sudden death.[89–92] To the best of the authors' knowledge, CPVT has not been described in dogs and cats.

Iterative Polymorphic Ventricular Tachycardia

Iterative PVT is characterised by paroxysms of sustained or non-sustained PVT alternating with sinus beats or sinus rhythm. This rhythm disturbance is more commonly observed in young German Shepherd dogs with familial ventricular arrhythmias and is discussed in more detail in chapter 22.

Bidirectional Ventricular Tachycardia (BVT)

BVT is a rare type of PVT characterised by an alternating beat-to-beat QRS axis on the ECG (Figure 11.21).[93] It may be seen with digitalis toxicity, CPVT and other conditions that predispose to delayed afterdepolarisations and triggered activity.[93] It is thought to be due to alternating ectopic foci located in the distal His–Purkinje system.[93,94] Alternatively, an ectopic focus above the ramification of the bundle of His with alternating conduction via the right and left bundle branches could also be possible.[95] The most common ECG pattern consists of right bundle branch block (RBBB) QRS morphology with a beat-to-beat alternation of the frontal QRS axis, although other patterns such as alternating RBBB and left bundle branch block (LBBB), or narrow QRS complexes with a beat-to-beat alternation of the QRS axis, have also been described.[96–98] Experiments in dogs showed BVT in 30 out of 200 dogs with experimentally induced ventricular arrhythmias[95] following adrenaline injection.

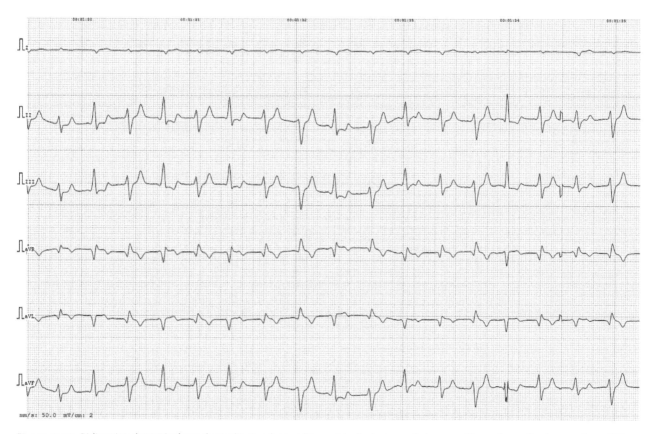

Figure 11.21 Bidirectional ventricular tachycardia. A polymorphic ventricular tachycardia is seen with an alternating beat-to-beat QRS axis suggestive of possible bidirectional ventricular tachycardia in a dog with digitalis toxicity. Note the alternating right and left bundle branch block conformations of the ventricular beats in the beginning of the trace. [7-year-old, female neutered, Saluki dog with digitalis toxicity] (50 mm/s, 5 mm/mV)

Ventricular Fibrillation

VF is characterised by rapid and disorganized activation of the ventricular myocardium, resulting in a pulseless terminal arrhythmia. The ventricular myocardium is depolarised by simultaneous and fragmented electrical wave fronts, causing it to quiver rather than contract. This is a terminal rhythm that requires immediate emergency treatment, such as cardiopulmonary resuscitation and electrical defibrillation (discussed further in this chapter).[99]

Electrocardiographic Findings

On the ECG, VF appears as undulations of different shapes and sizes without discernible P, QRS or T waves (Figure 11.22). It is typically preceded by VT lasting from a few to several beats.[100] A succession of different wave

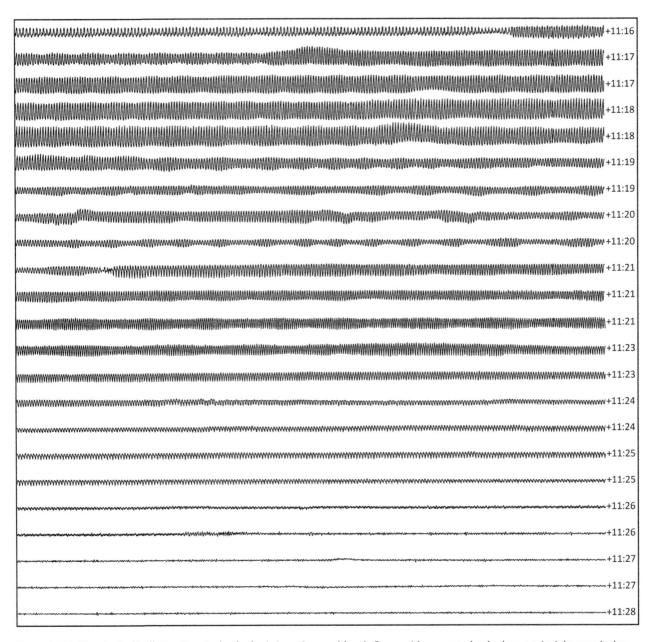

Figure 11.22 Ventricular fibrillation. Terminal arrhythmia in an 8-year-old male Boxer with suspected arrhythmogenic right ventricular cardiomyopathy (ARVC). Each line displays 30 s of a single-lead ambulatory ECG trace. Ventricular tachycardia is seen in the first line, with ventricular fibrillation occurring towards the end. The first stage of VF is seen until 11:19, with rapid wide deflections with a rate between 500 and 600 bpm. From 11:19 until 11:25, the amplitude, duration and morphology of these deflections become progressively smaller and irregular, corresponding to a fragmented activation of the ventricular myocardium (stage 2). Small rapid oscillations of the baseline follow until 11:26 (stage 3), and then become progressively less frequent until they eventually stop (stage 4). [8-year-old, male Boxer dog with ARVC]

appearances seen in experimental studies in dogs has led to the division of VF into four stages:[101]

Stage 1: Tachysystolic or undulatory stage. This stage includes rapid and wide ECG deflections with a rate between 500 and 600 bpm. It was later shown to be very rapid VT caused by figure-of-eight re-entry.[102,103]

Stage 2: Convulsive incoordination (11–40 s). During this stage, the ventricular myocardium is swept by progressively smaller and dissociated waves that still lead to relatively vigorous but uncoordinated muscle contraction. The ECG deflections become irregular in amplitude, duration and morphology, corresponding to a fragmented activation of the ventricular myocardium. The depolarisation rate is above 600 bpm.

Stage 3: Tremulous incoordination (up to 3 min). During this stage, there is a progressive reduction of the areas of contracting myocardium. On the ECG, oscillations of the baseline can be seen with a rate between 1100 and 1700 bpm.

Stage 4: Atonic fibrillation. At this stage, muscle contraction no longer occurs despite continued electrical activity on the ECG. The baseline oscillations become progressively smaller and less frequent (<400 bpm) until they finally disappear.

Underlying Mechanism

During VF, multiple 'wavelets' of electrical activity occur instead of one organized depolarisation wave that sweeps the whole ventricles and then stops. Pre-existing electrophysiological heterogeneities of adjacent cardiac cells (e.g. cells in different states of repolarisation) may allow the wavefront to be 'broken' into multiple depolarisation waves, thereby creating the necessary conditions for re-entry (e.g. spiral wave re-entry) and subsequently fibrillation.[100] Alternatively, heterogeneity may also be caused by an event that causes dynamic instability such as rapid pacing or a high-amplitude premature stimulus.[100] In the presence of sufficient heterogeneity, an appropriate trigger (e.g. VPC) may initiate the initial wavebreak and possibly lead to fibrillation. A sign of electrophysiological heterogeneity may be seen on the ECG as T wave alternans. This consists of variations of the amplitude of the T wave between subsequent beats caused by varying action potential duration of the cardiac cells. It can be used as a sign of vulnerability to ventricular arrhythmia and fibrillation.

Treatment

Medical Treatment

Class Ib (lidocaine, procainamide and mexiletine), class II (atenolol, propranolol and esmolol) and class III drugs (sotalol and amiodarone) are effective in the treatment of ventricular arrhythmias. In cases of sustained or incessant ventricular arrhythmia with significant haemodynamic effects (e.g. ventricular flutter), intravenous medication may be used initially to stabilize the patient and is later replaced by oral medication. Lidocaine, procainamide, esmolol, sotalol and amiodarone are examples of drugs that can be used intravenously in this setting. The choice of drug will depend on the underlying problem, potential side effects, drug availability and personal preference (see chapter 17 for more information on drug dosages and protocols). Lidocaine is usually the first choice for most clinicians. This must be done in the hospital setting with appropriate monitoring (at least continuous ECG and blood pressure) and care.

Once the patient is stable, oral medication can be started. Common choices include sotalol, mexiletine, amiodarone and also sotalol combined with mexiletine.

Electrical Defibrillation/Cardioversion

Given the potential for VF, ideally an electrical defibrillator should be available in every centre dedicated to the treatment of severe ventricular arrhythmias.

Electrical defibrillation is the non-synchronized delivery of an electrical shock to the heart to reset the rhythm, and it represents the most effective treatment for VF. The defibrillation shock stuns and depolarises the majority of the cardiac muscle that becomes temporarily unexcitable, causing disruption of the uncoordinated wavelets of VF and promoting the resumption of sinus rhythm.[104] Types of defibrillation include: *external*, where the shock is delivered to the heart through the thoracic wall; *internal*, where the shock is delivered through paddles applied directly on the heart; and *transvenous* through an implantable cardioverter defibrillator (ICD). The type of current used also differentiates defibrillation into *monophasic* and *biphasic*. Generally, newer defibrillators are biphasic and have been shown to be effective at lower energy levels compared to the monophasic defibrillators in both humans and dogs.[105,106]

During *external defibrillation*, the patient is placed in dorsal or lateral recumbency, and self-adhesive pads or hand-held defibrillation paddles are applied on opposite sides of the chest following application of conductive paste or gel.[107,108] Currently, one single shock is recommended as opposed to the three successive shocks that were routinely administered previously to minimize the interruption in chest compressions during cardiopulmonary resuscitation. Different energy dosages have been described in the literature. These include:

- 2–5 J/kg[106,107]
- 7 J/kg for patients <15 kg and 10 J/kg for patients >15 kg[107,108]
- 50 J for small dogs and cats, 100 J for medium-sized dogs and 200 J for large dogs.[45]

If the first shock is not effective, additional single shocks of increasing energy are delivered after 2 minutes of chest compressions.

Internal defibrillation is accomplished during open-chest cardiopulmonary resuscitation using special paddles and saline-soaked sponges that are placed between the paddles and the epicardium. The energy applied in this case is 1/10 of the energy used during external defibrillation (0.2–0.5 J/kg).[108]

ICDs are devices programmed to detect dangerous ventricular arrhythmias (life-threatening VT and fibrillation) and terminate them through the delivery of an electrical shock. They consist of a pulse generator and a transvenous lead equipped with one or two defibrillation coils. The technique of implantation is similar to the pacemaker implantation, with the lead placed transvenously into the right ventricle and the pulse generator in a subcutaneous 'pocket' over the left thorax at the region of the left ventricular apex. Only two reports of ICD implantation exist in veterinary literature, and currently their use in dogs is limited due to the technical difficulties and complications reported. Rapid sinus tachycardia during exercise or excitement, and over-sensing of T waves, may result in inappropriate shock delivery, and this complication occurred in both the reported cases.[109,110]

Electrical cardioversion is also a useful tool to convert dangerous ventricular rhythms (e.g. ventricular flutter) that fail to respond to medical treatment back to a more stable rhythm (see chapter 9 for more information on electrical cardioversion).

References

1 Yamada T. Idiopathic ventricular arrhythmias: relevance to the anatomy, diagnosis and treatment. J Cardiol. 2016;68:463–471.

2 Hoffmayer KS, Gerstenfeld EP. Diagnosis and management of idiopathic ventricular tachycardia. YMCD. 2013;38:131–158.

3 Qu Z, Weiss JN. Mechanisms of ventricular arrhythmias: from molecular fluctuations to electrical turbulence. Ann Rev Physiol. 2015;77:29–55.

4 Hayes JJ, Stewart RB, Green HL, Bardy GH. Narrow QRS ventricular tachycardia. Ann Intern Med. 1991;114:460–463.

5 Sundhu M, Yildiz M, Gul S, Syed M, Azher I, Mosteller R. Narrow complex ventricular tachycardia. Cureus. 2017;1–4. doi:10.7759/cureus.1423

6 Lerman BB, Stein KM, Markowitz SM. Mechanisms of idiopathic left ventricular tachycardia. J Cardiovasc Electrophysiol. 1997;8:571–583.

7 Paraskevaidis S, Theofilogiannakos EK, Konstantinou DM, Mantziari L, Kefalidis C, Megarisiotou A, et al. Schmaler QRS-Komplex bei idiopathischer (faszikulärer) linksventrikulärer Tachykardie. Herz. 2013;40:147–149.

8 Kraus MS, Moïse NS, Rishniw M, Dykes N, Erb HN. Morphology of ventricular arrhythmias in the boxer as measured by 12-lead electrocardiography with pace-mapping comparison. J Vet Intern Med. 2002; 16:153–158.

9 Park K, Kim Y, Marchlinski FE. Using the surface electrocardiogram to localize the origin of idiopathic ventricular tachycardia. Pacing Clin Electrophysiol. 2012;35:1516–1527.

10 Haqqani HM, Morton JB, Kalman JM. Using the 12-lead ECG to localize the origin of atrial and ventricular tachycardias: part 2-ventricular tachycardia. J Cardio Electrophysiol. 2009;20:825–832.

11 Penela D, De Riva M, Herczku C, Catto V, Pala S, Fernández-Armenta J, et al. An easy-to-use, operator-independent, clinical model to predict the left vs. right ventricular outflow tract origin of ventricular arrhythmias. Europace. 2015;17: 1122–1128.

12 Jadonath RL, Schwartzman DS, Preminger MW, Gottlieb CD, Marchlinski FE. Utility of the 12-lead electrocardiogram in localizing the origin of right ventricular outflow tract tachycardia. Am Heart J. 1995;130:1107–1113.

13 Santilli R, Perego M. In Elettrocardiografia del cane e del gatto (eds. Santilli R, Perego M, pp. 141–162). Amsterdam: Elsevier; 2009.

14 Robles de Medina EO, Bernard R, Coumel P, Damato AN, Fisch C, Krikler D, et al. Definition of terms related to cardiac rhythm. WHO/ISFC Task Force. Eur J Cardiol. 1978;8:127–144.

15 Smirk FH. R waves interrupting T waves. Br Heart J. 1949;11:23–36.

16 Gutierrez MR, Changfoot GH, Peretz DI. Significance of T wave interruption by premature beats as a cause of sudden death. CMAJ. 1968;98:144–149.

17 Lown B, Wolf M. Approaches to sudden death from coronary heart disease. Circulation. 1971;44:130–142.

18 Gunasekaran T, Sanders RA. Sudden cardiac death in a dog during Holter recording-R on T phenomenon. J Vet Cardiol. 2017;1–7. doi:10.1016/j.jvc.2017.08.003

19 Diana A, Fracassi F. ECG of the month. Accelerated idioventricular rhythm. J Am Vet Med Assoc. 2005;226:1488–1490.

20 Marriott HJ, Schwartz NL, Bix HH. Ventricular fusion beats. Circulation. 1962;26:880–884.

21 Sargent JMC, Dennis S, Fuentes VL. ECG of the month. J Am Vet Med Assoc. 2013;242:748–750.

22 Sharma E, Arunachalam K, Di M, Chu A, Maan A. PVCs, PVC-induced cardiomyopathy, and the role of catheter ablation. Crit Path Cardiol. 2017;16:76–80.

23 Akoum NW, Daccarett M, Wasmund SL, Hamdan MH. An animal model for ectopy-induced cardiomyopathy. Pacing Clin Electrophysiol. 2010;34:291–295.

24 Gopinathannair R, Etheridge SP, Marchlinski FE, Spinale FG, Lakkireddy D, Olshansky B. Arrhythmia-induced cardiomyopathies: mechanisms, recognition, and management. J Am Coll Cardiol. 2015;66:1714–1728.

25 Meurs KM. Arrhythmogenic right ventricular cardiomyopathy in the Boxer dog. Vet Clin NA Small Anim Pract. 2017;47:1103–1111.

26 Boutet BG, Saunders AB, Gordon SG. Clinical characteristics of adult dogs more than 5 years of age at presentation for patent ductus arteriosus. J Vet Intern Med. 2017;31:685–690.

27 Santilli RA, Bontempi LV, Perego M. Ventricular tachycardia in English bulldogs with localised right ventricular outflow tract enlargement. J Small Anim Pract. 2011;52:574–580.

28 Calvert CA, Jacobs GJ, Smith DD, Rathbun SL, Pickus CW. Association between results of ambulatory electrocardiography and development of cardiomyopathy during long-term follow-up of Doberman pinschers. J Am Vet Med Assoc. 2000;216:34–39.

29 Calvert CA, Pickus CW, Jacobs GJ, Brown J. Signalment, survival, and prognostic factors in Doberman pinschers with end-stage cardiomyopathy. J Vet Intern Med. 1997;11:323–326.

30 Aronson E, McCaw D. Congenital cardiac disease in dogs. Mod Vet Pract. 1984;65:687–690.

31 Santilli RA, Battaia S, Perego M, Tursi M, Grego E, Marzufero C, et al. Bartonella-associated inflammatory cardiomyopathy in a dog. J Vet Cardiol. 2017;19:74–81.

32 Thompson DJ, Cave NJ, Scrimgeour AB, Thompson KG. Haemangiosarcoma of the interventricular septum in a dog. NZ Vet J. 2011;59:332–336.

33 Romito G, Toaldo MB, Diana A, Cipone M. ECG of the month. J Am Vet Med Assoc. 2015;247:484–486.

34 Winter RL, Hariu CD, Saunders AB. ECG of the month. J Am Vet Med Assoc. 2010;236:961–963.

35 Sanders RA, Kurosawa TA. ECG of the month. J Am Vet Med Assoc. 2013;243:342–344.

36 Long VP, Bonilla IM, Vargas-Pinto P, Nishijima Y, Sridhar A, Li C, et al. Heart failure duration progressively modulates the arrhythmia substrate through structural and electrical remodeling. Life Sci. 2015;123:61–71.

37 Edmondson EF, Bright JM, Halsey CH, Ehrhart EJ. Pathologic and cardiovascular characterization of pheochromocytoma-associated cardiomyopathy in dogs. Vet Pathol. 2014;52:338–343.

38 Tappin S, Brown P, Ferasin L. An intestinal neuroendocrine tumour associated with paroxysmal ventricular tachycardia and melaena in a 10-year-old boxer. J Small Anim Pract. 2008;49:33–37.

39 Aona BD, Rush JE, Rozanski EA, Cunningham SM, Sharp CR, Freeman LM. Evaluation of echocardiography and cardiac biomarker concentrations in dogs with gastric dilatation volvulus. J Vet Emerg Crit Care. 2017;46:98–97.

40 Ajioka M, Sugiyama S, Ogawa K, Satake T, Ozawa T. Mechanism of cardiac arrhythmias induced by epinephrine in dogs with hypokalemia. J Am Coll Cardiol. 1986;8:1373–1379.

41 Gabriel Filho SJ, Ribeiro CA. ECG of the month: multiform ventricular tachycardia. J Am Vet Med Assoc. 2012;241:1288–1290.

42 Atlee JL, Bosnjak ZJ. Mechanisms for cardiac dysrhythmias during anesthesia. Anesthesiology. 1990;72:347–374.

43 Scruggs SM, Mama K, Bright JM, Zirofsky D. Accelerated idioventricular rhythm following propofol induction in a dog undergoing ocular surgery. Vet Anaesth Analg. 2010;37:385–386.

44 Pellegrino L. [Accelerated idioventricular rhythm (slow ventricular tachycardia) in patients with acute myocardial infarct and in patients with digitalis intoxication: clinical and electrocardiographic study]. Boll Soc Ital Cardiol. 1975;20:1785–1793.

45 Kittleson MD. In Small animal cardiovascular medicine (eds. Kittleson MD, Kienle RD, pp. 469–493). St. Louis: Mosby; 1998.

46 Kellum HB, Stepien RL. Third-degree atrioventricular block in 21 cats (1997–2004). J Vet Intern Med. 2006;20:97–103.

47 Tilley LP, Smith F. In Manual of canine and feline cardiology (eds. Tilley LP, Smith F, Oyama M, Sleeper MM, pp. 49–77). Amsterdam: Elsevier; 2008.

48 Ware WA. In Cardiovascular disease in small animal medicine (ed. Dukes-McEwan J, pp. 206–209). London: Manson/Veterinary Press; 2011.

49 Riera ARP, Barros RB, de Sousa FD, Baranchuk A. Accelerated idioventricular rhythm: history and chronology of the main discoveries. Indian Pacing Electrophysiol J. 2010;10:40–48.

50 Guglielmini C, Diana A, Civitella C, Diana D, Luciani A, Cipone M. Accelerated idioventricular rhythm in 9 dogs. Vet Res Commun. 2006;30:305–307.

51 Bonnemeier H, Ortak J, Wiegand UKH, Eberhardt F, Bode F, Schunkert H, et al. Accelerated idioventricular rhythm in the post-thrombolytic era: incidence, prognostic implications, and modulating mechanisms after direct percutaneous coronary intervention. Ann Noninvasive Electrocardiol. 2005;10:179–187.

52 Riva UR, Budriesi N, Fancinelli M, Labriola E. [An accelerated idioventricular rhythm and sports

activity: comments on a clinical case and a characterization of the arrhythmia]. Cardiologia. 1994;39:591–596.

53 Cote E, Jaeger R. Ventricular tachyarrhythmias in 106 cats: associated structural cardiac disorders. J Vet Intern Med. 2008;22:1444–1446.

54 Vassalle M, Knob RE, Cummins M, Lara GA, Castro C, Stuckey JH. An analysis of fast idioventricular rhythm in the dog. Circ Res. 1977;41:218–226.

55 Ilvento JP, Provet J, Danilo P, Rosen MR. Fast and slow idioventricular rhythms in the canine heart: a study of their mechanism using antiarrhythmic drugs and electrophysiologic testing. Am J Cardiol. 1982;49:1909–1916.

56 Ramsey I. BSAVA small animal formulary. London: British Small Animal Veterinary Association; 2014.

57 Moïse NS. In Textbook of canine and feline cardiology (eds. Fox PR, Sisson DD, Moise SN, pp. 331–385). Philadelphia: Saunders; 1999.

58 Rothfeld EL, Zucker IR. Multiform accelerated idioventricular rhythm. Angiology. 1974;25:457–461.

59 Willich T, Goette A. Update on management of cardiac arrhythmias in acute coronary syndromes. Minerva Cardioangiol. 2015;63:121–133.

60 Comerford TJ, Propert DB. Accelerated idioventricular rhythm in patients without acute myocardial infarction. Angiology. 1979;30:768–775.

61 Muir WW, Lipowitz AJ. Cardiac dysrhythmias associated with gastric dilatation-volvulus in the dog. J Am Vet Med Assoc. 1978;172:683–689.

62 Macintire DK, Snider TG. Cardiac arrhythmias associated with multiple trauma in dogs. J Am Vet Med Assoc. 1984;184:541–545.

63 Michaeli E, Rosén A. Depression of isoprenaline-induced idioventricular rhythm in man by beta-adrenergic receptor blocking agents. Acta Med Scand. 1968;183:401–406.

64 Sclarovsky S, Strasberg B, Fuchs J, Lewin RF, Arditi A, Klainman E, et al. Multiform accelerated idioventricular rhythm in acute myocardial infarction: electrocardiographic characteristics and response to verapamil. Am J Cardiol. 1983;52:43–47.

65 Josephson ME, Horowitz LN, Farshidi A, Spielman SR, Michelson EL, Greenspan AM. Recurrent sustained ventricular tachycardia. 4. Pleomorphism. Circulation. 1979;59:459–468.

66 Brugada J, Boersma L, Allessie M, Navarro-Lopez F. The complexity of mechanisms in ventricular tachycardia. Pacing Clin Electrophysiol. 1993;16:680–686.

67 Meurs KM, Stern JA, Reina-Doreste Y, Spier AW, Koplitz SL, Baumwart RD. Natural history of arrhythmogenic right ventricular cardiomyopathy in the boxer dog: a prospective study. J Vet Intern Med. 2014;28:1214–1220.

68 Brechenmacher C, Laham J, Iris L, Gerbaux A, Lenègre J. [Histological study of abnormal conduction pathways in the Wolff-Parkinson-White syndrome and Lown-Ganong-Levine syndrome]. Arch Mal Coeur Vaiss. 1974;67:507–519.

69 Basso C. Arrhythmogenic right ventricular cardiomyopathy causing sudden cardiac death in Boxer dogs: a new animal model of human disease. Circulation. 2004;109:1180.

70 Agullo-Pascual E, Cerrone M, Delmar M. Arrhythmogenic cardiomyopathy and Brugada syndrome: diseases of the connexome. FEBS Lett. 2014;588:1322–1330.

71 Corrado D, Basso C, Rizzoli G, Schiavon M, Thiene G. Does sports activity enhance the risk of sudden death in adolescents and young adults? J Am Coll Cardiol. 2003;42:1959–1963.

72 Corrado D, Link MS, Calkins H. Arrhythmogenic right ventricular cardiomyopathy. N Engl J Med. 2017;376:61–72.

73 Hayashi M, Murata M, Satoh M, Aizawa Y, Oda E, Oda Y, et al. Sudden nocturnal death in young males from ventricular flutter. Japan Heart J. 1985;26:585–591.

74 Gurevitz O, Viskin S, Glikson M, Ballman KV, Rosales AG, Shen W-K, et al. Long-term prognosis of inducible ventricular flutter: not an innocent finding. Am Heart J. 2004;147:649–654.

75 Kim J-B. Channelopathies. Korean J Pediatr. 2014;57:1–18.

76 Antzelevitch C. Ionic, molecular, and cellular bases of QT-interval prolongation and torsade de pointes. Europace. 2007;9:iv4–iv15.

77 Tan HL. Electrophysiologic mechanisms of the long QT interval syndromes and torsade de pointes. Ann Intern Med. 1995;122:701–714.

78 Eckardt L, Haverkamp W, Borggrefe M, Breithardt G. Experimental models of torsade de pointes. Cardiovasc Res. 1998;39:178–193.

79 Vos MA, Verduyn SC, Gorgels APM, Lipcsei GC, Wellens HJJ. Reproducible induction of early afterdepolarizations and torsade de pointes arrhythmias by d-sotalol and pacing in dogs with chronic atrioventricular block. Circulation. 1995;91:864–872.

80 Viskin S, Alla SR, Barron HV, Heller K, Saxon L, Kitzis I, et al. Mode of onset of torsade de pointes in congenital long QT syndrome. J Am Coll Cardiol. 1996;28:1262–1268.

81 Wilde AAM, Amin A. Channelopathies, genetic testing and risk stratification. Int J Cardiol. 2017;237:53–55.

82 Fernández-Falgueras A, Sarquella-Brugada G, Brugada J, Brugada R, Campuzano O. Cardiac channelopathies and sudden death: recent clinical and genetic advances. Biology. 2017;6:7–21.

83 Ware WA, Reina-Doreste Y, Stern JA, Meurs KM. Sudden death associated with QT interval prolongation and KCNQ1 gene mutation in a family of English Springer Spaniels. J Vet Intern Med. 2015;29:561–568.

84 Brugada R, Hong K, Cordeiro JM, Dumaine R. Short QT syndrome. CMAJ. 2005;173:1349–1354.

85 Brugada R, Hong K, Dumaine R, Cordeiro J, Gaita F, Borggrefe M, *et al*. Sudden death associated with short-QT syndrome linked to mutations in HERG. Circulation. 2004;109:30–35.

86 Priori SG, Pandit SV, Rivolta I, Berenfeld O, Ronchetti E, Dhamoon A, *et al*. A novel form of short QT syndrome (SQT3) is caused by a mutation in the KCNJ2 gene. Circ Res. 2005;96:800–807.

87 Antzelevitch C, Pollevick GD, Cordeiro JM, Casis O, Sanguinetti MC, Aizawa Y, *et al*. Loss-of-function mutations in the cardiac calcium channel underlie a new clinical entity characterized by ST-segment elevation, short QT intervals, and sudden cardiac death. Circulation. 2007;115:442–449.

88 Bellocq C, van Ginneken ACG, Bezzina CR, Alders M, Escande D, Mannens MMAM, *et al*. Mutation in the KCNQ1 gene leading to the short QT-interval syndrome. Circulation. 2004;109:2394–2397.

89 Francis J, Sankar V, Krishnan Nair V, Priori SG. Catecholaminergic polymorphic ventricular tachycardia. Heart Rhythm. 2005;2:550–554.

90 Leenhardt A, Denjoy I, Guicheney P. Catecholaminergic polymorphic ventricular tachycardia. Circ Arrhythm Electrophysiol. 2012;5:1044–1052.

91 Wall JJ, Iyer RV. Catecholaminergic polymorphic ventricular tachycardia. Pediatr Emerg Care. 2017;33:427–431.

92 Leenhardt A. Catecholaminergic polymorphic ventricular tachycardia. J Arrhythmia. 2011;27:JSE2–JSE2.

93 Baher AA, Uy M, Xie F, Garfinkel A, Qu Z, Weiss JN. Bidirectional ventricular tachycardia: ping pong in the His–Purkinje system. Heart Rhythm. 2011;8:599–605.

94 Cohen SI, Deisseroth A, Hecht HS. Infra-His bundle origin of bidirectional tachycardia. Circulation. 1973;47:1260–1266.

95 Mehta MC, Sharma VN. Experimental bidirectional ventricular tachycardia in the dog. Br Heart J. 1964;26:67–74.

96 Leenhardt A, Lucet V, Denjoy I, Grau F, Do Ngoc D, Coumel P. Catecholaminergic polymorphic ventricular tachycardia in children. Circulation. 1995;91:1512–1519.

97 Leenhardt A, Extramiana F, Milliez P, Denjoy I, Thomas O, Meddane M, *et al*. [Bidirectional ventricular tachycardias]. Arch Mal Coeur Vaiss. 2003;96(7):27–31.

98 Rothfeld EL. Bidirectional tachycardia with normal QRS duration. Am Heart J. 1976;92:231–233.

99 Jalife J. Ventricular fibrillation: mechanisms of initiation and maintenance. Ann Rev Physiol. 2000;62:25–50.

100 Weiss JN, Chen PS, Qu Z, Karagueuzian HS, Garfinkel A. Ventricular fibrillation: how do we stop the waves from breaking? Circ Res. 2000;87:1103–1107.

101 Wiggers CJ. Studies on ventricular fibrillation produced by electric shock. Am J Physiol. 1930;93:197–212.

102 Bonometti C, Hwang C, Hough D, Lee JJ, Fishbein MC, Karagueuzian HS, *et al*. Interaction between strong electrical stimulation and reentrant wavefronts in canine ventricular fibrillation. Circ Res. 1995;77:407–416.

103 Chen PS, Wolf PD, Dixon EG, Danieley ND, Frazier DW, Smith WM, *et al*. Mechanism of ventricular vulnerability to single premature stimuli in open-chest dogs. Circ Res. 1988;62:1191–1209.

104 Dosdall DJ, Fast VG, Ideker RE. Mechanisms of defibrillation. Ann Rev Biomed Eng. 2010;12:233–258.

105 van Alem AP, Post J, Koster RW. VF recurrence: characteristics and patient outcome in out-of-hospital cardiac arrest. Resuscitation. 2003;59:181–188.

106 Lee S-G, Moon H-S, Hyun C. The efficacy and safety of external biphasic defibrillation in toy breed dogs. J Vet Emerg Crit Care. 2008;18:362–369.

107 Cole SG, Otto CM, Hughes D. Cardiopulmonary cerebral resuscitation in small animals: a clinical practice review. Part II. J Vet Emerg Crit Care. 2003;13:13–23.

108 Plunkett SJ, McMichael M. Cardiopulmonary resuscitation in small animal medicine: an update. J Vet Intern Med. 2008;22:9–25.

109 Pariaut R, Saelinger C, Queiroz-Williams P, Strickland KN, Marshall HC. Implantable cardioverter-defibrillator in a German shepherd dog with ventricular arrhythmias. J Vet Cardiol. 2011;13:203–210.

110 Nelson OL, Lahmers S, Schneider T, Thompson P. The use of an implantable cardioverter defibrillator in a Boxer Dog to control clinical signs of arrhythmogenic right ventricular cardiomyopathy. J Vet Intern Med. 2006;20:1232–1237.

12

Clinical Approach to Arrhythmias and Intermittent Collapse
Ruth Willis

Introduction

The key message in this chapter is to always evaluate the patient, not just the electrocardiogram (ECG) trace. Some patients with severe arrhythmias may walk into the clinic looking reasonably well, whereas a similar arrhythmia in other patients may result in significant hypotension and collapse. Therefore, it is important to evaluate the heart rate and rhythm in the context of clinical findings – for example, if the ECG trace shows sinus bradycardia with a rate of 40 bpm, this may be physiological in a sleeping dog but pathological in a patient who is awake and ambulatory.

Arrhythmias detected during clinical examination may be:

- Normal variation, such as sinus arrhythmia or physiological sinus tachycardia
- Incidental finding, for example occasional single ventricular ectopic beats, as up to 50 single ventricular premature beats in a 24 h period are considered to be within acceptable limits.
- Potentially significant, especially if there are referable events in the history such as episode(s) of collapse or exercise intolerance
- Secondary to significant cardiac disease or congestive heart failure (e.g. atrial fibrillation)
- Secondary to systemic disease (e.g. gastric dilation and torsion).

Some breeds are predisposed to arrhythmias, such as Boxers, Dobermans, Great Danes (ventricular arrhythmias) and giant-breed dogs (atrial fibrillation). The finding of an arrhythmia in any of these breeds is much more likely to prompt further investigation.

Approach to Cases With a History of Intermittent Collapse

In patients who have experienced one or more episodes of collapse, a detailed history is vital to establish whether the event was a fit, faint or fall. In human patients, *syncope* is defined as a transient loss of consciousness due to transient global cerebral hypoperfusion followed by spontaneous complete recovery, and the same definition also seems appropriate for dogs and cats.[1]

Whilst some causes of syncope are benign, syncope can also be associated with life-threatening arrhythmias, and therefore further investigation is often advisable. One review showed that 1 in 20 human patients with syncope experienced a severe adverse event, including death, after initial evaluation in the emergency department.[2]

To obtain a detailed description of the events, perform clinical examination and discuss further investigation will typically take around 30–60 min, and it is important to allow sufficient time. Whilst the history will help to direct further investigation, there is a huge potential overlap between neurological and cardiac causes of collapse. Therefore, even when the history directs us in a particular direction, it is important to retain an open mind, especially as some bradyarrhythmias will induce hypoxic seizures. It is also possible to have episodes of pre-syncope when the signs are less marked – for example, events where the patient shows ataxia or a change in mentation rather than syncope.

Understandably, owners are generally alarmed and upset by these episodes that are often unexpected and can appear quite dramatic. This is especially relevant when we are asking questions relating to the duration of the event, as the perceived duration of the episode is often exaggerated. In patients who have experienced

Guide to Canine and Feline Electrocardiography, First Edition. Ruth Willis, Pedro Oliveira and Antonia Mavropoulou.
© 2018 John Wiley & Sons Ltd. Published 2018 by John Wiley & Sons Ltd.
Companion website: www.wiley.com/go/willis/electrocardiography

multiple episodes, it can be very helpful to ask owners to record a video of an event on a portable device such as their mobile phone. These videos are often very helpful in guiding further investigation.

Syncope is an uncommon presenting sign in cats and, when it occurs, may be associated with underlying cardiac or systemic disease (e.g. anaemia, intracranial disease etc.).

History in Cases With Intermittent Collapse

In cases with intermittent collapse, a very detailed history is key to formulating an appropriate plan for further investigation. Therefore, in addition to a normal general health history, in cases with intermittent collapse the history will typically include questions such as:

1) What was the dog or cat doing prior to the episode?
2) Did anything appear to provoke the event? For example, something that caused a sudden change in activity, such as the doorbell ringing whilst the dog was at rest?
3) Did the episode come on suddenly or gradually?
4) Did the patient remain standing or become recumbent?
5) If the patient became recumbent, then was he or she in sternal or lateral recumbency? Was their head on the floor (which could suggest a flaccid unconscious patient), or did the head remain raised off the ground?
6) Did the patient respond to your voice and presence during the event? (The purpose of this question is to determine whether there was loss of consciousness. Many owners associate their dog's eyes being open with consciousness and sometimes need to be told that dogs can be unconscious and unresponsive with their eyes open.)
7) Was there any limb movement during the event?
8) Did body position change during the event? For example, opisthotonus?
9) Was there any urination, defaecation or vomiting before, during or after the event?
10) How long did the event last? (Remember – an accurate measure of duration is rarely obtained!)
11) Was recovery from the event sudden or gradual?
12) What did the dog or cat do after the event?
13) *If multiple events are reported, ask*:
    a) How many events have there been?
    b) When was the first one, and how frequent are they?
    c) Do the episodes all look the same, or have they changed?
    d) Have you noticed any trigger – such as a link to feeding or a particular activity such as ball chasing?
    e) Has any treatment been given? If so, then what was the response?
    f) Have you obtained a video recording?

As it is vital to have an accurate description of the event(s), once the owners have described the event, it is sometimes useful to repeat back to them your understanding of what they have said and, if necessary, allow them to correct any errors.

Occasionally, dogs with significant arrhythmias will experience an event during a period of rest, and owners may describe the dog waking suddenly and sometimes vocalising as though distressed or in pain (see Figure 12.1). Whilst events that occur at rest are more likely to be seizures than episodes of syncope, an arrhythmia as the cause of the seizures cannot be completely discounted.

It is important to recognise that while syncope occurs intermittently, the threat of recurrence continuously impairs quality of life, with many owners becoming reluctant to allow their dog to perform normal activities such as exercise, play and competition work.[1]

Comparison to Human Syncope

Syncope is a common presenting sign in human patients, and, as in cats and dogs, the cause may be benign or a pre-emptive sign of a life-threatening event. In human medicine, scoring systems have been developed to stratify risk. However, due to different disease predilections between species, these scores may not be directly applicable to our patient group.[1–4]

Fits, Faints and Falling Over

Whilst the 'classic' fit and faint are described, dogs rarely show all the signs of one category, and the description may suggest elements from several categories. As a result, the decision on whether to investigate a fit or a faint is often made on the basis of 'best fit'. See Figure 12.2.

Differential Diagnosis of Syncope/ Intermittent Weakness

Table 12.1 shows some potential causes of intermittent syncope in dogs and cats.

Managing Owner Expectation

In cases with collapse, there is a long differential diagnosis list, as shown in Table 12.1. Whilst history is the key in choosing appropriate diagnostic tests, it is important

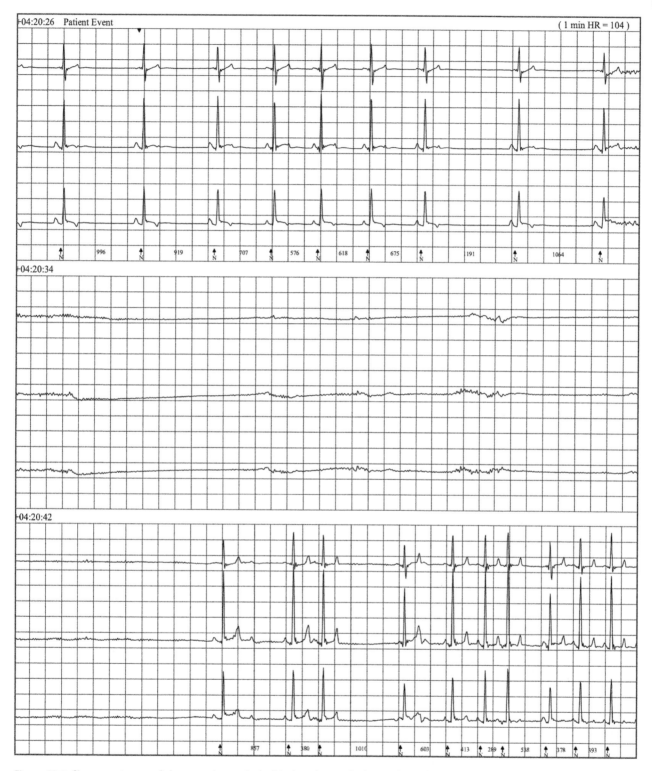

Figure 12.1 Sinus arrest, second-degree atrioventricular block and asystole during sleep. This ambulatory ECG trace is from a 12-year-old dog who the owners reported would frequently 'wake up screaming'. The trace shows that around the time of an episode, there was a sudden long (>10 s) pause in ventricular activity, possibly containing several consecutive unconducted P waves, followed by resumption of sinus rhythm with several supraventricular premature beats. [12-year-old, female neutered, Cavalier King Charles Spaniel dog with 'screaming' episodes]

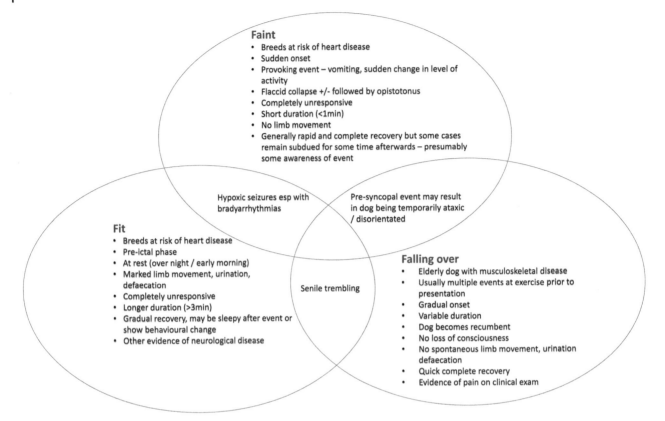

Figure 12.2 General features of fits, faints and falls, and overlap between these categories.

to warn owners that especially in cases with very infrequent collapse, investigation may carry a significant cost implication and there is still a possibility that it will not reveal a definitive diagnosis. If appropriate investigation does not reveal a definitive diagnosis, then the owners can be reassured that the prognosis is likely to be good except in breeds such as Boxers that are predisposed to malignant ventricular arrhythmias.[5]

Clinical Examination in Cases With Intermittent Collapse

The next step in the investigation of intermittent collapse is a thorough clinical examination, as this, in conjunction with the history, may help to rule in or rule out some of the disorders shown in Table 12.1.

Signs that would raise suspicion of a cardiac cause of collapse include:

- Signs of peripheral hypoperfusion, such as pale mucous membranes, prolonged capillary refill time (>2 s) and cold extremities
- Unexpectedly high or low heart rate
- Weak femoral or peripheral pulses or pulse deficit
- Abnormal respiratory rate or pattern
- Heart murmur

- Arrhythmia
- Gallop sound in cats
- Weak precordial impulse
- Absence of lung sounds in some or all of thorax, suggesting pleural effusion.

It is also appropriate to differentiate primary cardiac disease (e.g. ventricular ectopy associated with Doberman dilated cardiomyopathy) from cardiac changes secondary to systemic disease, such as ventricular ectopy secondary to thoracic trauma and associated myocardial contusions (see chapter 23).

Diagnostic Testing in Cases With Intermittent Syncope

In cases with intermittent syncope and history and clinical findings suggesting cardiac aetiology, further investigation may include the tests shown in Table 12.2.

Cardiac Biomarkers in Intermittent Collapse

Plasma *cardiac troponin* is a marker of myocardial damage and is often elevated in cases with significant acute cardiomyocyte damage or necrosis. A study comparing cardiac troponin I (cTnI) concentrations in dogs with

Table 12.1 Potential causes of intermittent syncope in dogs and cats

Cardiovascular

- Bradyarrhythmia
- Tachyarrhythmia
- Congenital causes of inadequate cardiac output (e.g. aortic, pulmonic or atrioventricular valve stenosis)
- Acquired causes of inadequate cardiac output (e.g. dilated cardiomyopathy, *Dirofilaria immitis*, severe atrioventricular valve incompetence and, less commonly, hypertrophic or restrictive cardiomyopathy)
- Impaired cardiac filling (e.g. pericardial effusion, constrictive pericardial disease and intracardiac mass)
- Drugs (e.g. vasodilators)
- Neurally mediated syncope, including tussive syncope
- Cyanotic heart disease (e.g. right to left shunting congenital disease)

Pulmonary

- Diseases causing severe hypoxaemia
- Pulmonary thromboembolism
- Pulmonary hypertension (e.g. *Angiostrongylus vasorum* infection)

Metabolic

- Hypoglycaemia
- Electrolyte abnormalities, especially potassium and calcium (see chapter 23)
- Hypoadrenocorticism (see chapter 23)

Haematological

- Anaemia
- Sudden haemorrhage

Neurological

- Seizure
- Brain tumour
- Cerebrovascular accident
- Trauma (see chapter 23)

Selected non-cardiac causes of collapse in dogs (see chapter 23)

- Exercise-induced collapse in Labradors
- Border collie collapse
- Epileptoid cramping syndrome in Border terriers
- L-2 hydroxyglutaric aciduria in Staffordshire Bull terriers
- Labrador myopathy

Note: It is important to note that this list is not exhaustive, but does contain some of the more common causes to be considered.

Table 12.2 Tests frequently performed in the investigation of intermittent syncope with history and clinical findings suggesting a cardiac aetiology

Test	Rationale
Haematology	Screening for abnormalities such as anaemia
Serum biochemistry	Screening for systemic disease and electrolyte abnormalities. May include cortisol and total thyroxine if hypoadrenocorticism and hypothyroidism are clinical concerns. See chapter 23 for further information on arrhythmias secondary to systemic disease.
Cardiac biomarkers	NTproBNP is a marker of myocardial stretch. Troponin is a marker of cardiomyocyte damage.
Parasite screening	In endemic areas, testing for *Dirofilaria immitus*, *Trypanosoma cruzi* and *Angiostronglyus vasorum* may be worthwhile.
Blood pressure	Hypotension may result in weakness or collapse. Hypertension could result in neurological signs.
Echocardiography	Screening for structural cardiac disease. Will also detect pleural effusion and some intrathoracic masses.
Resting ECG	Screening for persistent arrhythmias
Ambulatory ECG	Screening for intermittent arrhythmias
Thoracic radiographs	Assessing presence of congestive heart failure or lower respiratory tract disease
Physical manoeuvres	Assessing whether a vagal manoeuvre to increase parasympathetic tone or a precordial thump can interrupt a tachycardia

ECG, Electrocardiogram; NTproBNP, N-terminal pro-brain natriuretic peptide.

seizures and cardiogenic syncope showed that whilst there was a significant difference between groups, there was also considerable overlap, resulting in the conclusion that cTnI concentration cannot reliably distinguish syncope and seizures.[6]

Plasma *N-terminal pro-brain natriuretic peptide* (NTproBNP) is a marker of myocardial stretch, and therefore, in cases with arrhythmias without evidence of significant structural heart disease, it may be within the reference range. A large number of papers have been published on the utility of cardiac biomarkers and are summarised in a review article.[7]

Resting and Ambulatory ECGs

The main purpose of obtaining a resting ECG is to document heart rate and rhythm. In the investigation of arrhythmias, the greatest yield is likely to be in cases where a persistent (e.g. atrial fibrillation) or very frequent arrhythmia is detected. A normal resting ECG does not preclude an intermittent arrhythmia.[8] The use of ambulatory ECGs is discussed in chapter 15.

Logical Approach to Evaluation of the ECG

The key questions when presented with an ECG are:

1) What is the heart rate and rhythm?
2) Are any abnormalities present?
3) What is the significance of those abnormalities?

Interpretation of the ECG trace is described in chapter 4, and callipers are useful to determine whether the rhythm is regular.

See Table 4.4 for reference intervals for cat and dog electrocardiographic measurements.

Physiological Versus Pathological Rhythms

Physiological heart rhythms are described in chapter 5 and consist of:

- Sinus rhythm with heart rate appropriate for age and demeanour in dogs and cats
- Sinus arrhythmia in dogs
- Sinus tachycardia in dogs and cats.

Pathological arrhythmias are more likely to be clinically significant; examples include:

- Frequent single or multiple consecutive premature beats
- Accelerated idioventricular rhythm
- Ventricular, atrial or junctional tachycardia
- Prolonged sinus pauses
- Inappropriate heart rate for level of activity or demeanour
- Second-degree atrioventricular block (2AVB) during sinus rhythm
- High-grade 2AVB and also third-degree atrioventricular block (3AVB)
- Escape rhythm.

Primary Versus Secondary Arrhythmias

If an arrhythmia is detected, it is important to refer back to physical examination findings to determine if it is a primary arrhythmia or secondary to concurrent disease. For example, ventricular arrhythmias in dogs commonly occur secondary to systemic disease (see chapter 23). Likewise, bradyarrhythmias may occur secondary to concurrent conditions altering vagal tone, such as severe respiratory disease, intracranial disease, gastrointestinal disturbance and ocular disease (see chapter 23). However, it is likely that a thorough history and clinical examination would reveal evidence of trauma or these serious systemic disorders.

Physical Manoeuvres

In dogs presenting with incessant narrow-QRS complex tachycardia, physical interventions are sometimes employed in an attempt to interrupt the tachycardia (Figure 13.7). These manoeuvres are intended to raise vagal tone sufficiently to slow atrioventricular node conduction, thereby creating unfavourable conditions for re-entry and terminating the tachycardia. In dogs, *vagal manoeuvres* can be performed by placing pressure on the eyes[9] or neck in the area of the carotid sinus (caudodorsal to the larynx).[10] Pressure is applied unilaterally or bilaterally for up to 10 s, whilst heart rate is continually monitored. In humans, the gag reflex may alter vagal tone and temporary cessation of supraventricular tachycardia after vomiting has been described in a puppy.[11]

A precordial thump is delivered by placing a dog in right lateral recumbency, feeling for the left apex beat, and a fist is then used to strike the left apex. The energy delivered by the blow is transferred to the myocardium, and if a ventricular beat is generated as a response, then this may have the effect of temporarily terminating tachycardia. However, the guidelines for treatment of human out-of-hospital cardiac arrest do not currently recommend a precordial thump due to the risk of rhythm deterioration.[12]

Ice-water face immersion is commonly used in human patients, as stimulating the diver's reflex may result in bradycardia.[13] The face may be immersed or, in other cases, cold packs placed on the face. An unsuccessful attempt to use this technique was briefly described in a 4-month-old puppy.[11]

Case Examples

Case 1

Signalment: A 10-year-old, female, neutered English Springer Spaniel dog

History: The patient was presented for investigation of two episodes of collapse over the preceding 48 h. The first episode was not directly witnessed, but the owners were alerted by the sound of the dog falling down the stairs, and she was unresponsive for a short time when they found her lying at the foot of the stairs. The second event occurred after slight exertion and resulted in the dog becoming recumbent, with a brief period of extension of the front legs and neck followed by rapid and complete recovery. On reflection, the owners felt that over recent weeks the dog had shown episodes of being 'vacant', but she had remained standing and would readily respond if her name was called, suggesting that she was not losing consciousness.

Physical examination revealed:
- Alert and ambulatory
- Normal respiratory rate and effort
- Heart rate was 24 bpm, and the rhythm was irregular due to frequent long pauses.
- Reasonable cardiac output signs – mucous membranes were pink with capillary refill time of <2 s. Femoral pulse quality was good, and no pulse deficit was detected.
- No obvious jugular vein distension or palpable abdominal fluid thrill.
- No abnormalities were detected on abdominal palpation, or on musculoskeletal and brief neurological examination.

Given the bradycardia, it seemed logical to pursue this as the possible aetiology of the collapse episodes.

Investigation:
- Haematology and serum biochemistry (including electrolytes) revealed no clinically significant abnormalities.
- Resting ECG showed sinus rhythm with frequent and often prolonged sinus pauses not followed by an escape beat. An ambulatory ECG from a similar case is shown in Figure 12.3.
- Echo showed:
  - Mild generalised increase in cardiac chamber sizes which was attributed to the bradyarrhythmia
  - Mild thickening of the atrioventricular valves – typical for a dog of this age
  - Mild atrioventricular valve regurgitation.

Diagnosis: Sick sinus syndrome.

Treatment:
- Medical treatment with theophylline was instigated, and this resulted in a slight increase in heart rate,

but heart rate was still persistently below the accepted range.
- Permanent transvenous pacemaker implantation was performed, and this resulted in resolution of the clinical signs and a marked improvement in the dog's demeanour and ability to exercise.

Key point:

The 'classic' signs of syncope are more commonly associated with bradyarrhythmias than tachyarrhythmias.

Case 2

Signalment: An 8-year-old, female, entire Great Dane

History: The dog was referred for 1–2 episodes of ataxia. One of the episodes of ataxia occurred at exercise; the dog remained standing during the event, and recovery was spontaneous and rapid. The other episode occurred on slight exertion, and the owner described the dog briefly appearing unsteady without recumbency or loss of consciousness. The dog was generally keen to exercise and, prior to recent exercise restriction, was doing two long walks each week with a dog walker with no apparent exercise intolerance.

Physical examination demonstrated:
- Alert and in good body condition
- Respiratory rate and effort were normal at rest.
- Heart rate was 92 bpm, and the rhythm was slightly irregular.

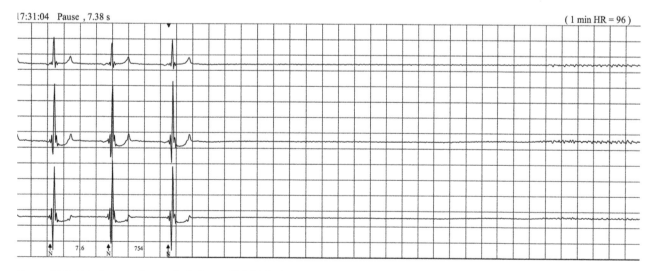

Figure 12.3 Sick sinus syndrome. Ambulatory ECG (Holter) trace showing three consecutive sinus beats with low-amplitude P waves followed by asystole for 7.38 s. No referable signs were observed during this pause. [12-year-old, female West Highland White terrier with a history of multiple episodes of syncope]

- Mucous membranes were pink with a capillary refill time (CRT) of <2 s.
- Femoral and peripheral pulses were strong with no deficit detected.
- Extremities felt warm on palpation.
- On auscultation, no abnormal cardiac or respiratory sounds were detected, but the rhythm was slightly more irregular than expected for sinus arrhythmia.

Investigation:
- *Resting ECG* showed atrial fibrillation with a slow ventricular response rate.
- *24 h ambulatory ECG* showed slow atrial fibrillation with a slow ventricular response rate (Figure 12.4).
- *Echocardiography* revealed normal cardiac chamber dimensions, and indices of systolic function were slightly depressed.

- *Thoracic radiographs* showed no evidence of congestive heart failure.
- *Haematology*, *serum biochemistry* and *total thyroxine assay* did not reveal evidence of systemic disease.

Provisional diagnosis: Slow atrial fibrillation combined with slight depression of systolic function were considered to be the likely cause of pre-syncope at exercise.

Comment:
- The loss of an organised atrial contraction during atrial fibrillation reduces ventricular filling, and this is exacerbated by the irregular heart rhythm resulting in a decrease in cardiac output. This slight drop in cardiac output may be tolerated at rest, but effects are likely to be more noticeable during periods of exercise.

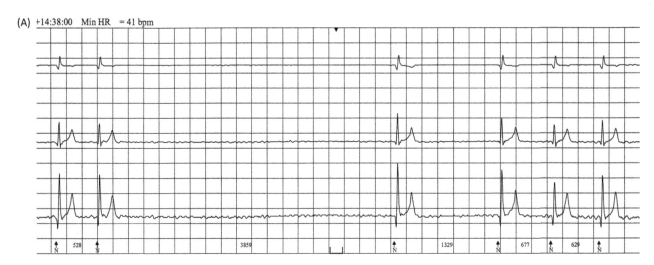

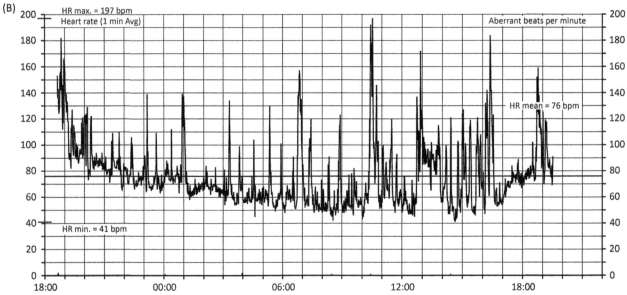

Figure 12.4 Slow atrial fibrillation. (A) Short section of trace from the 24 h ambulatory ECG recording, which showed that atrial fibrillation persisted throughout the recording and there was minimal ventricular ectopy. The ventricular rate during this section of trace was 41 bpm. (B) Tachogram from the same case illustrating that the mean ventricular rate over the 24 h period was 76 bpm. The maximum heart rate during exercise was 197 bpm, which is lower than generally seen in cases with atrial fibrillation. [8-year-old, female Great Dane dog]

- A 24 h ambulatory ECG recording was performed to document the mean ventricular rate during atrial fibrillation and showed a 24 h mean rate of 76 bpm (for more information on ambulatory ECGs and atrial fibrillation, see chapters 9 and 15).
- The relatively low mean ventricular rate suggests that a negative chronotrope is not required at present.
- In light of slightly reduced systolic function, treatment with the inodilator pimobendan was started, and this resulted in resolution of clinical signs.
- Rechecking echo and Holter was advised every 6–12 months in view of the risk of progression to a dilated cardiomyopathy phenotype.

Key point:

Atrial fibrillation tends to result in exercise intolerance or pre-syncope, rather than complete flaccid collapse with unconsciousness.

Case 3

Signalment: A 10-year-old, male, neutered Labrador Retriever crossbreed dog

History: The dog was presented for investigation of a heart murmur as well as a single episode of abnormal behaviour described as syncope. The heart murmur was first noted recently, and the dog had no history of signs referable to heart failure such as breathlessness, lethargy, anorexia or weight loss.

The episode occurred a few weeks before presentation, and prior to the event the dog had been exercising in bad weather. When the dog arrived home, he ate normally and, several hours later, was asleep immediately prior to the onset of signs. At the start of the event, the dog suddenly stood, and his owner was immediately aware that he did not look normal; the dog walked to another room and stood staring into space for some time. He was slightly ataxic and sat down briefly, but at no point was there recumbency or loss of consciousness, although he was described as looking tense and anxious which is out of character. Apart from some panting, breathing rate and effort were normal during the episode. The episode lasted for around 1 h before the dog settled and then slept through the night. The next day, he appeared completely normal.

Physical examination:
- The dog was alert, ambulatory and in good body condition.
- Respiratory rate and effort were normal at rest.

- Heart rate was 100 bpm, and the rhythm was regular.
- Normal cardiac output signs: Mucous membranes were pink with a CRT of <2 s, there was no obvious jugular distension or pulsation, the apex beat felt normal on palpation and femoral pulses were strong and regular with no deficit detected.
- There was no abdominal fluid thrill, and abdominal palpation felt unremarkable.
- Auscultation revealed a soft-grade 3/6 systolic murmur loudest over the left heart base, but no gallop sound or adventitious lung sounds were heard.
- There was reduced range of motion and possible pain on manipulation of both shoulders and elbows. No neck pain was elicited, but the dog did tense when ventral pressure was placed on his thoracic and lumbar spine.

The following investigation was performed:
- Haematology and serum biochemistry revealed no clinically significant abnormalities.
- ECG during echocardiography showed sinus rhythm.
- Echocardiography revealed normal cardiac chamber dimensions and good systolic function. There was mild thickening of the atrioventricular valves, typical for a dog of this age, and corresponding mild mitral and tricuspid regurgitation.
- Thoracic radiography revealed no significant abnormalities.
- A 24 h ambulatory ECG showed no abnormalities.

Provisional diagnosis or differential diagnoses:
- Murmur due to mild atrioventricular valve disease
- Aetiology of episode of behavioural change is unclear.

Comment: The aetiology of the episode of behavioural change remains unclear in this case, but the discussion with the owner was that it could be attributable to pain or perhaps a partial seizure. The outcome was that the owner was going to monitor the dog at home and call for advice if there were any further episodes of pain or behavioural change, as this might prompt imaging of the dog's brain and spine. Six months later, the dog has had no further events.

Key point:

Whilst the event was initially described as syncope, a detailed history was more suggestive of neurological disease or pain. In cases where there has been a single event, sometimes a reasonable approach may be to rule out potentially life-threatening cardiorespiratory conditions and then monitor to see if signs recur.

Case 4

Signalment: A 9-year-old, female, spayed Greyhound

History: The dog was presented for investigation of a heart murmur and arrhythmia that had been detected recently. Whilst the dog's exercise tolerance had decreased a little recently, this had been attributed to age, and the dog was still capable of an active lifestyle including vigorous exercise. No coughing or breathlessness was reported, but the owner reported that recently the dog was panting more after exercise than noted previously.

Physical examination demonstrated:
- The dog was alert and in good body condition.
- Heart rate was 96 bpm, and the rhythm was irregular due to frequent premature beats which did not seem typical of sinus arrhythmia.
- Mucous membranes were pink with a CRT of <2 s.
- No obvious jugular distension or pulsation.
- Femoral pulse quality was reasonable, but there was often a pulse deficit associated with the premature beats.
- Respiratory rate and effort were normal at rest, and tracheal palpation did not elicit a cough.
- On auscultation, there was a grade 1/6 systolic murmur loudest at the left heart base; no gallop sound or adventitious lung sounds were detected.
- As might be expected in an ex-racing greyhound, there was evidence of musculoskeletal disease, including mild discomfort on extension of the dog's left shoulder, during movement of both hips and also when ventral pressure was placed on her thoracolumbar spine.

Investigation:
- ECG during echo showed predominantly sinus rhythm interspersed with frequent single supraventricular premature beats followed by a short pause.
- Echocardiography revealed normal cardiac chamber dimensions and good systolic function. There was laminar flow in the aorta and pulmonary artery, and flow velocity was at the upper end of the accepted range which was attributed to the dog being slightly anxious.
- A 24 h ambulatory ECG recording showed 4040 supraventricular premature beats which generally occurred singly. Whilst supraventricular tachycardia was documented during the recording, the trace from around these times corresponded to baseline artefact and diary entries, suggesting exercise and excitement, and had the appearance of sinus tachycardia with a maximum instantaneous rate of 187 bpm. There were no features of pathological tachycardia such as sudden onset or offset, P' waves or electrical alternans.

Provisional diagnosis: Arrhythmia documented, but musculoskeletal disease was thought more likely to be the cause of the dog's reduced exercise tolerance.

Treatment recommendations: None for arrhythmia; trial therapy with non-steroidal anti-inflammatory drugs (NSAIDs).

Comment: The dog was rechecked 4 weeks later, and exercise tolerance was reported to have improved, so NSAID therapy was continued.

Key point:

Whilst an arrhythmia was documented, it was not thought to be the cause of exercise intolerance. Frequent supraventricular premature beats may precede the development of atrial fibrillation, so further monitoring is recommended.

Case 5

Signalment: A 2.5-year-old, male, neutered crossbreed dog

History: The dog was presented for investigation of an unwitnessed episode of collapse or seizure during a walk in the woods. He was otherwise healthy and exercising normally. There was no history of previous episodes such as this one or health issues.

Physical examination:
- The dog was alert and in good body condition.
- Heart rate was 100 bpm, and the rhythm was irregular due to occasional brief pauses.
- Mucous membranes were pink with a CRT of <2 s.
- No obvious jugular distension or pulsation.
- Femoral pulse quality was normal.
- Respiratory rate and effort were normal at rest, and tracheal palpation did not elicit a cough.
- Abnormalities were not detected on auscultation.
- Neurological examination was unremarkable.

Investigation:
- ECG showed a sinus rhythm with first-degree and occasional second-degree (Mobitz II) atrioventricular block.
- Echocardiography was unremarkable.
- An episode of seizure was recorded during a 24 h ambulatory ECG recording (Figure 12.5). This episode occurred at the time of patient discharge – the dog became very excited when he saw his owner, jumped into his lap, and then fell to the ground and had a tonic-clonic seizure. The episode lasted for several seconds and was quickly followed by full recovery. The Holter revealed sinus tachycardia

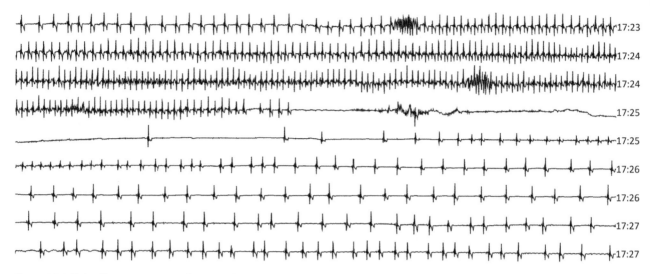

Figure 12.5 Episodic seizure activity due to prolonged sinus arrest. This extract from a Holter monitor shows the heart rhythm at the time of a tonic-clonic seizure episode in a young dog. This episode occurred at the time of discharge. The dog got very excited when he saw his owner, hence the baseline artefact and sinus tachycardia, and then had an episode of tonic-clonic seizure caused by prolonged brain hypoxia due to a 23 s period of sinus arrest, interrupted by a ventricular escape beat, and then another 6.7 s pause before slow recovery of a normal sinus rhythm. [2.5-year-old, male neutered, crossbreed dog with conduction system disease]

followed by a 23 s pause interrupted by a ventricular escape beat, and then another 6.7 s pause before slow resumption of sinus rhythm.

Diagnosis: Conduction system disease affecting the sinus node and atrioventricular node.

Treatment and follow-up: An artificial pacemaker was implanted, and the dog has been well since.

Key point:

Whilst the episode was a typical seizure, the cause was prolonged brain hypoxia due to a bradyarrhythmia. A cardiac aetiology should not be ruled out in a case with seizure episodes, particularly if there are signs of heart disease such as an irregular heart rhythm or heart murmur.

References

1 Moya A, Sutton R, Ammirati F, Blanc J-J, Brignole M, Dahm JB, *et al.* Guidelines for the diagnosis and management of syncope (version 2009). Eur Heart J. 2009;30:2631–2671.

2 Thiruganasambandamoorthy V, Kwong K, Wells GA, Sivilotti MLA, Mukarram M, Rowe BH, *et al.* Development of the Canadian Syncope Risk Score to predict serious adverse events after emergency department assessment of syncope. CMAJ. 2016;188:E289–E298.

3 Sheldon R, Rose S, Ritchie D, Connolly SJ, Koshman M-L, Lee MA, *et al.* Historical criteria that distinguish syncope from seizures. J Am Coll Cardiol. 2002;40:142–148.

4 Shen WK, Traub SJ, Decker WW. Syncope management unit: evolution of the concept and practice implementation. Prog Cardiovasc Dis. 2013;55:382–389.

5 Barnett L, Martin MWS, Todd J, Smith S, Cobb M. A retrospective study of 153 cases of undiagnosed collapse, syncope or exercise intolerance: the outcomes. J Small Anim Pract. 2011;52:26–31.

6 Dutton E, Dukes McEwan J, Cripps PJ. Serum cardiac troponin I in canine syncope and seizures. J Vet Cardiol. 2017;19:1–13.

7 Oyama MA. Using cardiac biomarkers in veterinary practice. Vet Clin North Am Small Anim Pract. 2013;43:1261–1272–vi.

8 Wess G, Schulze A, Geraghty N, Hartmann K. Ability of a 5-minute electrocardiography (ECG) for predicting arrhythmias in Doberman Pinschers with cardiomyopathy in comparison with a 24-hour ambulatory ECG. J Vet Intern Med. 2010;24:367–371.

9 Turner Giannico A, de Sampaio MOB, Lima L, Corona Ponczek C, De Lara F, Montiani-Ferreira F. Characterization of the oculocardiac reflex during compression of the globe in Beagle dogs and rabbits. Vet Ophthalmol. 2014;17:321–327.

10 Vatner SF, Franklin D, Van Citters RL, Braunwald E. Effects of carotid sinus nerve stimulation on blood-flow distribution in conscious dogs at rest and during exercise. Circ Res. 1970;27:495–503.

11 Atkins CE, Kanter R, Wright K, Saba Z, Baty C, Swanson C, *et al.* Orthodromic reciprocating tachycardia and heart failure in a dog with a concealed posteroseptal accessory pathway. J Vet Intern Med. 1995;9:43–49.

12 Smith J, Judge B. BET 1: Effectiveness of the precordial thump in restoring heart rhythm following out-of-hospital cardiac arrest. Emerg Med J. 2016;33:366–367.

13 Gallo LJ, Maciel BC, Manco JC, Marin Neto JA. Limitations of facial immersion as a test of parasympathetic activity in man. J Physiol. 1988;396:1–10.

13

Diagnostic Approach to Narrow-QRS Complex Tachycardia

Antonia Mavropoulou

Introduction

Narrow-QRS complex tachycardias are usually of supraventricular origin which is why they are commonly described as supraventricular tachycardias (SVTs). Their differentiation is a common diagnostic challenge as they may present with similar electrocardiographic features, especially when heart rate is significantly elevated (Figure 13.1). Despite their similarities, several features can be used for their differentiation. Twelve-lead electrocardiogram (ECG) obtained during sinus rhythm and during tachycardia may potentially reveal the mechanism of arrhythmia[1] and represents the first step for diagnosis. The same electrocardiographic criteria used in people can be applied in dogs[2] and potentially in cats with narrow-QRS tachycardia. Drug trials or vagal manoeuvers can help reveal the underlying rhythm by reducing conduction through the atrioventricular node (AVN), slowing the heart rate or interrupting the tachycardia. This can allow a much better recognition of the electrocardiographic waves and may facilitate the electrocardiographic diagnosis. However, despite the undoubted utility of the 12-lead ECG, in certain cases intracardiac electrophysiologic studies are necessary for a definitive diagnosis and treatment.[3,4]

Several algorithms have been published in human literature as a practical guide for clinicians,[5–7] but, to the best of the author's knowledge, they are lacking in the veterinary literature.

The purpose of this chapter is to review the electrocardiographic criteria used for the differentiation of narrow-QRS complex tachycardias and to propose a useful algorithm to help clinicians develop a stepwise approach to the differential diagnoses of narrow-QRS complex tachycardias (see Figure 13.2).

Stepwise Approach to the Differential Diagnosis of Narrow-QRS Complex Tachycardias

Step 1: Is this a Narrow-QRS Complex Tachycardia? QRS <70 ms in Dogs and <40 ms in Cats

As the name suggests, narrow-QRS complex tachycardias are characterized by a normal QRS complex duration (<70 ms in dogs[2] and <40 ms in cats). These rhythm disturbances usually arise above the bundle of His (i.e. sinus node, atrial tissue or atrioventricular [AV] junction) and may involve an accessory pathway as explained in chapter 10. Although infrequent, narrow-QRS ventricular tachycardia has also been reported in human[8] and veterinary literature,[9] and it should always be considered in the differential diagnosis, especially when treatment for SVT is unsuccessful. Nevertheless, they represent an exception to the rule and will not be discussed further here.

Step 2: Is the Rhythm Regular or Irregular?

An irregular rhythm is most commonly present in atrial fibrillation, atrial flutter (with variable AV nodal conduction) and multifocal atrial tachycardia (MAT). However, as the rate of the tachycardia increases, the irregularity of the rhythm may become less apparent, and it may be mistaken for a regular SVT.

A regular rhythm is most commonly seen in sinus tachycardia, macro-reentrant tachycardias (orthodromic atrioventricular reciprocating tachycardia [OAVRT], atrioventricular nodal reciprocating tachycardia [AVNRT] and atrial flutter with constant AV conduction) and junctional tachycardia.[10] Atrial fibrillation can also present with a regular rhythm in the case of third-degree AV block and a ventricular or junctional escape rhythm (see Figure 9.11).[5]

Guide to Canine and Feline Electrocardiography, First Edition. Ruth Willis, Pedro Oliveira and Antonia Mavropoulou.
© 2018 John Wiley & Sons Ltd. Published 2018 by John Wiley & Sons Ltd.
Companion website: www.wiley.com/go/willis/electrocardiography

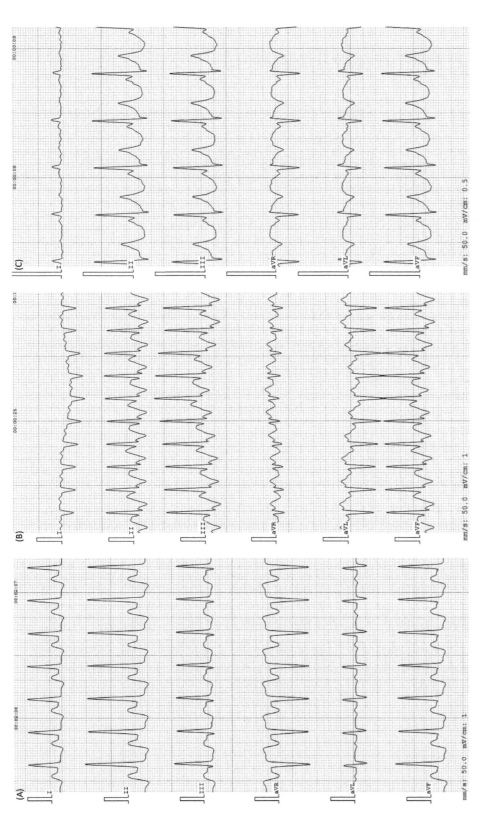

Figure 13.1 Different narrow-QRS tachycardias. These are three examples of different narrow-QRS tachycardias with similar electrocardiographic presentation that pose a diagnostic challenge. (A) A narrow-QRS (60 ms) tachycardia is seen with a rate of approximately 230 bpm and a regular rhythm. Obvious P or F waves are not seen and if present are likely superimposed on the QRS-T. The T wave appears biphasic in lead II with a negative component followed by a positive one. Assuming that both components form part of the T wave, the QTc would be 278 ms, which is abnormally long. This suggests that the positive component might actually be a superimposed P or F wave, although we cannot really be sure based on this trace alone. An additional trace of this case is shown in Figure 13.4. Differential diagnoses should include focal atrial tachycardia, atrial flutter (reverse typical or atypical as there is return to baseline), junctional tachycardia and atrioventricular reciprocating tachycardia. [11-year-old, male neutered, Cavalier King Charles Spaniel with chronic valvular degenerative disease and SVT] (50 mm/s; 10 mm/mV) (B) A narrow-QRS (50 ms) tachycardia is seen with a rate of approximately 240 bpm and a regular rhythm. A deflection that is negative in leads I, II, III and aVF and positive in aVR and aVL is seen on the ST segment, raising suspicion of a retrograde P'. Assuming that the deflection that follows is the T wave ending just before the next QRS, the QTc would be approximately 220–230 ms, which is within the normal range (150–240 ms). Alternatively, both deflections could be ascending and descending components of typical flutter (F) waves superimposed on the T wave. Additional traces of this case are shown in Figure 13.3. Differential diagnoses should include atrioventricular reciprocating tachycardia, atrial flutter, junctional tachycardia originating from the distal atrioventricular bundle with 1:1 retrograde P', and focal atrial tachycardia. [4-month-old, male Staffordshire Terrier with SVT] (50 mm/s; 10 mm/mV) (C) A narrow-QRS (50–60 ms) tachycardia is seen with a rate of approximately 180 bpm and a regular rhythm. Two deflections are seen between each QRS without an obvious return to baseline; they are positive in leads II, III and aVF and are negative in leads aVR and aVL, and one of them is partially buried in the QRS. The first deflection is likely to be (or include) the T wave with a QTc of 220–230 ms, which falls within the expected range. It is possible that a P or F wave may be superimposed in the T, suggesting an atrial depolarisation rate of 260 bpm with a 2:1 atrioventricular conduction. These findings are suspicious of atrial flutter; however, focal atrial tachycardia or atrioventricular reciprocating tachycardia may not be ruled out. Junctional tachycardia with isorhythmic atrioventricular dissociation of type 2 is unlikely at this rate as is a pre-excited tachycardia given that the QRS is normal in duration. See Figure 13.5 for more traces of this case. [8-year-old, female neutered, Bernese Mountain dog with SVT] (50 mm/s; 20 mm/mV)

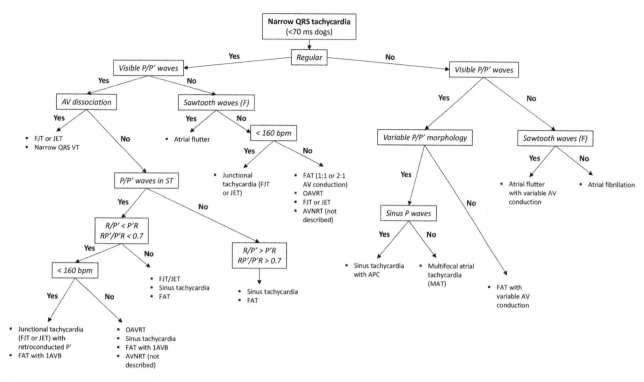

Figure 13.2 Algorithm for the diagnosis of narrow-QRS rhythms in dogs. APC = atrial premature complex; AVB = atrioventricular block; AVNRT = atrioventricular node reentrant tachycardia; FAT = focal atrial tachycardia; FJT = focal junctional tachycardia; JET = junctional ectopic tachycardia; MAT = multifocal atrial tachycardia; OAVRT = orthodromic atrioventricular reciprocating tachycardia; VT = ventricular tachycardia.

Step 3: What is the Ventricular Rate?

The ventricular rate does not allow a definitive diagnosis by itself as substantial overlap exists between different tachycardias in dogs[2] as described for humans.[3,11,12] Nevertheless, the ventricular rate tends to be higher in focal atrial tachycardia (FAT) (210–340 bpm)[2] and in atrial flutter with 1:1 AV conduction (270–360 bpm),[2,13] while it tends to be lower in OAVRT (190–270 bpm).[2] A heart rate of 100–160 bpm has been described in focal junctional tachycardia (FJT).[14] In atrial fibrillation, the rate is variable depending on the refractoriness of the AV node.[15,16] It commonly ranges between 120 and 260 bpm in dogs and between 200 and 280 bpm in cats. It is important to note that these ranges are not absolute and exceptions are common (e.g. FJT >160 bpm), which is why the ventricular rate is not a reliable indicator of the type of SVT.

Step 4: Identifying Sinus (P) or Ectopic (P′) Atrial Depolarisation Waves During Tachycardia

Identification of the P/P′ waves during tachycardia is essential for the diagnosis but is often challenging, especially when the heart rate is high (Figures 13.1, 13.3 and 13.4). Vagal manoeuvres or the use of drugs that slow AV conduction (e.g. calcium channel blockers, sotalol etc.) can help reveal the presence of P/P′ waves previously hidden within the QRS complexes or the T waves (Figures 13.5 and 13.6).[17,18] Their identification may be made easier when the QRS-T complexes of the SVT are compared to the QRS-T complexes during sinus rhythm. P/P′ waves may precede the QRS complex or may occur during the ascending or descending limb of the R wave, the ST segment or the T wave, and their position may provide information regarding the mechanism of the arrhythmia.

- In *sinus tachycardia*, P waves precede the QRS complex, have a normal morphology (like the P wave during normal heart rate) and have a normal PR interval.
- In *OAVRT*, P′ waves may be seen in the initial ST segment and are negative in leads II, III and aVF[2] (Figure 13.3; and see chapter 10).
- In *AVNRT*, distinct P′ waves are not identified as they occur during the QRS complex; however, careful comparison of the QRS complexes during sinus rhythm and tachycardia may allow identification of pseudo S or Q waves in leads II, III and aVF or r′ waves in V1 (see chapter 10).
- In *FAT*, P′ wave morphology depends on the location of the ectopic focus (see chapter 8).[7] In dogs, P′ waves have been most commonly described as positive in the

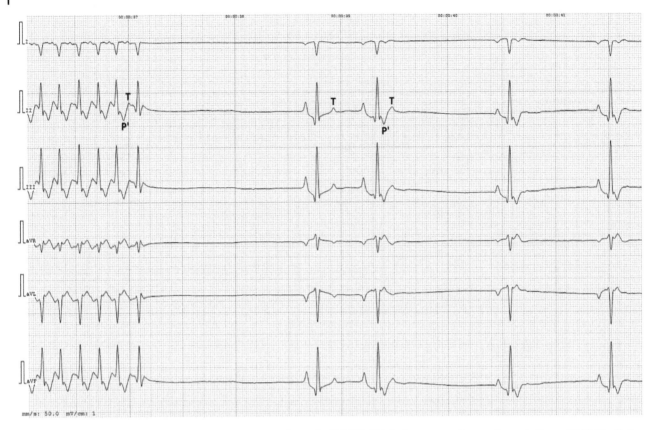

Figure 13.3 Orthodromic atrioventricular reciprocating tachycardia (OAVRT). This is the same patient as shown in Figure 13.1B. The first six beats correspond to narrow-QRS tachycardia as described in 13.1B. The tachycardia terminates abruptly and is followed by four sinus beats with respiratory sinus arrhythmia. By comparing the ST segment of the first sinus beat to the ST during tachycardia, and the other sinus beats, a retrograde P' (negative in leads II, III and aVF and positive in aVR and aVL) becomes apparent in the ST segment. This is consistent with OAVRT. [4-month-old, male, Staffordshire Bull Terrier dog with OAVRT confirmed with an electrophysiology study] (50 mm/s; 10 mm/mV)

inferior leads (II, III and aVF) located within the descending limb of the T wave.[2] Less often, FAT may present with negative P' waves in the inferior leads, but their position is usually different compared to the OAVRT and they do not cause distortion of the ST segment (Figure 13.4).[2]

- In *FJT*, sinus P waves may precede the QRS complexes with a constant PQ interval (isorhythmic AV dissociation with type 2 synchronization), or they may move back and forth across the QRS complexes (isorhythmic AV dissociation with type 1 synchronization). Alternatively, in the presence of 1:1 ventriculo-atrial conduction, negative P' waves inscribed in the descending branch of the QRS complex (pseudo S waves) may be seen in leads II, III and aVF.[14,19]
- In *atrial flutter* or *fibrillation*, P/P' waves not identified as the normal P waves are replaced by 'sawtooth' F waves in atrial flutter or f waves in atrial fibrillation (see chapters 8 and 9). Atrial fibrillation is usually easily identified due to the irregular pattern of ventricular activation. Diagnosis of typical atrial flutter is also relatively straightforward if the characteristic F waves

are visible with absence of the isoelectric line (although it may still be difficult in the case of 2:1 AV conduction) (Figure 13.5).[20–22] Diagnosis can be challenging in reverse typical or atypical flutter when the isoelectric line is interposed between the F waves,[13,23,24] and differentiation from other narrow-QRS complex tachycardias (e.g. FAT) can be difficult especially when AV conduction is 2:1 (see chapter 8). As a general rule, 2:1 conduction should be suspected whenever an F or P/P' wave is halfway between the QRS complexes, and it strongly suggests that another F or P/P' wave is buried within the QRS complex (the Bix rule).[25]

Step 5: What is the Relationship Between the P' Wave and the QRS Complex?

The relationship between the P' and QRS complex is another helpful tool to distinguish between the different types of SVT. The P' is located between two QRS in succession. Logic dictates that if the P' is closer to the next QRS (RP' > P'R), it is likely to have triggered it (e.g. FAT). Alternatively, if the P' is closer to the previous QRS

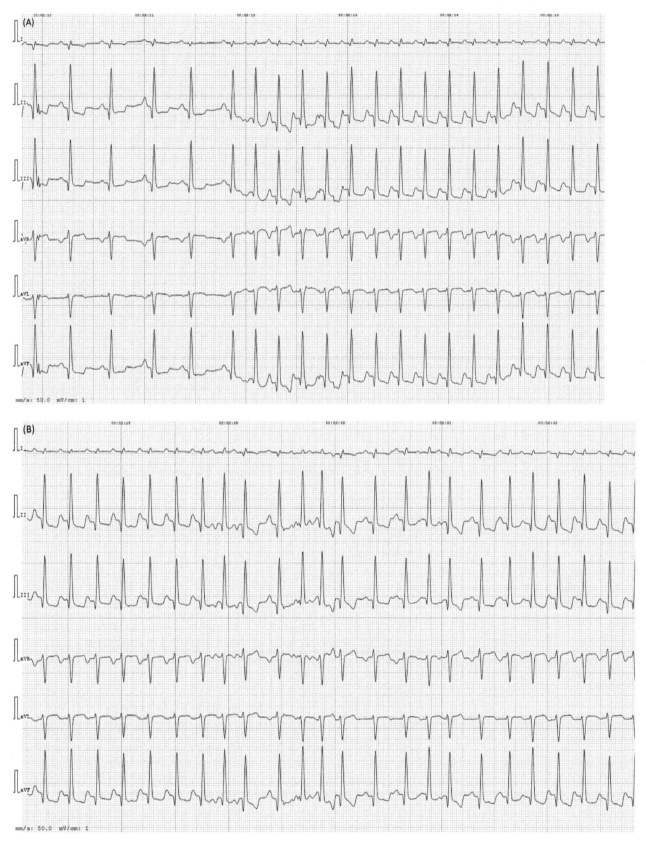

Figure 13.4 Focal atrial tachycardia. This is the same patient as shown in Figure 13.1A. (A) The first six beats are sinus with a normal P-QRS-T. The seventh beat is premature after which a narrow-QRS tachycardia is seen with sudden onset and a regular rhythm. Comparison of the T wave during sinus rhythm and tachycardia suggests that the positive deflection seen at the end of the T during tachycardia is indeed an ectopic P′ wave with a RP′>P′R consistent with focal atrial tachycardia. The sudden onset suggests a possible micro re-entrant mechanism for the tachycardia. The first beat is not preceded by the same P′ wave as seen during tachycardia, and instead a small deflection may be seen superimposed on the T wave, suggesting a possible different ectopic focus. Similar beats are seen during tachycardia in (B) rendering the rhythm irregular. These findings are suggestive of a multifocal tachycardia which would fit with the clinical presentation of chronic valvular degenerative disease with marked structural changes in this case. [11-year-old, male neutered, Cavalier King Charles Spaniel with chronic valvular degenerative disease and SVT] (50 mm/s; 10 mm/mV)

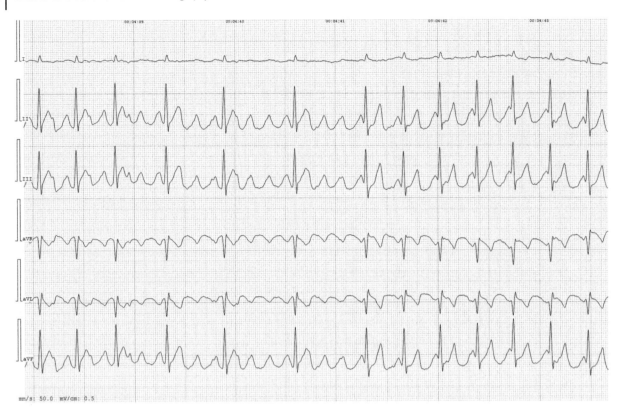

Figure 13.5 Atrial flutter. This is the same patient as shown in Figure 13.1C after administration of oral sotalol. Flutter waves are now visible, confirming a diagnosis of atrial flutter. [8-year-old, female neutered, Bernese Mountain dog with SVT] (50 mm/s; 20 mm/mV)

(RP' < P'R), it is possible that it was retro-conducted to the atria (e.g. OAVRT or FJT), particularly if the P' conformation is consistent with an origin on the floor of one of the atria. Studies in humans have shown that a short RP' interval (RP' < P'R) and a RP'/P'R <1 is more frequently seen in OAVRT, while long RP' interval (RP' > P'R) and a RP'/P'R >1 is more commonly seen in FAT.[1,6,11] Similar findings were described in dogs where the RP'/P'R was on average 0.6 ± 0.18 in the case of OAVRT and 1.45 ± 0.52 in the case of FAT.[2] A cut-off of 0.7 was proposed to distinguish OAVRT (RP'/P'R <0.7) and FAT (RP'/P'R >0.7).[2]

Step 6: Are there Instances of AV Block During Tachycardia?

The presence of second-degree AV block during tachycardia without its termination is diagnostic for the presence of an atrial rhythm in which the AV node and ventricles do not form part of the arrhythmia circuit (AV node-independent tachycardia). These include sinus tachycardia, FAT, MAT, junctional tachycardia (depending on origin), atrial flutter and atrial fibrillation (Figures 13.5, 13.6 and 13.7). On the contrary, OAVRT is not possible in cases of AV block, as the AV node forms part of the re-entrant circuit that sustains tachycardia and therefore a block would cause its termination.[2,11,26]

Step 7: Are there ST Segment Changes?

ST segment depression ≥1.5–2 mm in the inferior leads and ST elevation ≥1–1.5 mm in lead aVR during tachycardia have been reported in humans[11,12,27] and dogs.[2] It is more frequently observed in OAVRT in comparison to FAT or AVNRT. These distortions are caused not only by retrograde atrial activation (seen as P' waves at the beginning of the ST segment) but also by repolarisation changes or the effects of catecholamines during tachycardia.[28,29]

Step 8: Is Electrical Alternans Present?

Electrical alternans (defined as beat-to-beat oscillation of QRS complex amplitude ≥1 mm in at least one lead) is most commonly seen in dogs with OAVRT and less frequently detected during FAT.[2] Published reports in people yielded conflicting results, with some studies showing that electrical alternans was predictive of reentrant tachycardias and others failing to show an association between the type of tachycardia and this electrocardiographic finding.[11,30,31] These latter studies found that electrical alternans is a rate-dependent phenomenon independent of the type of tachycardia.[32,33] This feature should not be used as the sole characteristic to distinguish different types of SVT.

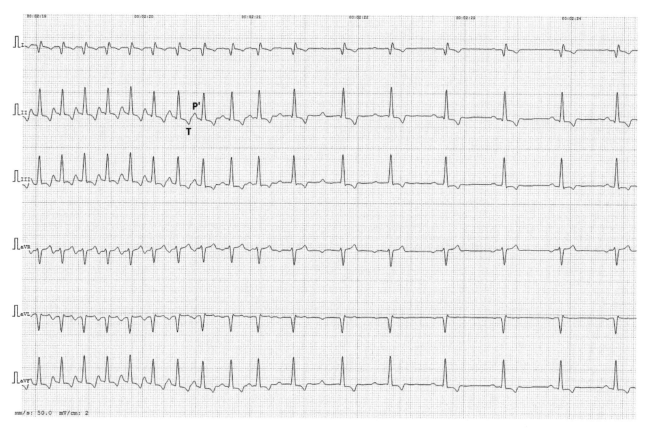

Figure 13.6 Vagal manoeuvre during tachycardia. This electrocardiographic trace was recorded from a dog with focal atrial tachycardia during a vagal manoeuvre. The initial part of the trace is similar to the one on Figure 13.1A. A narrow QRS (50 ms) is seen with a rate of approximately 280 bpm and a regular rhythm. From the seventh beat, the rate starts to decrease, and a P' separates from the T with a progressive increase in P'R interval until the P-QRS-T normalises with a sinus rhythm of approximately 120 bpm towards the end of the trace. The P' is similar in appearance to the presumed sinus P, suggesting either sinus tachycardia or focal atrial tachycardia originating from the roof of the right atrium. [10-year-old, female neutered, Labrador Retriever dog with suspicion of tachycardia-induced cardiomyopathy] (50 mm/s; 5 mm/mV)

Step 9: Is Cycle Length Alternans Present?

Cycle length alternans is defined as a beat-to-beat oscillation of the cycle length (RR intervals) ≥20 ms that can be seen during SVTs.[12] Cycle length irregularity is more commonly seen in dogs with FAT and less frequently in OAVRT,[2] but similarly to reports in people it is not a discriminator of the mechanism of arrhythmia.[11,12]

Step 10: Is there Evidence of Ventricular Pre-excitation During Sinus Rhythm?

Ventricular pre-excitation indicates the presence of an accessory pathway that allows antegrade conduction from the atria to the ventricles.[34] Its presence increases the likelihood of OAVRT.[18,35,36] However, in rare cases, other SVTs (e.g. FAT or atrial fibrillation) may occur in the presence of ventricular pre-excitation via an accessory pathway (see Figure 9.10), hence this possibility should also be considered.[2]

Step 11: How Does the Tachycardia Start and Terminate?

A gradual acceleration and deceleration of the rate at the onset and offset of tachycardia, respectively ('warm-up' and 'cool-down' phenomena), suggest that the underlying arrhythmia mechanism is enhanced or abnormal automaticity.[37,38] This may be seen with automatic atrial tachycardias (e.g. FAT, MAT and FJT) or sinus tachycardia. Alternatively, a sudden onset and offset of tachycardia are more likely to occur with triggered activity (e.g. FAT, MAT and FJT) or reentry (OAVRT, AVNRT and atrial flutter). This means that unfortunately, in cases of sudden onset and offset of tachycardia, all types of SVT are still possible, but if warm-up and cool-down phenomena are present, a reentrant tachycardia is not likely to be present.

The onset and offset of tachycardia should also be inspected for possible eliciting triggers such as premature ectopic beats (more common in reentrant tachycardias). A precordial thump may induce an ectopic beat, resulting

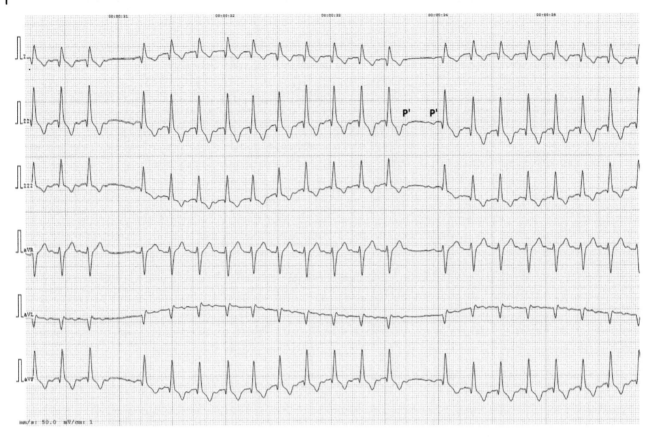

Figure 13.7 Atrioventricular block during tachycardia. This electrocardiographic trace shows a narrow-QRS tachycardia with a rate of approximately 200–220 bpm and an irregular rhythm. The QRS is normal (60 ms; MEA, 77°) and is preceded by an ectopic P′ wave with likely origin on the floor of the left atrium and a constant P′R interval of 90 ms. These findings are consistent with a focal atrial tachycardia. Two non-conducted P′ waves may be seen, indicating that the atrioventricular node and ventricles do not form part of the arrhythmia mechanism. [6-year-old, male Siberian Husky dog with focal atrial tachycardia confirmed with an electrophysiology study] (50 mm/s; 10 mm/mV)

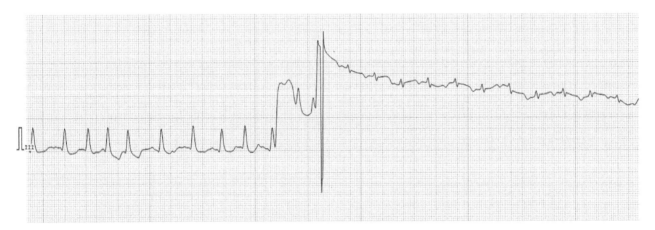

Figure 13.8 Precordial thump during tachycardia. This is the same patient as shown in Figures 13.1A and 13.4. The initial part shows an irregular narrow-QRS tachycardia that could be interpreted as possible atrial fibrillation or, in this case, multifocal atrial tachycardia as suspected based on the previous traces. The sharp deflection seen in the middle of the trace is a movement artefact caused by the precordial thump, and the rhythm that follows is sinus. Lead III was chosen as it was the one least affected by movement artefact. [11-year-old, male neutered, Cavalier King Charles Spaniel with chronic valvular degenerative disease and SVT] (50 mm/s; 10 mm/mV)

in tachycardia termination (Figure 13.8). Additionally, the presence of a P' wave at offset with an electrical axis consistent with an origin in the floor of one of the atria is suggestive of a retro-conducted P' during OAVRT.

References

1 Page RL, Joglar JA, Caldwell MA, Calkins H, Conti JB, Deal BJ, *et al*. 2015 ACC/AHA/HRS guideline for the management of adult patients with supraventricular tachycardia. Heart Rhythm. 2016;13:e136–e221.

2 Santilli RA, Perego M, Crosara S, Gardini F, Bellino C, Moretti P, *et al*. Utility of 12-lead electrocardiogram for differentiating paroxysmal supraventricular tachycardias in dogs. J Vet Intern Med. 2008;22:915–923.

3 Kalbfleisch SJ, el-Atassi R, Calkins H, Langberg JJ, Morady F. Differentiation of paroxysmal narrow QRS complex tachycardias using the 12-lead electrocardiogram. J Am Coll Cardiol. 1993;21:85–89.

4 Katritsis DG, Josephson ME. Differential diagnosis of regular, narrow-QRS tachycardias. Heart Rhythm. 2015;12:1667–1676.

5 Buttà C, Tuttolomondo A, Di Raimondo D, Milio G, Miceli S, Attanzio MT, *et al*. Supraventricular tachycardias: proposal of a diagnostic algorithm for the narrow complex tachycardias. J Cardiol. 2013;61:247–255.

6 Borloz MP, Mark DG, Pines JM, Brady WJ. Electrocardiographic differential diagnosis of narrow QRS complex tachycardia: an ED-oriented algorithmic approach. Am J Emerg Med. 2010;28:378–381.

7 Buttà C, Tuttolomondo A, Giarrusso L, Pinto A. Electrocardiographic diagnosis of atrial tachycardia: classification, P-wave morphology, and differential diagnosis with other supraventricular tachycardias. Ann Noninvasive Electrocardiol. 2015;20:314–327.

8 Hayes JJ, Stewart RB, Green HL, Bardy GH. Narrow QRS ventricular tachycardia. Ann Intern Med. 2011;114:460–463.

9 Stern JA, Doreste YR, Barnett S, Lahmers SM, Baumwart RD, Seino KK, *et al*. Resolution of sustained narrow complex ventricular tachycardia and tachycardia-induced cardiomyopathy in a Quarter Horse following quinidine therapy. J Vet Cardiol. 2012;14:445–451.

10 Katritsis DG, Josephson ME. Differential diagnosis of regular, narrow-QRS tachycardias. Heart Rhythm. 2015;12:1667–1676.

11 Erdinler, I, Okmen, E, Oguz, E, Akyol, A, Gurkan, K, Ulufer, T. Differentiation of narrow QRS complex tachycardia types using the 12-lead electrocardiogram. Ann Noninvasive Electrocardiol. 2002;7:120–126.

12 Zhong YM, Guo JH, Hou AJ, Chen SJ, Wang Y, Zhang HC. A modified electrocardiographic algorithm for differentiating typical atrioventricular node re-entrant tachycardia from atrioventricular reciprocating tachycardia mediated by concealed accessory pathway. Int J Clin Pract. 2006;60:1371–1377.

13 Santilli RA, Ramera L, Perego M, Moretti P, Spadacini G. Radiofrequency catheter ablation of atypical atrial flutter in dogs. J Vet Cardiol. 2014;16:9–17.

14 Perego M, Ramera L, Santilli RA. Isorhythmic atrioventricular dissociation in Labrador Retrievers. J Vet Intern Med. 2012;26:320–325.

15 Rankin AC, Workman AJ. Rate control in atrial fibrillation: role of atrial inputs to the AV node. Cardiovasc Res. 1999;44:249–251.

16 Garrigue S, Tchou PJ, Mazgalev TN. Role of the differential bombardment of atrial inputs to the atrioventricular node as a factor influencing ventricular rate during high atrial rate. Cardiovasc Res. 1999;44:344–355.

17 Nattel S, Gersh BJ, Opie LH. In Drugs for the heart (eds. Opie LH, Gersh BJ, pp. 272–331). Amsterdam: Elsevier; 2013.

18 Atkins CE, Kanter R, Wright K, Saba Z, Baty C, Swanson C, *et al*. Orthodromic reciprocating tachycardia and heart failure in a dog with a concealed posteroseptal accessory pathway. J Vet Intern Med. 1995;9:43–49.

19 Rosen KM. Junctional tachycardia: mechanisms, diagnosis, differential diagnosis, and management. Circulation. 1973;47:654–664.

20 Santilli RA, Perego M, Perini A, Carli A, Moretti P, Spadacini G. Radiofrequency catheter ablation of cavo-tricuspid isthmus as treatment of atrial flutter in two dogs. J Vet Cardiol. 2001;12:59–66.

21 Bun S-S, Latcu DG, Marchlinski F, Saoudi N. Atrial flutter: more than just one of a kind. Eur Heart J. 2015;36:2356–2363.

22 Inama G, Pedrinazzi C, Durin O, Agricola P, Romagnoli G, Gazzaniga P. Usefulness and limitations of the surface electrocardiogram in the classification of right and left atrial flutter. J Cardiovasc Med (Hagerstown). 2006;7:381–387.

23 Shah D. ECG manifestations of left atrial flutter. Curr Opin Cardiol. 2009;24:35–41.

24 Cosio FG, Martín-Peñato A, Pastor A, Núñez A, Goicolea A. Atypical flutter: a review. Pacing Clin Electrophysiol. 2003;26:2157–2169.

25 Nikolić G. The Bix rule. Heart Lung J Acute Crit Care. 2008;37:321–322.

26 Obel OA, Camm AJ. Supraventricular tachycardia: ECG diagnosis and anatomy. Eur Heart J. 1997;18:2–11.

27 Ho Y-L, Lin L-Y, Lin J-L, Chen M-F, Chen W-J, Lee Y-T. Usefulness of ST-segment elevation in lead aVR during tachycardia for determining the mechanism of

narrow QRS complex tachycardia. Am J Cardiol. 2003;92:1424–1428.

28 Riva SI, Della Bella P, Fassini G, Carbucicchio C, Tondo C. Value of analysis of ST segment changes during tachycardia in determining type of narrow QRS complex tachycardia. J Am Coll Cardiol. 1996;27:1480–1485.

29 Nelson SD, Kou WH, Annesley T, de Buitleir M, Morady F. Significance of ST segment depression during paroxysmal supraventricular tachycardia. J Am Coll Cardiol. 1988;12:383–387.

30 Kalbfleisch SJ, El-Atassi R, Calkins H, Langberg JJ, Morady F. Differentiation of paroxysmal narrow QRS complex tachycardias using the 12-lead electrocardiogram. J Am Coll Cardiol. 1993;21: 85–89.

31 Green M, Heddle B, Dassen W, Wehr M, Abdollah H, Brugada P, *et al*. Value of QRS alteration in determining the site of origin of narrow QRS supraventricular tachycardia. Circulation. 1998;68:368–373.

32 Morady F, DiCarlo LA, Baerman JM, de Buitleir M, Kou WH. Determinants of QRS alternans during narrow QRS tachycardia. J Am Coll Cardiol. 1987;9:489–499.

33 Kay GN, Pressley JC, Packer DL, Pritchett EL, German LD, Gilbert MR. Value of the 12-lead electrocardiogram in discriminating atrioventricular nodal reciprocating tachycardia from circus movement atrioventricular tachycardia utilizing a retrograde accessory pathway. Am J Cardiol. 1987;59:296–300.

34 Hill BL, Tilley LP. Ventricular preexcitation in seven dogs and nine cats. J Am Vet Med Assoc. 1985;187:1026–1031.

35 Wright KN, Mehdirad AA, Giacobbe P, Grubb T, Maxson T. Radiofrequency catheter ablation of atrioventricular accessory pathways in 3 dogs with subsequent resolution of tachycardia-induced cardiomyopathy. J Vet Intern Med. 1999;13:361–371.

36 Santilli RA, Spadacini G, Moretti P, Perego M, Perini A, Tarducci A, *et al*. Radiofrequency catheter ablation of concealed accessory pathways in two dogs with symptomatic atrioventricular reciprocating tachycardia. J Vet Cardiol. 2006;8:157–165.

37 Vera Z, Mason DT. Reentry versus automaticity: role in tachyarrhythmia genesis and antiarrhythmic therapy. Am Heart J. 1981;101:329–338.

38 García Cosío F, Pastor Fuentes A, Núñez Angulo A. Arrhythmias (IV). Clinical approach to atrial tachycardia and atrial flutter from an understanding of the mechanisms. Electrophysiology based on anatomy. Rev Esp Cardiol (Engl. ed.). 2012;65:363–375.

14

Diagnostic Approach to Wide-QRS Complex Tachycardia
Antonia Mavropoulou

Introduction

Wide-QRS complex tachycardias (WCTs) represent a diagnostic challenge that has important implications for the acute management of the arrhythmia and for prognosis. It may be of supraventricular or ventricular origin, and differential diagnoses based on the 12-lead electrocardiogram (ECG) can be divided into four categories:[1,2]

1) Ventricular tachycardia
2) Supraventricular tachycardia (SVT) with bundle branch block (BBB) (due to anatomic damage of the conduction system or due to functional block/rate-dependent block)
3) SVT with intraventricular conduction delay due to ventricular hypertrophy and/or dilation
4) SVT with atrioventricular (AV) conduction via an accessory pathway (pre-excited SVT or antidromic AV reentrant tachycardia).

Even though most of these tachycardias are of ventricular origin (an estimated approximately 80% of total WCTs in people),[3] the correct diagnosis and differentiation from the other types are very important. Inappropriate treatment can lead to arrhythmia and/or haemodynamic deterioration, and may have severe clinical implications.

A definitive diagnosis often requires intracardiac electrophysiologic studies; however, the 12-lead ECG remains the cornerstone and the most widely available test used for their differential diagnosis. Over the years, various electrocardiographic criteria and many algorithms have been developed in human medicine, and some of them may be applicable to veterinary cardiology; however, validation studies in dogs and cats are lacking, and caution is advised when using some of these criteria in veterinary patients.

Stepwise Approach to the Differential Diagnosis of Wide-QRS Complex Tachycardias

Step 1: Is this a Wide-QRS Complex Tachycardia?

A WCT is a rhythm characterized by tachycardia and QRS complexes with a duration >70 ms in dogs and >40 ms in cats.

Step 2: Is the Rhythm Regular or Irregular?

WCT can be either regular or irregular.
Regular WCTs include:

- Monomorphic ventricular tachycardia (VT)
- Regular SVTs with wide QRS complexes due to aberrant intraventricular conduction.

Irregular WCTs of ventricular origin include:

- Polymorphic VT and torsades de pointes (see chapter 11)
- Irregular SVTs include atrial fibrillation and atrial flutter with variable AV conduction. Fast atrial fibrillation with an intraventricular conduction disturbance can present with a relatively regular rhythm resembling monomorphic or polymorphic VT, and may represent a real diagnostic challenge (see chapter 9).

Step 3: Is there Atrioventricular Dissociation?

P waves may be difficult to distinguish during WCT but, when visible, they can provide useful information and may indicate AV dissociation. The lack of communication between atria and ventricles causes irregular and inconsistent PR intervals, and the P wave is usually seen 'marching' through the QRS complexes. Fusion and capture beats (see chapter 11) are also features of AV dissociation and, when present, have additional diagnostic value (Figure 14.1).

Guide to Canine and Feline Electrocardiography, First Edition. Ruth Willis, Pedro Oliveira and Antonia Mavropoulou.
© 2018 John Wiley & Sons Ltd. Published 2018 by John Wiley & Sons Ltd.
Companion website: www.wiley.com/go/willis/electrocardiography

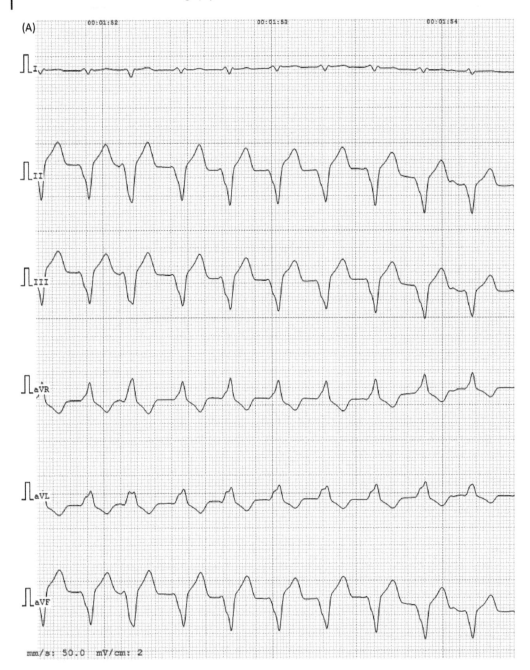

Figure 14.1 Ventricular tachycardia. (A) A wide-QRS tachycardia is seen with a rate of approximately 210 bpm and a slightly irregular rhythm. The QRS duration is 80 ms (normal < 70ms) with a right bundle branch block morphology. Obvious P waves are not seen except in the very last beat with a PR interval of approximately 100 ms, raising suspicion of sinus or supraventricular tachycardia with concomitant right bundle branch block. (B) This trace was recorded from the same patient after administration of lidocaine. The first and fourth beats present a normal QRS (60 ms; MEA: 80°) and are preceded by a normal P wave (40 ms; MEA: 60°) with a normal PR interval (100 ms). These are sinus beats without right bundle branch block, suggesting that the wide-QRS tachycardia is in fact ventricular in origin. Additionally, a fusion beat (*) may also be seen which is again suggestive of ventricular tachycardia. [8-year-old, male, crossbreed dog with intrathoracic hemangiosarcoma] (50 mm/s; 5 mm/mV)

AV dissociation usually indicates a ventricular rhythm (VT). Less frequently, a WCT with AV dissociation may be associated with a junctional tachycardia with aberrant intraventricular conduction; however, this situation is rare.[4,5]

If P waves are consistently coupled with the QRS complexes, then SVT with an intraventricular conduction disturbance and SVT with ventricular pre-excitation via an accessory pathway are potential differential diagnoses (Figure 14.2). Less frequently, VT with ventriculo-atrial

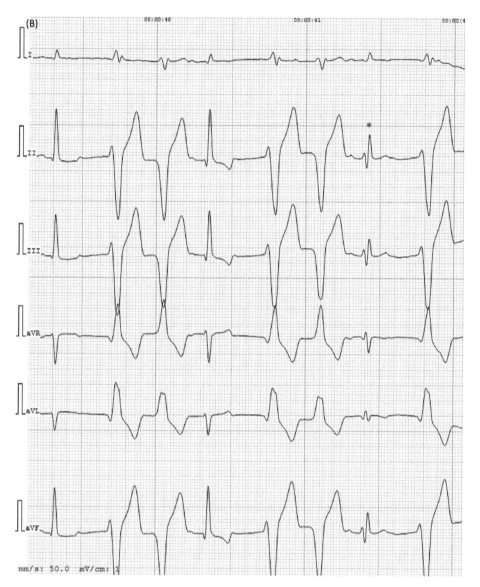

Figure 14.1 (Cont'd)

conduction of the impulses may occur, and this is likely to result in negative P waves shortly before or after the QRS complex.

Step 4: Look at QRS Morphology During Sinus Rhythm

The ECG trace during sinus rhythm can show signs of a pre-existing bundle branch block (see chapter 7) or ventricular pre-excitation (see chapter 10), and it may help to correctly interpret the WCT.

Step 5: Is there QRS Concordance in the Precordial Leads?

QRS concordance exists when the QRS complexes have the same polarity, either all positive or all negative, in all precordial leads (V1 to V6), and when present it is suggestive of a VT.[2] This was thought to be particularly true in the case of negative concordance (negative QRS complexes in all precordial leads), in which the tachycardia originates from the apex of the left ventricle; however, more recent reports in human patients showed that other conditions (i.e. SVT in patients with aberrancy or morphological abnormalities of the chest, e.g. pectus excavatum) may present negative concordance and mimic VT.[6–9] Less consistently, a positive concordance (positive QRS complexes in the precordial leads) has been associated with a VT of left posterior wall origin but also with an SVT with a left posterior accessory pathway.

Precordial concordance for VT is reported to have a high specificity (>90%) but low sensitivity (20%) in human patients, and its absence is not a reliable criterion

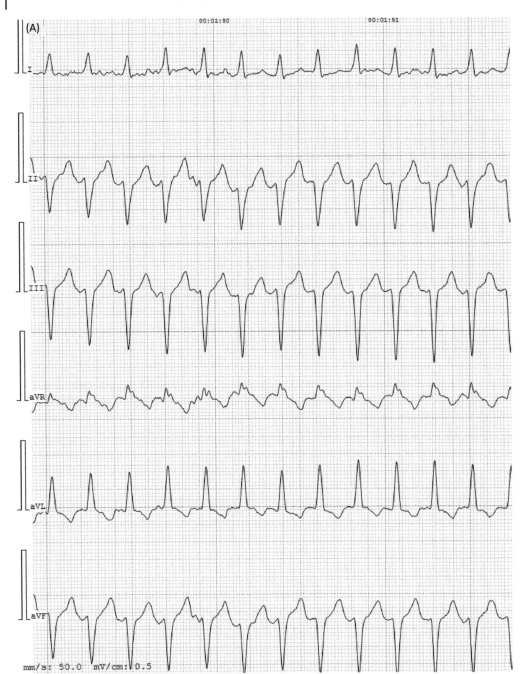

Figure 14.2 Sinus tachycardia with right bundle branch block in a cat. (A) A wide-QRS tachycardia is seen with a heart rate of approximately 270 bpm and a regular rhythm. The QRS duration is 80 ms (normal <40 ms) with a right bundle branch block morphology. Obvious P waves are not visible, perhaps with the exception of a small wave between the end of the T wave of the fourth beat and the QRS of the fifth beat. If this was indeed a P wave, the PR interval would be 50 ms, which is shorter than normal, suggesting that it may not be associated with the QRS and that ventricular tachycardia should be the main differential. Alternatively, a pre-excited rhythm might be present. (B) This trace was recorded from the same patient when he was calmer. A wide-QRS rhythm is still seen with a rate of approximately 180 bpm. Normal P waves (30 ms; MEA: 60°) are now seen preceding each QRS with a normal PR interval (70–80 ms), revealing a sinus rhythm with right bundle branch block instead of ventricular tachycardia. [14-year-old, male neutered Persian cat with lymphoplasmacytic rhinitis] (50 mm/s; 20 mm/mV)

to rule out VT.[7] This has not been reported in dogs or cats, and therefore care must be taken when considering QRS concordance for the differential diagnosis of WCT in our patients.

Other Criteria

The following criteria are widely used in human medicine for the differentiation of WCTs. However, to the best of the authors' knowledge, their validity has not been tested in veterinary patients, and their applicability remains uncertain.

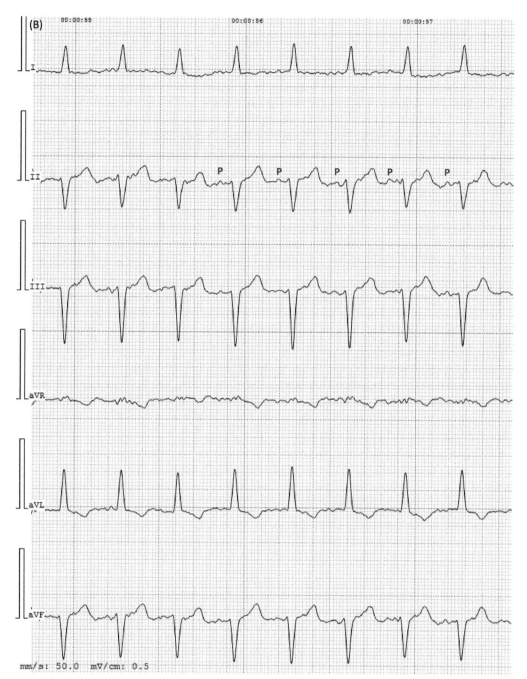

Figure 14.2 (Cont'd)

How Wide are the QRS Complexes?

Generally, the wider the QRS complexes, the greater the chance the tachycardia is of ventricular origin due to the longer cell-to-cell transmission of the impulse.[7]

Paradoxically, QRS complexes that are narrower during WCT than during sinus rhythm also favour diagnosis of VT.[2,7] Usually, the origin of the tachycardia in these cases is close to the interventricular septum, resulting in a more synchronous activation of the ventricles and consequently a narrower QRS complex.[10]

What is the Morphology of the QRS Complexes During Tachycardia?

The morphology of the QRS complexes during tachycardia in the standard and precordial leads can help differentiate between the different WCTs.

The following criteria favour VT over SVT in humans:[11–14]

- The absence of an RS pattern in all precordial leads.
- An interval of >100 ms from the onset of the QRS to the nadir of the S wave in precordial leads with an RS

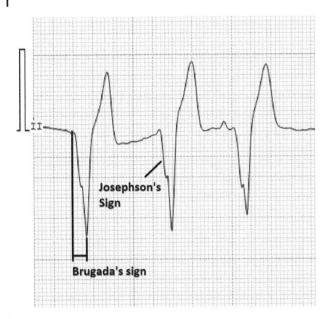

Figure 14.3 Possible Josephon's and Brugada's signs. Both of these signs are suggestive of ventricular tachycardia in humans but have not been studied or validated in dogs or cats. Brugada's sign consists of an interval >100 ms (upper limit of QRS in a human) from the start of the QRS to the nadir of the S wave. Given that this is an example from a dog, that distance is not >100 ms, as the upper limit of the QRS in dogs is only 70 ms. In this case, that distance is 73 ms, although conclusions cannot be drawn without studies to assess this in dogs. Josephon's sign corresponds to a notch in the descending limb of the S wave. [6-year-old, male Boxer dog with myocardial disease] (50 mm/s; 20 mm/mV)

morphology (Brugada's sign) (Figure 14.3). It is important to point out that 100 ms is the upper limit of normal for the QRS in a human, in contrast to 70 ms in dogs and 40 ms in cats. This criterion has not been studied or validated in our patients.

- The presence of a notch in the descending limb of the S wave (close to the nadir of the S wave), known as Josephson's sign (Figure 14.3).
- Morphologic criteria focusing on V1, V2 and V6:
  - When the tachycardia presents a right bundle branch block (RBBB) configuration with a qR, R, Rr' and RS morphology of the QRS complexes in V1 and an R/S ratio <1 in V6
  - When the tachycardia presents a left bundle branch block (LBBB) configuration with an initial R wave ≥30 ms or an interval of ≥70 ms from the onset of the QRS complex to the nadir of the S wave in V1 or V2, notching of the descending limb of the S wave in V1 or V2 (Figure 14.3) or an initial q wave in V6.
- The following features in aVR: initial R wave, initial r or q wave >40 ms, notching of the descending branch of a predominantly negative QRS complex and a ratio Vi/Vt ≤1, where Vi is the voltage during the initial 40 ms and Vt is the voltage during the terminal 40 ms of the QRS complex.

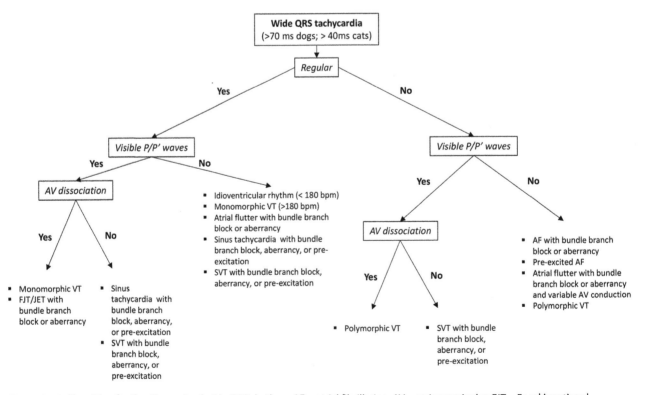

Figure 14.4 Algorithm for the diagnosis of wide-QRS rhythms. AF = atrial fibrillation; AV = atrioventricular; FJT = Focal junctional tachycardia; JET = Junctional ectopic tachycardia; SVT = supraventricular tachycardia; VT = ventricular tachycardia.

What is the QRS Axis?

The following QRS main electrical axis during WCT favours the diagnosis of VT:[3]

- Right superior axis (−90 to ±180)
- RBBB configuration with left axis deviation (> − 30°)

- LBBB pattern with right axis deviation (> + 90°)
- QRS axis shift >40° between sinus rhythm and WCT
- RBBB pattern with a normal axis.

Figure 14.4 provides an algorithm for diagnosing wide-QRS rhythms.

References

1 Alzand BSN, Crijns HJGM. Diagnostic criteria of broad QRS complex tachycardia: decades of evolution. Europace. 2011;13:465–472.

2 Vereckei A. Current algorithms for the diagnosis of wide QRS complex tachycardias. Curr Cardiol Rev. 2014;10:262–276.

3 Akhtar M, Shenasa M, Jazayeri M, Caceres J, Tchou PJ. Wide QRS complex tachycardia: reappraisal of a common clinical problem. Ann Intern Med. 1988;109:905–912.

4 Akhtar M. Reentrant junctional tachycardias. Pacing Clin Electrophysiol. 1990;13:2133–2139.

5 Wang K, Benditt DG. AV dissociation: an inevitable response. Ann Noninvasive Electrocardiol. 2011;16:227–231.

6 Kappos KG, Andrikopoulos GK, Tzeis SE, Manolis AS. Wide-QRS-complex tachycardia with a negative concordance pattern in the precordial leads: are the ECG criteria always reliable? Pacing Clin Electrophysiol. 2006;29:63–66.

7 Pellegrini CN, Scheinman MM. Clinical management of ventricular tachycardia. Curr Prob Cardio. 2010;35:453–504.

8 Volders PGA, Timmermans C, Rodriguez L-M, van Pol PEJ, Wellens HJJ. Wide QRS complex tachycardia with negative precordial concordance: always a ventricular origin? J Cardiovasc Electrophysiol. 2003;14:109–111.

9 Pappas LK, Efremidis M, Letsas KP, Gavrielatos GD, Alexanian IP, Sideris A, Kardaras F. Wide QRS complex supraventricular tachycardia with negative precordial concordance. Am Heart Hosp J. 2009;7:67–68.

10 Sousa PA, Pereira S, Candeias R, >de Jesus I. The value of electrocardiography for differential diagnosis in wide QRS complex tachycardia. Rev Port Cardiol. 2014;33:165–173.

11 Wellens HJ, Bär FW, Lie KI. The value of the electrocardiogram in the differential diagnosis of a tachycardia with a widened QRS complex. Am J Med. 1978;64:27–33.

12 Brugada P, Brugada J, Mont L, Smeets J, Andries EW. A new approach to the differential diagnosis of a regular tachycardia with a wide QRS complex. Circulation. 1991;83:1649–1659.

13 Vereckei A, Duray G, Szénási G, Altemose GT, Miller JM. New algorithm using only lead aVR for differential diagnosis of wide QRS complex tachycardia. Heart Rhythm. 2008;5:89–98.

14 Kindwall KE, Brown J, Josephson ME. Electrocardiographic criteria for ventricular tachycardia in wide complex left bundle branch block morphology tachycardias. Am J Cardio. 1988;61:1279–1283.

15

Ambulatory Electrocardiographic Recordings
Ruth Willis

Introduction

An ambulatory electrocardiogram (ECG) is a recording of the heart rate and rhythm whilst a patient performs normal activities, often over a prolonged period of time. A number of different types of devices are available and will be discussed in more detail in this chapter.[1–3] Ambulatory ECGs are useful as a patient's heart rate and rhythm recorded in the consulting room may not be representative of heart rate and rhythm at home, and there are a number of situations where an ambulatory ECG recording can provide useful information regarding the diagnosis and treatment of cardiac disease.[4,5]

Common Indications for Obtaining an Ambulatory ECG

1) Intermittent collapse with a history suggestive of an intermittent arrhythmia
2) Exercise intolerance with a history suggestive of an intermittent arrhythmia
3) Detection of arrhythmia, especially in a predisposed breed
4) Assessment of drug efficacy – for example, assessing ventricular rate control in atrial fibrillation
5) Screening for disease in breeds at risk of arrhythmias – for example, in breeding dogs.

Types of Monitor for Obtaining an Ambulatory ECG

There are two broad categories of devices – those that record short sections of trace (loop recorders), and those that record for the entire duration whilst they are connected to the patient.

Loop Recorders

1. Event Recorder

These monitors are also known as *loop recorders* and continually record and overwrite a short section of ECG trace. Whilst these monitors facilitate a longer recording duration, they do not store the entire recording, and therefore storage of the areas of interest depends on manual activation by the owner or automatic activation. Activation stores a short section of trace around the time of events that may be detected automatically or pre-defined by the operator. Manual activation by the owner requires pressing a button on the monitor, or a remote control, to ensure that a section of ECG from around the time of the event is captured.

If the monitor is configured to automatically detect events, these events are detected by abnormal beat timing compared to several preceding R-R intervals, and these complexes are then designated as narrow or wide-QRS beats. Therefore, in systems using automatic activation, it is essential that complexes are correctly identified by the software and also that the selected sections are manually reviewed to ensure correct complex designation.[6] Some systems have a pre-determined number of ECG loops that can be stored (e.g. 20 min of recording time), and when the memory allocation to a certain category is full, a new event replaces an existing record only if it is more severe – for example, a sinus pause of 3 s duration would result in over-writing of shorter pauses. As a result, the total number of each event during the recording may not be elucidated.[6]

Easy access to the manual activation button is advantageous in human patients but may not be in dogs, as pressure on the monitor (e.g. when a dog is rolling or sleeping in dorsal recumbence) can result in inadvertent manual activation. This may be problematic as, on some monitors, events stored in the manual recording memory cannot be replaced by automatically detected events.

In all ambulatory systems, careful electrode position may be required as large T waves may result in incorrect designation of QRS complexes as wide rather than narrow.[6]

> *Advantages*: Long recording duration making device suitable for intermittent collapse; non-invasive
> *Disadvantages*: Some patients may not tolerate a longer recording interval; some systems require manual activation by owner.

2. Smart Phone Technology

Devices are available that can be attached to a smart phone and record a single-lead ECG (see Figures 15.1 and 15.2). A bipolar electrode case fits onto the smart phone and records electrical activity at the body surface, and then the software in the case saves and transmits this single-lead ECG. An application on the smart phone transforms the transmitted electrical signal to ultrasound, and then the smart phone's microphone receives the ultrasound signal and can then transmit the data in a wireless PDF format. If additional electrodes are used, the smart phone technology can then generate a 12-lead ECG from these data.[7]

> *Advantages*: Can be applied rapidly to patient during the event; patient does not need to wear device
> *Disadvantages*: The rhythm that caused the event may have converted back to normal by the time the device is placed on the patient and activated.

3. Implantable Loop Recorder

These loop recorders are implanted subcutaneously and allow a longer monitoring period of months to years which may be useful in cases of patients who collapse infrequently. As might be expected given the recording period, only short sections of the ECG trace are stored in response to automatic or manual activation by the owners, and the device then stores a loop of ECG from around the time of activation. When setting the criteria for automatically detected events, it is important to account for the marked sinus arrhythmia and sinus pauses often seen in resting dogs, as otherwise the auto-activation events could all be recorded whilst the dog is sleeping and has a physiological sinus bradycardia. As the device is implanted subcutaneously on the left hemi-thorax[8] or abdomen,[2] it is usually well tolerated, and there is no requirement for external vests or jackets (see Figure 15.3). The device records a single channel of ECG using electrodes situated at either end of the device. Once an event has been recorded, it can be downloaded non-invasively using a device such as the ones used for pacemaker interrogation and programming. There have been multiple reports in the use of these devices in both cats and dogs.[2,8–11] In one retrospective study involving 23 dogs undergoing investigation of intermittent weakness or collapse, an event occurred during the monitoring period of 13/23 cases and, of the cases that showed signs, recordings of diagnostic value were obtained in 11 of these 13 cases. In the two remaining patients, the signs described were more suggestive of neurological disease.[9]

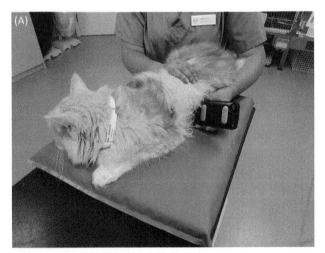
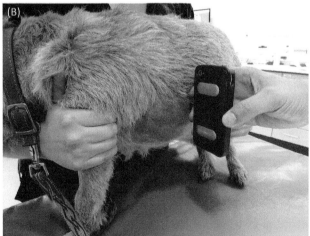

Figure 15.1 Smart phone ECG. (A) The device is ready to be placed on a cat. If the patient is unclipped, then copious amounts of surgical spirit need to be applied to ensure adequate electrical contact. (B) The device is about to be placed on a dog. As this patient has previously been clipped for echocardiography, less surgical spirit is required to ensure good electrode contact. Images courtesy of Jon Wray.

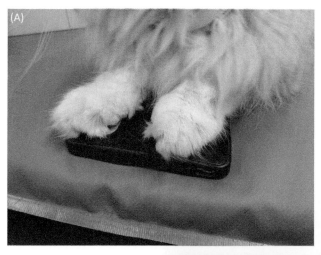
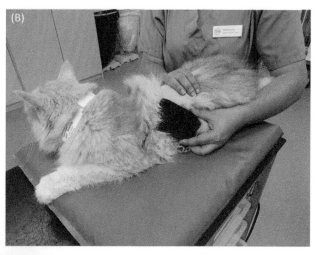
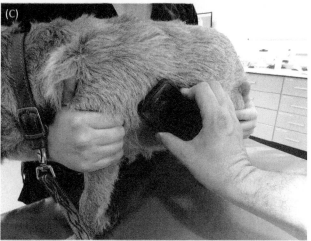

Figure 15.2 Smart phone ECG placement. (A) The cat's paws may be placed on the electrodes to obtain a trace, or alternatively the device may be placed on the cat's thorax as shown in (B); the hair is parted and soaked with surgical spirit. (C) Placement of the device on the left side of the thorax with the electrodes in close contact with the skin. Images courtesy of Jon Wray.

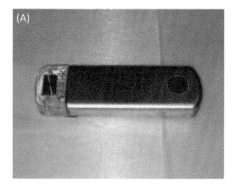
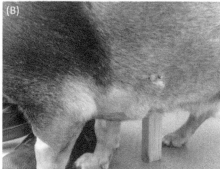
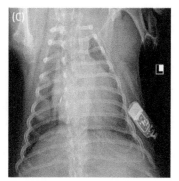

Figure 15.3 (A) Implantable loop recorder (ILR). (B) Implant site. The device is implanted under the skin on the thorax. (C) Radiograph showing the ILR in place.

Advantages
- Usually well tolerated due to small size
- Long recording period
- If further syncopal episodes occur, there is a good probability of obtaining a diagnosis.[2]

Disadvantages
- Sedation or general anaesthesia is required to implant and remove device.
- Device needs to be removed prior to cremation.
- Risk of surgical complications, such as infection and seroma formation, skin erosion and device migration
- Specialist equipment required to interrogate
- Cost
- Patients with device in place should not undergo magnetic resonance imaging (MRI), defibrillation, electrosurgical cautery, radiofrequency ablation or lithotripsy.
- Activation device should not be used close to sources of electromagnetic energy (e.g. mobile phones).

Heart Rate Monitors

Wearable heart rate monitors are widely available and popular for use in humans as performance or fitness-monitoring devices. These devices have many forms – some monitor heart rate using a belt around the thorax, whilst others are contained within watches worn on the wrist. Some of these devices have been used in dogs as a form of telemetric ambulatory ECG, mainly in research rather than clinical settings.[12] Movement of the electrodes during vigorous exercise can result in mis-sensing of the R wave and incorrect calculations of heart rate. One such device has been tested in dogs in the standing position and also at trot on a treadmill, but this may not replicate the normal activity of dogs in their home environment.[12,13]

Continuous Recorders

1. Holter Monitors

These devices are worn externally for the duration of the recording; they are therefore non-invasive and are currently the most widely available and common means of obtaining an ambulatory ECG. Early systems were large and used a cassette tape,[1,3] but modern digital systems are much smaller and lighter (Figure 15.4). These monitors differ from loop recorders in that the ECG for the entire recording duration is stored; therefore, they provide more information than the loop recorders, such as mean heart rate and also ventricular beat counts.

The use of these devices has been described in cats[14–17] and dogs.[18] In dogs, the device is worn on the dog's back,

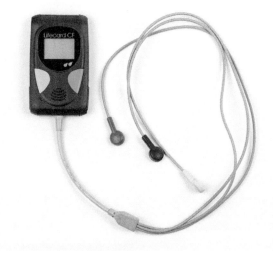

Figure 15.4 Digital Holter monitor.

and there are numerous methods for keeping the monitor in place, ranging from specially designed dog vests or jackets to the use of copious quantities of cohesive bandage (Figure 15.5).[3]

Many owners are understandably concerned about whether the recording will be diagnostic if their pet does not collapse or show signs whilst wearing the monitor. To conclusively determine whether a dysrhythmia is responsible for the signs observed by the owner, an ECG must be obtained during a collapse episode; however, useful information can still be obtained even if the dog does not show clinical signs during the recording.

Placement of Holter Monitor

Careful skin preparation is vital to obtain a diagnostic recording. The hair needs to be closely clipped, and then the skin cleaned and wiped with alcohol-based solution to remove grease and then dried prior to application of electrodes. The required number of electrodes are then attached, and sometimes the electrode glue is re-enforced with tissue glue to ensure electrodes remain *in situ* for the duration of the recording. Whilst numerous systems are available for holding the monitor in place, elasticated vests are generally more comfortable for the patients than adhesive bandage. The monitors are splash-proof but not waterproof, so dogs cannot swim whilst wearing the monitor.

Advantages
- Entire trace is recorded, so it can produce quantitative data such as a ventricular beat count.
- Non-invasive
- Usually well tolerated
- Equipment readily available.

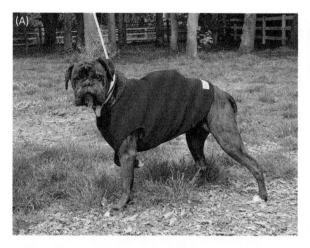
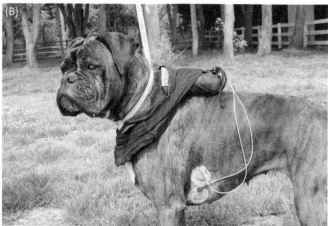

Figure 15.5 Digital Holter monitoring placement. (A) Digital Holter monitor on a dog. (B) The vest has been partially removed to show the monitor held within a pocket on the dog's back and to highlight electrode positioning on the left hemithorax. With this system, an additional electrode is placed on the right hemithorax.

Disadvantages
- Some animals will behave differently whilst wearing the equipment.
- As the device is worn externally, there is a risk of damage to the equipment.
- Dogs cannot swim whilst wearing the device.

Ambulatory ECGs in Cats

It is possible to obtain an ambulatory ECG from a cat using a Holter monitor (Figure 15.6). As mentioned in the figure caption, a large cat with a placid temperament may tolerate wearing the monitor like a dog, providing that it can be kept indoors during the recording. However, some cats will not tolerate wearing the monitor and must be hospitalised, sometimes with a 24h recording being obtained as two 12h sessions, with an overnight rest period to minimise patient stress. The obvious limitation of the latter approach is that the cat's behaviour may not be normal whilst hospitalised.[15]

Holter parameters in normal cats and also cats with asymptomatic hypertrophic cardiomyopathy have been described.[15,19]

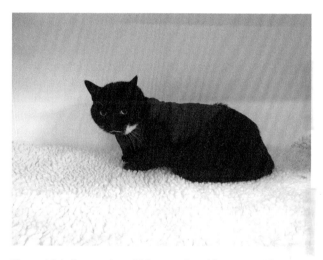

Figure 15.6 Cat wearing a Holter monitor. A large cat with a placid temperament may tolerate wearing the monitor like a dog providing that it can be kept indoors for the duration of the recording. However, many cats will not tolerate wearing the monitor and have to be hospitalised sometimes, with a 24h recording being obtained as two 12h sessions with an overnight period of rest to minimise patient stress. This is obviously a limitation as the heart rate rhythm is not recorded during the patient's normal activities in the home environment.

2. Telemetry

Telemetry provides a wireless connection between a monitor on the patient and a nearby computer. The device size and appearance are similar to those of a Holter monitor, and the equipment settings can be adjusted to automatically store events such as tachycardia or bradycardia. The benefit of this type of equipment is that these devices are generally well tolerated, and heart rate and rhythm can be monitored in real time.

Being able to assess heart rate and rhythm in real time is the key advantage of these systems over other ambulatory ECG systems; however, the range of these devices is limited, and therefore they are often used in an intensive care setting (Figure 15.7).

Advantage: Heart rate and rhythm can be monitored remotely in real time.
Disadvantage: Limited range, so patient needs to remain relatively close to the receiver station; availability of equipment.

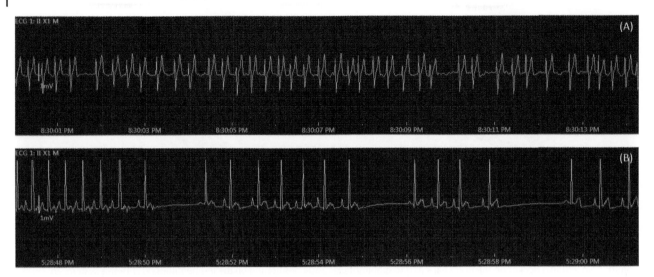

Figure 15.7 Sample traces obtained using telemetry. (A) Rapid atrial fibrillation. (B) Sinus pauses.

3. Other Wearable Devices (adhesive patch)

In human patients, more compact devices with built-in adhesive patches are sometimes used for longer recording periods, and these devices are designed mainly to detect paroxysmal atrial fibrillation. Clinical evaluation is underway, and therefore data from canine patients with naturally occurring disease are currently lacking. Whilst the small size of the device is appealing from the perspective of patient comfort, it could also result in inadvertent device damage or ingestion. Only a single lead of ECG trace (whereas a Holter monitor will produce 2–3 leads, depending on the recording duration) makes them good for the detection of intermittent dysrhythmias but, depending on ectopic complex morphology, may make them unsuitable for producing a ventricular ectopic beat count. See Figure 15.8 for an example of a dog (Great Dane) wearing one of these devices on the left hemi-thorax.

Advantages
- Small device, so more comfortable to wear, thereby facilitating longer recordings
- Device is splash-proof.

Disadvantages
- Small device more susceptible to patient damage
- Only single lead of ECG, making them better for detection of intermittent arrhythmias than full quantitative analysis as would be obtained using a Holter monitor.

Analysis of Holter Recordings

Analysis of the recording is performed using commercial software supplemented with manual review to ensure that as many QRS complexes as possible are detected and also that they are correctly designated as being either narrow or wide-QRS complexes.

Artefact Count

Artefact describes the sections of trace that were not of diagnostic quality. Whilst often ignored, the artefact count on the trace should be assessed as this gives an indication of the reliability of the quantitative analysis. If there is intermittent partial or complete loss of electrode contact, a high artefact count may be unavoidable, and this should be mentioned in the report as it will have the effect of reducing the total beat count and possibly the mean heart rate. Arrhythmias occurring during these periods will also not be documented. After automated analysis has occurred, the operator should manually check the entire recording and make adjustments to lower the artefact count. Once you are familiar with the software, this can be done in a number of ways, such as by adjusting the sensitivity of R wave sensing and also by templating some normal and abnormal complexes.

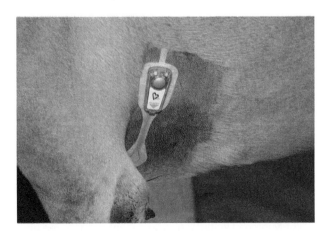

Figure 15.8 Adhesive patch device. A small adhesive patch device placed over the left precordial impulse of a Great Dane to monitor heart rate and rhythm for up to 7 consecutive days.

Total Beat Count

The total beat count is the number of QRS complexes that occurred during the recording. The total beat count per minute is used to calculate the mean heart rate during each minute of the recording, and this can then be plotted against time to provide a tachogram. Large T waves can result in T waves being designated as R waves and, if this occurs frequently, overestimation of the total beat count.

Tachogram and Mean Heart Rate

Mean heart rate on a 24 h ambulatory ECG is the average heart rate over the entire 24 h period (see Figure 15.9). Mean heart rate is influenced by numerous factors, such as patient temperament, fitness, level of activity, drugs and also concurrent cardiac and/or systemic disease. In dogs, the 24 h mean heart rate is usually in the range of 65–90 bpm but, for example, in a dog with sick sinus syndrome the mean heart rate will tend to be below the accepted range with minimal variability.

Aberrant Beat Count

Aberrant beats are beats with a different QRS morphology from the sinus beats – the majority of these beats are likely to be ventricular, but the possibility of supraventricular complexes with aberrant conduction may also merit consideration in some cases. Aberrant beats may be detected by the software during analysis, but manual review of the entire recording is required to ensure that beats are being classified correctly. This is especially important in cats and Dobermans, as the QRS complex morphology of the aberrant beats may be relatively similar to that of the sinus beats. If beats are being misclassified, then manual adjustments can be made to the analysis criteria in one or more leads, and also some analysis systems will allow templating of abnormal QRS complexes in one or more leads. After making these changes, it is important to review the trace to ensure that over-sensing has not occurred, as this would result in a falsely elevated aberrant beat count.

The report should provide a total aberrant beat count and an indication of whether there was complex ventricular ectopy (e.g. couplets, triplets or ventricular tachycardia). This information is reported in the initial summary table and, in more detail, on the lower line of the tachogram and in the tables highlighting the times during the recording when each event occurred.

Some analysis software will sub-classify the single aberrant beats according to the R-R interval between the aberrant beat and the preceding sinus beat. The R-on-T aberrant beats are those that occur with the shortest R-R interval compared to the previous beats, whereas premature aberrants have a slightly longer R-R compared to the preceding sinus beats and isolated aberrants are escape beats that occur after a sinus pause. Occasional isolated aberrants during periods of low heart rate are common in dogs and unlikely to be clinically significant; however, if these beats are occurring during sinus rhythm, then this could suggest sinus node dysfunction or conduction block (see chapter 7).

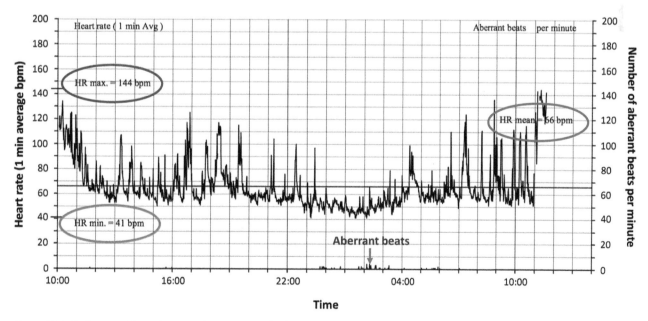

Figure 15.9 Tachogram. The tachogram shows time on the horizontal axis and heart rate on the left vertical axis. The maximum heart rate is highlighted in red, the minimum heart rate in green and the mean heart rate in blue. The right-hand vertical axis shows the number of aberrant beats that, during this recording, tended to occur overnight and are highlighted by an arrow.

Heart Rate Variability

Heart rate variability (HRV) analysis is a beat-to-beat analysis designed to investigate the influence of the autonomic nervous system on heart rhythm and arrhythmias – for further information, see chapter 16.

Holter Findings in Normal Dogs

Heart Rate

Maximum, minimum and mean heart rates from 24 h ambulatory ECGs have been published in healthy small and large-breed dogs, and findings are summarised in Table 15.1. In a large colony of beagles used for research, higher mean and minimum heart rates were reported in female dogs[20] similar to findings reported in human patients.[21]

In a study involving 60 apparently healthy dogs with body weights varying from 2 to 80 kg, the minimum, mean and maximum heart rates were not found to be influenced by body size.[24] A larger study evaluating 5000 healthy dogs found that the mean difference in heart rate between dogs weighing 5 and 55 kg was only 10.5 bpm which was considered unlikely to be clinically significant.[25] Another study highlighted the effects of breed and temperament on heart rate, with terriers, spitz breeds, bull terriers and spaniels having higher heart rates.[26]

The effects of age, body weight and temperament on heart rate were investigated in approximately 400 dogs, and it was reported that dogs <1 year old had higher heart rates than older individuals, and the dog's temperament had a greater influence on heart rate than body weight.[27]

General Ambulatory ECG Parameters

Some general ambulatory ECG parameters in normal dogs are summarised in Table 15.2.[20]

Table 15.2 Normal ambulatory ECG findings in dogs

Parameter	
Heart rhythm	Sinus and sinus arrhythmia
Sinus pauses	Occasional 4–6 s pauses at rest
1AVB	Only at low heart rates
2AVB	Occasional low-grade 2AVB during periods of low heart rate
SVT	Sinus tachycardia with rate of 240 bpm during periods of exercise or excitement; during intense exercise, the instantaneous rate may reach >300 bpm for short periods
Escape beats	Occasional examples during low heart rates

1AVB, First-degree atrioventricular block; 2AVB, second-degree atrioventricular block; 3AVB, third-degree atrioventricular block; bpm, beats per minute; SVT, supraventricular tachycardia.

Changes in Complex Morphology

Regular changes in T wave morphology are a common finding on ambulatory ECG recordings from dogs (Figure 15.10). The traces were obtained from the same dog 2 h apart and show changes in the P-QRS-T morphology. This is attributed to changes in patient body position rather than pathological change.

Ventricular Ectopy in Normal Dogs

The frequency of ventricular ectopy on 24 h ambulatory ECG recordings has also been published for normal dogs of several breeds, as shown in Table 15.3.

The general conclusion of these studies is that in normal dogs, up to 50 single ventricular premature beats over 24 h would generally be considered to be within acceptable limits. Cases exceeding this threshold or showing complex ventricular ectopy such as couplets, triplets or ventricular tachycardia would be considered abnormal, and further investigation may be indicated to screen for concurrent cardiac and/or systemic disease. It is important to note that there can be considerable

Table 15.1 Heart rates in normal dogs: minimum, maximum and mean heart rates reported in several studies using normal dogs of different breeds

	Breed			
	CKCS (n = 21)[22]	wD (n = 16)[22]	CT (n = 13)[22]	Large breed (n = 34)[23]
Maximum heart rate (bpm)	191.7 ± 35.9	167.4 ± 20.6	184.8 ± 22.8	171 (130–240)
Minimum heart rate (bpm)	51.7 ± 7.5	41.8 ± 6.6	45.3 ± 7.2	39 (29–52)
Mean heart rate (bpm)	82.4 ± 12.8	67.3 ± 7.5	74.9 ± 10.3	66 (52–86)

CKCS, Cavalier King Charles Spaniel; wD, wire-haired Dachshund; CT, Cairn Terrier.

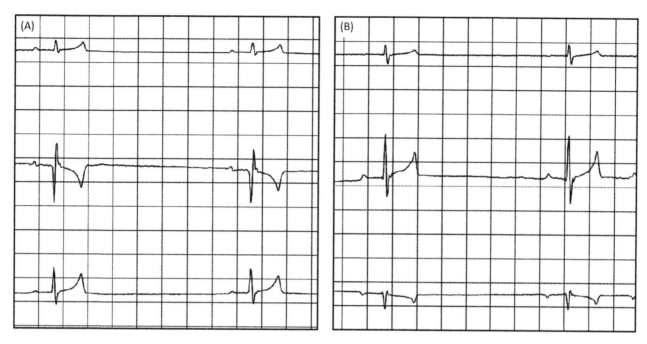

Figure 15.10 *T wave morphology.* (A) Ambulatory ECG trace showing changes in T wave morphology attributable to changes in body position at different times (A and B) during the same recording. (B) Regular changes in T wave morphology are a common finding on ambulatory ECG recordings from dogs.

Table 15.3 Frequency of ventricular ectopy in normal dogs of different breeds

Breed	Frequency of ventricular ectopy on 24 h ambulatory ECG
Boxers[28]	<91 VPCs/24 h
Boxers[29]	<50 VPCs/24 h
Dobermans[30]	<50 VPCs/24 h
Beagles[20]	<9
Large-breed dogs[23]	0–24

ECG, Electrocardiogram; VPC, ventricular premature contraction.

day-to-day variation in the frequency and complexity of ventricular ectopy in dogs.[31] For further information on ventricular ectopy in dogs with cardiomyopathy, see chapter 20.

Changes in the Frequency of Ventricular Ectopy with Age

In human patients, it has been reported that the frequency of ventricular ectopy tends to increase with increasing age,[32] and similar findings have been reported in a small group of cats, with 7–15-year-old cats showing more ventricular ectopy than 1–6-year-old individuals.[17] In this study, 67% of apparently normal older cats also showed complex ventricular ectopy.[17] In dogs, the frequency of ventricular ectopy has been shown to be positively correlated to increasing age.[28]

Normal Holter Findings in Cats

Figure 15.11 shows examples of feline ECG complex morphology seen on ambulatory ECGs, and Table 15.4 summarises 24 h ambulatory ECG (Holter) findings from studies using normal cats.

In cats, higher heart rates in females were documented in one study.[15] However, this contrasts with another study where entire male cats were reported to have significantly higher heart rates than female cats and neutered male cats.[17] Telemetry has been used to compare cats' heart rates at home with their heart rates in a hospital environment, either resting in a kennel or being restrained. In these 16 apparently healthy young cats, the mean heart rate during restraint for echocardiography was 187 + 25 bpm, whilst in a quiet room in the teaching hospital it was significantly lower at 150 + 23 bpm and, when the cats were at home, heart rate was 132 + 19 bpm which was a significant reduction.[33]

Diurnal Variation in Dogs and Cats

Diurnal variation in heart rate results in a lower heart rate overnight during periods of rest compared to during waking hours. This phenomenon has been observed in human patients[34] and also occurs in dogs and cats.[17,20]

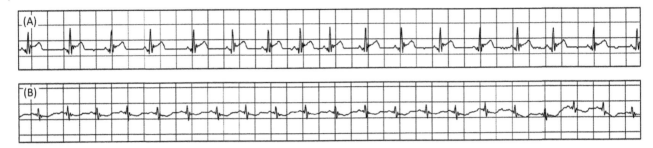

Figure 15.11 Feline ECG complex morphology seen on ambulatory ECGs. These traces are from two different cats and illustrate the variation in P waves and QRS complexes often seen in this species. (A) Distinct P, QRS and T complexes are seen; (B) lower amplitude P waves and QRS complexes are present that can make interpretation challenging. Nonetheless, the rhythm is regular, and there is consistently a small positive deflection before each narrow-QRS complex which is likely to be a P wave, hence the rhythm diagnosis of sinus rhythm.

Table 15.4 24 h ambulatory ECG findings in normal cats

	Cats (*n* = 20)[15]	Cats (*n* = 23)[17]	Cats (*n* = 15)[19]
Normal rhythms	Sinus with occasional sinus arrhythmia at rest	Sinus with occasional sinus arrhythmia at HR <160 bpm	
Maximum HR	267 bpm	235 ± 25 bpm	233 ± 21 bpm
Minimum HR	F = 117 bpm M = 97 bpm	131 ± 23 bpm	134 ± 28 bpm
Mean HR (bpm)	157 bpm	168 bpm	170 ± 25 bpm
Ventricular ectopy	0–59 single beats Higher count seen in one cat due to periods of accelerated idioventricular rhythm	Median 3 (0–146) per 24 h	Mean 4 per 24 h
Complex ectopy	None	None	Rare (20%, 3 cats)
Supraventricular premature beats	Uncommon (mean 3 ± 2 per 24 h recording)	Uncommon (1 example seen)	Rare (1 per 24 h)
Sinus pauses	Rare (<1 s duration)		
1AVB	Rare		
2AVB	Single example observed		
SVT HR >240 bpm	Mean of 19 (±7.2) min during a 24 h recording		
Bradycardia HR <99 bpm	Rare		
Escape beats	None		

1AVB, First-degree atrioventricular block; 2AVB, second-degree atrioventricular block; bpm, beats per minute; F, female; HR, heart rate; M, male; SVT, supraventricular tachycardia.

Ambulatory ECGs in the Assessment of Anti-arrhythmic Treatment Efficacy

In human patients, one study showed that the extent of spontaneous variation in arrhythmia frequency that occurred in individual patients from day to day was 23%, between 8 h periods within a single day was 29%, and from hour to hour was 48%.[35] In Boxers with >500 VPCs/24h, the variability in the frequency of ventricular ectopy measured by consecutive 24 h Holter recordings for 7 days was up to 80%.[31] A study using German Shepherd dogs with inherited ventricular arrhythmias showed a similar trend in that, when comparing two control 24 h ambulatory ECG (Holter) recordings, changes in the frequency of ventricular ectopy of up to 61% were considered within the limits of spontaneous variability.[36]

In Boxers, the grade of arrhythmia (see chapter 20) appeared to be less variable than the frequency of VPCs, but if the frequency of ventricular ectopy is lower, then the variability tends to be higher.[31] As might be expected, increasing numbers of 24 h ambulatory ECG recordings for an individual dog reduce the confidence interval for the day-to-day variability.[36]

As a result of this spontaneous variability, it has been stated that if two 24h ambulatory ECG monitoring periods are being compared, a reduction in the frequency of ventricular ectopy of 80–90% may be necessary before we can be confident that any change is drug induced.[35] Another study (in human patients) reported similar results – when comparing a 24h test period with a 24h control period, a 65% decrease in mean hourly frequency of ventricular tachycardia and a 75% reduction in the frequency of couplets are required to demonstrate therapeutic efficacy rather than a reduction due to spontaneous variation alone.[37]

A study conducted in human patients using similar methodology to drug trials except that no medication was given showed that without medication, 65% of human patients in the study had a reduction in VPCs of >50% during the 6h monitoring period. This study highlights the need for careful interpretation of anti-arrhythmic drug response, as whilst none of the subjects in this study received anti-arrhythmic medication, 65% of them would have been classed as responders on the basis of the ECG changes alone.[38]

Holter monitoring has been used to assess the efficacy of treatment of German Shepherd dogs (GSDs) with inherited ventricular arrhythmias,[36] and also for evaluation of treatment efficacy in dogs with atrial fibrillation.[39] In the GSD study, a crossover design was used to investigate drug efficacy in a research colony of GSDs, but this crossover design would probably not be appropriate for clinical cases.[36]

For further information on the use of ambulatory ECGs in monitoring the effectiveness of anti-arrhythmic therapy in atrial fibrillation, see chapter 9; and for further information on diagnosis and treatment of arrhythmias associated with canine cardiomyopathies, see chapter 20.

References

1 Hall LW, Dunn JK, Delaney M, Shapiro LM. Ambulatory electrocardiography in dogs. Vet Rec. 1991;129:213–216.

2 James R, Summerfield N, Loureiro J, Swift S, Dukes McEwan J. Implantable loop recorders: a viable diagnostic tool in veterinary medicine. J Small Anim Pract. 2008;49:564–570.

3 Petrie J-P. Practical application of holter monitoring in dogs and cats. Clin Tech Small Anim Pract. 2005;20:173–181.

4 Meurs KM, Spier AW, Wright NA, Hamlin RL. Comparison of in-hospital versus 24-hour ambulatory electrocardiography for detection of ventricular premature complexes in mature Boxers. J Am Vet Med Assoc. 2001;218:222–224.

5 Wess G, Schulze A, Geraghty N, Hartmann K. Ability of a 5-minute electrocardiography (ECG) for predicting arrhythmias in Doberman Pinschers with cardiomyopathy in comparison with a 24-hour ambulatory ECG. J Vet Intern Med. 2010;24:367–371.

6 Eastwood JM, Elwood CM. Assessment of an ECG event recorder in healthy dogs in a hospital environment. J Small Anim Pract. 2003;44:161–168.

7 Baquero GA, Banchs JE, Ahmed S, Naccarelli GV, Luck JC. Surface 12 lead electrocardiogram recordings using smart phone technology. J Electrocardiol. 2015;48:1–7.

8 Willis R, McLeod K, Cusack J, Wotton P. Use of an implantable loop recorder to investigate syncope in a cat. J Small Anim Pract. 2003;44:181–183.

9 MacKie BA, Stepien RL, Kellihan HB. Retrospective analysis of an implantable loop recorder for evaluation of syncope, collapse, or intermittent weakness in 23 dogs (2004–2008). J Vet Cardiol. 2010;12:25–33.

10 Santilli RA, Ferasin L, Voghera SG, Perego M. Evaluation of the diagnostic value of an implantable loop recorder in dogs with unexplained syncope. J Am Vet Med Assoc. 2010;236:78–82.

11 Ferasin L. Recurrent syncope associated with paroxysmal supraventricular tachycardia in a Devon Rex cat diagnosed by implantable loop recorder. J Feline Med Surg. 2009;11:149–152.

12 Essner A, Sjostrom R, Ahlgren E, Lindmark B. Validity and reliability of Polar(R) RS800CX heart rate monitor, measuring heart rate in dogs during standing position and at trot on a treadmill. Physiol Behav. 2013;114–115:1–5.

13 Essner A, Sjostrom R, Ahlgren E, Gustas P, Edge-Hughes L, Zetterberg L, et al. Comparison of Polar® RS800CX heart rate monitor and electrocardiogram for measuring inter-beat intervals in healthy dogs. Physiol Behav. 2015;138:247–253.

14 Ferasin L, van de Stad M, Rudorf H, Langford K, Hotston MA. Syncope associated with paroxysmal atrioventricular block an ventricular standstill in a cat. J Small Anim Pract. 2002;43:124–128.

15 Ware WA. Twenty-four-hour ambulatory electrocardiography in normal cats. J Vet Intern Med. 1999;13:175–180.

16 Goodwin JK, Lombard CW, Ginex DD. Results of continuous ambulatory electrocardiography in a cat with hypertrophic cardiomyopathy. J Am Vet Med Assoc. 1992;200:1352–1354.

17 Hanas S, Tidholm A, Egenvall A, Holst BS. Twenty-four hour Holter monitoring of unsedated healthy cats in the home environment. J Vet Cardiol. 2009;11:17–22.

18 Goodwin JK. Holter monitoring and cardiac event recording. Vet Clin North Am Small Anim Pract. 1998;28:1391–1407–viii.

19 Jackson BL, Lehmkuhl LB, Adin DB. Heart rate and arrhythmia frequency of normal cats compared to cats with asymptomatic hypertrophic cardiomyopathy. J Vet Cardiol. 2014;16:215–225.

20 Ulloa HM, Houston BJ, Altrogge DM. Arrhythmia prevalence during ambulatory electrocardiographic monitoring of beagles. Am J Vet Res. 1995;56:275–281.

21 Stramba-Badiale M, Locati EH, Martinelli A, Courville J, Schwartz PJ. Gender and the relationship between ventricular repolarization and cardiac cycle length during 24-h Holter recordings. Eur Heart J. 1997;18:1000–1006.

22 Rasmussen CE, Vesterholm S, Ludvigsen TP, Häggström J, Pedersen HD, Moesgaard SG, et al. Holter monitoring in clinically healthy Cavalier King Charles Spaniels, Wire-haired Dachshunds, and Cairn Terriers. J Vet Intern Med. 2011;25:460–468.

23 Meurs KM, Spier AW, Wright NA, Hamlin RL. Use of ambulatory electrocardiography for detection of ventricular premature complexes in healthy dogs. J Am Vet Med Assoc. 2001;218:1291–1292.

24 Lamb AP, Meurs KM, Hamlin RL. Correlation of heart rate to body weight in apparently normal dogs. J Vet Cardiol. 2010;12:107–110.

25 Hezzell MJ, Dennis SG, Humm K, Agee L, Boswood A. Relationships between heart rate and age, bodyweight and breed in 10,849 dogs. J Small Anim Pract. 2013;54:318–324.

26 Bodey AR, Michell AR. Epidemiological study of blood pressure in domestic dogs. J Small Anim Pract. 1996;37:116–125.

27 Ferasin L, Ferasin H, Little CJL. Lack of correlation between canine heart rate and body size in veterinary clinical practice. J Small Anim Pract. 2010;51:412–418.

28 Stern JA, Meurs KM, Spier AW, Koplitz SL, Baumwart RD. Ambulatory electrocardiographic evaluation of clinically normal adult Boxers. J Am Vet Med Assoc. 2010;236:430–433.

29 Meurs KM, Spier AW, Miller MW, Lehmkuhl L, Towbin JA. Familial ventricular arrhythmias in boxers. J Vet Intern Med. 1999;13:437–439.

30 Wess G, Schulze A, Butz V, Simak J, Killich M, Keller LJM, et al. Prevalence of dilated cardiomyopathy in Doberman Pinschers in various age groups. J Vet Intern Med. 2010;24:533–538.

31 Spier AW, Meurs KM. Evaluation of spontaneous variability in the frequency of ventricular arrhythmias in Boxers with arrhythmogenic right ventricular cardiomyopathy. J Am Vet Med Assoc. 2004;224:538–541.

32 Rossi A. Twenty-four-hour electrocardiographic study in the active very elderly. Cardiology. 1987;74:159–166.

33 Abbott, JA. Heart rate and heart rate variability of healthy cats in home and hospital environments. J Feline Med Surg. 2005;7:195–202.

34 Dickinson DF, Scott O. Ambulatory electrocardiographic monitoring in 100 healthy teenage boys. Br Heart J. 1984;51:179–183.

35 Morganroth J, Michelson EL, Horowitz LN, Josephson ME, Pearlman AS, Dunkman WB. Limitations of routine long-term electrocardiographic monitoring to assess ventricular ectopic frequency. Circulation. 1978;58:408–414.

36 Gelzer ARM, Kraus MS, Rishniw M, Hemsley SA, Moïse NS. Combination therapy with mexiletine and sotalol suppresses inherited ventricular arrhythmias in German shepherd dogs better than mexiletine or sotalol monotherapy: a randomized cross-over study. J Vet Cardiol. 2010;12:93–106.

37 Michelson EL, Morganroth J. Spontaneous variability of complex ventricular arrhythmias detected by long-term electrocardiographic recording. Circulation. 1980;61:690–695.

38 Winkle RA. Antiarrhythmic drug effect mimicked by spontaneous variability of ventricular ectopy. Circulation. 1978;57:1116–1121.

39 Gelzer ARM, Kraus MS, Rishniw M, Moise NS, Pariaut R, Jesty SA, et al. Combination therapy with digoxin and diltiazem controls ventricular rate in chronic atrial fibrillation in dogs better than digoxin or diltiazem monotherapy: a randomized crossover study in 18 dogs. J Vet Intern Med. 2009;23:499–508.

16

Heart Rate Variability
Domingo Casamian-Sorrosal

Introduction

Heart rate variability (HRV) is a numerical means of describing the oscillations in the heart rate or R-R interval between consecutive heart beats. Fluctuation in heart rate is a fundamental and intrinsic characteristic of normal cardiac function. As described in chapter 2, both the sympathetic and parasympathetic nervous systems are key determinants of these fluctuations in heart rate and rhythm. Cardiac chronotropy can be represented in two ways – in other chapters, the term *heart rate* is used and provides an estimate of heart rate normalised to time, hence the unit is beats per minute; however, this chapter focuses on the variation in R-R interval (measured in milliseconds) between consecutive heart beats. The terms NN and R-R are both used in the literature, but for clarity this chapter will use R-R as this term is used elsewhere. Figure 16.1 shows the relationship between heart rate and R-R interval.

Changes in heart rate are largely mediated by changes in sympathetic or parasympathetic nervous activity acting on the sinoatrial node. However, although sympathetic and parasympathetic systems exert opposing chronotropic actions, the effects are not symmetrical. Vagal stimulation of the sinoatrial node is mediated via synaptic release of acetylcholine, and the effects of this are almost immediate and short-acting due to rapid turnover of acetylcholine. Therefore, vagal control of the heart is modulated on a beat-by-beat basis (short latency). Sinus arrhythmia provides a good example of the parasympathetic nervous system exerting beat-to-beat control on heart rate.[2] In contrast, sympathetic stimulation of the sinoatrial node increases heart rate via noradrenaline release, and noradrenaline is reabsorbed and metabolised more slowly than acetylcholine; therefore, the effects of sympathetic stimulation are regarded as slower onset and longer lasting than parasympathetic stimulation (long latency).[3] Sympathetic stimulation results in reduced HRV, and, conversely, increased HRV is associated with parasympathetic dominance.

Whilst in humans high HRV has been associated with a healthy cardiovascular system, it is important to remember that in all species, the interactions between autonomic nervous system, heart rate, blood flow, baroreceptor sensitivity and cerebral autoregulation are highly complex. Therefore, care should be taken not to over-interpret single HRV measurements in this complex milieu.

Measurement of Heart Rate Variability

Several methods for HRV quantification have been described. A key step is to identify normal beats (normal R waves) and the intervals between consecutive R waves. Although the P wave is a closer graphic representation of the sinus node activity and therefore the P-P interval would be preferred, the majority of analysers do not reliably detect P waves and therefore the R-R interval is used as a surrogate of P-P. The presence of ventricular or supraventricular ectopy can invalidate HRV calculations, and therefore these beats must be removed from analysis.[4]

Measurement of the R-R intervals is the basis of HRV analysis as these time intervals are then used to construct a waveform that varies in amplitude and frequency (Figure 16.2).[4,5] The length of the electrocardiogram (ECG) trace required for HRV analysis depends on the methodology used and may vary from short (e.g. 20 R-R intervals) to long (e.g. 24 h) periods.[4] In general, beat-to-beat HRV occurs every few seconds and is classified as short-term or high-frequency variability, whereas long-term or low-frequency HRV occurs over longer periods.[4] It is important to be aware of potential limitations of different methodologies; for example, short-term recordings may fail to detect very-low-frequency oscillations, and data from long-term recordings are more likely to be influenced by external environmental conditions.[3] Although many variables within different methods and recording times correlate, it is important to always compare the results with recordings obtained using consistent methodology over a similar recording period. Specialized software is usually required for analysis; however, some time domain methods are simpler and can be performed manually.[4,6]

Linear Methods of Calculating HRV

Time Domain

This is a relatively simple and reproducible means of assessing HRV by comparing R-R intervals at various points in time, and Figure 16.3 shows an example from a normal dog. In this method, indexes of HRV are expressed in units of time (milliseconds). Correct calculation of time domain indexes requires that ectopic beats, unsensed beats, and artefact are excluded from the analysis, and therefore a good-quality recording is required.

The parameters commonly calculated are shown in Table 16.1.

It is important to note that SDNN, SDANN and SDNNi require long-term recordings of at least 18 h for accurate assessment,[7] and also it is inappropriate to compare SDNNs from recordings of different durations.[8] In human patients, rMSSD and pNN50 have been shown to quantify the modulation in R-R interval driven by ventilation. If shorter recordings are used for analysis, then

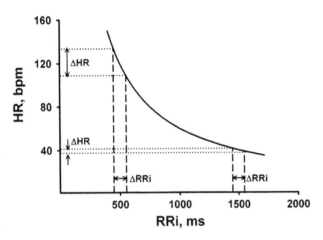

Figure 16.1 This figure shows the inverse relationship between heart rate (HR) and R-R interval (R-Ri). Note the hyperbolic relationship and therefore the same change in R-Ri (100 ms) can result in a marked changes in HR. With permission from Draghici AE, Taylor JA. The physiological basis and measurement of heart rate variability in humans. J Physiol Anthropol. 2016;35:22.[1]

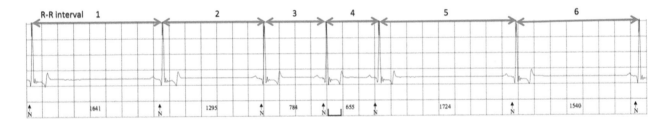

Ambulatory ECG trace from 6 year old male Doberman Pinscher

R-R inteval	R-R interval duration (ms)
1	1641
2	1295
3	768
4	655
5	1724
6	1540

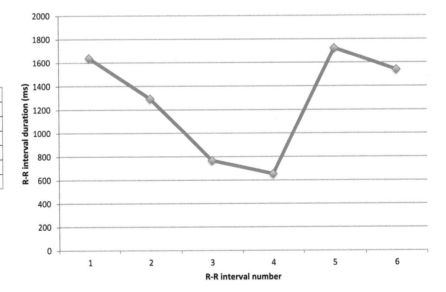

Figure 16.2 Changes in R-R interval during sinus arrhythmia. The ECG shows sinus arrhythmia and this physiological variation of instantaneous heart rate is the basis of heart rate variability. This variation in R-R interval can be used to construct a wave, which varies in amplitude and frequency.

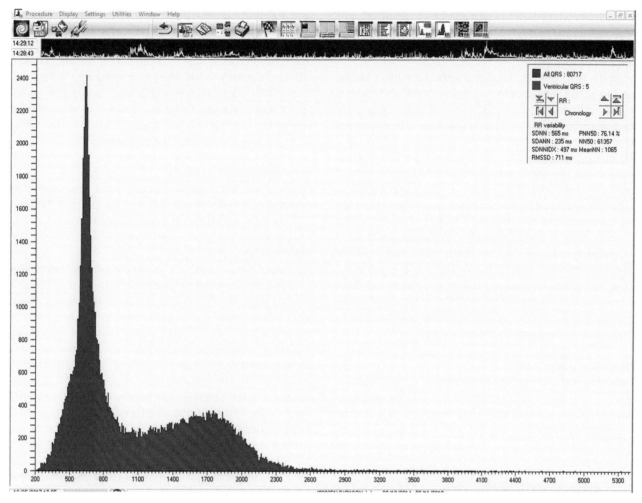

Figure 16.3 Example of a 24 h time domain analysis from a normal dog. An R-R interval distribution histogram can be seen. R-R interval lengths are plotted on the *x*-axis versus the numbers of the intervals falling within each interval range (or bin) on the *y*-axis. Note that normal dogs do not show a Gaussian distribution of R-R intervals. The upper right corner shows results of several statistical time-domain variables. *Source*: Courtesy of Yolanda Martinez Pereira, University of Edinburgh, UK.

Table 16.1 Time domain indexes

Parameter	Definition	Unit	Parameter assessed
Mean NN	Mean R-R of all intervals	Milliseconds	
SDNN	Standard deviation of all normal R-R intervals during the entire recording	Milliseconds	Overall autonomic tone
SDANN	Standard deviation of the mean R-R interval calculated for each short (usually 5 min) segment of the entire recording	Milliseconds	Total variability
SDNNi or SDNN index	Standard deviation of the mean of all normal R-R intervals measured in successive 5 min periods	Milliseconds	High and low-frequency variations
rMSSD or RMSSD	Square root of the mean of the sum of the squares of the differences between successive normal R-R intervals over the entire 24 h recording	Milliseconds	High-frequency variations (parasympathetic tone)
SDSD	Standard deviation of differences between adjacent R-R intervals	Milliseconds	High-frequency variations (parasympathetic tone)
pNN50	% of adjacent R-R intervals with a difference in duration of >50 ms	%	High-frequency variations (parasympathetic tone)

Source: With permission from Task Force of the European Society of Cardiology and the North American Society of Pacing and Electrophysiology. Heart rate variability: standards of measurement, physiological interpretation and clinical use. Circulation. 1996;93(5):1043–1065.

measurements estimate high-frequency variations in heart rate.[8]

Geometric Measures

From the time domain data, geometrical methods can be used to present the data in a different format and thereby derive additional parameters. Most of these geometric methods require the R-R interval sequence to be converted to a discrete scale that permits the construction of a smoothed histogram. Thus, R-R interval distribution histograms are plotted with the R-R interval lengths plotted on the *x*-axis versus the numbers of the intervals falling within each interval (or bin) on the *y*-axis. Most experience has been obtained with the length of the bins on the *x*-axis of approximately 8 ms (precisely 7.8125 ms = 1/128 s).[8] If the patient's heart rate was constant, only a single tall bar would be seen, but, due to the variation in R-R intervals, these histograms are typically bell shaped but do not show a Gaussian distribution.[9] The variance (or spread of distribution) of R-R intervals against the mean will increase in proportion to the length of the recording.[8]

Poincaré or Lorenz Plots

Time domain analysis has been used to create Poincaré plots (also called Lorenz graphs) which illustrate short-term HRV by plotting an R-R interval (R-R$_{(n)}$) on the *x*-axis versus the following R-R interval (RR$_{(n+1)}$) on the *y*-axis (Figure 16.4).[4] The Poincaré plot can reveal not only the more global autonomic influence but also the short-term beat-to-beat impact on rhythm.[10] On Poincaré graphs, when the R-R interval changes minimally or increases and decreases very slowly (i.e. low HRV), the points would all appear along a 45° imaginary line, which starts at the origin and divides the graph. Short R-R intervals following long R-R intervals fall below the dividing line, and long RR intervals following short RR intervals appear above this line.[4]

Other Geometrical Measures

Other geometrical methods have been described that detect low-frequency change, and the derived parameters are shown in Table 16.2 and Figure 16.5.

Vasovagal Tonus Index

Vasovagal tonus index (VVTI) is a time domain indicator of the higher frequency elements of HRV that can be calculated manually. VVTI can be calculated from a standard ECG recorded with a paper speed of 25 or 50 mm/s, although 50 mm/s will give better temporal resolution. ECGs are recorded in the standard manner with the dog in right lateral recumbency after a variable period of adaptation to the environment, depending on the animal's character. The R-R interval durations are measured with a ruler to the nearest quarter of a millimetre (equivalent to the nearest 10 ms). VVTI is calculated as the natural logarithm of the variance of the R-R intervals for 20–60 consecutive QRS complexes (VVTI20 and VVTI60, respectively). Non-sinus rhythms and ectopic beats should not be included in the analysis.[11,12] The short sampling interval favours detection of high-frequency oscillations such as those caused by variations in parasympathetic tone.[6]

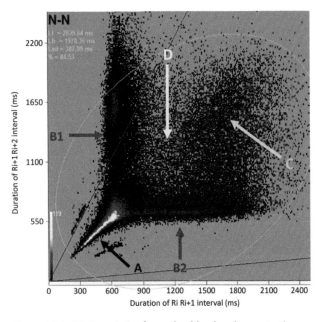

Figure 16.4 A Poincaré plot from a healthy dog demonstrating common features. (A) Stalk representing short–short R-R intervals. (B1) Arm representing short-long R-R intervals. (B2) Arm representing long-short R-R intervals. (C) Cluster representing long–long R-R intervals. (D) Zone of lower density representing a range of R-R intervals occurring infrequently. *Source*: Journal of Veterinary Cardiology (2018) vol. 20 (1) pp. 20–32.

Calculation of VVTI is performed as follows:

$$VVTI = LN[VAR(Z1 - Z20)]$$
$$or\ VVTI = LN[VAR(Z1 - Z60)]$$

where:
LN: natural logarithm
VAR: variance
Z1: first R-R
Z20: subsequent 20 R-R intervals
Z60: subsequent 60 R-R intervals.

Heart Rate Turbulence

Heart rate turbulence (HRT) describes the small short-term fluctuations in sinus cycle length following a ventricular premature beat.[13] The haemodynamic disturbances caused by a ventricular premature complex (VPC) provide insights into the regulation of the

Table 16.2 Geometric measures of HRV

Parameter	Definition	Units
Triangle index or HRV triangular index	Total number of R-R intervals divided by the maximum of the density distribution of the histogram measured on a discrete scale with bins of 1/128 s = total number of R-R / maximum number of N-N of equal length	
Triangular interpolation of NN interval histogram (TINN)	Baseline width of the distribution measured as a base of a triangle approximating the R-R	Milliseconds

N-N, Time in milliseconds between two consecutive R waves (same as R-R).

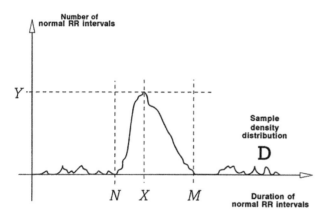

Figure 16.5 How the geometric measures of HRV are calculated from the R-R interval histogram. To perform geometric measures on the R-R interval histogram, the sample density distribution D is constructed, which assigns the number of equally long R-R intervals to each value of their lengths. The most frequent R-R interval length X is established, that is, $Y = D(X)$ is the maximum of the sample density distribution D. The HRV triangular index is the value obtained by dividing the area integral of D by the maximum Y. When the distribution D with a discrete scale is constructed on the horizontal axis, the value is obtained according to the formula HRV index = (total number of all R-R intervals)/Y. For the computation of the TINN measure, the values N and M are established on the time axis and a multilinear function q constructed such that $q(t) = 0$ for $t \leq N$ and $t \geq M$ and $q(X) = Y$, and such that the integral $\int 0 + \infty$ (D(t) − q(t))2 dt is the minimum among all selections of all values N and M. The TINN measure is expressed in milliseconds and given by the formula TINN = $M − N$.[8]

autonomic nervous system.[15] After a ventricular premature beat, heart rate increases for 1–2 beats and then decelerates for a few beats before returning to baseline.[14] HRT indexes show a modest correlation with HRV.[15]

The effect on HRV is described in terms of turbulence onset (TO) and turbulence slope (TS). TO is the amount of sinus acceleration following a VPC; TS is the rate of sinus deceleration that follows this sinus acceleration. TS is calculated over 24 R-R intervals encompassing the VPC, with >2 before and <20 after. If these measurements are taken for all VPCs over a 24 h period, then a mean can be calculated for TO and TS for each patient.[15] Abnormal HRT is a predictor of mortality in human patients post myocardial infarction,[16] but the utility of

this parameter in clinical canine and feline heart disease is yet to be elucidated.

Other Time Domain Methods for Calculation of Canine Parasympathetic Activity

The canine index of parasympathetic activity (CIPA) has been reported in dogs[17,18] and utilizes a microprocessor-controlled device (the Neuroscope; Medifit Instruments, Essex, UK) to derive real-time measurements of heart rate and parasympathetic activity. The software analyses the changes occurring in several subsequent R-R intervals and compares them against a pre-existing algorithm to calculate the CIPA.[18] A similar and more recent index used in dogs is the parasympathetic tone activity (PTA) index which is calculated using the increase of parasympathetic tone induced by each respiratory cycle to measure the 'relative quantity' of parasympathetic tone from an established algorithm.[19]

Frequency Domain Analysis of Heart Rate Variability

Spectral analysis of heart rate partitions HRV into frequency components using complex mathematical algorithms. Power spectral density analysis provides data on how power (R-R variance) distributes as a function of frequency.

To be suitable for this form of analysis, the ECG should satisfy certain technical requirements:

- Sampling frequency range of 250–500 Hz
- Ectopic beats, arrhythmias, missing data and noise effects should be filtered and omitted.
- Recording duration must be >10× the wavelength of the lower frequency band; therefore, recordings of 1 min can assess only high-frequency components of HRV, 2 min are required for low-frequency components and 5 min recordings are preferred.

Frequency domain indexes are expressed in Hertz (the number of cycles per second) and are divided into four categories as shown in Table 16.3 and Figure 16.6. Two additional measures (low frequency/high frequency

Table 16.3 Frequency domain indexes

Variable	Approximate frequency	Description
High frequency (HF)	0.15–0.4 Hz	Respiratory sinus arrhythmia, mostly due to vagal activity
Low frequency (LF)	0.04–0.15 Hz	Mayer wave oscillations associated with both sympathetic and parasympathetic activity
Very low frequency (VLF)	0.0033–0.04 Hz	Changes over 20 s–5 min; associated with changes in renin–angiotensin aldosterone system, thermoregulation and peripheral vasomotor tone*
Ultralow frequency (ULF)	<0.003 Hz	Changes between 5 min and 24 h; associated with changes in renin–angiotensin aldosterone system, thermoregulation and peripheral vasomotor tone**
LF/HF		Interaction between the sympathetic and parasympathetic nervous systems
Total power	<0.4 Hz	Variance of all R-R intervals over the temporal segment

*More recent studies suggest VLF variation is generated by stimulation of afferent sensory neurones within the heart.[20]
**ULF frequency components of heart rate variability are also influenced by physical activity.[21]
Note: The units for these measurements are ms^2 apart from LF/HF, which is a ratio and therefore does not have a unit.
Source: With permission from Task Force of the European Society of Cardiology and the North American Society of Pacing Electrophysiology. Heart rate variability: standards of measurement, physiological interpretation, and clinical use. Circulation. 1996;93:1043–1065.

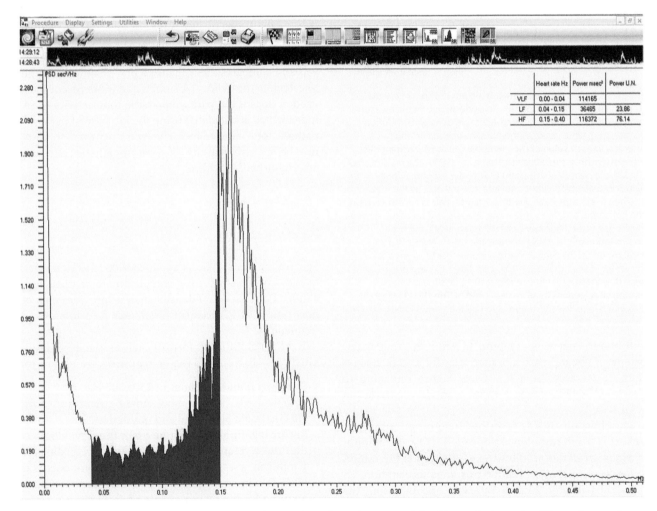

Figure 16.6 Example of a 24 h frequency domain analysis study performed in a normal dog. The x-axis shows the different frequencies, and the y-axis their relative intensity (power). A numerical representation of the different spectral components (with their corresponding frequency range) can be observed at the top right of the picture. The shaded area represents the low frequency band. The area under the power spectral curve (power) in a particular frequency band is considered to be a measure of HRV at that frequency. VLF, Very low frequency; LF, low frequency; HF, high frequency. *Source*: Courtesy of Yolanda Martinez Pereira, University of Edinburgh, UK.

[LF/HF] and power) may be derived from these data, as shown in Table 16.3.

Time Domain and Frequency Domain Approximate Correlates

Whilst direct comparisons between different methodologies may not be possible, conceptually it may be useful to know which time and frequency domain parameters correlate, as is shown in Table 16.4. A study in Dobermans with pre-clinical dilated cardiomyopathy (DCM) showed similar correlation of these parameters.[22]

Non-linear Methods for Calculating HRV

These methods use complex mathematics to model the entire system rather than a single element.[23] The clinical significance of this methodology has not been elucidated in dogs.

Physiological Influences on HRV

A number of physiological variations in HRV have been observed in normal dogs including:

- Diurnal variation – Indices pertaining to parasympathetic tone are higher overnight (midnight to 6 a.m.) in studies involving Dobermans, Dachshunds and laboratory-housed Beagles.[24–27]
- Age – Increasing age resulting in reduced parasympathetic activity in humans;[3] in dogs, a similar trend has been proposed.[11,24]
- Breed – Brachycephalic dogs have higher VVTI than other breeds,[6] and VVTI was lower in Cavalier King Charles Spaniel (CKCS) than in other breeds.[11]

Table 16.4 Time domain and frequency domain approximate correlates

Time domain variable	Approximate frequency domain correlate
SDNN	Total power
HRV triangle index	Total power
TINN	Total power
SDANN	ULF
SDNN index	Mean of 5 min total power
RMSSD	HF
SDSD	HF
NN50 count	HF
pNN50	HF
Differential index	HF

Source: With permission from Task Force of the European Society of Cardiology and the North American Society of Pacing Electrophysiology. Heart rate variability: standards of measurement, physiological interpretation, and clinical use. Circulation. 1996;93:1043–1065.

A study investigating HRV in clinically healthy small-breed dogs considered to be at varying risk of developing mitral valve disease (MVD) has been reported. In this study, CKCS were considered to be at high risk of MVD, wire-haired Dachshunds (wD) were considered to be at moderate risk of MVD, and Cairn Terriers (CT) at low risk of MVD. These dogs had ten HRV parameters assessed from ambulatory ECG recordings, and 15/27 Holter-derived HRV variables were significantly associated with breed. During Holter recording, the minimum and mean heart rates were higher in CKCS compared with wD. CKCS had significantly lower values than wD, CT or both in 10 out of 13 HRV variables.[28]

- Sex – A study in young, healthy Dachshunds showed high HRV in male dogs compared to females.[24]

HRV in Canine Heart Disease

HRV in Congestive Heart Failure

Several studies using various methods of calculating HRV have investigated HRV in canine congestive heart failure. HRV has been showed to be lower in patients with congestive heart failure due to DCM,[6,12,29] MVD,[6,11,29–31] arrhythmogenic right ventricular cardiomyopathy[32] and tachycardia-induced cardiomyopathy.[33] A trend towards increasing HRV after therapy of congestive heart failure has also been observed.[29]

Heart Rate Variability in Doberman DCM

The correlation between time and frequency domain parameters has been investigated in normal Dobermans and compared to Dobermans with pre-clinical DCM. This study showed good correlation between time domain and frequency domain parameters in a pattern similar to that shown in Table 16.4. HRV tended to decrease in dogs with more advanced pre-clinical disease, but this difference did not reach significance.[22] When similar parameters were investigated using a different software programme and including Dobermans with more advanced disease, reduced HRV was detected in the dogs with most advanced myocardial failure.[34] As changes in HRV have only been detected in more advanced disease, HRV analysis has not been shown to be a sensitive tool in screening for DCM.[34] This is likely to be at least partly because the profound sinus arrhythmia seen in dogs renders HRV relatively insensitive.

Heart Rate Variability and Mitral Valve Disease

A reduction in HRV in dogs with degenerative atrioventricular valve disease has been documented in multiple studies.[6,29,30,35] In cases with early myxomatous disease resulting in mitral valve prolapse, the effect on HRV variables is variable.[24,28] However, in dogs with more advanced disease, the effect is more consistent – for example, a study using advanced ECG parameters showed a correlation between the total spectral power of R-R interval variability and the severity of mitral regurgitation.[36]

HRV was measured using VVTI in 81 CKCS to investigate if it could be used to evaluate the severity of mitral regurgitation and to predict decompensation. Twenty-two of the dogs were clinically normal, and 59 had mitral regurgitation caused by chronic valvular disease of varying severity. HRV was reduced among dogs with severe left atrial and ventricular dilatation and clinical signs of congestive heart failure.[30]

A longitudinal study reviewing 853 ECGs from 257 dogs with degenerative MVD was used to investigate the effects of advancing cardiac disease on heart rate and VVTI. The dogs who died or were euthanised as a result of cardiac or non-cardiac disease were compared to dogs who were still alive at least 6 months after their last ECG was recorded. In the dogs who died, there was an increase in HR and decrease in VVTI evident at least 18 months before death. In the dogs who died or were euthanised due to cardiac disease, there was a further decrease in VVTI approximately 1 year before death. In this study, VVTI was proposed as a biomarker for cardiac mortality but also for all-cause mortality.[11]

Another study investigated HRV in small-breed dogs with advanced atrioventricular valve disease with and without a history of syncope.[37] This study recruited 43 dogs and used time and frequency domain HRV parameters to compare syncopal and non-syncopal dogs. The results showed that eight HRV parameters representing parasympathetic influence were lower in dogs with a history of syncope, perhaps suggesting that altered autonomic tone or baroreceptor reflex disruption predisposes dogs to these syncopal events.[37]

A study comparing time domain HRV parameters in dogs with myxomatous atrioventricular valve disease, with and without evidence of heart failure, showed a high correlation between the echocardiographic evaluation of disease severity and the reduction in HRV variables pertaining to parasympathetic tone.[31]

HRV in Sick Sinus Syndrome

Dogs with sick sinus syndrome have also been shown to have significant decrease in HRV,[38] and specific geometrical patterns on tachograms and Poincaré plots can be observed.[39]

HRV and Prognosis in Cardiac Disease

HRV has also been studied as a prognostic factor in dogs for different cardiac diseases. In dogs with DCM, lower VVTI values were found in dogs with more advanced heart failure and also VVTI was positively correlated with survival time.[12]

As mentioned earlier in this chapter, a study showed that dogs with degenerative MVD have an increase in heart rate and decrease in HRV over a year before death, with greater changes in those dogs dying or euthanized due to cardiac disease.[11] However, to date, HRV has not been found to be a useful prognostic tool in dogs with ventricular arrhythmias due to arrhythmogenic right ventricular cardiomyopathy.[32]

Non-cardiac Applications for HRV

HRV analysis has also been studied in dogs with non-cardiac disease. As is the case in humans, HRV is decreased in dogs with diabetes mellitus, particularly if the diabetes mellitus is poorly controlled.[40]

HRV has been studied in certain behavioural conditions – for example, HRV was shown to be a predictor of dogs' emotional state.[41,42] HRV has been used as an indicator of stress, with studies showing increased HRV (assumed to indicate reduced stress) in kennelled dogs played music.[43] In both laboratory and companion dogs, analysis of HRV variables during periods of exposure to a standardised recording of thunder was suggestive of sympathetic stimulation during periods of thunder.[44]

Recent studies have been very encouraging in the use of HRV (the PTA index) as a marker of nociception during anaesthesia.[19]

Heart Rate Variability in Cats

In a research setting, a crossover trial investigating the effects of atenolol on HRV in anaesthetised cats showed that it was possible to measure HRV in anaesthetised cats.[45] In another study, anaesthetised cats were subjected to chronic intermittent hypoxia and showed changes in HRV spectral indexes towards the low-frequency band and also alteration of the LF/HF ratio.[46] Spectral analysis of sympathetic discharge has also been investigated in decerebrate artificially ventilated cats.[47,48]

In clinical studies, VVTI has been used to assess the effects of physiological and behavioural stress in cats.[49] Another study compared heart rates of cats at home to heart rates during rest in a quiet room in the hospital and heart rates during echocardiography. Significant differences in HRV profiles between these settings suggested that sympathetic tone was higher and parasympathetic tone lower whilst cats were in the hospital.[50]

References

1 Draghici AE, Taylor JA. The physiological basis and measurement of heart rate variability in humans. J Physiol Anthropol. 2016;35:22.

2 Hayano J, Yasuma F, Okada A, Mukai S, Fujinami T. Respiratory sinus arrhythmia: a phenomenon improving pulmonary gas exchange and circulatory efficiency. Circulation. 1996;94:842–847.

3 Xhyheri B, Manfrini O, Mazzolini M, Pizzi C, Bugiardini R. Heart rate variability today. Prog Cardiovasc Dis. 2012;55:321–331.

4 Calvert CA. Heart rate variability. Vet Clin North Am Small Anim Pract. 1998;28:1409–1427– viii.

5 Rajendra Acharya U, Paul Joseph K, Kannathal N, Lim CM, Suri JS. Heart rate variability: a review. Med Biol Eng Comput. 2006;44:1031–1051.

6 Doxey S, Boswood A. Differences between breeds of dog in a measure of heart rate variability. Vet Rec. 2004;154:713–717.

7 Kleiger RE, Stein PK, Bosner MS, Rottman JN. Time domain measurements of heart rate variability. Cardiol Clin. 1992;10:487–498.

8 Task Force of the European Society of Cardiology and the North American Society of Pacing and Electrophysiology. Heart rate variability: standards of measurement, physiological interpretation and clinical use. Circulation. 1996;93:1043–1065.

9 Moïse NS, Gladuli A, Hemsley SA, Otani NF. 'Zone of avoidance': RR interval distribution in tachograms, histograms, and Poincare plots of a Boxer dog. J Vet Cardiol. 2010;12:191–196.

10 Climent AM, de la Salud Guillem M, Husser D, Castells F, Millet J, Bollmann A. Poincare surface profiles of RR intervals: a novel noninvasive method for the evaluation of preferential AV nodal conduction during atrial fibrillation. IEEE Trans Biomed Eng. 2009;56:433–442.

11 Lopez-Alvarez J, Boswood A, Moonarmart W, Hezzell MJ, Lotter N, Elliott J. Longitudinal electrocardiographic evaluation of dogs with degenerative mitral valve disease. J Vet Intern Med. 2014;28:393–400.

12 Pereira YM, Woolley R, Culshaw G, French A, Martin M. The vasovagal tonus index as a prognostic indicator in dogs with dilated cardiomyopathy. J Small Anim Pract. 2008;49:587–592.

13 Watanabe MA. Heart rate turbulence: a review. Indian Pacing Electrophysiol J. 2003;3:10–22.

14 Schmidt G, Malik M, Barthel P, Schneider R, Ulm K, Rolnitzky L, et al. Heart-rate turbulence after ventricular premature beats as a predictor of mortality after acute myocardial infarction. Lancet. 1999;353:1390–1396.

15 Bauer A, Malik M, Schmidt G, Barthel P, Bonnemeier H, Cygankiewicz I, et al. Heart rate turbulence: standards of measurement, physiological interpretation, and clinical use: International Society for Holter and Noninvasive Electrophysiology Consensus. J Am Coll Cardiol. 2008;52:1353–1365.

16 Schmitt KE, Tyrrell WD, Pasieka G. Characterization and clinical significance of ventricular premature complexes in Irish Wolfhounds. In ACVIM Forum Proceedings, Seattle, June 2013.

17 Little CJ, Julu PO. Investigation of heart rate variability in a dog with upper respiratory tract obstruction. J Small Anim Pract. 1995;36:502–506.

18 Little CJ, Julu PO, Hansen S, Reid SW. Real-time measurement of cardiac vagal tone in conscious dogs. Am J Physiol. 1999;276:H758–H765.

19 Mansour C, Merlin T, Bonnet-Garin J-M, Chaaya R, Mocci R, Ruiz CC, et al. Evaluation of the parasympathetic tone activity (PTA) index to assess the analgesia/nociception balance in anaesthetised dogs. Res Vet Sci. 2017;115:271–277.

20 Murphy DA, Thompson GW, Ardell JL, McCraty R, Stevenson RS, Sangalang VE, et al. The heart reinnervates after transplantation. Ann Thorac Surg. 2000;69:1769–1781.

21 Serrador JM, Finlayson HC, Hughson RL. Physical activity is a major contributor to the ultra low frequency components of heart rate variability. Heart. 1999;82:e9.

22 Calvert CA, Wall TM. Correlations among time and frequency measures of heart rate variability recorded by use of a Holter monitor in overtly healthy Doberman pinschers with and without echocardiographic evidence of dilated cardiomyopathy. Am J Vet Res. 2001;62:1787–1792.

23 Tan CO, Cohen MA, Eckberg DL, Taylor JA. Fractal properties of human heart period variability: physiological and methodological implications. J Physiol. 2009;587:3929–3941.

24 Olsen LH, Mow T, Koch J, Pedersen HD. Heart rate variability in young, clinically healthy Dachshunds: influence of sex, mitral valve prolapse status, sampling period and time of day. J Vet Cardiol. 1999;1:7–16.

25 Calvert CA, Wall TM. Correlations among time and frequency measures of heart rate variability recorded by use of a Holter monitor in overtly healthy Doberman pinschers with and without echocardiographic evidence of dilated cardiomyopathy. Am J Vet Res. 2001;62:1787–1792.

26 Calvert CA, Wall M. Evaluation of stability over time for measures of heart-rate variability in overtly healthy Doberman Pinschers. Am J Vet Res. 2002;63:53–59.

27 Matsunaga T, Harada T, Mitsui T, Inokuma M, Hashimoto M, Miyauchi M, *et al.* Spectral analysis of circadian rhythms in heart rate variability of dogs. Am J Vet Res. 2001;62:37–42.

28 Rasmussen CE, Vesterholm S, Ludvigsen TP, Häggström J, Pedersen HD, Moesgaard SG, *et al.* Holter monitoring in clinically healthy Cavalier King Charles Spaniels, Wire-haired Dachshunds, and Cairn Terriers. J Vet Intern Med. 2011;25:460–468.

29 Boswood A, Murphy A. The effect of heart disease, heart failure and diuresis on selected laboratory and electrocardiographic parameters in dogs. J Vet Cardiol. 2006;8:1–9.

30 Häggström J, Hamlin RL, Hansson K, Kvart C. Heart rate variability in relation to severity of mitral regurgitation in Cavalier King Charles spaniels. J Small Anim Pract. 1996;37:69–75.

31 Oliveira MS, Muzzi RAL, Araujo RB, Muzzi LAL, Ferreira DF, Nogueira R, *et al.* Heart rate variability parameters of myxomatous mitral valve disease in dogs with and without heart failure obtained using 24-hour Holter electrocardiography. Vet Rec. 2012;170:622.

32 Spier AW, Meurs KM. Assessment of heart rate variability in Boxers with arrhythmogenic right ventricular cardiomyopathy. J Am Vet Med Assoc. 2004;224:534–537.

33 Piccirillo G, Ogawa M, Song J, Chong VJ, Joung B, Han S, *et al.* Power spectral analysis of heart rate variability and autonomic nervous system activity measured directly in healthy dogs and dogs with tachycardia-induced heart failure. Heart Rhythm. 2009;6:546–552.

34 Calvert CA, Wall M. Effect of severity of myocardial failure on heart rate variability in Doberman pinschers with and without echocardiographic evidence of dilated cardiomyopathy. J Am Vet Med Assoc. 2001;219:1084–1088.

35 Rasmussen CE, Falk T, Zois NE, Moesgaard SG, Häggström J, Pedersen HD, *et al.* Heart rate, heart rate variability, and arrhythmias in dogs with myxomatous mitral valve disease. J Vet Intern Med. 2012;26:76–84.

36 Spiljak Pakkanen M, Domanjko Petric A, Olsen LH, Stepancic A, Schlegel TT, Falk T, *et al.* Advanced electrocardiographic parameters change with severity of mitral regurgitation in Cavalier King Charles Spaniels in sinus rhythm. J Vet Intern Med. 2012;26:93–100.

37 Rasmussen CE, Falk T, Domanjko Petric A, Schaldemose M, Zois NE, Moesgaard SG, *et al.* Holter monitoring of small breed dogs with advanced myxomatous mitral valve disease with and without a history of syncope. J Vet Intern Med. 2014;28:363–370.

38 Bogucki S, Noszczyk-Nowak A. Short-term heart rate variability in dogs with sick sinus syndrome or chronic mitral valve disease as compared to healthy controls. Pol J Vet Sci. 2017;20:167–172.

39 Gladuli A, Moïse NS, Hemsley SA, Otani NF. Poincaré plots and tachograms reveal beat patterning in sick sinus syndrome with supraventricular tachycardia and varying AV nodal block. J Vet Cardiol. 2011;13:63–70.

40 Pirintr P, Chansaisakorn W, Trisiriroj M, Kalandakanond-Thongsong S, Buranakarl C. Heart rate variability and plasma norepinephrine concentration in diabetic dogs at rest. Vet Res Commun. 2012;36:207–214.

41 Katayama M, Kubo T, Mogi K, Ikeda K, Nagasawa M, Kikusui T. Heart rate variability predicts the emotional state in dogs. Behav Proc. 2016;128:108–112.

42 Wormald D, Lawrence AJ, Carter G, Fisher AD. Reduced heart rate variability in pet dogs affected by anxiety-related behaviour problems. Physiol Behav. 2017;168:122–127.

43 Bowman A, Dowell FJ, Evans NP. The effect of different genres of music on the stress levels of kennelled dogs. Physiol Behav. 2017;171:207–215.

44 Franzini de Souza CC, Maccariello CEM, Dias DPM, Almeida NADS, de Medeiros MA. Autonomic, endocrine and behavioural responses to thunder in laboratory and companion dogs. Physiol Behav. 2017;169:208–215.

45 Khor KH, Shiels IA, Campbell FE, Greer RM, Rose A, Mills PC. Evaluation of a technique to measure heart rate variability in anaesthetised cats. Vet J. 2014;199:229–235.

46 Rey S, Tarvainen MP, Karjalainen PA, Iturriaga R. Dynamic time-varying analysis of heart rate and blood pressure variability in cats exposed to short-term chronic intermittent hypoxia. Am J Physiol Regul Integr Comp Physiol. 2008;295:R28–R37.

47 Montano N, Lombardi F, Gnecchi Ruscone T, Contini M, Finocchiaro ML, Baselli G, *et al.* Spectral analysis of sympathetic discharge, R-R interval and systolic arterial pressure in decerebrate cats. J Auton Nerv Syst. 1992;40:21–31.

48 Lombardi F, Montano N, Finocchiaro ML, Ruscone TG, Baselli G, Cerutti S, *et al.* Spectral analysis of sympathetic discharge in decerebrate cats. J Auton Nerv Syst. 1990;30(Suppl.):S97–S99.

49 Conti LM, Champion T, Guberman UC, Mathias CH, Fernandes SL, Silva EG, *et al.* Evaluation of environment and a feline facial pheromone analogue on physiologic and behavioral measures in cats. J Feline Med Surg. 2017;19:165–170.

50 Abbott JA. Heart rate and heart rate variability of healthy cats in home and hospital environments. J Feline Med Surg. 2005;7:195–202.

17

Anti-arrhythmic Drugs
Joel Freitas da Silva

> **Important note about anti-arrhythmic medications**
>
> No drugs are licensed for the treatment of arrhythmias in dogs or cats. Therefore, clinicians are encouraged to reflect carefully on the available evidence for treatment efficacy and also to obtain fully informed consent from owners prior to using any anti-arrhythmic medication.

Introduction

Anti-arrhythmic drugs are used in veterinary medicine with the goals of improving clinical signs and prolonging survival. Although the benefits of treating acute, symptomatic arrhythmias may be obvious, assessing the efficacy of chronic treatment of arrhythmias is more challenging. Apparent improvements in the number or complexity of asymptomatic ventricular arrhythmias may not necessarily translate into improved survival or lower risks of sudden death, and, in some instances, survival may even be negatively affected.[1] Unfortunately, there is a paucity of clinical trials in veterinary medicine that precludes the development of evidence-based guidelines for the use of anti-arrhythmic drugs. Many clinical decisions are currently based on studies with low levels of evidence and personal experience. Technological advances such as device-based or ablative therapies are likely to change the way arrhythmias are managed in companion animals in future.

Drug Classification

Anti-arrhythmic drugs are commonly classified according to their basic mechanism of action in four classes – the Vaughan Williams classification. However, this classification is hampered by the weak link between the drug actions, arrhythmia mechanism and treatment efficacy. A more complex classification system – the Sicilian Gambit[2] – has been proposed to review and complement the original classification, but, as this system has not gained widespread acceptance in the veterinary field, the Vaughan Williams classification is used in this chapter and summarised in Table 17.1.

Class I

Class I anti-arrhythmic drugs block membrane sodium (Na^+) channels, depressing phase 0 of the action potential and thereby slowing conduction velocity. As spontaneous depolarisation of nodal cells relies on calcium rather than sodium, class I drugs affect cardiomyocytes more than nodal cells. By suppressing spontaneous depolarisation of cardiomyocytes, class I drugs may interrupt re-entrant arrhythmias by creating a more electrically homogeneous environment.

Class I agents are subdivided into three classes (IA, IB and IC) that differ in their electrophysiological properties, especially in the way they affect repolarisation – see Figure 17.1.

Class IA

Class IA includes *quinidine, procainamide* and *disopyramide*. Like other Class I drugs, they depress the action potential upstroke (phase 0), slowing velocity conduction in atrial, ventricular and Purkinje cells. Unlike other class I drugs, they increase action potential duration and prolong the refractory period, and therefore could be considered to also have a mild class III action – see Table 17.2. By slowing conduction and lengthening the refractory period, these drugs may interrupt re-entrant or triggered arrhythmias. However, it is important to highlight that both these electrophysiological effects may also be pro-arrhythmic.

Table 17.1 Summary of Vaughan Williams anti-arrhythmic drug classification

Class	Channel effects	Effect on repolarisation time	Drug examples
IA	Moderate sodium channel block	Prolongs	Quinidine, procainamide
IB	Sodium channel block (weaker than class IA drugs)	Shortens	Lidocaine, mexiletine
IC	Strong sodium channel block	Unchanged	Flecainide, propafenone
II	I_f (depolarising current in pacemaker cells)	Unchanged	β-blockers
III	Repolarising potassium currents	Marked prolongation	Sotalol, amiodarone
IV	AV node calcium block	Unchanged	Dilitazem, verapamil
IV-like	K channel opener	Unchanged	Adenosine

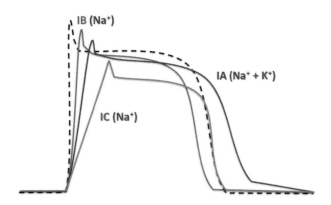

Figure 17.1 Effects of class I anti-arrhythmic drugs on the cardiomyocyte action potential. (Black dotted line) Normal cardiomyocyte action potential. All class I drugs delay depolarisation to various degrees. This is translated as a decrease in the slope of the rapid depolarisation stage. (Red line) Administration of a *class IA drug* (e.g. quinidine) prolongs depolarisation due to moderate Na^+ channel blockade but also increases the effective repolarisation period (ERP) due to effects on K^+ channels. (Blue line) Administration of a *class IB drug* (e.g. lidocaine) prolongs depolarisation slightly due to weak Na^+ channel blockade and reduces the ERP. (Green line) Administration of a *class IC drug* (e.g. flecainide) markedly prolongs depolarisation due to strong Na^+ channel blockade without an effect on ERP. Na^+, Sodium; K^+, potassium.

Table 17.2 Summary of the electrocardiogram (ECG) changes induced by class IA anti-arrhythmic drugs

	Quinidine	Procainamide
Sinus node discharge rate	Mild to moderate increase	Low doses: Increased High dose: Depressant effect
PR interval	Normal	Normal
QRS duration	Mild increase	Normal or increased
QT interval	Increase	Normal or increased

Quinidine and procainamide are two drugs belonging to this group. In addition to their electrophysiological effects, they also have indirect (vagolytic) effects resulting in increased heart rate and enhanced atrioventricular node (AVN) conduction. These drugs have been used for the treatment of ventricular and supraventricular tachyarrhythmias. Quinidine has been used for conversion of atrial fibrillation,[3] but it is not currently recommended for this purpose, especially in dogs with structural heart disease.

Intravenous (IV) procainamide may be used for emergency treatment of life-threatening ventricular arrhythmias. Oral procainamine has been used for chronic treatment of ventricular arrhythmias in dogs,[4] although the reduction in the severity of ventricular arrhythmias was inconsistent, and adverse effects were common. Procainamide has been used to treat orthodromic atrioventricular reciprocating tachycardia in dogs, as it can decrease conduction velocity of the accessory pathway(s).[5] Adverse effects of class IA drugs include gastrointestinal disturbances, weakness, hypotension, cardiac depression and QT prolongation; however, these effects are seen less frequently with procainamide compared to quinidine. Class 1A drugs can be pro-arrhythmic by increasing ventricular rate in atrial fibrillation, promoting ventricular arrhythmias or causing atrioventricular (AV) block at higher doses. Quinidine also increases the risk of digoxin toxicity.

Class IA anti-arrhythmic drugs have lost importance over the years in favour of safer and more efficacious drugs. They currently have limited application in veterinary medicine.

Class IB

Class IB drugs inhibit the fast sodium channel whilst shortening the action potential duration in healthy tissue – see Figure 17.1 and Table 17.3. They possess fast onset/offset kinetics and bind more avidly to open or inactivated channels. Drugs from this class display *use dependence* which means that the degree of effect is higher in cells that are depolarising more rapidly (e.g. during tachycardia). These properties

Table 17.3 Summary of the ECG changes induced by class IB anti-arrhythmic drugs

	Class IB drugs: Lidocaine, mexiletine, tocainide
Sinus node discharge rate	None or mild increase
PR interval	Normal
QRS duration	Normal
QT interval	Normal or decreased

are desirable when treating tachyarrhythmias as these drugs will be more effective at higher heart rates. Class IB drugs also act selectively in diseased tissue, where they cause a profound decrease in conduction velocity, thereby interrupting re-entrant circuits.[6] Lidocaine does not alter atrial refractoriness or conduction velocity, which may at least partly explain the ineffectiveness of lidocaine at treating supraventricular arrhythmias.[7]

Lidocaine

Lidocaine is widely used as a first-line emergency treatment for haemodynamically unstable ventricular arrhythmias. Lidocaine may be effective in the treatment of re-entrant, automatic or triggered ventricular arrhythmias[8] due to multiple electrophysiological effects, including:

1) Marked depression of the phase 0 in diseased tissue,[6] thereby slowing conduction with little effect on healthy tissue[9]
2) Shortening of the action potential duration and, to a lesser extent, the effective refractory period as shown in Figure 17.1. Lidocaine binds to the sodium channel whilst it is in the inactivated state, and, as the channel recovers from inactivation, the lidocaine unbinds. However, the sodium channel remains refractory during the time between channel activation and lidocaine unbinding, resulting in a period of post-repolarisation refractoriness.[10]
3) Reducing dispersion of refractoriness by shortening the refractory period
4) Minimal effect on sinus node discharge or AVN conduction at therapeutic doses, and no anticholinergic effect
5) Minimal myocardial depressant effects, and therefore safer for use in patients with structural heart disease in comparison to other anti-arrhythmic drugs.

Lidocaine binding is dependent on extracellular potassium concentration – hypokalaemia promotes recovery of sodium channels from the inactivated state, thereby reducing lidocaine binding and drug efficacy.

Whilst lidocaine is more commonly used for ventricular arrhythmias, there are also rare reports of it being effective in converting acute, vagally mediated atrial fibrillation in dogs[11] and also termination of supraventricular tachycardia in dogs.[12]

Pharmacokinetics

After IV administration, lidocaine is rapidly de-ethylated by liver microsomes and extensively distributed to extravascular tissues. Therefore, repeated doses or a continuous rate infusion is necessary to maintain therapeutic concentrations. Liver disease or reduced liver blood flow decreases drug clearance, thereby increasing the half-life. Lidocaine is not suitable for oral administration due to extensive first-pass effect and the formation of toxic metabolites.

Dose

In dogs, lidocaine is administered as bolus(es) of 2–4 mg/kg IV over 1–3 min that can be repeated up to a cumulative dose of 8 mg/kg.[13] A continuous rate infusion can be used after the initial bolus(es) at a rate of 25–100 μg/kg/min. The onset of anti-arrhythmic effects occurs within minutes and lasts for less than 10–15 min after administration.[14] Cats are more sensitive to the effects of lidocaine, and lower doses should be used in this species: 0.25–2 mg/kg IV slowly in 0.25–0.5 mg/kg bolus(es), followed by a constant rate IV infusion of 0.01–0.04 mg/kg/min.[13]

Adverse Effects

Slow boluses of lidocaine have minimal adverse hemodynamic effects, but high doses may cause vasodilation and reductions in systolic function, and may exacerbate conduction abnormalities. Adverse effects include drowsiness and depression, agitation, muscle twitching, nystagmus and seizures.[15] Transient nausea and vomiting may occur. Cats are more likely to show adverse reactions at lower doses than dogs, and this drug should be used with caution in this species.

Interactions

Cimetidine and propranolol may prolong clearance of lidocaine. In cases also receiving hepatic enzyme inducers (e.g. barbiturates), the dose of lidocaine should be increased.

Mexiletine

Mexiletine is a class Ib anti-arrhythmic that shares electrophysiological characteristics with lidocaine but without an extensive first-pass effect; therefore, it is administered orally for chronic treatment of ventricular arrhythmias. Efficacy has been demonstrated in Boxers[4,16,17] and German Shepherds[18] with ventricular arrhythmias (see chapters 20 and 22). Mexiletine causes minimal depression of systolic function, and, like lidocaine, efficacy is impaired by hypokalaemia. The efficacy of mexiletine may be increased by combination with other anti-arrhythmic drugs, including atenolol[4] or sotalol.[18] Availability of this drug has been limited at times in both the UK and several European countries.

Pharmacokinetics

Mexiletine is well absorbed after oral administration and has good bioavailability. Mexiletine is mainly excreted in the urine and approximately 10% is metabolised in the liver, with a plasma half-life of 3–4 h in the dog.[19]

Dose

Recommended dose in dogs is 4–10 mg/kg PO q8–12h.[13] A maximum dose of 8 mg/kg PO q12h is recommended if used in conjunction with sotalol.[18]

Adverse Effects

Gastrointestinal disturbances (vomiting, diarrhoea and decreased appetite) may be seen with mexiletine and can be minimised by administering medication with food. Less common adverse effects include lethargy, ataxia, tremors, convulsions, nystagmus and disorientation. Rarely, bradycardia, hypotension, jaundice and hypotension have been reported.

Interactions

Several drugs may interfere with absorption and elimination of mexiletine: antacids, aluminium–magnesium, opioids and atropine may delay mexiletine absorption; urinary acidifying agents and acetazolamide may accelerate renal excretion of mexiletine, while alkalinising drugs and cimetidine may reduce it.

Sotalol prolongs the effects of mexiletine, thereby allowing twice-daily administration of both drugs.[20]

Tocainide

Tocainide is another analogue of lidocaine that, similarly to mexiletine, does not suffer extensive first-pass metabolism. The dose in dogs is 15–20 mg/kg PO q8h, and this drug has been used for treatment of ventricular tachyarrhythmias in Dobermans with pre-clinical dilated cardiomyopathy.[21] However, adverse effects including gastrointestinal signs, neurotoxicity and ocular and renal toxicity limit the use of this drug in dogs.[21]

Class IC

This class includes drugs such as flecainide, propafenone and encainide. These drugs markedly reduce phase 0 of the action potential, causing a significant reduction in conduction velocity, especially in the His–Purkinje fibres

Table 17.4 Summary of the ECG changes induced by class IC anti-arrhythmic drugs

	Class IC drugs: Propafenone
Sinus node discharge rate	Decreased
PR interval	Normal or increased
QRS duration	Normal
QT interval	Normal or decreased

(see Figure 17.1 and Table 17.4). At higher doses, propafenone has some mild β-blocking properties, thereby slowing the rate of spontaneous depolarisation within the sinus node and also slowing AVN conduction. Additionally, these drugs may variably prolong action potential duration by delaying inactivation of the slow sodium channel and inhibition of the rapid repolarising channel (I_{Kr}). This depressant effect on conduction velocity combined with prolongation of the action potential duration may contribute to the pro-arrhythmic tendencies of these drugs, and these effects would be enhanced by high heart rates and/or structural heart disease. These drugs have been shown to increase mortality in people with underlying structural heart disease[22] but are used in human patients for treatment of supraventricular tachyarrhythmias, including paroxysmal atrial fibrillation and Wolff–Parkinson–White syndrome.[7] They are rarely used for treatment of supraventricular tachycardias in dogs, but flecainide has been used for life-threatening ventricular arrhythmias when benefits are likely to outweigh pro-arrhythmia risks.

Class II

β-blockers (or β-adrenergic antagonists) have been used extensively in veterinary medicine for various purposes, including to treat arrhythmias, to alleviate obstructive heart disease (e.g. subaortic stenosis,[23] pulmonic stenosis[24] and hypertrophic obstructive cardiomyopathy)[25,26] and systemic hypertension[27] and to mitigate the cardiac effects of excessive catecholamines[28] or thyrotoxicosis[29,30] (see chapter 23).

The efficacy of β-blockade depends on several factors:

- The type of receptors targeted by a specific drug
- The level of adrenergic stimulation
- The density and sensitivity of β-receptors.

Therefore, the extent of β-blockade does not correlate well with serum levels, and doses need to be tailored to each patient and clinical situation. β-blockers may be sub-classified according to their varying affinity for adrenergic receptors: first-generation drugs have a non-selective β-blocker effect, whilst second-generation drugs are β1 selective. The latter are usually preferred as non-selective β-blockers may exhibit undesirable effects of β2 blockade, including bronchoconstriction, increased vascular resistance or reduced insulin release in hyperglycaemia. Third-generation β-blockers (e.g. carvedilol) have a non-selective effect on both β and α1 receptors, resulting in vasodilation in addition to β-blockade effects.

β-blockers have little or no direct electrophysiological effect and exert their anti-arrhythmic effects indirectly by reducing the cardiac effects of adrenergic stimulation, as described in chapter 2 (see Figure 2.6). Briefly, these drugs inhibit the pacemaker current (I_f) and the inward Ca current (I_{Ca-L}).

The adverse effects of β-blockade are related to excessive attenuation of sympathetic tone in cases with cardiovascular disease. Although β-blockers may have beneficial anti-arrhythmic effects, myocardial function may depend on adrenergic stimulation, and catastrophic consequences may occur in patients with unstable cardiovascular function if these drugs are used inappropriately.

β-receptors vary in density and sensitivity in different clinical situations – β-receptors may be 'down-regulated' in chronic heart failure (receptor density and sensitivity decrease) and 'up-regulated' with chronic β-blockade (receptor density and sensitivity increase). The latter effect is of clinical importance, as catecholamine sensitivity may be caused by sudden withdrawal of β-blockade.[14]

Atenolol

Atenolol is the most commonly used β-blocker in dogs and cats. The anti-arrhythmic effects of atenolol result from cardioselective β1 adrenergic receptor blockade. Atenolol administration results in a reduction in heart rate, delayed AVN conduction and a prolonged refractory period in myocardial cells – see Table 17.5.

Indications for the use of atenolol include supraventricular and ventricular arrhythmias, but its efficacy is often low when used alone. However, atenolol combined with mexiletine has been shown to be effective for the treatment of ventricular arrhythmias in Boxers.[4] In the treatment of atrial fibrillation, monotherapy with atenolol

Table 17.5 Summary of the ECG changes induced by class II anti-arrhythmic drugs

	Class II drugs
Sinus node discharge rate	Decreased
PR interval	Normal or increased
QRS duration	Normal
QT interval	Normal

may not provide adequate ventricular rate control, but, when used in conjunction with other drugs such as digoxin, it may be more efficacious.[31]

Atenolol is more commonly used as a sole agent in cats to treat arrhythmias associated with thyrotoxicosis[29] or secondary to structural heart disease (e.g. hypertrophic obstructive cardiomyopathy).

Pharmacokinetics

Atenolol is water soluble and has high bioavailability in both cats and dogs. It is eliminated unchanged in the urine, and renal impairment may delay clearance of this drug. It has a longer half-life in dogs (5–6 h) than cats (3.5 h).

Dose

Recommended doses in dogs vary between 0.25 and 1 mg/kg PO q12h, and in cats between 6.25 and 12.5 mg/cat PO q12–24h, starting at a low dose and titrating to effect.

Atenolol syrup allows accurate dose titration in small patients.

Adverse Effects

Adverse effects of atenolol include bradycardia, myocardial depression, AV block, hypotension and syncope. Respiratory (bronchoconstriction) and central nervous system adverse effects are less likely than with propranolol due to $β_1$ selectivity and because atenolol does not readily cross the blood–brain barrier due to low lipophilicity.

Interactions

- Do not administer with α-adrenergic agonists (e.g. dexmedetomidine).
- Hypotensive effect is enhanced by anaesthetic agents, phenothiazines, anti-hypertensive drugs, diuretics and diazepam.
- Combination with calcium channel antagonists is generally contraindicated due to risk of bradycardia, hypotension, heart failure and AV block.
- Metabolism of atenolol is increased by:
  - Thyroid hormones, and therefore dose adjustment may be required in hyperthyroid cats on medication to reduce circulating total thyroxine.
  - Drugs that enhance hepatic metabolism (e.g. barbituates).
- Atenolol may block the bronchodilatory effect of theophylline.
- Atenolol may enhance the hypoglycaemic effect of insulin.

Propranolol

Propranolol is the prototype β-adrenergic receptor blocker. It is a non-selective, competitive blocker of $β_1$ and $β_2$ adrenergic receptors that causes reduction of the heart rate, slows AVN conduction and increases the AVN refractory period – see Table 17.5. Propranolol may be indicated for the treatment of supraventricular and ventricular arrhythmias in dogs and cats, for termination of supraventricular arrhythmias dependent on the AVN and for rate control in atrial fibrillation. In recent years, propranolol has been used less frequently as selective β-blockers (e.g. atenolol) have gained popularity.

Pharmacokinetics

Propranolol is lipophilic, suffers an extensive first-pass effect resulting in low oral bioavailability and has a shorter half-life then atenolol (1.5–2 h). Oral bioavailability is increased with high doses, resulting in saturation of hepatic enzymes, and its half-life is increased by reduced hepatic blood flow, for example in cases with right-sided heart failure.

Dose

In the emergency treatment of catecholamine-induced arrhythmias (e.g. phaechromocytoma), doses of 0.02–0.08 mg/kg IV are reported in dogs, with lower doses advised for patients in heart failure. This would be followed by 0.2–0.8 mg/kg PO q8–12h. Doses for IV administration are about 1/10 of the oral doses due to the first-pass effect with oral dosing.

In cats, a lower IV dose of 0.02–0.06 mg/kg IV slowly to effect is recommended.

Recommended oral doses of propranolol start from 0.1–0.5 mg/kg PO q8h in dogs and 2.5 mg/cat PO q 8–12h in cats, with titration to effect up to 1.5 mg/kg PO q8h in dogs and 10 mg PO q8h in cats. Propranolol has been used at doses of 0.1–0.5 mg/kg PO q8h for treatment of atrial fibrillation. Higher doses up to 2 mg/kg PO q8h have been suggested for the treatment of supraventricular or ventricular arrhythmias, but more efficacious drugs are available for the treatment of these arrhythmias.

Adverse Effects

Propranolol has little negative inotropic effect at lower doses, but care is needed at higher doses and especially if administered intravenously. Depression of myocardial function may cause deterioration of the cardiovascular function and have potential serious consequences in patients with congestive heart failure. Non-cardiac adverse reactions are uncommon and mainly related to $β_2$ blockade, and therefore include vasoconstriction, bronchoconstriction and inhibition of insulin release.

Similar to other β-blockers, propranolol may exacerbate AV block and reduce the rate of subsidiary pacemakers; therefore, it is contraindicated in cases of AV block and sinus node dysfunction.

Hypotensive effects are enhanced by drugs that depress myocardial activity, including anaesthetic agents, phenothiazines, anti-hypertensive drugs, diuretics and diazepam.

Interactions

- Oral aluminium hydroxide preparations reduce propranolol absorption.
- Cimetidine may decrease the metabolism of propranolol.
- Hepatic enzyme induction by phenobarbital or phenytoin may increase the metabolism of propranolol.
- Propanolol reduces lidocaine clearance, so it increases the risk of lidocaine toxicity.
- In diabetic patients, insulin requirement may be lowered as propranolol may enhance the hypoglycaemic effects of insulin.

Esmolol

Esmolol is a β1-selective blocker with ultra-short action due to rapid metabolism by red blood cell esterases.[32] A steady state is achieved within 5–30 min, depending on if a loading dose is used, and its effects disappear within 20 min post infusion.

Similar to other β-blockers, esmolol decreases the heart rate, depresses AV nodal conduction and decreases myocardial oxygen demand.

Esmolol is indicated for acute treatment of supraventricular tachycardia in cats and dogs and to reduce high ventricular rates in atrial fibrillation. It may also be used to treat ventricular arrhythmias, but other drugs (such as class I or class III) are usually better choices in dogs. The short duration of action can be useful to assess the likely effectiveness of using β-blockers.

Dose

Esmolol is administered to dogs as a continuous rate infusion of 25–200 µg/kg/min starting with low doses and titrating to effect.[13] A loading bolus of 0.05–0.5 mg/kg IV over 5 min can be used to achieve a steady state more quickly in dogs.[13]

Adverse Effects

This drug may cause myocardial depression, depending on the dose and loading bolus, and high doses should be avoided in patients with significant myocardial or valvular dysfunction. Adverse effects include bradycardia, AV block, hypotension, syncope, hypoglycaemia, bronchospasm and diarrhoea. Depression and lethargy are thought to be secondary to esmolol's lipophilicity, allowing central nervous system penetration. Esmolol can reduce glomerular filtration and therefore exacerbate pre-existing renal dysfunction.

Interactions

The hypotensive effects of esmolol are enhanced by agents that depress myocardial function, including anaesthetics, phenothiazines, antihypertensives, diuretics and diazepam. Use with calcium channels blockers is discouraged due to risk of bradycardia, hypotension and severe AV block which may be fatal. Concurrent use of digoxin increases the likelihood of bradycardia, especially as esmolol increases serum digoxin levels by up to 20%. Concurrent use of morphine and esmolol increases serum esmolol concentration by up to 50%. The bronchodilatory effect of theophylline is blocked by esmolol.

Metoprolol

Metoprolol is a β1-selective β-blocker. It has been anecdotally reported as effective in some types of automatic atrial tachycardia. It has also been used in arrhythmias induced by chocolate toxicity (see chapter 23), as it does not reduce renal excretion of methylxanthines.[33]

Class III

Class III drugs lengthen the action potential duration by inhibiting repolarising potassium current (I_K), thereby delaying repolarisation and prolonging the refractory period – reflected in the resting electrocardiogram (ECG) as lengthening of the QT interval (see Table 17.6). However, the most commonly used drugs belonging to this family – sotalol and amiodarone – are not pure class III drugs and possess additional electrophysiological properties belonging to other anti-arrhythmic drug classes. The use of these drugs in veterinary patients has increased significantly in recent years.

Sotalol

Sotalol is a class III anti-arrhythmic drug with additional non-selective β-blocker effects. It prolongs the action potential by increasing the atrial, AV, nodal, accessory pathway and ventricular refractoriness and ventricular repolarisation.[34] At low doses, β-blockade predominates, and significant class III effects are achieved only at higher doses.[35] Sotalol shows *reverse-use dependence*, which is a less desirable property – at higher heart rates, the prolongation of the action potential is diminished, causing a reduction in anti-arrhythmic effects.

Table 17.6 Summary of the ECG changes induced by common class III anti-arrhythmic drugs

	Amiodarone	Sotalol
Sinus node discharge rate	Decreased	Decreased
PR interval	Normal	Normal or increased
QRS duration	Normal	Increased
QT interval	Increased	Increased

Sotalol is used in dogs to treat supraventricular and ventricular arrhythmias, and to provide rate control in atrial fibrillation and atrial flutter. It is widely accepted as the first-line drug to treat ventricular arrhythmias in Boxers, as the ability of this drug to reduce ventricular arrhythmias has been demonstrated when administered alone[4,16] or in combination with mexiletine.[17] This drug is also effective in German Shepherd dogs with inherited ventricular arrhythmias in combination with mexiletine.[18] The combination of sotalol and mexiletine reduced the frequency of ventricular ectopy in German Shepherds with inherited arrhythmias, although neither drug used alone was effective, and dogs receiving only sotalol actually showed an increase in the number of runs of ventricular tachycardia.[18]

The combination of sotalol and mexiletine is particularly interesting, as the latter attenuates action potential prolongation by sotalol and reduces the frequency of early afterdepolarisations; therefore, concurrent use of mexiletine and sotalol results in a marked reduction in spontaneous and triggered activity. Sotalol also increases mexiletine concentrations.[18]

Pharmacokinetics

The commercially available sotalol is a racemic mixture of *d*- and *l*-sotalol. The *d*-enantiomer has almost exclusive class III properties, whereas the *l* enantiomer combines class III and non-selective β-blocker (class II) properties. The combination of these two enantiomers likely contributes to the safety and efficacy of this drug, as *d*-sotalol, which has pure class III properties, increased the mortality in human patients recovering from myocardial infarction.[36]

Following oral administration, sotalol is rapidly and almost completely absorbed and has high bioavailability.[37,38] Protein binding is minimal, and the drug is almost completely (up to 90%) eliminated unchanged in the urine;[38] hence, its clearance is reduced in patients with impaired renal function. Peak effect occurs 2–4 h after oral administration.

Dose

Doses range from 1.5 to 3.5 mg/kg PO q12h[4] in dogs, and doses of 2 mg/kg PO q12h or 10–20 mg PO q12h have been used in cats. Another source reports 0.5–3 mg/kg PO q12h in dogs.[13] It is advisable to start with lower doses in case of myocardial dysfunction.

Adverse Effects

Some of the adverse effects of sotalol are related to QT prolongation and its pro-arrhythmic potential. *Torsades de pointes* may occur in the presence of hypokalaemia or bradycardia, or in genetically predisposed people. However, although this pro-arrhymic effect of sotalol has been reported in canine models of torsades de pointes, it has not been documented in clinical cases with naturally occurring disease.[39,40] Negative inotropy and chronotropy are adverse effects related to the β-blockade, and therefore this drug should be used with caution in patients with severe systolic dysfunction or a concurrent bradyarrhythmia. The effects of sotalol on myocardial function appear to be less marked than those of propranolol. The negative inotropic effect is thought to be partially offset by prolongation of the action potential caused by the class III effect. Other possible adverse reactions include hypotension, bradycardia, lethargy, nausea and vomiting.[14] Incidences of aggressive behaviour have also been anecdotally reported.

Interactions

- Concurrent administration of sympathomimetics (e.g. terbutaline and phenylpropanolamine) reduces the efficacy of both drugs.
- The myocardial depressant effect of drugs such as anaesthetics is enhanced by concurrent sotalol administration.
- The hypotensive effects of drugs such as hydralazine or phenothiazine are enhanced by concurrent sotalol administration.
- Sotalol may prolong the hypoglycaemic effects of insulin therapy.

Amiodarone

Amiodarone is often referred to as a *wide-spectrum anti-arrhythmic*. This drug has unique properties combining effects of all four classes of anti-arrhythmic drugs, and it can be used to treat a wide range of arrhythmias. It is classified as a class III but additionally is a strong Na^+ blocker (class I) with ancillary calcium blocker (Class IV) and also α_1 and β-adrenergic receptor blocker (Class II) properties. The electrophysiological effects of amiodarone are prolongation of the action potential and effective refractory period in both atrial and ventricular tissues, thereby reducing repolarisation heterogeneity, and also slowing of AVN and accessory pathway conduction. Amiodarone exhibits use dependence and therefore is more efficacious at higher heart rates.[41]

Amiodarone is indicated for the treatment of supraventricular and ventricular arrhythmias, and it has the unusual advantage of causing minimal depression of myocardial contractility. Amiodarone has been used for ventricular rate control in atrial fibrillation and also for conversion of atrial fibrillation back to sinus rhythm.[42] The slowing of conduction velocity in accessory pathway tissue means that amiodarone may be efficacious in the treatment of AV re-entrant tachycardias.

IV amiodarone can be used for acute treatment of ventricular or supraventricular tachyarrhythmias, including acute atrial fibrillation in dogs.[43] Adverse reactions, including pruritus, erythema, subcutaneous oedema, urticaria, agitation, tachypnoea and hypotension, are frequent in formulations containing the co-solvents benzyl alcohol and polysorbate 80,[44,45] but a formulation free of these solvents is now available.[46]

Pharmacokinetics

Amiodarone has complex pharmacokinetics. It is highly lipid soluble, the intestinal absorption is slow and incomplete (30–50%) and there is slow and extensive distribution into myocardium adipose tissue, lungs and liver. The concentration of the active metabolite N-desethylamiodarone also increases with chronic administration, further contributing to amiodarone's complex pharmacokinetics. Steady serum and tissue concentrations are reached after several weeks. Amiodarone elimination also decreases with chronic administration; its plasma half-life after a single dose is 7.5 h but increases to 3.2 days after repeated administrations.[47] The therapeutic range in dogs is not well defined but may be between 0.5 and 2 mg/ml.[48] It is rapidly eliminated from plasma after discontinuation,[47] but accumulation in peripheral stores (e.g. myocardium and adipose) results in very slow elimination that can last for weeks. This may be inconvenient or problematic if treatment interruption is required.

Dose

In dogs, amiodarone is often started with an oral loading dose of 8–10 mg/kg PO q12h for one week, followed by 5–10 mg/kg PO q24h.[49] A dose of 5–7.5 mg/kg PO q24h without a loading dose has also been reported in dogs.[48] Another source reports an oral loading dose for dogs of 10–15 mg/kg PO q12h, followed by 7.5 mg/kg PO q12h for 14 days and then 5–7.5 mg PO q24h.[13]

An aqueous solution of amiodarone can be used intravenously with dogs at a dose of 2 mg/kg. It is administered as a bolus over 10 min, followed by a continuous rate infusion at 0.8 mg/kg/h for 6 h, and then reduced to 0.4 mg/kg/h.[46]

Adverse Effects

The major limitation of this drug is its potential toxicity. In dogs, hepatopathy (with symptomatic or asymptomatic increased hepatic enzyme activity) and thyroid dysfunction are the main concerns, but gastrointestinal disorders, neutropenia and anaemia may also occur.[51] According to one report, adverse reactions were common in Doberman Pinschers, consisting mainly of dose-related and reversible hepatic toxicity.[52] However, another study including dogs of different breeds reported that adverse reactions were infrequent.[48] In light of potential hepatotoxicity, blood should be taken to assess hepatic parameters and bile acids regularly during treatment – for example, prior to starting therapy, after 1 and

3 months of treatment and then every 3 months or sooner if there is clinical concern.

Amiodarone may also cause thyroid dysfunction, and multiple mechanisms for this adverse effect have been proposed:

- Amiodarone and/or N-desethylamiodarone may inhibit peripheral conversion from thyroxine (T4) to triiodothyronine (T3).
- Inhibition of cellular uptake of T4 and T3
- Inhibition of T3 binding to nuclear receptors.

The second and third mechanisms are considered more important than the first. However, despite the reduction in T4 levels seen in dogs receiving amiodarone, clinical hypothyroidism is uncommon.

Interactions
- Amiodarone may increase serum levels of anti-coagulants, β-blockers, calcium channel blockers, ciclosporin, digoxin, lidocaine, methotrexate, quinidine and theophylline.
- Cimetidine increases serum levels of amiodarone.

Dronedarone

Dronedarone is a non-ionidated analogue of amiodarone developed for the treatment of atrial fibrillation and atrial flutter in human patients. Like amiodarone, drone-darone acts as a blocker of potassium, calcium and sodium channels and has anti-adrenergic effects.[53] At present, limited data are available in veterinary medicine regarding this drug – one study in healthy dogs showed that dronedarone at a dose of 20 mg/kg PO q12h produced negative dromotropy with minimal effect on cardiac function,[54] and IV administration is capable of producing negative dromotropy, inotropy and lusitropy in anesthetised dogs.[55,56]

Other Class III Drugs

Bretylium, ibutilide and dofetilide are other class III drugs but are rarely used in veterinary medicine. Bretylium is potentially indicated in life-threatening ventricular arrhythmias if other drugs fail or if there is risk of ventricular fibrillation. Ibutilide and dofetilide are purer class III agents used in people for conversion of atrial flutter and atrial fibrillation, but little is known about their efficacy and safety in veterinary patients.

Class IV

Calcium channel blockers reduce calcium ion influx across cell membranes in different tissues. The anti-arrhythmic and vascular effects of these compounds are related to blockade of slow L-type channels. These channels are involved in excitation–contraction coupling in cardiac tissue and in vascular smooth muscle contraction.

Table 17.7 Summary of the ECG changes induced by diltiazem

	Diltiazem
Sinus node discharge rate	Decreased
PR interval	Normal or increased
QRS duration	Normal
QT interval	Normal

Calcium channel blockers are sub-classified as follows:

1) *Dihydropyridines* (e.g. amlodipine, nifedipine) have predominantly vascular effects and no significant electrophysiological effect.
2) *Non-dihydropyidines* (e.g. verapamil and diltiazem) have anti-arrhythmic and vascular effects. They are particularly useful in cases with arrhythmias involving tissues dependent on inward calcium current (e.g. the sinus node and the AVN).

Diltiazem and verapamil are the most commonly used calcium channel blockers in veterinary medicine. They reduce the rate of depolarisation of the pacemaker cells on the sinus node and, more importantly, reduce conduction velocity in the sinus node and AVN – see Table 17.7. These drugs also produce some degree of vasodilation, although to a much lesser extent than dihydropyridines. This effect may be responsible for the lack of reduction of heart rate seen with these drugs, and in some situations it may even cause an increase in heart rate (verapamil) due to reflex autonomic response.[57] The effects on the AV node are of clinical interest in supraventricular arrhythmias because AV node–dependent re-entrant arrhythmias may be interrupted or AV conduction slowed, resulting in a lower ventricular rate.

Calcium channel blockers reduce contractility and should be used with caution in patients with myocardial dysfunction. These drugs are also contraindicated in patients with conduction disturbances (AV block), bradycardia or other types of sinus dysfunction (sick sinus syndrome). Adverse effects include bradycardia, hypotension, lethargy and anorexia.

Diltiazem

Diltiazem is a benzothiazepine-type calcium channel blocker that slows AV conduction. It also causes mild peripheral and coronary vasodilation.[58]

Diltiazem is commonly used to terminate or reduce the ventricular response rate to supraventricular arrhythmias. For many veterinary cardiologists, diltiazem is the drug of choice for rate control in atrial fibrillation either alone or in combination with digoxin. The combination of diltiazem and digoxin has been shown to be more effective than either drug alone in the management of atrial fibrillation.[59]

Pharmacokinetics

Diltiazem achieves its peak effect within 2 h of oral administration, and it has a duration of action of at least 6 h.[58] Diltiazem is metabolised in the liver with production of active metabolites[58] that prolong its effects, and enterohepatic circulation accounts for a second peak in plasma concentration 3–4 h after dosing.[60]

Modified-release formulations are often used in dogs to reduce frequency of administration. These formulations show highly variable pharmacokinetics in cats[61] that may result in inefficiency or adverse effects; therefore, more frequent administration of a short-acting formulation is recommended in this species.

Dose

Acute treatment of supraventricular tachyarrhythmias: IV administration in doses of 0.05–0.25 mg/kg over 1–5 min and repeated in 5 min intervals if required. The dose can be increased with caution up to a total dose of 0.75 mg/kg.[14,62,63] Doses recommended for cats are 0.125–0.35 mg/kg in a slow IV bolus.[64] A different source reports a lower dose of 0.05–0.25 mg/kg IV over 1–2 min.[13] Bolus administration can be followed by a continuous rate infusion at 2–6 µg/kg/min in both species.

Chronic treatment of supraventricular tachyarrhythmias: in dogs, 1–4 mg/kg PO q8h with regular tablets or 3–5 mg/kg PO q12h if modified-release tablets are used.[49,59,62] Higher doses should be avoided in patients with systolic dysfunction. Doses of 1–2.5 mg/kg PO q8h are recommended for cats.[63,64]

Adverse Effects

Adverse effects of diltiazem include nausea, anorexia, vomiting, diarrhoea, bradycardia or conduction disturbances (AV block). Diltiazem has limited negative inotropic effect, but caution is advised in patients with heart failure. Diltiazem is contraindicated in patients with bradycardia, conduction disturbances or sick sinus syndrome.

Interactions

- Concurrent administration of diltiazem and β-adrenergic blockers can result in marked negative inotropic and chronotropic effects; therefore, it is not recommended.
- Calcium salts and vitamin D administration may reduce effectiveness of diltiazem.
- Cimetidine inhibits metabolism of diltiazem.

- Diltiazem administration has a variable effect on digoxin levels.
- Diltiazem enhances the effect of theophylline.
- Diltiazem may displace highly protein-bound agents from plasma proteins.
- Diltiazem may increase intracellular vincristine concentrations.

Verapamil

Verapamil, a phenylalkylamine, is the prototype calcium channel blocker. Similarly to diltiazem, it has the potential to reduce sinus rate, and it slows AVN conduction and prolongs AVN refractoriness. Due to its effects on the AVN, verapamil is mainly used intravenously for acute treatment of supraventricular arrhythmias to terminate re-entrant arrhythmias or to slow the ventricular response rate.

Pharmacokinetics

Despite good absorption after oral administration, verapamil has low bioavailability due to extensive first-pass effect. Half-life after IV administration varies between 1.7 and 3.7 h.[58]

Dose

In dogs, IV doses range from 0.05 to 0.15 mg/kg, administered as bolus(es) of 0.05 mg/kg slowly over 10–30 min with ECG monitoring. Administration can be repeated up to four times at 5–10 min intervals at a reduced dose of 0.025 mg/kg IV q5 min.[13,65] CRI at 2–10 µg/kg/min can be used for continued effect in dogs. Recommended oral dose in the dog is 0.5–1.0 mg/kg PO q8h[58] or up to 3.0 mg/kg PO q8h, according to another source.[13]

In cats, a dose of 0.025 mg/kg may be given by slow IV injection over 5 min and can be repeated q5 min up to eight times.

Adverse Effects

Adverse effects of verapamil and precautions during its use are similar to those of diltiazem. Hypotension, bradycardia and AV block can occur, and careful monitoring during administration is vital. Profound cardiovascular depression may result with co-administration of verapamil with β-blockers or lidocaine.[66] Verapamil also increases digoxin concentration.

Interactions

- Broadly similar to diltiazem
- Not recommended to combine with β-blockers, due to potential for negative chronotropic and inotropic effects
- Co-administration with sodium channel blockers may result in cardiovascular depression and hypotension.

- Calcium salts and vitamin D administration may reduce effectiveness of verapamil.
- Cimetidine inhibits metabolism of verapamil.
- Verapamil administration may increase serum digoxin concentrations.
- Verapamil enhances the effect of theophylline.
- Verapamil may increase intracellular vincristine concentrations.

Other Anti-arrhythmic Agents

Cardiac Glycosides: Digoxin

Currently, digitalis glycoside use in veterinary medicine is almost exclusively reserved for rate control in atrial fibrillation. It has been used historically to treat other supraventricular arrhythmias and as an inotropic agent. The inotropic effects of digoxin result from Na^+/K^+ ATPase pump inhibition, leading to increased intracellular sodium concentrations. Sodium exchanges with extracellular calcium via the Ca^{2+}/Na^+ exchanger lead to a higher intracellular calcium concentration. The increase in intracellular calcium concentration exerts a mild positive inotropic effect. However, increased intracellular calcium concentration also has potential pro-arrhythmic effects.

The main anti-arrhythmic effects of digoxin are mediated by sympathetic inhibition and parasympathomimetic effects. These effects result in:

- A reduction in heart rate
- A decrease in AV node conduction velocity
- Prolongation of AV node refractoriness
- Depression of atrial automaticity.[67]

Digoxin is more effective in reducing the ventricular rate in atrial fibrillation when combined with diltiazem[59] or β-blockers.

Dose
Recommended digoxin dose for dogs is 2.5–3 μg/kg PO q12h. For patients weighing more than 20 kg, the dose can be calculated using the body surface area at 0.22 mg/m^2. A maximum dose of 0.25 mg/dog should not be exceeded. Digoxin is rarely used in cats, but when used a dose of 1/8 to a 1/4 of a 0.125 mg tablet PO q48h is given with careful monitoring for signs of toxicity. The alcohol-based elixir is usually poorly tolerated by feline patients.[64]

Adverse Effects
Digitalis toxicity may result in neurologic, gastrointestinal or cardiac signs. A narrow therapeutic-toxic window and poor correlation between dose and serum concentration may facilitate digoxin toxicity, and therefore serum concentration monitoring is strongly recommended. Trough serum concentration is measured at least 6–8 h after the last administration and more than 6 days after the beginning of treatment. Serum concentrations of 0.8–1.2 ng/mL are currently recommended.[68] Dosing should be primarily based on the clinical response, with lower doses being preferred as long as a desired clinical effect is achieved (e.g. an adequate decrease in ventricular rate in atrial fibrillation), and the recommended therapeutic range should not be exceeded to prevent toxicity. Gastrointestinal signs such as diarrhoea, vomiting and anorexia may be the first signs of toxicity. Cardiac toxicity may manifest as conduction disorders leading to AV block, bundle branch block and atrial or ventricular re-entrant arrhythmias. Triggered arrhythmias (delayed afterdepolarisations – see chapter 6) may occur due to increased intracellular calcium concentration.

Interactions
- Reduced digoxin absorption from the gastrointestinal tract is seen if there is concurrent administration of antacids, chemotherapy agents (e.g. cyclophosphamide, cytarabine, doxorubicin and vincristine) and cimetidine.
- Increased serum levels and reduced elimination are seen with concurrent administration of amiodarone, antimuscarinics, diazepam, erythromycin, loop and thiazide diuretics, oxytetracycline, quinidine and verapamil.
- Spironolactone has a variable effect on digoxin levels.

Adenosine

Adenosine is an endogenous nucleoside used in human patients to terminate supraventricular arrhythmias. It acts by slowing AVN conduction, restoring sinus rhythm in arrhythmias that depend on the AVN. Adenosine requires rapid IV administration,[14] ideally using a central vein, and it appears to be ineffective in dogs, even at higher doses than those used in people.[69] Esmolol, diltiazem or verapamil are preferred in dogs for this purpose.

Omega-3 Fatty Acids

The use of omega-3 fatty acids has been advocated as adjuvant therapy for prevention and treatment of ventricular arrhythmias. One study in Boxer dogs with arrhythmogenic cardiomyopathy showed reduction of the number of ventricular premature complexes (VPCs) with a combination of eicosapentaenoic acid (EPA) and docosahexaenoic acid (DHA), suggesting a beneficial effect in this breed,[70] but, as yet, there are no veterinary studies strongly supporting the efficacy of omega-3 fatty acids as anti-arrhythmics.

Magnesium

Magnesium is necessary for normal Na^+/K^+ ATPase pump function and also for normal potassium channel function. Magnesium may act as a physiological calcium channel blocker, and IV administration may result in slowing of heart rate and in minimal PR interval prolongation. Hypomagnesaemia has been reported as a risk factor for ventricular arrhythmias due to shortening of action potential amplitude and duration, and also decreased resting membrane potential, thereby predisposing to spontaneous automaticity. If hypomagnesaemia is documented, then administration of magnesium chloride (0.3 mEq/kg) over 10 min should be followed by a constant rate infusion of 0.2 mEq/kg/h to maintain serum magnesium concentrations of 1.5–2.4 mEq/L.

Treatment of Bradyarrhythmias

Anticholinergic drugs such as atropine are used in diagnosis and treatment of bradyarrhythmias, as described in chapter 7. Propantheline is a member of this group, and the dose for dogs is 0.2–0.5 mg/kg PO q8–12h. Vagolytic drugs can cause adverse effects, including mydriasis, constipation, dry mouth and keratoconjunctivitis sicca.

Sympathomimetic drugs may also be useful in the treatment of bradyarrhythmias. Isoproterenol has been reported for treatment of severe bradyarrhythmias in dogs anaesthetised for pacemaker implantation. Isoproterenol is a non-selective pure β-agonist drug which increases the rate of discharge of the sinus node and also subsidiary pacemakers. A dose of 0.05–0.2 μg/kg/min is recommended in dogs, but, due to the risk of tachyarrhythmias, the dose should be titrated and the lowest effective dose used.

β2-agonist drugs have been used in the treatment of bradyarrhythmias. Terbutaline may be effective in the treatment of vagally mediated sinus bradycardia. The dose in dogs is 1.25–5 mg/dog PO q8–12h; if administered parenterally, a dose of 0.01 mg/kg is given intramuscularly, intravenously or subcutaneously q4h. The dose in cats is 0.312–1.25 mg/cat PO q8–12h, or 0.01 mg/kg is given intramuscularly, intravenously or subcutaneously q4h. Adverse effects include restlessness, panting, gastrointestinal upsets and fine tremor.

Theophylline is a methyl xanthine derivative that causes inhibition of phosphodiesterase and prostaglandin production, regulates calcium flux and intracellular calcium distribution and antagonises adenosine. Theophylline has a modest positive chronotrophic and inotropic effect on cardiac tissue. The dose in dogs is 20 mg/kg PO q24h. Adverse effects include restlessness, panting, nausea, vomiting, diarrhoea, polydipsia, polyuria, twitching and convulsions.

References

1 Ruskin JN. The cardiac arrhythmia suppression trial (CAST). N Engl J Med. 1989;321:386–388.

2 Rosen MR, Schwartz PJ. The 'Sicilian Gambit': a new approach to the classification of antiarrhythmic drugs based on their actions on arrhythmogenic mechanisms. Euro Heart J. 1991;12:1112–1131.

3 Pyle RL. Conversion of atrial fibrillation with quinidine sulfate in a dog. J Am Vet Med Assoc. 1967;151:582–589.

4 Meurs KM, Spier AW, Wright NA, Atkins CE, DeFrancesco TC, Gordon SG, et al. Comparison of the effects of four antiarrhythmic treatments for familial ventricular arrhythmias in Boxers. J Am Vet Med Assoc. 2002;221:522–527.

5 Atkins CE, Kanter R, Wright K, Saba Z, Baty C, Swanson C, et al. Orthodromic reciprocating tachycardia and heart failure in a dog with a concealed posteroseptal accessory pathway. J Vet Intern Med. 1995;9:43–49.

6 Allen JD, Brennan FJ, Wit AL. Actions of lidocaine on transmembrane potentials of subendocardial Purkinje fibers surviving in infarcted canine hearts. Circ Res. 1978;43:470–481.

7 Nattel S, Gersh BJ, Opie LH. In Drugs for the heart (eds. Opie LH, Gersh BJ, pp. 272–331). Amsterdam: Elsevier; 2013.

8 Gorgels AP, van den Dool A, Hofs A, Mulleneers R, Smeets JL, Vos MA, et al. Comparison of procainamide and lidocaine in terminating sustained monomorphic ventricular tachycardia. Am J Cardiol. 1996;78:43–46.

9 Armstrong EJ, Armstrong AW, Clapham DE. In Principles of pharmacology: the pathophysiologic basis of drug therapy (eds. Golan DE, Tashjian AH, p. 412). Philadelphia: Wolters Kluwer Health/Lippincott Williams & Wilkins; 2012.

10 Bigger JTJ, Mandel WJ. Effect of lidocaine on the electrophysiological properties of ventricular muscle and purkinje fibers. J Clin Invest. 1970;49:63–77.

11 Pariaut R, Moïse NS, Koetje BD, Flanders JA, Hemsley SA, Farver TB, et al. Lidocaine converts acute vagally associated atrial fibrillation to sinus rhythm in German Shepherd dogs with inherited arrhythmias. J Vet Intern Med. 2008;22:1274–1282.

12 Johnson MS, Martin M, Smith P. Cardioversion of supraventricular tachycardia using lidocaine in five dogs. J Vet Intern Med. 2006;20:272–276.

13 Ramsey I. BSAVA small animal formulary. London: British Small Animal Veterinary Association; 2014.

14 Moïse NS. In *Textbook of canine and feline cardiology* (eds. Fox PR, Sisson DD, Moise SN, pp. 331–385). Philadelphia: Saunders; 1999.

15 Plumb DC. Plumb's veterinary drug handbook. Hoboken: Wiley Blackwell; 2011.

16 Caro-Vadillo A, Garcia-Guasch L, Carreton E, Montoya-Alonso JA, Manubens J. Arrhythmogenic right ventricular cardiomyopathy in boxer dogs: a retrospective study of survival. Vet Rec. 2013;172:268.

17 Prosek R, Estrada A, Adin D. Comparison of sotalol and mexiletine versus stand alone sotalol in treatment of Boxer dogs with ventricular arrhythmias. J Vet Intern Med. 2006;20(3):748.

18 Gelzer ARM, Kraus MS, Rishniw M, Hemsley SA, Moïse NS. Combination therapy with mexiletine and sotalol suppresses inherited ventricular arrhythmias in German shepherd dogs better than mexiletine or sotalol monotherapy: a randomized cross-over study. J Vet Cardiol. 2010;12:93–106.

19 Miller MW, Adams HR. In Veterinary pharmacology and therapeutics (eds. Riviere JE, Papich MG, pp. 575–602). Hoboken: Wiley-Blackwell; 2009.

20 Scollan KF, Sisson DD. Mexiletine serum levels with twice daily dosing in combination with sotalol in healthy dogs. J Vet Intern Med. 2014;28:711–744.

21 Calvert CA, Pickus CW, Jacobs GJ. Efficacy and toxicity of tocainide for the treatment of ventricular tachyarrhythmias in Doberman pinschers with occult cardiomyopathy. J Vet Intern Med. 1996;10:235–240.

22 Cardiac Arrhythmia Suppression Trial, I. Preliminary report: effect of encainide and flecainide on mortality in a randomized trial of arrhythmia suppression after myocardial infarction. N Engl J Med. 1989;321:406–412.

23 Eason BD, Fine DM, Leeder D, Stauthammer C, Lamb K, Tobias AH. Influence of beta blockers on survival in dogs with severe subaortic stenosis. J Vet Intern Med. 2014;28:857–862.

24 Francis AJ, Johnson MJS, Culshaw GC, Corcoran BM, Martin MWS, French AT. Outcome in 55 dogs with pulmonic stenosis that did not undergo balloon valvuloplasty or surgery. J Small Anim Pract. 2011;52:282–288.

25 Jackson BL, Adin DB, Lehmkuhl LB. Effect of atenolol on heart rate, arrhythmias, blood pressure, and dynamic left ventricular outflow tract obstruction in cats with subclinical hypertrophic cardiomyopathy. J Vet Cardiol. 2015;17(Suppl. 1):S296–S305.

26 Schober KE, Zientek J, Li X, Fuentes VL, Bonagura JD. Effect of treatment with atenolol on 5-year survival in cats with preclinical (asymptomatic) hypertrophic cardiomyopathy. J Vet Cardiol. 2013;15:93–104.

27 Taylor SS, Sparkes AH, Briscoe K, Carter J, Sala SC, Jepson RE, *et al.* ISFM consensus guidelines on the diagnosis and management of hypertension in cats. J Feline Med Surg. 2017;19:288–303.

28 Edmondson EF, Bright JM, Halsey CH, Ehrhart EJ. Pathologic and cardiovascular characterization of pheochromocytoma-associated cardiomyopathy in dogs. Vet Pathol. 2015;52:338–343.

29 Henik RA, Stepien RL, Wenholz LJ, Dolson MK. Efficacy of atenolol as a single antihypertensive agent in hyperthyroid cats. J Feline Med Surg. 2008;10:577–582.

30 Trepanier LA. Medical management of hyperthyroidism. Clin Tech Small Anim Pract. 2006;21:22–28.

31 Jung SW, Sun W, Griffiths LG, Kittleson MD. Atrial fibrillation as a prognostic indicator in medium to large-sized dogs with myxomatous mitral valvular degeneration and congestive heart failure. J Vet Intern Med. 2016;30:51–57.

32 Reynolds RD, Gorczynski RJ, Quon CY. Pharmacology and pharmacokinetics of esmolol. J Clin Pharmacol. 1986;26(Suppl. A):A3–A14.

33 Smith FWK, Schrope DP, Sammarco CD. In Manual of canine and feline cardiology (eds. Smith FWK, Tilley LP, Oyama MA, Sleeper MM, pp. 239–274). Amsterdam: Elsevier: 2016.

34 Fitton A, Sorkin EM. Sotalol: an updated review of its pharmacological properties and therapeutic use in cardiac arrhythmias. Drugs. 1993;46:678–719.

35 Gomoll AW, Lekich RF, Bartek MJ, Comereski CR, Antonaccio MJ. Comparability of the electrophysiologic responses and plasma and myocardial tissue concentrations of sotalol and its d stereoisomer in the dog. J Cardiovasc Pharmacol 1990;16:204–211.

36 Waldo AL, Camm AJ, deRuyter H, Friedman PL, MacNeil DJ, Pauls JF, *et al.* Effect of d-sotalol on mortality in patients with left ventricular dysfunction after recent and remote myocardial infarction. The SWORD Investigators. Survival With Oral d-Sotalol. Lancet. 1996;348:7–12.

37 Funck-Brentano C. Pharmacokinetic and pharmacodynamic profiles of d-sotalol and d,l-sotalol. Eur Heart J. 1993;14(Suppl. H):30–35.

38 Schnelle K, Garrett ER. Pharmacokinetics of the β-adrenergic blocker sotalol in dogs. J Pharm Sci. 1973;62:362–375.

39 Davy JM, Weissenburger J, Ertzbischoff O, Lainee P, Chezalviel F, Poirier JM, *et al.* Sotalol-induced torsades de pointe in the conscious dog with atrioventricular block: role of hypokalemia. Arch Mal Coeur Vaiss. 1988;81:1117–1124.

40 Chezalviel-Guilbert F, Davy JM, Poirier JM, Weissenburger J. Mexiletine antagonizes effects of sotalol on QT interval duration and its proarrhythmic effects in a canine model of torsade de pointes. J Am Coll Cardiol. 1995;26:787–792.

41 Kodama I, Kamiya K, Toyama J. Amiodarone: ionic and cellular mechanisms of action of the most promising class III agent. Am J Cardiol. 1999;84:20R–28R.

42 Saunders AB, Miller MW, Gordon SG, Van De Wiele CM. Oral amiodarone therapy in dogs with atrial fibrillation. J Vet Intern Med. 2006;20:921–926.

43 Oyama MA, Prosek R. Acute conversion of atrial fibrillation in two dogs by intravenous amiodarone administration. J Vet Intern Med. 2006;20:1224–1227.

44 Oyama MA, Prošek R. Acute conversion of atrial fibrillation in two dogs by intravenous amiodarone administration. J Vet Intern Med. 2006;20:1224–1227.

45 Cober RE, Schober KE, Hildebrandt N, Sikorska E, Riesen SC. Adverse effects of intravenous amiodarone in 5 dogs. J Vet Intern Med. 2009;23:657–661.

46 Levy NA, Koenigshof AM, Sanders RA. Retrospective evaluation of intravenous premixed amiodarone use and adverse effects in dogs (17 cases: 2011–2014). J Vet Cardiol. 2016;18:10–14.

47 Brien JF, Jimmo S, Brennan FJ, Armstrong PW, Abdollah H. Disposition of amiodarone and its proximate metabolite, desethylamiodarone, in the dog for oral administration of single-dose and short-term drug regimens. Drug Metab Dispos. 1990;18:846–851.

48 Pedro B, López-Alvarez J, Fonfara S, Stephenson H, Dukes-McEwan J. Retrospective evaluation of the use of amiodarone in dogs with arrhythmias (from 2003 to 2010). J Small Anim Pract. 2012;53:19–26.

49 Plumb DC. Plumb's veterinary drug handbook. Chichester: John Wiley & Sons; 2015.

50 Pedro B, López-Alvarez J, Fonfara S, Stephenson H, Dukes-McEwan J. Retrospective evaluation of the use of amiodarone in dogs with arrhythmias (from 2003 to 2010). J Small Anim Pract. 2012;53:19–26.

51 Bicer S, Nakayama T, Hamlin RL. Effects of chronic oral amiodarone on left ventricular function, ECGs, serum chemistries, and exercise tolerance in healthy dogs. J Vet Intern Med. 2002;16:247–254.

52 Kraus MS, Thomason JD, Fallaw TL, Calvert CA. Toxicity in Doberman Pinchers with ventricular arrhythmias treated with amiodarone (1996–2005). J Vet Intern Med. 2009;23:1–6.

53 Patel C, Yan GX, Kowey PR. Dronedarone. Circulation. 2009;120:636–644.

54 Saengklub N, Youngblood B, Del Rio C, Sawangkoon S, Hamlin RL, Kijtawornrat A. Short-term effects of oral dronedarone administration on cardiac function, blood pressure and electrocardiogram in conscious telemetry dogs. J Vet Med Sci. 2016;78:977–985.

55 Saengklub N, Limprasutr V, Sawangkoon S, Buranakarl C, Hamlin RL, Kijtawornrat A. Acute effects of intravenous dronedarone on electrocardiograms, hemodynamics and cardiac functions in anesthetized dogs. J Vet Med Sci. 2016;78:177–186.

56 Djandjighian L, Planchenault J, Finance O, Pastor G, Gautier P, Nisato D. Hemodynamic and antiadrenergic effects of dronedarone and amiodarone in animals with a healed myocardial infarction. J Cardiovasc Pharmacol. 2000;36:376–383.

57 Millard RW, Grupp G, Grupp IL, DiSalvo J, DePover A, Schwartz A. Chronotropic, inotropic, and vasodilator actions of diltiazem, nifedipine, and verapamil: a comparative study of physiological responses and membrane receptor activity. Circ Res. 1983;52:I29–I39.

58 Cooke KL, Snyder PS. Calcium channel blockers in veterinary medicine. J Vet Intern Med. 1998;12:123–131.

59 Gelzer ARM, Kraus MS, Rishniw M, Moïse NS, Pariaut R, Jesty SA, et al. Combination therapy with digoxin and diltiazem controls ventricular rate in chronic atrial fibrillation in dogs better than digoxin or diltiazem monotherapy: a randomized crossover study in 18 dogs. J Vet Intern Med. 2009;23:499–508.

60 Piepho RW, Bloedow DC, Lacz JP, Runser DJ, Dimmit DC, Browne RK. Pharmacokinetics of diltiazem in selected animal species and human beings. Am J Cardiol. 1982;49:525–528.

61 Wall M, Calvert CA, Sanderson SL, Leonhardt A, Barker C, Fallaw TK. Evaluation of extended-release diltiazem once daily for cats with hypertrophic cardiomyopathy. J Am Anim Hosp Assoc. 2005;41:98–103.

62 Kittleson MD, Kienle RD. Drugs used to treat cardiac arrhythmias. In Small animal cardiovascular medicine (pp. 517–518). St. Louis: Mosby; 1998.

63 Kraus MS, Gelzer ARM. In Manual of canine and feline cardiology (eds. Smith FWK, Tilley LP, Oyama MA, Sleeper MM, pp. 313–329). Amsterdam: Elsevier; 2016.

64 Côté E, Meurs KM, Sleeper MM, MacDonald KA. In Feline cardiology (pp. 439–468). Hoboken: John Wiley & Sons, Inc.; 2011. doi:10.1002/9781118785782.ch30

65 Kittleson M, Keene B, Pion P, Woodfield J. Verapamil administration for acute termination of supraventricular tachycardia in dogs. J Am Vet Med Assoc. 1988;193:1525–1529.

66 Kapur PA, Matarazzo DA, Fung DM, Sullivan KB. The cardiovascular and adrenergic actions of verapamil or diltiazem in combination with propranolol during halothane anesthesia in the dog. Anesthesiology. 1987;66:122–129.

67 Muir WM III, Sams RA, Moise SN. In Textbook of canine and feline cardiology (eds. Fox PR, Sisson D, Moise SN, pp. 307–330). Philadelphia: Saunders; 1999.

68 Trepanier LA. Applying pharmacokinetics to veterinary clinical practice. Vet Clin North Am Small Anim Pract. 2013;43:1013–1026.

69 Wright KN. In Kirk's current veterinary therapy (eds. Bonagura JD, Twedt DC, pp. 722–727). Philadelphia: Elsevier Saunders; 2009.

70 Smith CE, Freeman LM, Rush JE, Cunningham SM, Biourge V. Omega-3 fatty acids in Boxer dogs with arrhythmogenic right ventricular cardiomyopathy. J Vet Intern Med. 2007;21:265–273.

18

Pacemaker Therapy
Simon Swift

Introduction

A pacemaker is a small device composed of a generator and a lead that sits in close contact with the right ventricular endo- and myocardium. It is capable of sensing electrical activity in the myocardium and delivering low-energy electrical impulses to trigger depolarisation when appropriate. Pacemakers have been used for heart rate and rhythm control in dogs since a Basenji was paced in 1967.[1] Pacemakers are used for long-term palliation of the symptoms of bradyarrhythmias in dogs and cats, but also have been used in other species.[2,3] This chapter focuses on the use of pacemakers for the treatment of symptomatic bradyarrhythmias.

Indications

Common arrhythmias that require pacemaker therapy include:

- High-grade second-degree atrioventricular block (2AVB)
- Third-degree atrioventricular block (3AVB)
- Sick sinus syndrome (SSS)
- Persistent atrial standstill
- Neurocardiogenic (vasovagal) syncope.

Patients with occasional 2AVB may not be symptomatic or require treatment. This is especially true with Mobitz type 1 (also known as Wenckebach where there is gradual increasing of the PR interval prior to the blocked P wave), which is usually associated with high vagal tone. These patients may respond to a vagolytic agent such as propantheline. Frequent 2AVB Mobitz type 2 with a fixed P-R interval is more concerning as it suggests conduction system disease. If several consecutive P waves are not conducted, this is termed *high grade* (see chapter 7) and is often associated with clinical signs such as syncope.[4] Some dogs with high-grade 2AVB may progress to complete atrioventricular (AV) block, thereby meriting evaluation for pacemaker placement.[5]

3AVB is usually associated with a slow escape rhythm, with the rate depending on the site of origin. Dogs usually display referable clinical signs such as severe exercise intolerance and episodes of syncope. However, in occasional cases, for example an older dog with concurrent illness (e.g. orthopedic issues resulting in reduced mobility), the bradycardia is an incidental finding. Owners should be warned that patients with 3AVB are at risk of sudden death if the escape rhythm fails.[4] Labradors are one of the most commonly presented breeds, although English Springer Spaniels have a younger age onset.[6–9] These patients rarely respond to an atropine response test (see chapter 7).

West Highland white terriers, Cairn terriers and miniature Schnauzers are the most common breeds seen with SSS.[10] Incidence increases with age, and some dogs live with mild forms of the disease for years without showing referable clinical signs or requiring therapy. Detection of long sinus pauses in a predisposed breed should raise suspicion of SSS, and care should be taken if administration of sedative drugs or opioids is required as this can precipitate an acute crisis due to long pauses requiring emergency pacing. Cocker spaniels have been reported to be predisposed to 2AVB, 3AVB and SSS.[7,11]

Persistent atrial standstill due to myocardial disease is an indication for pacing and is usually seen in young dogs. However, the client should be aware that while this may help the acute problem of bradycardia, the long-term outcome due to the atrial myocardial dysfunction will not change, although there have been reports of dogs living for extended periods following pacemaker implantation.[12,13]

Neurocardiogenic syncope may be associated with bradycardia and/or vasodilation; as a result, patients may be only partially responsive to pacemaker implantation.

Cats that require pacemaker implantation usually have 3AVB. Cats often have a fast escape rhythm (100–140 bpm)

Guide to Canine and Feline Electrocardiography, First Edition. Ruth Willis, Pedro Oliveira and Antonia Mavropoulou.
© 2018 John Wiley & Sons Ltd. Published 2018 by John Wiley & Sons Ltd.
Companion website: www.wiley.com/go/willis/electrocardiography

and so are usually only treated if they are symptomatic.[14] Although sudden death is a concern in untreated cats, there is no evidence that pacemaker implantation prolongs survival.[14]

Assessment of the Patient

A thorough physical examination should be performed to look for any disease that might necessitate further investigation or influence treatment. A resting or ambulatory ECG recording is needed to confirm the arrhythmia. An ambulatory ECG recording is often indicated if the bradycardia is intermittent and cannot be identified on a resting ECG. An echocardiogram is usually required to assess myocardial function, chamber size and myocardial remodelling that may be associated with the bradyarrhythmia. It is uncommon for a cause of AV block to be identified. Routine haematology and biochemistry can help identify any concurrent disease that may preclude pacemaker placement. A troponin level may help indicate cases of myocarditis. In dogs with myocarditis, the AV block may resolve as the myocarditis improves[15] in up to 13% of cases.[5] Further evaluation depends on clinical signs. Urinalysis and culture can be helpful if there is a concern for urinary tract infection, and abdominal ultrasonography and thoracic radiography may be indicated in the older patient to screen for significant comorbidities. However, if the patient is experiencing frequent syncope, intervention should not be unduly delayed.

Conditions that increase the likelihood of an adverse event include infection of any organ, myocarditis, severe cardiac disease, neoplasia, pro-thrombotic disease or any other severe concurrent disease (e.g. renal, liver, central nervous system etc.). Ideally, a disease which may affect long-term outcome (e.g. Chagas disease)[16] or require alternative therapy (e.g. tick-borne diseases)[17] should be addressed first.

Physics of Pacing

The pacemaker consists of a battery or generator and a lead that delivers the current to the heart. The pacemaker delivers a shock directly to the myocardium, causing it to depolarise and hence contract. To maximise battery life, the voltage (V) should be adjusted to the minimum possible to allow depolarisation but with a safety margin to ensure it does occur. Generally, the voltage is set to twice the minimum that will cause depolarisation. In addition, the duration that the current is applied can also be changed. A curve can be drawn of the strength (amplitude) against the duration of the impulse, and this is the strength–duration curve (Figure 18.1).

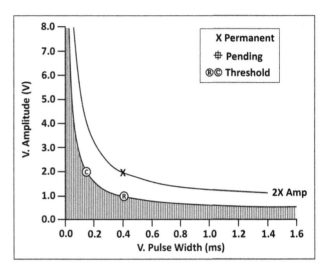

Figure 18.1 Strength duration curve. The strength (pulse amplitude in V) of the impulse is plotted against its duration (pulse width in milliseconds). Values that fall in the shaded area under the curve will fail to capture the myocardium and will not result in depolarisation. The rheobase (®) refers to the lowest voltage that results in consistent capture at infinitely long pulse duration. In other words, it corresponds to the lowest voltage necessary to trigger myocardial depolarisation at the longest pulse duration possible (in clinical practice, 2 ms). The chronaxie (©) is the minimum pulse width able to trigger depolarisation at double the strength of the rheobase (in this example, 0.15 ms). The energy consumed by a pulse at chronaxie is the minimal effective amount. To optimize battery life whilst accounting for a safety margin, the pulse amplitude was set to 2 V × 0.4 ms in this example. Modern pacemaker units use automatic threshold capture management algorithms that adjust these parameters automatically to maximize battery life.

Values on or above the curve will result in capture. It is used to optimise the settings of the pacemaker.

The *rheobase* refers to the lowest voltage that results in capture at infinitely long pulse duration. *Chronaxie* is the pulse width that corresponds to twice the rheobase in the strength–duration curve. It approximates the point of stimulation threshold.

Lead repositioning is recommended if the amplitude required to capture the heart is >0.5 V or the pulse duration exceeds 0.2 ms.

A programmer or interrogator is a computer that interfaces with the pulse generator, allowing the settings to be assessed and changed after implantation. The thresholds for the strength–duration curve can be calculated. Typically, the programmer does this automatically, incrementally decreasing the energy of the pacemaker until capture is lost. The threshold is equal to the last voltage that caused a depolarisation before capture was lost (Figure 18.2). When pacemakers are first implanted, this is usually low at 0.5–0.75 V, but may increase over the first few months due to exit block occurring as a result of fibrosis around the tip of the lead.

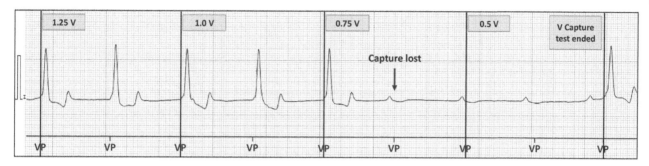

Figure 18.2 Capture test to determine the thresholds for the strength duration curve. The aim of this test is to determine the lowest voltage and pulse width that result in myocardial depolarisation and then to plot the strength duration curve. The voltage test is performed first to determine the rheobase. The paced rate during the test is set to a higher value than the intrinsic rhythm (if present) to avoid interference; in this case, it was set to 90 bpm. This may be challenging in cases with tachyarrhythmias that may effectively render this test impossible to perform. A starting voltage must be chosen, and once the test starts, the programmer automatically decreases the voltage (keeping the pulse width constant), whilst the operator monitors the electrocardiogram for loss of capture (normally, a button must be pressed throughout the test, and the test stops either when the operator stops pressing the button or when the lowest voltage possible is reached). In this case, the starting voltage was 1.75 V, and 0.25 decrements occurred every two beats. Loss of capture occurred on the second beat at 0.75 mV, and therefore 1.0 mV was considered the rheobase. The test may then be repeated to determine the minimum pulse duration that results in myocardial depolarisation at double the voltage at rheobase (chronaxie). [6-year-old, female neutered, Labrador Retriever with 3AVB and a VVIR pacemaker] (50 mm/s, 20 mm/mV)

Impedance

The programmer also calculates the impedance of the pacing system. Impedance is the resistance to current flow and is largely a function of the lead electrode radius, with smaller radii generating higher resistance. Ohm's law dictates that the higher the resistance, the lower the current will be, and therefore the longer the battery life. Impedance is usually in the region of 250–1200 Ohms. If the value falls outside this range, it is suggestive of poor lead positioning and requires redirection of the lead. Very high impedances can also suggest a loose-set screw or lead fracture, and low impedance indicates a failure of conductor insulation. Typically, impedance falls over the first 2 weeks after implantation before rising to about 15% above implantation values.

Sensitivity (or sensing)

The *sensitivity* of the pacemaker refers to the ability of the system to detect deflections on the ECG. The pacemaker uses the cardiac lead as an electrode to monitor the intrinsic activity. It is extremely important that a pacemaker can detect intrinsic complexes and inhibit its function. Inappropriate sensing (under-sensing) could allow depolarisation of the pacemaker on an intrinsic T wave that may precipitate ventricular fibrillation and sudden death (Figure 18.3). Over-sensing could result in the pacemaker detecting T or even P waves and interpreting those as R waves, inhibiting its function (Figure 18.4). The sensing function is similar to a brick wall extending upwards from the baseline of the ECG, and the complexes are visualised above the wall. The wall needs to be high enough that it hides the P and T waves but not so high that it conceals intrinsic R waves. If a dog

has ventricular ectopic beats, then this adds a further complication as they often have a different morphology and polarity from intrinsic complexes, making their R waves smaller. The *refractory period* refers to the period following a paced or intrinsic complex during which the pacemaker can sense signals, but these do not reset the pacing interval. At the start of the refractory period, there is a blanking period during which the pacemaker is blind to signals (see Box 18.1). The length of these can be varied to improve function.

Pacemaker Terminology

Pacemaker systems are described by a five-letter generic code,[19] although only the first four are relevant for the systems commonly used in veterinary medicine, as illustrated in Table 18.1. The first letter indicates which chamber is paced, and the second indicates which chamber is sensed. These may be none (O), the atrium (A), the ventricle (V) or both (dual [D]). The third letter describes how the pacemaker behaves in response to a sensed intrinsic beat. A lack of response (O) means that the system is working in asynchronous mode and that pacing occurs regardless of whether intrinsic beats occur. This mode carries the risk of ventricular fibrillation if a pacing impulse is delivered during the vulnerable period (peak of T wave) of an intrinsic beat. In triggered mode (T), pacing occurs if an intrinsic beat is sensed. This mode is used in dual-chamber systems or systems with atrial sensing (floating atrial electrode) where sensed intrinsic atrial activity triggers ventricular depolarisation (e.g. in cases with 3AVB). Most commonly, the system is set for inhibited mode (I), in which sensed intrinsic cardiac

Box 18.1 Common pacemaker settings in single-chamber systems

Lower rate interval (LRI)
The lowest rate at which the pacemaker is set to pace.
(normally set to 60-80 bpm)

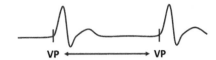

Upper sensor rate interval
Highest paced rate (shortest interval) that is set in response to exercise in rate-responsive mode. In most units the rate of heart rate increase (reaction time) and decrease (recovery time) can also be modified.
(typically set to 130-140 bpm)

Hysteresis
To favour the patient's own intrinsic rhythm a rate that is lower than the LRI may be allowed - Hysteresis rate. For example, if the LRI is set at 60 bpm and the hysteresis rate is set at 50 bpm an intrinsic rhythm will be allowed to fall to 50 bpm even if this is lower than the set LRI. If the rate falls below the hysteresis rate the pacemaker starts pacing at the LRI.
(typically set to 10 bpm less than LRI)

Sleep
Some units allow setting a lower LRI during rest. This may be done by setting a lower LRI during a set time period (e.g. 10pm to 8am) or by recognizing a period of inactivity in rate-responsive mode.
(typically set to 40-50 bpm)

Sensitivity
Any deflections with an amplitude below the set sensitivity are ignored. The aim is to avoid T and P waves from being mistaken with intrinsic QRS.
(normally set to 2.8-5 mV)

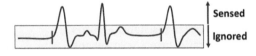

Refractory period (RP)
Interval initiated by a paced or sensed event designed to prevent inhibition by cardiac (e.g. R wave of paced beat, T wave) or non-cardiac events (e.g. noise). Events sensed during this period do not affect the lower rate interval but start another refractory period
(normally set to last 20-30ms longer than the QT interval)

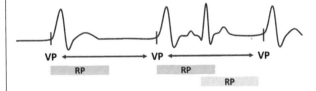

Blanking period (BP)
Interval at the beginning of the refractory period in which the pacemaker ignores any signals, cardiac or non-cardiac. The aim is to avoid oversensing of the pacing stimulus or depolarization.
(typically 100ms in single-chamber systems)

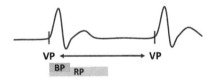

activity inhibits pacing so that the pacemaker does not interfere with the native intrinsic rhythm. The fourth letter indicates whether rate modulation is activated (R) or not (O). This refers to the ability of the pacemaker to increase the rate in response to exercise. Most pacemakers have a piezoelectric crystal that acts as an accelerometer, detecting motion and increasing heart rate accordingly. Other units use minute ventilation that unfortunately may not be useful in dogs as they pant to lose heat. The fifth letter refers to anti-tachycardia

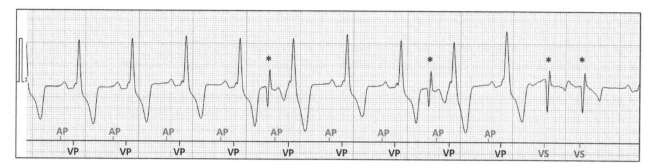

Figure 18.3 Example of under-sensing. This trace was recorded from a dog with sick sinus syndrome fitted with a pacemaker set to DDDR mode. Pacing is occurring in both the right atrium and ventricle. The paced rate during the trace is 120 bpm as the pacemaker sensor was being tested during interrogation. The atrial and ventricular marker channels are represented in the bottom of the trace where atrial-paced (AP), ventricular-paced (VP) and ventricular-sensed (VS) signals can be seen. Intrinsic beats (*) can be seen with a narrow QRS, of which the first two were not sensed by the pacemaker that kept pacing at the same rate in both the atrium and ventricle. [10-year-old, male neutered, crossbreed dog with sick sinus syndrome and a DDDR pacemaker] (50 mm/ms, 20 mm/mV)

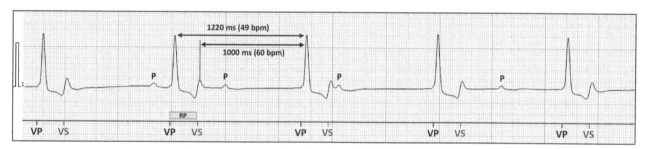

Figure 18.4 Over-sensing of T waves. This electrocardiogram was recorded from a dog with third-degree atrioventricular block (3AVB) after pacemaker implantation. The pacemaker was set to pace in VVI mode at 60 bpm (lower rate interval [LRI] = 1000 ms), the ventricular refractory period (RP) was set to 250 ms and sensitivity to 2.0 mV. The paced rate is approximately 49 bpm instead of the set 60 bpm, and closer analysis of the electrocardiogram reveals that the interval between each T wave and QRS is 1000 ms, which corresponds to the LRI (60 bpm). This suggests that the T waves are being sensed outside the ventricular RP and are being mistaken for intrinsic depolarisations, and this results in resetting the pacemaker each time a T wave is sensed. On the bottom of the picture, the marker channel of the pacemaker is represented as seen using the programmer. Pacemaker impulses are represented as VP (ventricular paced), and impulses sensed outside the RP are represented as VS (ventricular sensed). Analyses of the marker channel confirmed that T waves were being sensed outside of the RP. The QT interval is approximately 300 ms, which means that part of the T wave falls outside of the RP (represented by the green box). Increasing the RP to 320 ms was successful in preventing over-sensing. Additionally, increasing the sensitivity threshold to 3.0 mV (lowering pacemaker sensitivity) resulted in the T waves being ignored completely. [7-year-old, female neutered, Labrador Retriever with 3AVB and a VVIR pacemaker] (50 mm/s, 20 mm/mV)

Table 18.1 Pacemaker system generic code adapted for veterinary medicine

I: Chamber paced	II: Chamber sensed	III: Response to sensing	IV: Rate modulation
O = None	O = None	O = None	O = None
A = Atrium	A = Atrium	T = Triggered	R = Rate modulation
V = Ventricle	V = Ventricle	I = Inhibited	
D = Dual (A + V)	D = Dual (A + V)	D = Dual (T + I)	

Note: Pacemaker systems commonly used in veterinary medicine may be described by a four-letter system in which the first letter corresponds to the paced chamber, the second corresponds to the sensed chamber, the third indicates the response to sensing and the fourth indicates whether rate modulation is available and activated. In dogs, the most commonly used systems are VVI, in which the ventricle (right) is both paced and sensed, whilst pacing is inhibited in response to a sensed beat; and VVIR if rate-responsive mode is activated. *Source*: Modified from The Revised NASPE/BPEG Generic Code for Antibradycardia, Adaptive-Rate, and Multisite Pacing (2002).[19]

pacing or, more recently, to multisite pacing such as biventricular pacing.

Pacemakers used in dogs are usually set in VVI mode initially, and this is changed to VVIR after the lead has fully embedded.

Temporary Pacing

Temporary pacing is used to control rate either prior to permanent pacemaker implantation or during a procedure in a patient with SSS. For patients with 3AVB, induction of anaesthesia can represent the most dangerous time as drugs and physiological changes around the time of induction of anaesthesia could suppress the escape focus. However, if temporary pacing has been placed, this can be performed with minimal concern and the permanent pacemaker implanted without haste. The two most commonly used methods involve a temporary transvenous lead and external patches.[20] Transoesophageal pacing has been used and may be appropriate in patients with intact AV conduction, but not in patients with AV block as the impulse stimulates the atria via the oesophagus and is unable to reach the ventricles.[21–23] In emergency situations, percussive pacing (rhythmically applied mechanical stimuli – fist blows on the precordium – that induce depolarisation, resulting in myocardial contractions and thus ventricular ejection) may be more effective than chest compressions.[24]

1) *Temporary external pacing*: Pacing patches are applied to the chest wall over the heart on the thorax bilaterally (Figure 18.5). Paediatric patches are commonly used for our patients, although adult-sized patches may be useful in giant-breed dogs. They are attached to an external pacing generator that is able to

detect the ECG. If the heart rate falls below a set threshold chosen by the operator, pacing will start. Asynchronous pacing is also possible if necessary (e.g. if the pacing generator mistakenly interprets P waves as QRS in the case of 3AVB), although not without risk (e.g. pacing may happen on a T wave, triggering ventricular fibrillation). The amplitude of the electrical impulse delivered is important, as if insufficient it will not achieve ventricular pacing. The minimum estimated amount of energy should be chosen initially and titrated upwards whilst observing the ECG for evidence of capture (QRS following pacing stimulus), although this can be difficult to visualise due to muscle artefact following external pacing. Therefore, observing the pulse oximeter and capnography curves, or invasive pressure curve if available, is also useful to confirm the ventricular contraction. For guidance purposes, the following output energies are often a good starting point: (A) in cats or small dogs, 25–35 mA; (2) in medium-sized dogs, 50–70 mA; (3) in large-breed dogs, 80–90 mA; and (4) in giant-breed dogs, 90–100 mA. It is important to note that these are just guidelines based on experience and may not be true for each individual patient, as chest conformation and body condition significantly influence the amount of energy necessary to successfully trigger ventricular depolarisation.

Advantages of external pacing

- Easy and quick to set up without the need for specific skills, such as peripheral venous access and cardiac catheterisation, to place an internal pacing lead.

Disadvantages of external pacing

- While this system is effective, it often causes generalised muscle contractions, and the resulting movement may complicate surgery. This can be avoided

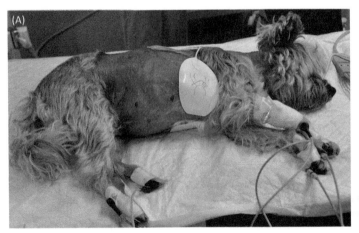
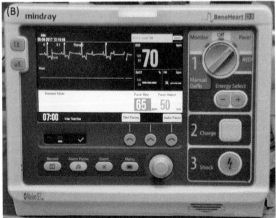

Figure 18.5 Temporary external pacing. (A) For optimal function, the pacing patches should be placed on each side of the chest close to the apex of the heart (sternum). (B) Example of external pacing monitor. The machine is set to pace at a rate of 65 ppm with an output of 50 mA. The patient's electrocardiogram is displayed on the monitor, and white markers appear above each sensed QRS. If intrinsic cardiac activity is not sensed, it will start pacing at the set rate. It is important to check that QRS and not P are sensed and also that a QRS occurs after a paced beat; otherwise, the pacing output will need to be increased until capture is seen.

by paralysing the patient once general anaesthesia has been induced, although this requires specialised anaesthetic skills and mechanical ventilation.

- The external pacemaker must be able to detect intrinsic complexes. In the case of 3AVB, P waves may be mistakenly interpreted as ventricular depolarisations (QRS) and therefore inhibit pacing. Selecting a different electrocardiographic lead and adjusting the sensitivity (making the waves smaller) may be sufficient to solve this problem. If not, asynchronous pacing may be necessary whilst being mindful of the risk of triggering ventricular fibrillation if a pacing impulse is delivered during the vulnerable period (peak of the T wave).

- Human patients often complain of chest pain after external pacing. So for veterinary patients, pain relief should be administered for a period after this procedure, the length depending on the duration of the external pacing.

2) *Temporary internal pacing*: A temporary pacing lead is introduced via a peripheral vein to allow the rate to be controlled. Typically, the right saphenous or left jugular vein is used. A 4 F micro-introducer is used to access the vein and then sized up to a 5 or 6 F introducer. The temporary lead is then guided fluoroscopically into the right ventricle. Some leads have a small balloon at the tip that can help guidance. Once the lead is in place, a temporary pacing box is used to control the rate (Figure 18.6). The settings can be changed to allow the rate, sensing and energy to be adjusted.

Permanent Pacemaker Implantation

Equipment

The equipment required includes a pacing lead, a pulse generator and a programmer that is able to interface with the generator.

The programmer is used to interrogate and program the pacemaker, changing and assessing the rate, sensitivity and current setting. It can also download any history stored on the pacemaker, such as episodes of tachycardia and heart rate. The data retrieval and programming are performed using telemetry attached via a wire to the programmer. Each pacemaker manufacturer has its own programmer, and the functionality of each system is slightly different.

The pulse generators vary depending on the manufacturer. Small single-lead systems are available but dual-lead generators can also be implanted (Figure 18.7). If a dual-lead generator is implanted and used as a single-lead system, the spare port on the generator must be plugged. Multi-lead generators are larger, and this can be problematic in smaller dogs. Batteries are made of lithium–iodine, and battery life is usually up to 8–10 years in newly implanted pacemakers. Generators can be donated and re-used, but their battery life may be limited.

The generator also senses intrinsic complexes. The *refractory period* refers to the period following a paced or intrinsic complex, during which the pacemaker can sense signals but these do not reset the pacing interval. At the start of the refractory period, there is a blanking period

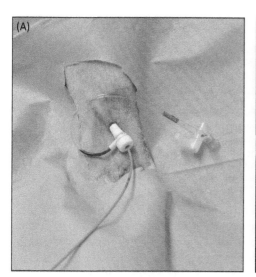
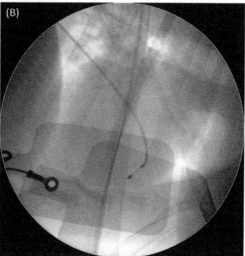
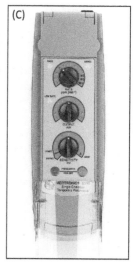

Figure 18.6 Temporary internal pacing. (A,B) Temporary pacing lead introduced via the saphenous vein up to the right ventricle in a dog. (C) Single-chamber temporary pacing box. At each corner on the top, there is a flash light indicator to signal when a paced impulse is delivered (green light on the left) and when an intrinsic beat is sensed (yellow light on the right). Using the top dial, the desired pacing rate can be chosen, in this case from 30 up to 180 bpm. Normally, during pacemaker implantation it is set for 60–80 bpm, but higher values can be used if necessary to maintain blood pressure, depending on the individual patient's cardiovascular function. The middle dial is used to select the energy output from 0.1 to 20 mA. This setting is titrated up to the minimum amount of energy necessary to trigger ventricular depolarisation whilst analyzing the ECG trace for paced QRS complexes. The bottom dial allows control of the sensitivity.

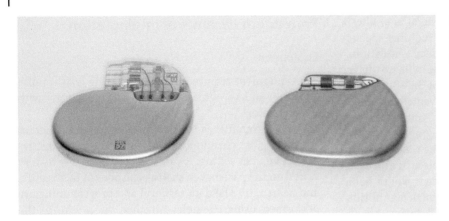

Figure 18.7 Pacemaker generators. The unit on the left is a dual-chamber unit (two lead slots), and the unit on the right is a single-chamber unit (one lead slot).

during which the pacemaker is blind to signals (see Box 18.1). The length of these can be varied to improve function.

There are many different pacing leads available, and choice may be determined by operator preference and device availability. The canine heart paced at 70 bpm will contract approximately 36 million times per year, so the lead must be flexible and resist fatigue. Lead length can vary, but exact length is not critical as an overlong lead can be coiled around the generator. The lead tip is platinum–iridium and steroid eluting to reduce exit block at the implantation site.[25,26] A small radius increases current density, thereby increasing the likelihood of depolarisation, whilst a large surface area increases sensing impedance. As both these properties are advantageous, leads tend to have a small radius with a large surface area. The different leads include:

- *Epicardial leads*: These are sutured directly to the epicardium with a hook, button electrode (Figure 18.8) or screw thread ending. Although they can be attached thoracoscopically, a transdiaphragmatic approach is usually taken. These leads tend to be used in small dogs and cats. This is because in cats, the use of endocardial leads has been associated with an increased risk of chylothorax.[27] Epicardial leads are also used if a lead infection develops on an endocardial lead. The generator is embedded in the abdomen.
- *Endocardial leads*: These are introduced via the right jugular vein and guided fluoroscopically into the right ventricle. They are normally steroid eluting: the silicone matrix is impregnated with dexamethasone that is released to surrounding tissues to decrease the immediate inflammatory response and development of exit block. There are two methods for securing these leads to the endocardium: active and passive fixation leads. The choice of leads is a matter of individual preference, as there is no evidence that either system is superior. Many cardiologists prefer active leads in more active dogs and in dogs with right ventricular enlargement.

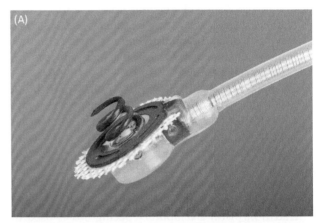

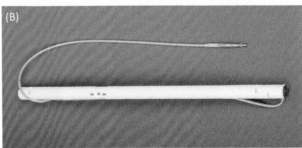

Figure 18.8 Epicardial lead. (A) The tip of the lead may be seen. There is a screw that is screwed into the heart muscle, and then the tip is secured with suture material to the surface of the heart. (B) The lead comes mounted in an implant device designed to allow the screwing of the lead tip into the muscle. Photo by Nat Whitley.

- *Passive fixation* (Figure 18.9A) leads have fine plastic tines or anchors that key into the trabecular muscle of the heart. They are usually covered by reactive tissue in 3–6 months.
- *Active fixation* (Figure 18.9B) leads deploy a screw thread at the lead tip. This can be exteriorised manually using a spanner device on the lead, or the lead tip can be covered with mannitol that dissolves in the body to expose the screw thread. With the retractable helix, the screw can be withdrawn for repositioning of the lead.

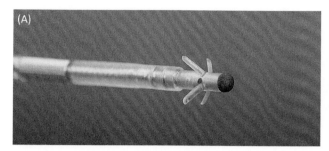 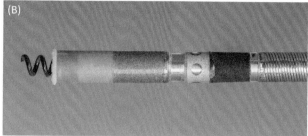

Figure 18.9 Endocardial leads. (A) Passive fixation. There are fine plastic tines or anchors at the tip of the lead that key into the muscular trabeculae of the heart. These are usually covered by reactive tissue in 3–6 months. (B) Active fixation. There is a screw at the end of the lead that is screwed into the heart muscle. Photo by Nat Whitley.

- *Atrial and ventricular leads*: Ventricular leads are straight, and a stiffening wire can be used to guide them from the right atrium, across the tricuspid valve and into the right ventricle. The wire is bent to allow the lead to cross the tricuspid valve, but once in the right ventricle, it is replaced with a straight wire to allow correct positioning, especially if an active lead is deployed. Atrial leads (Figure 18.10) have a natural J shape to allow them to sit in the right auricle. Again, a straight stiffening wire is used to access the right atrium, then the wire is withdrawn so the lead can curve back into the right auricle.
- *Polarity of the lead*: To complete the electrical circuit, two electrodes are necessary. In bipolar leads, both electrodes, with the distal as the cathode (negative electrode), are situated towards the lead tip, allowing a small circuit within the heart. Bipolar leads are less susceptible to electromechanical interference. Unipolar leads use the generator body as the positive anode and the lead tip as the negative cathode. This allows for a finer pacing lead but can cause muscle fasciculation over the generator that some patients find distressing. A larger pacing spike is seen on the surface ECG with unipolar leads (Figure 18.11).
- *Single lead with atrial sensing*: This is a single ventricular pacing lead that has a pair of atrial sensing electrodes at a set distance from the tip. As these are made for humans, this gap is usually too long for dogs, so a loop may need to be deployed in the right atrium to allow the sensing electrodes to be situated correctly.[28]

Dual-chamber Pacing

Humans with a single-chamber pacemaker may develop *pacemaker syndrome*, an ill-defined syndrome due to AV asynchrony that contributes to increased morbidity and mortality. Symptoms are due to a combination of decreased cardiac output, loss of atrial contribution to ventricular filling and loss of total peripheral resistance response, and they include heart failure, exercise intolerance and weakness, seizure, dizziness and arrhythmias.

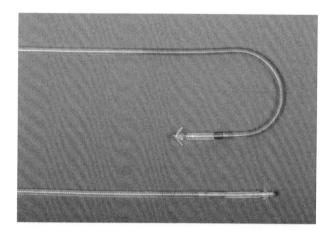

Figure 18.10 Atrial and ventricular leads. Ventricular leads are straight. Atrial leads have a natural J shape designed to allow them to sit in the right auricle. Photo by Nat Whitley.

Cannon A waves in the jugular veins may be seen where the atria contract against closed AV valves. This can occur intermittently or regularly if retrograde ventriculo-atrial conduction occurs. This is corrected by using an atrial sensing/ventricular pacing (VDD) system or a dual-chamber (DDD) one to synchronise AV contraction. It is unknown whether this syndrome occurs in veterinary patients, but studies examining if dogs with dual-chamber systems lived longer have failed to show benefits that would offset the longer surgical implantation time and higher cost of a dual-lead system.[29–31] However, cardiac output is more efficient in dogs with dual-chamber pacing.[26]

Dual-chamber pacing offers the advantages of restoring AV synchrony and augmenting cardiac output in a more physiological manner, and it has been performed in dogs.[30,32] The second lead is implanted in the right auricular appendage and has a J shape. Programming and adjustment are more complicated, with both leads able to sense and pace. After atrial pacing, both atrial and ventricular leads have a brief blanking period when sensing is disabled to avoid confusion with the pacing spike and subsequent after-potential. After a set period, the AV interval, the ventricular lead depolarises. At this

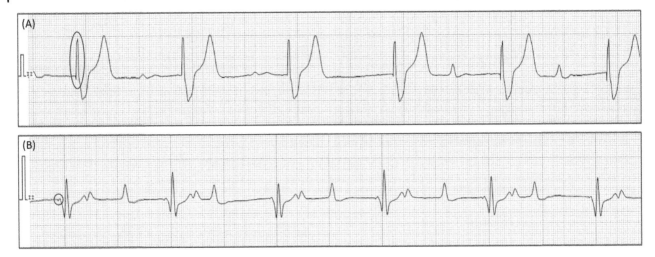

Figure 18.11 Unipolar versus bipolar pacing. These traces were taken from the same patient with the pacemaker set to pace in unipolar and bipolar modes. (A) Unipolar pacing (50 mm/s, 10 mm/mV). In unipolar mode, the tip lead functions as the cathode (negative electrode) and the anode (positive electrode) is the surface of the generator. The electrical impulse flows from the cathode, through the heart and body tissues and back to the generator, completing the electrical circuit. On the electrocardiogram, a large pacing spike is produced (red oval area) due to the fact that the electrical current flows through a larger area of tissue to complete the electrical circuit, in contrast to bipolar pacing. (B) Bipolar pacing (50 mm/s, 20 mm/mV). In bipolar mode, both electrodes are present in close vicinity (≈1 cm) in the extremity of the lead. For this reason, the electrical current must travel a very short distance to complete the circuit, causing a much smaller, almost imperceptible, pacing spike (red circle). [6-year-old, female neutered, Labrador Retriever with 3AVB and VVIR pacemaker]

time, the atrial lead has a post-ventricular atrial refractory period (PVARP), during which all events are ignored so the atrial lead does not detect the ventricular depolarisation (far-field sensing) or retrograde AV conducted atrial complexes. At this time, the ventricular lead also has a ventricular refractory period which should stop sensing of a T wave and resetting the rate. The total atrial refractory period (TARP) is a sum of the AV interval and the PVARP. The upper rate limit at which AV conduction can be maintained in a 1:1 manner is the *maximum tracking rate* (MTR) which is determined by the TARP. If atrial rates exceed the MTR, the pacemaker responds with a Wenckebach pattern.

AAI pacemakers may be appropriate in SSS, but DDD pacemakers are preferred in AV block. Specific problems include:

Hysteresis: This refers to the ability of the pacemaker to have a longer interval following a sensed complex, allowing more intrinsic rhythm (e.g. the paced rate may be 70 bpm) but following a sensed beat; the interval can be 1200 ms (50 bpm) before a paced beat is delivered. This can also help reduce pacemaker syndrome.

Cross-talk: This refers to the ability of a lead to sense a paced event in another chamber and inhibit its action. For example, a ventricular lead may sense an atrial paced complex, especially if a unipolar lead is used with a larger spike, and interpret that as an intrinsic ventricular complex, inhibiting its action. As this would be disastrous, algorithms prevent it from happening; for example, a blanking occurs in the ventricular lead after the atrial depolarisation period to prevent it from detecting the atrial complex, followed by a noise sampling period (during which a sensed or paced event will restart the refractory period but will not reset the pacing interval) allowing ventricular pacing.

Pacemaker-mediated tachycardia (PMT): This 'endless loop' occurs because of retrograde AV conduction stimulating an atrial complex that is sensed, triggering a ventricular depolarisation. If VA conduction occurred rapidly, it is likely to fall in the PVARP, so this is more likely to occur in cases with slow VA conduction and can occur in patients with 3AVB. To prevent this, the PVARP should be extended. In addition, pacemakers are designed to terminate PMT by not sensing every sixth atrial complex when running near the upper rate limit.

Automatic mode switching: It is important, in cases of rapid atrial or supraventricular tachyarrhythmias, that not all complexes are transmitted to the ventricles. The pacemaker detects this and switches from an atrial tracking mode to a non-tracking mode with a back-up rhythm, often with rate smoothing.

Dual Versus Single-chamber Pacing

As the advantages of dual pacing are clear in human medicine, it seems likely that this should be the case in veterinary medicine as well, but to date, studies have failed to demonstrate a benefit of dual-chamber pacemakers.[29] Implantation takes longer, as would be expected, but there seems to be little increased risk of infection or lead dislodgement. Unfortunately, until studies demonstrate a benefit, it is difficult to justify the increased expense of the extra lead and generator.

Pacemaker Implantation

Once temporary pacing has been established, the patient can be safely anaesthetised and placed in left lateral recumbency. The right jugular vein is usually chosen to negate the potential complication of a persistent left cranial vena cava diverting the pacemaker lead. The jugular vein is exteriorised and stabilised with ligatures (Figure 18.12A). The vein is opened, and the lead introduced with a straight stiffening wire. A vein pick can be helpful to open the vein for lead introduction (Figure 18.12B). The lead is advanced into the right atrium under fluoroscopic guidance. The wire is then removed and curved to allow the lead to pass ventrally through the tricuspid valve into the right ventricle. Once

in place, the curved wire is replaced with a straight wire, so the lead can be pushed against the ventricular myocardium while the screw is deployed in the case of active leads. Gentle traction on the lead will help determine how securely the lead is attached. In the case of passive leads, the lead is pushed into the apex of the right ventricle with a straight stiffening wire and left in place. Optimum position is in the right ventricular apex angled towards the diaphragm, although in dogs with severe mitral regurgitation or dilated cardiomyopathy, positioning the lead in the right ventricular outflow tract may be preferable.

Once the lead is thought to be in the correct position, the thresholds and setting of the pacemaker should be checked with the programmer. If the values are abnormal, the lead should be repositioned. Fluoroscopy of the entire system is then indicated to ensure that there is sufficient slack in the lead to allow for normal head movements. The lead is then sutured in the jugular vein using non-absorbable sutures (Figure 18.12C). Many leads have an anchoring sleeve, and using this in the jugular vein may enhance lead stability.[33]

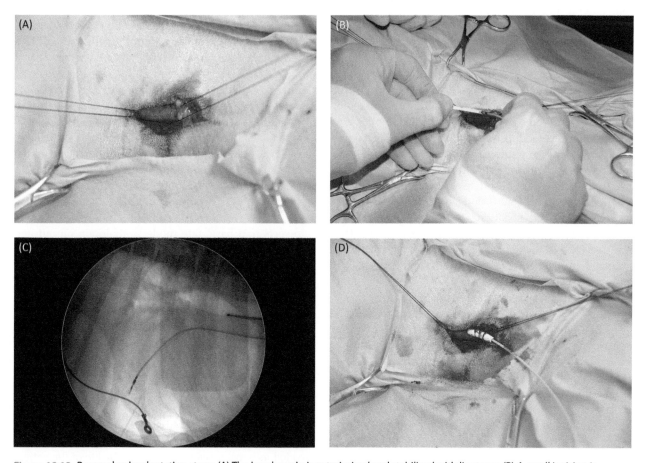

Figure 18.12 Pacemaker implantation steps. (A) The jugular vein is exteriorized and stabilized with ligatures. (B) A small incision is performed on the vein, and a vein pick is used to help introduce the lead. (C) The lead is positioned in the ventricle with fluoroscopic guidance. (D) After the lead is in position in the ventricle, the lead is sutured to the jugular vein using the anchoring sleeve with non-absorbable sutures.

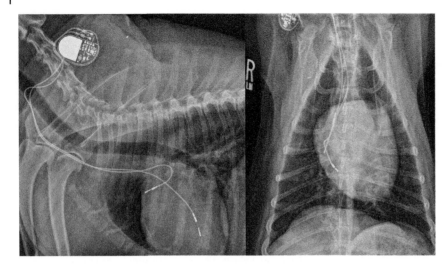

Figure 18.13 Chest radiographs to document lead position. It is important that radiographs are taken after pacemaker implantation, documenting the location and position of the generator and lead. This is used as a reference for the future in case of lead dislodgement/fracture or other possible complications involving the lead and the generator. In this case, lateral and sagittal radiographic views of the chest document the position of a dual-chamber unit in the neck and corresponding atrial and ventricular lead positions inside the heart.

A separate pocket is then created for the generator. This is usually in the dorsal cervical area under the cutaneous trunci muscle, although some cardiologists place the generator over the thoracic wall. The pocket should not be overlarge, as this may encourage seroma formation. Lateral and dorsoventral radiographs should be obtained to document final lead position (Figure 18.13).

Aftercare

The neck should be covered with a light-pressure support dressing to reduce the risk of seroma formation and protect the generator in the short term. Antibiotics are usually administered intravenously for the first 24 h only. Some cardiologists continue these orally for 10–14 days, but there is no evidence that this reduces the risk of infection. Patients are hospitalised for the first 24–48 h to reduce the risk of lead dislodgement, and very active patients may need sedation. The owners should be advised to rest the dogs for at least 4 weeks to allow the lead to embed in the endocardium. This is followed by a gradual return to exercise over the next 2–3 weeks. A leash and collar should never be used due to the risk of lead fracture, and blood samples should never be taken from the right jugular vein. The neck bandage is changed every 2–4 days, and, if no seroma is present when the sutures are removed, the bandage does not need to be replaced. If a seroma is present, the neck dressing should be replaced and activity restricted until it resolves. The seroma should not be drained as this increases the risk of infection.

Patients should be re-examined in one month and the pacemaker interrogated. At that point, the voltage threshold may be decreased and the rate responsive program activated. An initial revisit at 6 months can be followed by yearly rechecks to optimise function and battery life.

Follow-up

During the revisits, the following parameters should be assessed and recorded:

- *Threshold testing*: To assess correct pulse duration and voltage amplitude
- *Sensitivity testing*: To check the pacemaker is identifying the intrinsic complex appropriately. This is more difficult in dogs with 3AVB as they often become pacemaker dependent, so even if the rate is slowed, an intrinsic rhythm does not emerge. If T waves are sensed as R waves, the sensitivity can be increased (made less sensitive) or the refractory period can be extended. However, if the refractory period is too long, intrinsic complexes can cause multiple restarts of the refractory period, and the generator may switch to asynchronous pacing (noise reversion).
- *Battery life*: This is performed automatically. When the battery reaches the end of its life, the pacemaker reverts to a basic rate mode to maintain output and warn that the end of the battery life is approaching, which should prompt replacement.
- *Lead impedance*: This is performed automatically and indicates the resistance of the circuit. Trends can be evaluated over time.

Complications

It has been shown that the rate of complications is related to the experience of the cardiologist and team.[34] For that reason, it is recommended that pacemakers should be implanted by experienced clinicians. Complications can be divided into major (which can affect the life of the patient or require a major intervention) and minor ones.[6–8]

Major complications that can be present in 13–33% of patients:[6–8]

- *Lead dislodgement:* Lead dislodgement is more common in the postoperative period, before the lead becomes fully embedded in the heart muscle, but may also occur several months or even years after implantation. It may occur for several reasons, including excessive patient movement (e.g. neck pulling), trauma and poor implantation technique. This is a well-described complication in human and veterinary medicine, and it includes different lead dislodgement syndromes.[35]
  - *Twiddler's syndrome:* The lead twists over itself as the generator flips over in its pocket. This can eventually cause the lead to be pulled out of the endocardium. To prevent this, the generator should be fixed to the cutaneous trunci muscle with non-absorbable suture, using the existing hole on top of the generator.
  - *Reel syndrome:* The lead retracts as the generator flips over its sagittal axis (Figure 18.14). To prevent this, the generator should be fixed to the cutaneous trunci muscle with non-absorbable suture, using the existing hole on top of the generator.

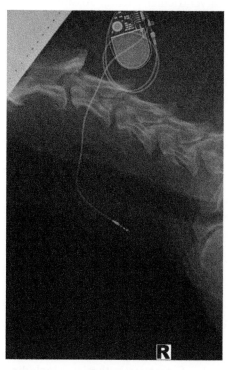

Figure 18.14 Lead dislodgement seen on a neck radiograph. The lead can be seen 'tucked' in the generator pocket in loops, whilst the tip is positioned in the neck. This suggests that the generator rotated over its sagittal axis, retracting the lead in loops around it – *reel syndrome*. This occurred 10 days after pacemaker implant. This was an unusual case in which the suture used to secure the generator to the cutaneous trunci muscle was still in place in the generator but not attached to the muscle, suggesting that it had torn through it, possibly due to a trauma. [12-year-old, female neutered, Northern Inuit with 3AVB]

  - *Ratchett syndrome:* The lead retracts without generator rotation due to progressive dislodgement at its fixation sites and protector sleeves. This may happen, for example, with a sudden pull on the neck. To prevent this, the patient should be rested until the lead has time to properly embed, and the lead should be fixated as well as possible with non-absorbable suture to the jugular vein.
- *Pacemaker infection:* This can occur at any time, and treatment with antibiotics is usually unsuccessful at resolving the infection. The pacemaker and lead need to be removed, and after a suitable period, another system needs to be implanted. If a transvenous system was used initially, it should be replaced by an epicardial one.
- *Over-sensing that can result in syncope:* The P wave is sensed as a QRS wave, and the pacemaker function is suppressed. The sensitivity should be reduced (higher mV) to avoid sensing of P waves.
- *Noise reversion (inappropriate asynchronous pacing):* If the pacemaker repeatedly senses impulses within the set refractory period, it may switch to asynchronous pacing as a protective measure. This was developed to avoid noise being mistaken for cardiac events, leading to inappropriate suppression of pacing and possible death. However, in dogs, this may occur if tachycardia coexists with bradycardia, as at faster rates, a shorter QT and taller T waves may lead to sensing of the T waves during the refractory period. In fact, this is more commonly seen with SSS than with 3AVB.[36] (to avoid this, the sensitivity should be adjusted to avoid sensing of T waves as much as possible in the first place. Additionally, the refractory period may also be shortened, and this may be particularly useful in case ectopic beats are sensed instead of T waves.) Concomitant treatment of tachyarrhythmias with anti-arrhythmic drugs is also recommended. In systems functioning in AAI mode or dual-chamber pacing, the trigger for noise reversion may be sensing of ventricular R and T waves by the atrial lead or the ventricular pacing artefact itself. To avoid this, sensing must be disabled for the atrial lead by setting a blanking period that should last approximately 20–30 ms longer than the pacing spike to the R wave interval.[36]
- *Bleeding*
- *Ventricular fibrillation*
- *Pacemaker failure or malfunction:*
  - *Output failure:* The pacemaker is no longer able to generate impulses (e.g. battery depletion).
  - *Failure to capture* (Figure 18.15): The impulse does not cause myocardial depolarisation. This may be caused by lead displacement or fracture, electrolyte imbalances, myocardial infarction or exit block in which fibrosis around the lead prevents the impulse from reaching excitable myocardial cells.

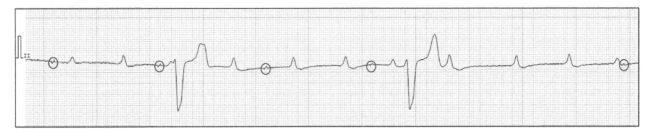

Figure 18.15 Failure to capture. This trace was recorded from a dog with a VVI pacemaker implanted for treatment of third-degree atrioventricular block (3AVB). The underlying rhythm is a ventricular escape rhythm with a rate of 30–40 bpm and 3AVB. Pacing spikes (red circles) may be seen without causing ventricular depolarisation, signalling lack of capture. In this case, this was caused by inappropriate impulse amplitude and duration attributed to the possible development of fibrosis around the lead tip, causing exit block. An increase in amplitude and duration was successful in achieving capture. Most modern generators have auto-capture features that are able to adjust these settings automatically on a daily basis; however, in this case this feature was not activated. [12-year-old, female neutered, Labrador Retriever with 3AVB] (50 mm/s, 10 mm/mV)

— *Pacemaker-mediated arrhythmias*:
  ◦ *PMT* is a macro re-entry tachycardia that may occur with systems functioning in AAI or dual-chamber pacing modes. A continuous cycle occurs in which a paced beat is retroconducted to the atria via the AV node and is sensed as native atrial activity, triggering another ventricular paced beat.
  ◦ *Sensor-induced tachycardia* is an inappropriately high-paced rhythm caused by malfunction of the sensors responsible for increasing the heart rate in response to exercise, tachypnoea, hypercapnia or acidaemia in rate-responsive systems. The maximum rate cannot exceed the pacemaker's upper rate limit.
  ◦ *Runaway pacemaker* is a potentially life-threatening malfunction related to battery depletion in older pacemaker models. The pacemaker may deliver paroxysms of pacing spikes at a very high rate that may trigger ventricular fibrillation, or alternatively low-amplitude impulses may fail to capture the ventricle and result in bradycardia or asystole.[37]
- *Cardiac perforation*[38]
- *Others*: Thrombus formation around the pacemaker lead, tricuspid stenosis[39] and cranial vena cava syndrome[40–42] or caudal vena cava syndrome.[43]

Minor complications, which can be present in 11–31% of dogs:

- *Seroma*: Should not be drained; instead, rest and a pressure bandage should be applied until it resolves.
- *Muscle twitching*: Usually a feature of unipolar programming, with the muscle overlying the generator being stimulated. This can be controlled by changing to bipolar mode or reducing the amplitude. Alternatively, the owner can be reassured that this problem often resolves spontaneously.

- *Arrhythmias* that do not impact life
- *Minor sensing issues*
- *Changes in QRS morphology* during pacemaker interrogation can be caused by anodal stimulation.[44]
- *Pacemaker syndrome*: This includes shortness of breath, syncope and even congestive heart failure associated with ventricular pacing. Possible mechanisms include the lack of AV synchrony with decreased ventricular filling, vagal reflex from increased atrial pressure when the atria contract against a closed AV valve, and cannon A waves stimulating cardiopulmonary baroreceptors.[47] It has not been documented in dogs.

Outcome

Results are usually excellent, with over 95% of dogs surviving pacemaker implantation and 1 year survival of 70–86%. However, 3 and 5-year survivals are 45 and 39%, respectively, due to the underlying cardiac disease or age of the patients.[7,8] Despite this, owner satisfaction is high at around 80%.[7]

Other Implantable Devices

In people, implantable cardiac defibrillators are also used for control of tachyarrhythmias, including serious supraventricular and ventricular tachycardias. Although use of these devices has been reported in dogs, their usefulness has been limited by the difficulty in adapting algorithms that can differentiate between an excited dog with large T waves and one in ventricular tachycardia.[45,46] It is likely that these treatments will become more viable in the future as technology improves.

References

1 Buchanan JW. First pacemaker in a dog: a historical note. J Vet Intern Med. 2003;17:713–714.

2 Ranjan R, *et al.* Diagnostic imaging and pacemaker implantation in a domestic goat with persistent left cranial vena cava. J Vet Cardiol. 2014;16:45–50.

3 van Loon G, Fonteyne W, Rottiers H, Tavernier R, Deprez P. Implantation of a dual-chamber, rate-adaptive pacemaker in a horse with suspected sick sinus syndrome. Vet Rec. 2002;151:541–545.

4 Schrope DP, Kelch WJ. Signalment, clinical signs, and prognostic indicators associated with high-grade second- or third-degree atrioventricular block in dogs: 124 cases (January 1, 1997–December 31, 1997). J Am Vet Med Assoc. 2006;228:1710–1717.

5 Santilli RA, Porteiro Vázquez DM, Vezzosi T, Perego M. Long-term intrinsic rhythm evaluation in dogs with atrioventricular block. J Vet Intern Med. 2016;30:58–62.

6 Wess G, Thomas WP, Berger DM, Kittleson MD. Applications, complications, and outcomes of transvenous pacemaker implantation in 105 dogs (1997–2002). J Vet Intern Med. 2006;20:877–884.

7 Oyama MA, Sisson DD, Lehmkuhl LB. Practices and outcome of artificial cardiac pacing in 154 dogs. J Vet Intern Med. 2001;15:229–239.

8 Johnson MS, Martin MWS, Henley W. Results of pacemaker implantation in 104 dogs. J Small Anim Pract. 2007;48:4–11.

9 Fonfara S, *et al.* English springer spaniels with significant bradyarrhythmias: presentation, troponin I and follow-up after pacemaker implantation. J Small Anim Pract. 2010;51:155–161.

10 Moneva-Jordan A, *et al.* Sick sinus syndrome in nine West Highland white terriers. Vet Rec. 2001;148:142–147.

11 Ward JL, *et al.* Outcome and survival in canine sick sinus syndrome and sinus node dysfunction: 93 cases (2002–2014). J Vet Cardiol. 2016;18:199–212.

12 Thomason JD, Kraus MS, Fallaw TL, Calvert CA. Survival of 4 dogs with persistent atrial standstill treated by pacemaker implantation. Can Vet J. 2016;57:297–298.

13 Schmitt KE, Lefbom BK. Long-term management of atrial myopathy in two dogs with single chamber permanent transvenous pacemakers. J Vet Cardiol. 2016;18:187–193.

14 Kellum HB, Stepien RL. Third-degree atrioventricular block in 21 cats (1997–2004). J Vet Intern Med. 2006;20:97–103.

15 Shih AC, *et al.* Effect of routine cardiovascular catheterization on cardiac troponin I concentration in dogs. J Vet Cardiol. 2009;11(Suppl. 1):S87–S92.

16 Saunders AB, *et al.* Bradyarrhythmias and pacemaker therapy in dogs with Chagas disease. J Vet Intern Med. 2013;27:890–894.

17 Trafny DJ, *et al.* Cardiac troponin-I concentrations in dogs with bradyarrhythmias before and after artificial pacing. J Vet Cardiol. 2010;12:183–190.

18 Coates S, Thwaites B. The strength-duration curve and its importance in pacing efficiency: a study of 325 pacing leads in 229 patients. Pacing Clin Electrophysiol. 2000;23:1273–1277.

19 Bernstein AD, *et al.* The revised NASPE/BPEG generic code for antibradycardia, adaptive-rate, and multisite pacing. North American Society of Pacing and Electrophysiology/British Pacing and Electrophysiology Group. Pacing Clin Electrophysiol. 2002;25:260–264.

20 Lee S, Nam S-J, Hyun C. The optimal size and placement of transdermal electrodes are critical for the efficacy of a transcutaneous pacemaker in dogs. Vet J. 2010;183:196–200.

21 DeFrancesco TC, Hansen BD, Atkins CE, Sidley JA, Keene BW. Noninvasive transthoracic temporary cardiac pacing in dogs. J Vet Intern Med. 2003;17:663–667.

22 Sanders RA, Green HW3, Hogan DF, Trafney D, Batra AS. Efficacy of transesophageal and transgastric cardiac pacing in the dog. J Vet Cardiol. 2010;12:49–52.

23 Sanders RA, Green HW3, Hogan DF, Sederquist K. Use of transesophageal atrial pacing to provide temporary chronotropic support in a dog undergoing permanent pacemaker implantation. J Vet Cardiol. 2011;13:227–230.

24 Iseri LT, Allen BJ, Baron K, Brodsky MA. Fist pacing, a forgotten procedure in bradyasystolic cardiac arrest. Am Heart J. 1987;113:1545–1550.

25 Estrada AH, *et al.* Evaluation of pacing site in dogs with naturally occurring complete heart block. J Vet Cardiol. 2009;11:79–88.

26 Maisenbacher HW, Estrada AH, Prosek R, Shih AC, Vangilder JM. Evaluation of the effects of transvenous pacing site on left ventricular function and synchrony in healthy anesthetized dogs. Am J Vet Res. 2009;70:455–463.

27 Ferasin L, van de Stad M, Rudorf H, Langford K, Hotston MA. Syncope associated with paroxysmal atrioventricular block an ventricular standstill in a cat. J Small Anim Pract. 2002;43:124–128.

28 Bulmer BJ, Oyama MA, Lamont LA, Sisson DD. Implantation of a single-lead atrioventricular synchronous (VDD) pacemaker in a dog with naturally occurring 3rd-degree atrioventricular block. J Vet Intern Med. 2002;16:197–200.

29 Lichtenberger J, Scollan KF, Bulmer BJ, Sisson DD. Long-term outcome of physiologic VDD pacing versus non-physiologic VVI pacing in dogs with high-grade atrioventricular block. J Vet Cardiol. 2015;17:42–53.

30 Bulmer BJ, *et al.* Physiologic VDD versus nonphysiologic VVI pacing in canine 3rd-degree atrioventricular block. J Vet Intern Med. 2006;20:257–271.

31 Genovese DW, Estrada AH, Maisenbacher HW, Heatwole BA, Powell MA. Procedure times, complication rates, and survival times associated with single-chamber versus dual-chamber pacemaker implantation in dogs with clinical signs of bradyarrhythmia: 54 cases (2004–2009). J Am Vet Med Assoc. 2013;242:230–236.

32 Weder C, Monnet E, Ames M, Bright J. Permanent dual chamber epicardial pacemaker implantation in two dogs with complete atrioventricular block. J Vet Cardiol. 2015;17:154–160.

33 Djani DM, *et al.* Congestive heart failure caused by transvenous pacemaker lead prolapse and associated right ventricular outflow tract obstruction in a dog. J Vet Cardiol. 2016;18:391–397.

34 Ward JL, *et al.* Complication rates associated with transvenous pacemaker implantation in dogs with high-grade atrioventricular block performed during versus after normal business hours. J Vet Intern Med. 2015;29:157–163.

35 Pachon M, Arias MA, Puchol A, Jerez-Valero M, Rodriguez-Padial L. Malignant ventricular arrhythmias during surgical procedures for pacemaker generator replacement: description of two cases. Rev Esp Cardiol (Engl ed). 2012;65:1136–1138.

36 Moïse NS, Estrada A. Noise reversion in paced dogs. J Vet Cardiol. 2002;4:13–21.

37 Prosek R, Sisson DD, Oyama MA. Runaway pacemaker in a dog. J Vet Intern Med. 2004;18:242–244.

38 Achen SE, Miller MW, Nelson DA, Gordon SG, Drourr LT. Late cardiac perforation by a passive-fixation permanent pacemaker lead in a dog. J Am Vet Med Assoc. 2008;233:1291–1296.

39 Connolly DJ, Neiger-Aeschbacher G, Brockman DJ. Tricuspid valve stenosis caused by fibrous adhesions to an endocardial pacemaker lead in a dog. J Vet Cardiol. 2007;9:123–128.

40 Mulz JM, Kraus MS, Thompson M, Flanders JA. Cranial vena caval syndrome secondary to central venous obstruction associated with a pacemaker lead in a dog. J Vet Cardiol. 2010;12:217–223.

41 Murray JD, O'Sullivan ML, Hawkes KCE. Cranial vena caval thrombosis associated with endocardial pacing leads in three dogs. J Am Anim Hosp Assoc. 2010;46:186–192.

42 Van De Wiele CM, Hogan DF, Green HW3, Parnell NK. Cranial vena caval syndrome secondary to transvenous pacemaker implantation in two dogs. J Vet Cardiol. 2008;10:155–161.

43 Stauthammer C, Tobias A, France M, Olson J. Caudal vena cava obstruction caused by redundant pacemaker lead in a dog. J Vet Cardiol. 2009;11:141–145.

44 Oyama MA, *et al.* Anodal stimulation in two dogs with transvenous permanent bipolar pacemakers. J Vet Cardiol. 2016;18:398–404.

45 Pariaut R, Saelinger C, Queiroz-Williams P, Strickland KN, Marshall HC. Implantable cardioverter-defibrillator in a German shepherd dog with ventricular arrhythmias. J Vet Cardiol. 2011;13:203–210.

46 Nelson OL, Lahmers S, Schneider T, Thompson P. The use of an implantable cardioverter defibrillator in a Boxer Dog to control clinical signs of arrhythmogenic right ventricular cardiomyopathy. J Vet Intern Med. 2006;20:1232–1237.

47 Moses HW, Mullin JC. In A practical guide to cardiac pacing (6th ed., pp. 171–172). Philadelphia: Lippincott Williams & Wilkins; 2007.

19

Electrophysiology Studies and Catheter Ablation

Pedro Oliveira and Martin Lowe

Introduction

In this chapter, we will discuss when and how to perform an electrophysiology study (EP study) and catheter ablation for the definitive diagnosis and treatment of cardiac arrhythmias. It is not our intent to provide a detailed description of all aspects of invasive cardiac electrophysiology (EP) but rather an overview of the topic in veterinary medicine.

What is an Electrophysiology Study and Catheter Ablation?

During an EP study, cardiac catheterization is used to obtain intracardiac electrocardiograms (ECGs) from specific areas in the heart. This allows a direct assessment of the propagation of cardiac electrical impulses revealing the underlying mechanism of cardiac arrhythmias, or simply to test the function of the various components of the cardiac conduction system (e.g. sinus node and atrioventricular node [AVN]). Once the underlying arrhythmia mechanism is known, catheter ablation can be used to target the abnormal electrical impulse and destroy the structures involved. This is performed by applying localized energy via the tip of a special catheter causing tissue necrosis. The target for ablation may be a localized area such as an ectopic focus or accessory pathway (AP), or a larger area involved in a re-entrant circuit (e.g. the cavotricuspid isthmus in typical atrial flutter).

Indications for an EP Study and Catheter Ablation

The main advantages of an EP study and catheter ablation are that a definitive diagnosis of the arrhythmia mechanism and a definitive treatment (cure) may be achieved. In human medicine, these procedures have become widespread and are the first-line treatment for many cardiac arrhythmias. Unfortunately, in veterinary medicine, this is not the case, and only a few centres worldwide routinely perform these procedures. The need for dedicated and expensive facilities as well as highly specialized skills makes it very difficult to set up an EP laboratory. Hopefully, this will change in the future, and it will be easier for our patients to benefit from these diagnostic and treatment modalities. Additional disadvantages include the need for general anaesthesia and the overall cost in comparison to medical treatment. However, it is worth considering that in some cases, lifelong medical treatment and regular monitoring end up being more expensive than the procedure itself.

Cardiac Arrhythmias in which EP Study and Ablation May be Beneficial

- Atrioventricular reciprocating tachycardia (accessory pathways)[1–3]
- Atrial tachycardia[4]
- Atrial flutter[5,6]
- Pre-excited atrial fibrillation
- Atrioventricular nodal reciprocating tachycardia (humans)
- Atrial fibrillation (humans)
- Ventricular arrhythmias (humans)

The Electrophysiology Laboratory

The following equipment is necessary in an interventional EP laboratory (and see Figure 19.1):

1) A *fluoroscopy unit* to guide catheter placement and manipulation within the heart. This may be a fixed or a mobile C-arm unit with a radiographic table. All staff members must wear appropriate protective clothing and radiation dosimeters.
2) A *multichannel data acquisition system* to record surface and intracardiac ECGs as well as blood pressure.

Guide to Canine and Feline Electrocardiography, First Edition. Ruth Willis, Pedro Oliveira and Antonia Mavropoulou.
© 2018 John Wiley & Sons Ltd. Published 2018 by John Wiley & Sons Ltd.
Companion website: www.wiley.com/go/willis/electrocardiography

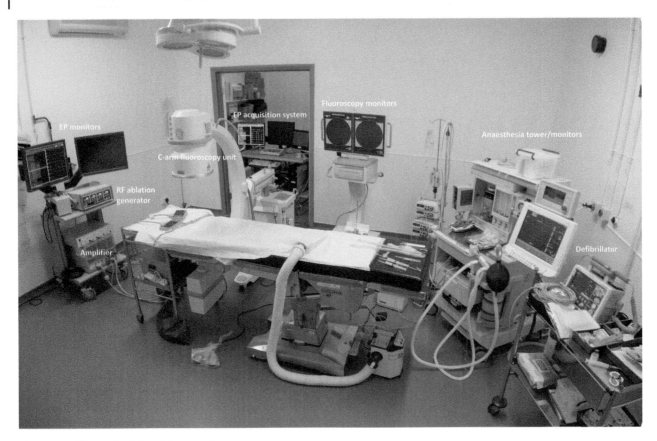

Figure 19.1 Electrophysiology laboratory layout.

It should be able to record all 12 surface leads and at least eight intracardiac leads.

3) A *cardiac stimulator* used to deliver pacing impulses via the EP catheters. It may be a separate unit or may be part of the acquisition system. Various pacing modes are used during an EP study (see below).

4) *Electrophysiology catheters* (see below)

5) An *ablation unit* used for catheter ablation

6) Standard *anaesthetic equipment and consumables*

7) A *defibrillator and cardioversion unit*

8) Temporary pacing facilities may also be useful as a back-up for the cardiac stimulator in cases that become pacing-dependent. It may also be necessary to implant a permanent pacemaker in such cases.

Staffing necessary to perform the following tasks:

1) Invasive procedures such as vascular access, catheter placement and manipulation (cardiologist/ electrophysiologist)

2) Operation of the acquisition system, cardiac stimulator and ablation generator (cardiac physiologist)

3) General anaesthesia and patient care (anaesthetist/ nurse)

4) Operation of the fluoroscopy unit and general support such as opening catheters etc. (theatre nurse).

Overview of a Standard Electrophysiology Study

Patient Preparation

General anaesthesia is required for our patients, and therefore a pre-anaesthetic assessment (e.g. blood analysis) and appropriate fasting period are necessary. Antiarrhythmic drugs should be discontinued whenever possible for at least four half-lives (2–3 days for most drugs). This may prove challenging in patients that are not stable off the drugs, or with amiodarone due to its long half-life.

The jugular and/or femoral veins are used for vascular access, and therefore these areas should be clipped and ready for antiseptic skin preparation.

During the procedure, the patient is positioned in dorsal recumbency.

Anaesthesia

The anaesthetic plan is tailored to each patient but is not necessarily different from other routine procedures. In our EP laboratory, most patients receive a premedication with an opioid (methadone or butorphanol) either alone or in combination with acepromazine (intramuscular or intravenous administration). Intravenous alfaxolone or propofol are our preferred induction agents, and this is followed by gaseous anaesthesia with isofluorane via an endotracheal tube.

We routinely use electrocardiography, pulse oximetry, capnography and both non-invasive and invasive blood pressure as monitoring tools. We find that invasive blood pressure is very important in our patients as pacing manoeuvres or cardiac arrhythmias can have a very significant haemodynamic effect.

The following injectable drugs are made available for all cases: adrenaline, atropine, lidocaine, procainamide, diltiazem (or verapamil), esmolol and amiodarone.

An external defibrillator must also be available, and if the risk of ventricular fibrillation is considered high, external pads are positioned on both sides of the chest beforehand to avoid interference with the sterile field.

Vascular Access

During an EP study, up to four catheters may be present inside the heart at any given time. It is important to take into account the size of the patient and the size and number of the required catheters to properly plan the vascular access. One vascular access sheath is necessary for each catheter. We routinely use three catheters, of which two are introduced via the left jugular vein (two 6Fr vascular access sheaths) and one via the right femoral vein (one 7Fr vascular access sheath). Percutaneous access may be used, although we prefer the modified Seldinger technique with exposure of the vessel, as it is easier to control post-procedure haemorrhage. Both vessels are repaired after the procedure and remain fully functional.

Electrophysiology Catheters and their Placements

Various catheters may be used during an EP study (Figures 19.2 and 19.3). A distinction is made between diagnostic catheters and catheters for mapping and ablation.

Diagnostic catheters are usually 5Fr or 6Fr and commonly carry two (quadripolar) or five (decapolar) electrode pairs (Figure 19.2). Each pair records one intracardiac lead and can also be used for pacing. A selection of electrode interspacing is available to register signals over a very localized area (2 mm) or a larger area (5–10 mm) within the chamber. In our experience, 2 or 5 mm electrode interspacing is more appropriate for our patients. Additionally, the tip may be fixed or steerable to simplify catheter manipulation (Figure 19.2).

Catheters for mapping and ablation are slightly larger (7Fr or 8 Fr) and have a variety of deflectable tip shapes. Most commonly, a 4 mm tip is present with three ring electrodes (Figure 19.3).

Additional, more specialized catheters exist, but these are normally sufficient to perform routine EP studies and catheter ablation.

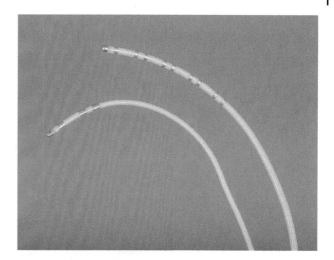

Figure 19.2 Diagnostic electrophysiology catheters. A 6Fr quadripolar (QUAD) 2 mm spaced catheter (lower) and a 6Fr decapolar (DECA) 2-8-2 mm spaced (upper) catheter with fixed tips can be seen.

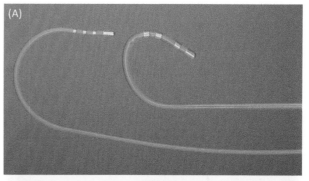

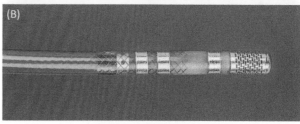

Figure 19.3 Mapping/radiofrequency ablation electrophysiology catheters. (A) 5 Fr and 7Fr bidirectional deflectable 4 mm tip ablation catheters. (B) 8Fr bidirectional deflectable irrigated 4 mm tip ablation catheter. Saline solution is injected through the small openings on the tip of irrigated catheters to provide active cooling; this reduces the likelihood of thrombus and char formation, and enables the creation of larger lesions.

Ideally, a standard EP study would include four catheters: (1) a quadripolar catheter (2 or 5 mm spacing) positioned in contact with the right atrial wall (high right atrium [HRA]), (2) a quadripolar catheter (2 or 5 mm spacing) positioned with the tip in contact with the right ventricular apex (right ventricle [RV]), (3) a decapolar catheter (2-8-2 mm spacing) positioned inside the coronary sinus (CS) and (4) a quadripolar catheter (2 mm spacing) positioned at the level of the atrioventricular junction (straddling the tricuspid annulus on the atrial side) to record His (H) electrograms.

Given the size of our patients in comparison to an adult human, we routinely use three catheters instead of four for our EP studies (Figure 19.4). A decapolar (2-8-2 mm spacing) and a quadripolar (normally 2 mm spacing) are inserted via the jugular access site, and the ablation catheter is used as the third diagnostic electrode via the femoral access site. The decapolar catheter is

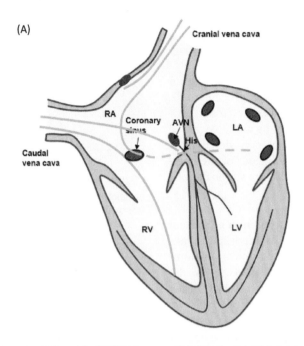

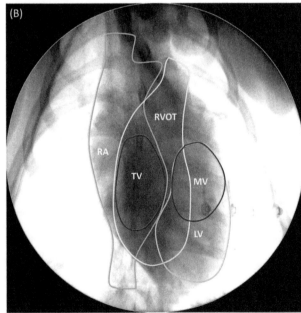

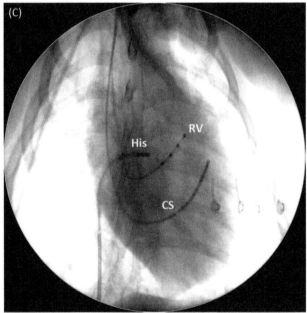

Figure 19.4 Catheter positioning during an electrophysiology study. (A) This diagram illustrates the position of the catheters in a standard four-catheter study. One catheter is positioned against the wall of the right atrium, another is close to the atrioventricular junction (His catheter), another is located inside the coronary sinus (CS) and finally another catheter is positioned inside the right ventricle (RV). (B) Ventrodorsal radiographic view of the chest of a dog during an electrophysiology study. The positions of the various chambers and structures are illustrated. The green line represents the position of the right atrium (RA); the yellow line represents the position of the RV and right ventricular outflow tract (RVOT); the orange line represents the position of the left ventricle (LV); and the red circular lines represent the tricuspid (TV) and the mitral (MV) valves. (C) The position of the three catheters is shown inside the heart in the same patient. One catheter is positioned inside the CS, another is located in the RV towards the RVOT and the other is positioned close the atrioventricular junction (His).

positioned inside the CS, and the remaining catheters are positioned interchangeably at the HRA, His or V positions as necessary. Access to the CS may prove challenging or impossible in smaller patients.

Basic EP Study Protocol

To understand an EP study, it is necessary to take into account the position of each catheter and the underlying rhythm or pacing manoeuvre being undertaken. Figure 19.5 illustrates the electrograms displayed during sinus rhythm in an EP study. At least three approximately orthogonal surface ECG leads (normally, I, aVF and V1) are displayed on the top of the trace. These are very useful to identify the underlying rhythm.

A basic EP study protocol at our EP lab includes the following steps:

1) *Measurement of the spontaneous sinus rate and basic intervals*: With catheters positioned at HRA, H and V,

the conduction intervals are measured across the cardiac conduction system. This may be useful in establishing whether the cause of a short PR is the presence of pre-excitation, or alternatively if a long PR interval is due to a delay in the compact node or the His–Purkinje system. An example of the various measurements can be seen in Figure 19.5.

2) *Ventricular extrastimulus testing*: Since the majority of EP studies in our patients are aimed at the diagnosis of supraventricular arrhythmias, it is advantageous to start by performing ventricular pacing manoeuvres before attempting atrial pacing, as the latter is more likely to induce atrial arrhythmias, including atrial fibrillation. Ventricular pacing also has the advantage of disclosing the presence of an AP at an early stage. The basic concept is that a ventricular pacing stimulus that is conducted retrogradely to the atria (VA conduction) has to travel up the Purkinje–His and AVN to reach the atria unless an AP is present. During

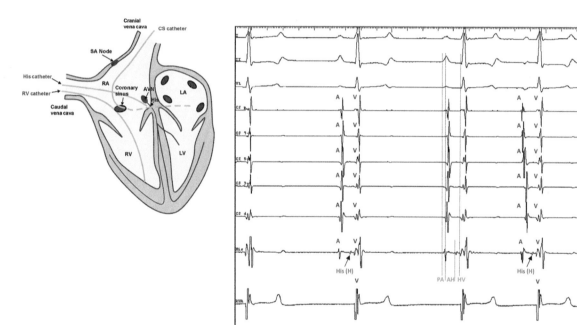

Figure 19.5 Intracardiac electrograms during sinus rhythm and basic intervals. The illustration on the left shows the position of each catheter inside the heart. A decapolar catheter is positioned inside the coronary sinus (CS catheter) and records both atrial (A) and ventricular (V) electrograms along the left heart chambers. A quadripolar catheter is positioned in the area adjacent to the atrioventricular node (His catheter). It records atrial (A) and ventricular (V) electrograms as well as a His potential (H) originating from the tissue adjacent to the His bundle. Finally, a third catheter is positioned in the apex of the right ventricle (RVA). This electrode records ventricular (V) electrograms. These electrograms may be seen in the figure on the right. Leads I, II and V1 of the surface electrocardiographic leads are shown on the top for clarity. Basic intervals may be measured during the electrophysiology study, illustrating the conduction of the electrical impulse through the heart as follows: PA is the interval between the earliest atrial impulse (atrial electrogram on a high right atrial catheter [not present in this case] or the onset of the P wave on the surface electrocardiogram) and the atrial electrogram on the His catheter; it represents the time it takes for the impulse to travel from one fixed point in the atrium to another, and if prolonged suggests a delay in intra-atrial conduction. AH is the interval between the atrial and His electrograms on the His catheter; it represents the time it takes for the impulse to travel over the atrioventricular node. HV is the interval between the His electrogram and the earliest recorded ventricular activation; it represents the time it takes for the impulse to travel through the His–Purkinje system. The sum of PA, AH and HV corresponds to the PR interval on the surface electrocardiogram. Unfortunately, reference values are not yet available in dogs. SA, Sinoatrial node; LA, left atrium; LV, left ventricle; RA, right atrium; RV, right ventricle; AVN, atrioventricular node; His, bundle of His. [1-year-old, male Cocker Spaniel dog]

the study, the earliest site of atrial retrograde activation is assessed. If the impulse travels up the AVN, this would be at the His catheter, signalling a "normal" (concentric) pattern of retrograde activation (Figure 19.6). If an AP is present, allowing the impulse to reach the atria via a route other than the AVN, the earliest site of retrograde atrial activation will be seen elsewhere (e.g. HRA with a right-side AP and distal CS with a left-side AP). This is termed an *eccentric retrograde activation pattern* (Figure 19.6). A concentric retrograde activation pattern that is non-decremental or shows discontinuity may also signal the presence of an AP with the atrial insertion at or close to the junctional area. If VA conduction is completely absent, atrioventricular reentrant tachycardia (AVRT) or AV nodal re-entry can be ruled out.

- *How is the ventricular extrastimulus test done?*

  A train of eight paced beats (S1) is delivered at a fixed cycle (400–600 ms) and is followed by a premature beat (S2) with a progressively shorter coupling interval (usually, from 400 ms to as low as 200 ms). The aim is to achieve a steady state of the cardiac tissue with the S1 beats and induce tissue refractoriness with an S2 that is premature enough. When tissue refractoriness occurs, either ventricular capture does not occur or VA conduction is interrupted at some point (Purkinje–His–AVN).

- *Why?*
  - Test retrograde conduction over Purkinje–His–AVN.
  - Detect an AP.
  - Induce arrhythmia.
- *What happens?*
  The VA interval of S2 becomes progressively larger than the VA interval of S1 with shorter coupling intervals until block occurs (no A after V).

3) *Atrial extrastimulus testing*: After ventricular pacing manoeuvres are performed, atrial pacing can be done.

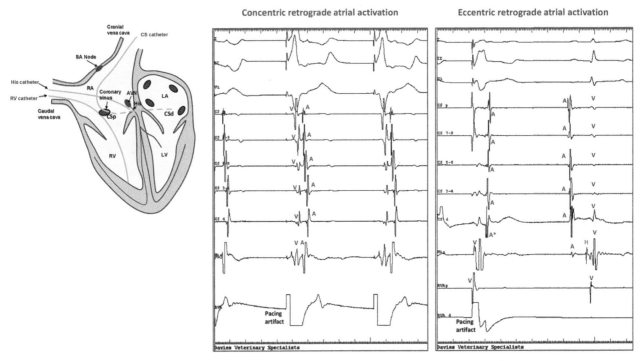

Concentric retrograde atrial activation Eccentric retrograde atrial activation

Figure 19.6 Retrograde atrial activation pattern. The illustration on the left shows the position of each catheter inside the heart. A decapolar catheter is positioned inside the coronary sinus (CS catheter) and records both atrial (A) and ventricular (V) electrograms along the left heart chambers. A quadripolar catheter is positioned in the area adjacent to the atrioventricular node (His catheter). It records A and V electrograms as well as a His potential (H) originating from the tissue adjacent to the His bundle. Finally, a third catheter is positioned in the apex of the right ventricle (RVA). This electrode records V electrograms. Concentric and eccentric retrograde atrial activation are illustrated on the right. A pacing stimulus is delivered on the apex of the right ventricle (pacing artefact on RV catheter), and the retrograde impulse conduction may be followed. With *concentric retrograde atrial activation*, the impulse travels up the Purkinje–His to reach the atria retrogradely via the atrioventricular node. The earliest atrial impulse is seen at the His catheter and is followed by CSp before progressively heading towards CSd as the impulse travels from the right atrium to the left atrium. [1-year-old, male Cocker Spaniel with focal atrial tachycardia] With *eccentric retrograde atrial activation*, the earliest atrial impulse is not seen at the His catheter, signalling that the impulse did not reach the atria via the atrioventricular node. In this example from a dog with a left-sided accessory pathway, the earliest atrial activation (A*) is seen at CSd. The impulse subsequently travels progressively towards CSp from the left atrium to the right atrium. In this case, an atrial wave is not seen on the His catheter due to retrograde block at the level of the atrioventricular node, but if present it would appear after or at the same time as CSp. SA, Sinoatrial node; LA, left atrium; LV, left ventricle; RA, right atrium; RV, right ventricle; AVN, atrioventricular node; His, bundle of His; CSp, coronary sinus proximal electrode; CSd, coronary sinus distal electrode. [3-year-old, male Labrador Retriever with orthodromic atrioventricular reciprocating tachycardia]

The technique is the same as for ventricular extrastimulus pacing with a train of eight beats at a fixed cycle (S1) followed by an extrastimulus (S2) with a progressively shorter coupling interval. Tissue refractoriness occurs when the atrium is no longer captured or when AV conduction is interrupted.

- *Why?*
  - Observe dynamic properties of conduction over the AVN and His–Purkinje (e.g. decremental conduction – see chapter 2).
  - Observe refractory periods of the AVN and right atrial myocardium.
  - Detect gross abnormalities of intra-atrial and intraventricular conduction.
  - Demonstrate dual AV nodal physiology or APs.
  - Induce arrhythmias.
- *What happens?*
  An AH or AV interval of S2 becomes progressively larger than an AH or AV interval of S1 with shorter coupling intervals until block occurs (no H or V after A).

4) *Incremental pacing*: Another pacing manoeuvre that can be useful is incremental pacing (atrial or ventricular). This consists in pacing continuously at a rate just above the spontaneous rhythm that is progressively increased (e.g. at progressively shorter coupling intervals between successive paced beats). It can be used to measure impulse conduction and tissue refractoriness during steady-state conditions as well as recovery of normal function. Arrhythmias may also be induced or terminated.

Additional comments: Sinus node function tests can also be performed if abnormal function is suspected (e.g. sick sinus syndrome); however, this is not a common indication for an EP study in our patients.

Basic intervals

Record the cycle length immediately preceding the complex to be measured during stable rhythm:

1) *PA interval*: From P or earliest atrial electrogram to A on His catheter (first intrinsic deflection); indicates the time it takes for intra-atrial conduction

2) *AH interval*: From atrial electrogram (intrinsic deflection) on His catheter to His electrogram (earliest onset); indicates the time it takes for an impulse to travel through the AVN; varies with autonomic tone or drugs; decremental conduction

3) *HV interval*: From onset of His electrogram to earliest ventricular activation (normally beginning of QRS on the surface ECG); represents the time taken for conduction over His–Purkinje.

PA + AH + HV = PR interval and indicate, respectively, how much time is spent in atrial conduction, AV node and His–Purkinje.

Radiofrequency Catheter Ablation

The most common type of catheter ablation uses radiofrequency (RF) energy delivered through a small electrode that heats the tissue to the point of necrosis. Alternating electrical current is delivered between the catheter tip and an indifferent electrode (a grounding patch attached to the skin of the patient). The temperature delivered usually ranges from 50 to 90 °C with a target between 50 and 60 °C. Tissue temperatures of at least 50 °C are necessary to cause irreversible damage to the tissue.[7] Injury is caused through resistive heating of the superficial layers of tissue in contact with the catheter via oscillations of ions produced directly by the electrical current. This only affects tissue in close contact with the tip of the catheter (1–2 mm).[8] Deeper lesions are obtained through conductive heating as heat propagates from this small area to adjacent tissue (normally, up to 5–7 mm).[7–9] The size of the lesion will depend on the duration of the ablation and the resistance (impedance) to heat propagation. During this process, heat is also transmitted to the surrounding blood with risk of coagulation and potential serious side effects. To avoid this, the surface temperature is monitored. Coagulation of the blood around the catheter tip may cause an increase in impedance and a less effective ablation. The use of irrigated catheters circumvents this problem by cooling the electrode tip via injection of saline solution as ablation is taking place (Figure 19.3B). This is particularly useful when targeting structures located deep in the myocardium, as a larger lesion size is made possible whilst reducing the likelihood of thrombus and char formation.[10–12]

Other forms of energy may be used for ablation, such as cryothermal energy (cryoablation), ultrasound, laser and microwaves.[13]

Risks and Complications

RF ablation is considered very safe and effective in human medicine. Possible complications may be associated with: (1) vascular access and catheter manipulation (blood vessel/cardiac structure damage, pericardial effusion, pneumothorax, haemorrhage/haematoma, etc.), (2) during energy delivery (atrioventricular block, thromboembolism, pericarditis, vessel/cardiac/oesophageal wall damage) or (3) other (infection, radiation exposure).[14] Major complications with contemporary ablation techniques have been reported in 0.8 to 6.0% of cases depending on the type of procedure performed.[15] The risk of complications was found to be lower for supraventricular tachycardias (SVTs; 0.8%) in comparison to atrial fibrillation (5.2%) and ventricular tachycardia (3.4% without structural disease and 6.0% with structural disease). The occurrence of procedure-related deaths is very low at around 0.1%, with myocardial infarction and thromboembolic events occurring in up to 0.5% of cases with SVT.[15–17] This information is lacking in veterinary medicine. A complication rate of 6.2% was reported in a well-established veterinary EP lab but without mention of the type of complications encountered.[18] Thus far, in our EP laboratory, we have encountered one complication in 14 cases during RF ablation consisting of a skin burn caused by inadvertent detachment of the RF grounding patch from the patient's skin. Induction of atrial fibrillation during atrial pacing manoeuvres was observed in two cases, with spontaneous conversion in one and successful electrical cardioversion in the other.

Success Rates

The overall success rate of RF ablation is high.

Ablation of AVRT and Accessory Pathways

In human medicine, acute success for treatment of AVRT is typically achieved in over 90% of cases. The rate of success is higher for left-sided free wall APs (96% with 2–5% recurrence) and lower for right-sided free wall APs (90% with 9–16.7% recurrence).[19] Ablation of septal APs is normally achieved in 93–98% of the cases, with recurrence in approximately 12–15% of cases but ranging from 6 to 50% for caudal-septal (posteroseptal) pathways.[20,21] A 1% risk of complete AV block with mid-septal pathways has been reported during ablation of mid-septal pathways, although transient block may be seen in up to 5% of cases. In veterinary medicine, an acute success rate of 98% with 4.5% recurrence has been reported.[18] In the author's EP laboratory, an acute success rate was observed in all cases treated so far with one recurrence (1/12).

Ablation of Focal Atrial Tachycardia

In humans, a success rate ranging from 69 to 100% has been reported for ablation of focal atrial tachycardia (FAT), with a low recurrence rate of up to 7%.[22] In veterinary medicine, an acute success rate of 79% has been reported with recurrence in 2% of cases.[18]

Ablation of Atrial Flutter

In the case of cavotricuspid isthmus–dependent atrial flutter, a success rate of 90–95% may be achieved with use of large (8–10 mm) or irrigated-tip catheters with a recurrence rate of 6.7%.[23,24] With smaller catheters (4–6 mm), the reported acute success rate is lower at 78–92% with a recurrence rate of 14%.[23,24] Most recurrences occur within 6 months from the procedure.[24] An acute success rate of 100% with recurrence in up to 15% of cases has been reported in veterinary medicine.[5,6,18]

Procedure and Technical Aspects

RF energy is produced by a generator and is delivered by a steerable catheter with a thermocoupled tip (Figure 19.3). The temperature of the tip, the power output and the impedance are constantly monitored during RF ablation. A sudden increase in impedance may be observed from boiling of blood at the interface between the catheter and be heard as a 'tissue pop'. RF ablation should be stopped immediately in this instance; the same should occur if catheter displacement occurs during ablation. Different temperature, energy and time combinations may be used, but normally a maximum of 65 °C and 75 W applied for 60 s should not be exceeded.

EP Study and RF Ablation Examples

Orthodromic Atrioventricular Reciprocating Tachycardia (OAVRT)

Step 1. Is there an Accessory Pathway?

The existence of pre-excitation (Figure 19.7) or eccentric retrograde activation during sinus rhythm (Figure 19.8), ventricular or para-Hisian pacing confirms the presence of an AP.

Step 2. Is the Accessory Pathway Involved in the Tachycardia?

AVRT typically starts when a beat is blocked at the AP, conducts to the ventricle via the AVN and normal conduction system, and then returns to the atria retrogradely via the AP starting macro re-entry. Atrial extrastimulus testing can be used to initiate AVRT (Figure 19.9) during the EP study, and the sequence of events can be examined. Observing tachycardia termination is also useful, as most commonly AVN-dependent tachycardias such as AVRT often terminate with AV block, and therefore the last intracardiac signal is an atrial signal. However, block at the AP may also occur. Tachycardia termination during AVRT may be achieved by a ventricular paced beat that is delivered when the His bundle is refractory and that does not reach the atria. The impulse is blocked at both the AVN and AP, proving that the ventricle and therefore an AP are part of the re-entry circuit.

Step 3. Locating the AP (mapping)

Once an AP and its involvement in the tachycardia mechanism are confirmed, the ablation catheter is used to find its location. Using the other catheters as reference, the aim is to find the site where earliest atrial activation occurs during tachycardia or ventricular pacing (Figure 19.10), or the site where earliest ventricular activation occurs during sinus rhythm and atrial pacing for AP that are capable of anterograde conduction (Figure 19.11). The mapping catheter is positioned on the tricuspid or mitral annulus, depending on whether a right or left AP is present, and is moved along the annulus to determine in which direction the earliest activation occurs. As it comes closer to the location of the AP, the A and V signals become fused and are hard to distinguish.

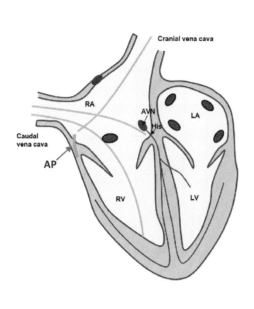

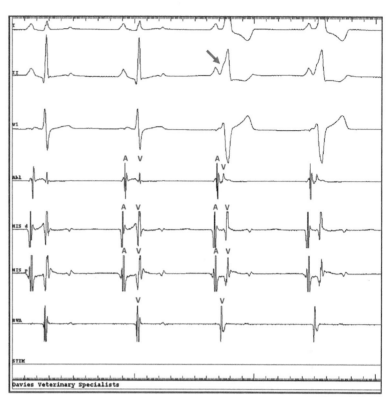

Figure 19.7 Ventricular pre-excitation. The illustration on the left shows the position of the catheters inside the heart, and the corresponding intracardiac signals are displayed on the right. The ablation catheter (Abl) is positioned in the tricuspid annulus close to the accessory pathway (AP); another catheter is positioned close to the atrioventricular junction (His); and, finally, a third catheter is positioned at the apex of the right ventricle (RVA). The first two beats are conducted normally via the conduction system, and the last two beats exhibit ventricular pre-excitation. Atrial signals (A) and ventricular signals (V) may be seen on the ablation and His catheters in correspondence to the P wave and QRS on the surface ECG. A ventricular signal is only seen on the RVA catheter in correspondence to the QRS. In the absence of pre-excitation, an interval is seen between A and V that corresponds to the delay in conduction via the atrioventricular node. In the pre-excited beats, ventricular depolarisation (V) is first seen at the site of the ablation and RVA catheters with a V shortly after the A on the ablation catheter. At the site of the His catheter, the normal gap between A and V is seen as the impulse travels through the atrioventricular node. Note that ventricular activation (V) is seen first at RVA and then His, in contrast with the normally conducted beats. This means that the impulse reached the right ventricular apex via the accessory pathway before the normally conducted impulse exited the atrioventricular node. A delta wave (arrow) may be seen on the surface ECG in the pre-excited beats. LA, Left atrium; LV, left ventricle; RA, right atrium; RV, right ventricle; AVN, atrioventricular node; His, bundle of His; AP, accessory pathway. [3-year-old, male neutered, Labrador Retriever with OAVRT]

Step 4. RF Ablation of the Atrial or Ventricular Insertion of the AP

When the site of the AP is located, ablation is performed whilst examining the intracardiac signals. Loss of conduction through the AP is signalled by a loss of A and V fusion and termination of tachycardia, or development of AV block during ventricular pacing, or loss of pre-excitation, depending on whether ablation is performed during tachycardia or sinus rhythm (Figure 19.12).

Step 5. Was the AP Successfully Ablated?

To ensure that the AP was successfully ablated, the EP study is repeated approximately 30 min after ablation. This includes ventricular and atrial extrastimulus testing to look for eccentric atrial retrograde conduction and tachycardia initiation. The purpose of waiting before repeating the EP study is to allow for recovery of function of any reminiscent AP tissue that might still be present

but unable to function due to inflammation caused by ablation – in other words, tissue that was damaged by ablation but not completely destroyed and that might recover function.

Focal Atrial Tachycardia and Atrial Flutter

Step 1. Ventricular Extrastimulus Testing

The absence of eccentric retrograde atrial activation during ventricular extrastimulus testing suggests that an accessory pathway is not present and that another supraventricular arrhythmia should be investigated. Concentric retrograde atrial activation is seen in most patients during ventricular pacing, although in some there is absence of ventriculo-atrial conduction. During tachycardia, the delivery of premature ventricular paced beats with the intent of causing AVN refractoriness (block) does not terminate FAT or atrial flutter, as they

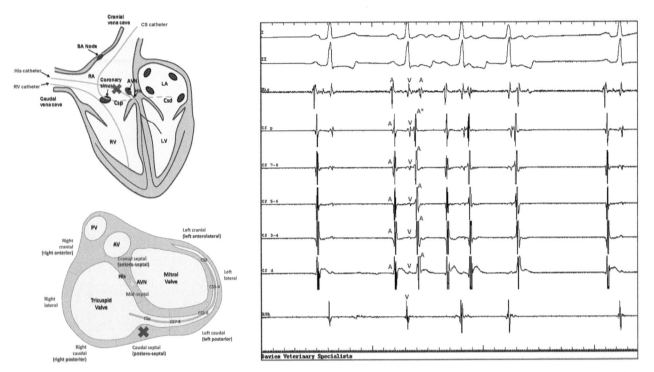

Figure 19.8 Eccentric retrograde atrial activation. The illustration on the left shows the position of the catheters inside the heart, and the corresponding intracardiac signals are displayed on the right. One catheter is positioned in the coronary sinus (CS), another catheter is positioned close to the atrioventricular junction (His) and a third catheter is positioned at the apex of the right ventricle (RVA). The first, second, third and fifth beats are sinus beats, and the fourth beat was a result of macro re-entry. Notice the presence of eccentric retrograde atrial activation on the second, third and fourth beats (the presence of A after V) with the earliest atrial signal at CSp rather than His, as this is the electrode that is closest to the accessory pathway (red cross on the illustrations on the left). On the fourth beat, ventricular activation (V) follows the previous retrograde eccentric atrial activation signalling macro re-entry. SA, Sinoatrial node; LA, left atrium; LV, left ventricle; RA, right atrium; RV, right ventricle; AVN, atrioventricular node; His, bundle of His; PV, pulmonic valve; AV, aortic valve; CSp, coronary sinus proximal electrode; CSd, coronary sinus distal electrode. [1-year-old, male Rottweiler dog with OAVRT]

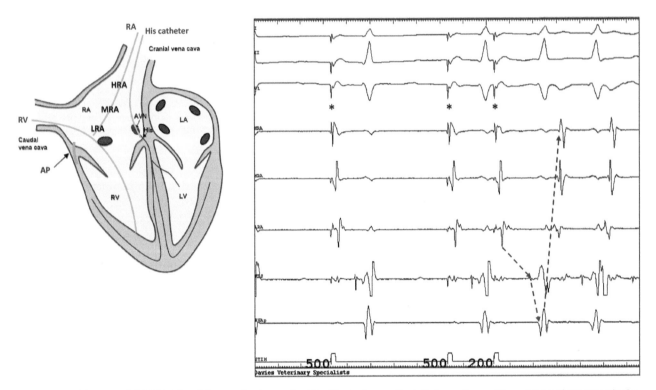

Figure 19.9 Initiation of OAVRT with atrial extrastimulus testing. The illustration on the left shows the position of the catheters inside the heart, and the corresponding intracardiac signals are displayed on the right. Catheters are positioned in the right atrium (HRA, high right atrium; MRA, middle right atrium; LRA, low right atrium), close to the atrioventricular junction (His), and at the apex of the right ventricle (RVA). The end of a train of eight paced beats (S1) with an interval of 500 ms is seen with a premature beat (S2) with a coupling interval of 200 ms. The pacing impulses (*) are delivered via the HRA catheter. Note that the premature beat has resulted in an atrioventricular conduction delay (longer AH interval) and is followed by retrograde eccentric atrial activation and subsequent His and ventricular activation initiating re-entry. LA, Left atrium; LV, left ventricle; RA, right atrium; RV, right ventricle; AVN, atrioventricular node; His, bundle of His; AP, accessory pathway. [6-month-old, male Staffordshire Bull Terrier with OAVRT]

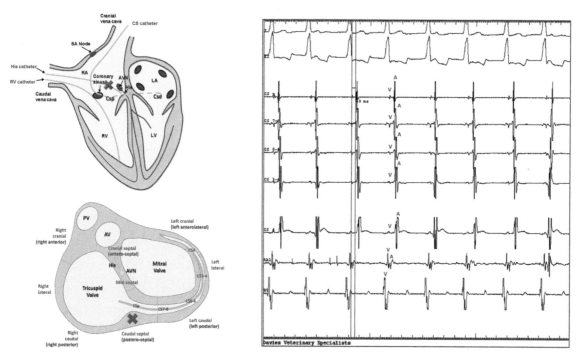

Figure 19.10 Accessory pathway mapping during tachycardia. The illustration on the left shows the position of the catheters inside the heart, and the corresponding intracardiac signals are displayed on the right. One catheter is positioned inside the coronary sinus (CS – decapolar), another catheter is positioned at the apex of right ventricle (RVA) and the ablation catheter is positioned along the annulus of the tricuspid valve in an attempt to locate the exact position of the accessory pathway using the CS catheter as reference. The earliest site of atrial activation is investigated (distance from A at the ablation catheter in relation to earliest A in the CS catheter which in this case occurs at CSp, as this is the electrode that is closest to the accessory pathway). SA, Sinoatrial node; LA, left atrium; LV, left ventricle; RA, right atrium; RV, right ventricle; AVN, atrioventricular node; His, bundle of His; PV, pulmonic valve; AV, aortic valve; CSp, coronary sinus proximal electrode; CSd, coronary sinus distal electrode. [1-year-old, male Rottweiler dog with OAVRT]

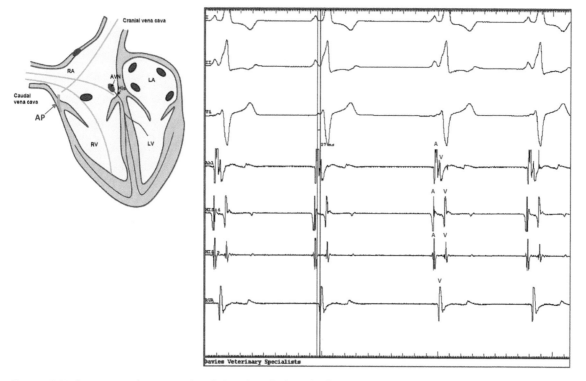

Figure 19.11 Accessory pathway mapping during sinus rhythm. The illustration on the left shows the position of the catheters inside the heart, and the corresponding intracardiac signals are displayed on the right. One catheter is positioned close to the atrioventricular junction (His), another catheter is positioned at the apex of the right ventricle (RVA) and the ablation catheter is positioned along the annulus of the tricuspid valve to locate the exact position of the accessory pathway. During sinus rhythm with pre-excitation, the earliest site of ventricular activation is at the level of the accessory pathway and occurs before the impulse reaches the RVA catheter. The earliest site of ventricular activation is investigated (distance from the beginning of V at the ablation catheter in relation to the beginning of V in the RVA catheter) and will signal the position of the pathway. LA, Left atrium; LV, left ventricle; RA, right atrium; RV, right ventricle; AVN, atrioventricular node; His, bundle of His; AP, accessory pathway. [1-year-old, male Rottweiler dog with OAVRT]

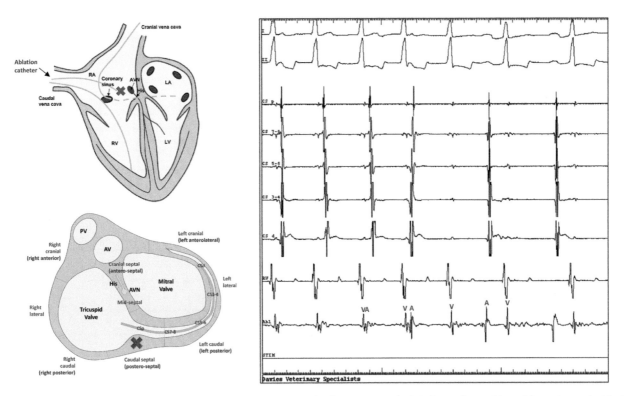

Figure 19.12 Radiofrequency ablation of the accessory pathway. The illustration on the left shows the position of the catheters inside the heart, and the corresponding intracardiac signals are displayed on the right. One catheter is positioned inside the coronary sinus (CS – decapolar), another catheter is positioned at the apex of the right ventricle (RVA) and the ablation catheter is now positioned over the accessory pathway. At the tip of the ablation catheter, fusion of the ventricular (V) and atrial (A) signals is seen during tachycardia. After the fourth beat, retrograde atrial activation is no longer seen (no atrial signals on the CS catheter after V or QRS), and the V and A signals on the ablation catheter become separated. This was the moment where conduction through the accessory pathway was interrupted with successful ablation and tachycardia termination with a return to sinus rhythm. LA, Left atrium; LV, left ventricle; RA, right atrium; RV, right ventricle; AVN, atrioventricular node; His, bundle of His; PV, pulmonic valve; AV, aortic valve. [1-year-old, male Rottweiler dog with OAVRT]

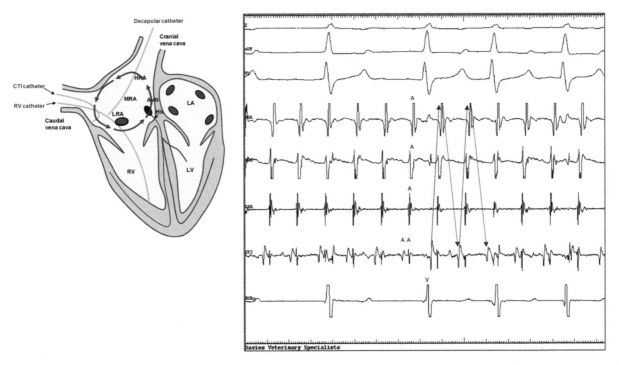

Figure 19.13 Intracardiac signals recorded during atrial flutter. The illustration on the left shows the position of the catheters inside the heart, and the corresponding intracardiac signals are displayed on the right. One catheter is positioned inside the right atrium (HRA, high right atrium; MRA, middle right atrium; LRA, low right atrium), another catheter is positioned at the apex of the right ventricle (RVA) and another catheter is positioned over the cavotricuspid isthmus (CTI). The flutter waves on the surface electrocardiogram are barely visible, but the intracardiac signals show an atrial activation with an anticlockwise direction from CTI to LRA, MRA, HRA and back to CTI. A double potential is seen at CTI as both the descending and ascending wavefronts spreading across the atrium are recorded with a line of block at this point. The cycle length of the atrial activation is 125 ms (480 bpm) with a 3:1 to 4:1 atrioventricular conduction (125–200 bpm). LA, Left atrium; LV, left ventricle; RV, right ventricle; AVN, atrioventricular node; His, bundle of His. [8-year-old, male Northern Inuit dog with atrial flutter and focal atrial tachycardia secondary to structural heart disease]

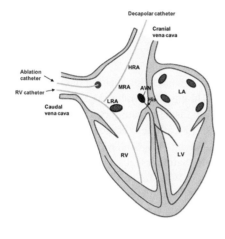

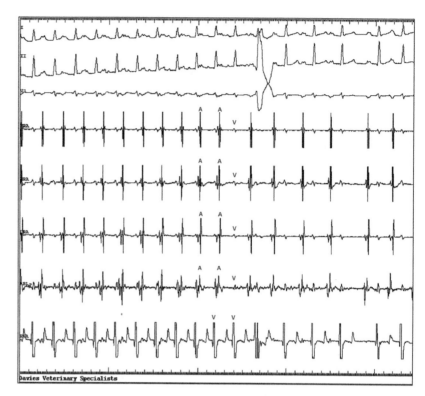

Figure 19.14 Intracardiac signals recorded at the moment of RF ablation of focal atrial tachycardia. The illustration on the left shows the position of the catheters inside the heart, and the corresponding intracardiac signals are displayed on the right. One catheter is positioned inside the right atrium (HRA, high right atrium; MRA, middle right atrium; LRA, low right atrium), another catheter is positioned at the apex of the right ventricle (RVA) and the ablation catheter is positioned over the atrial ectopic focus in the right atrium. From beats 1 to 11, focal atrial tachycardia is seen with a cycle length of 220 ms (272 bpm) and 1:1 atrioventricular conduction. The ectopic P' may be seen just after the QRS on the surface ECG, with the corresponding atrial signals (A) recorded on the right atrium and ablation catheters. On beat 11, atrial signals are no longer seen, and only a far-field ventricular signal is seen on these catheters (V). This was the moment at which successful ablation of the ectopic focus was achieved, and a sinus rhythm may be seen from beat 12 onwards. LA, Left atrium; LV, left ventricle; RV, right ventricle; AVN, atrioventricular node; His, bundle of His. [3-year-old, male neutered, Hamilton Hound dog with multifocal atrial tachycardia]

are independent from AVN conduction. This may also be tested by administering drugs that slow AVN conduction (e.g. diltiazem, verapamil and adenosine in humans).

Step 2. Atrial Extrastimulus Testing or Incremental Atrial Pacing

Initiation of FAT or atrial flutter may be achieved with atrial extrastimulus testing or incremental atrial pacing. The atrial activation pattern may then be examined during tachycardia. In typical atrial flutter, the re-entrant circuit is present in the right atrium (Figure 19.13). The wavefront travels in a circle along the tricuspid annulus and CS, up the interatrial septum, across the roof of the right atrium and then downwards and laterally between the tricuspid valve and the crista terminalis to reach the cavotricuspid isthmus (see chapter 8). In FAT, the earli-

est atrial activation site during tachycardia is investigated by moving the ablation catheter along the atrial wall and using the CS catheter as reference.

Step 3. RF Ablation

- *Atrial flutter*: In typical flutter, ablation of the cavotricuspid isthmus is performed to interrupt the re-entrant circuit.
- *FAT*: In FAT, ablation is performed at the site of earliest atrial activation during tachycardia (Figure 19.14).

Step 4. EP Study

EP study is repeated approximately 30 min after RF ablation.

Recommended Reading

Murgatroyd F, Krahn A, Klein GJ, Yee RK, Skanes AC. Handbook of cardiac electrophysiology: a practical guide to invasive EP studies and catheter ablation. London: Remedica; 2002.

References

1 Wright KN, Mehdirad AA, Giacobbe P, Grubb T, Maxson T. Radiofrequency catheter ablation of atrioventricular accessory pathways in 3 dogs with subsequent resolution of tachycardia-induced cardiomyopathy. J Vet Intern Med. 1999;13:361–371.

2 Wright KN. Interventional catheterization for tachyarrhythmias. Vet Clin North Am Small Anim Pract. 2004;34:1171–1185.

3 Santilli RA, Spadacini G, Moretti P, Perego M, Perini A, Tarducci A, *et al*. Radiofrequency catheter ablation of concealed accessory pathways in two dogs with symptomatic atrioventricular reciprocating tachycardia. J Vet Cardiol. 2006;8:157–165.

4 Santilli RA, Perego M, Perini A, Moretti P, Spadacini G. Electrophysiologic characteristics and topographic distribution of focal atrial tachycardias in dogs. J Vet Intern Med. 2010;24:539–545.

5 Santilli RA, Perego M, Perini A, Carli A, Moretti P, Spadacini G. Radiofrequency catheter ablation of cavo-tricuspid isthmus as treatment of atrial flutter in two dogs. J Vet Cardiol. 2010;12:59–66.

6 Santilli RA, Ramera L, Perego M, Moretti P, Spadacini G. Radiofrequency catheter ablation of atypical atrial flutter in dogs. J Vet Cardiol. 2014;16:9–17.

7 Haines DE, Watson DD. Tissue heating during radiofrequency catheter ablation: a thermodynamic model and observations in isolated perfused and superfused canine right ventricular free wall. Pacing Clin Electrophysiol. 1989;12:962–976.

8 Murgatroyd FD, Krahn AD, Klein GJ, Yee R, Skanes AC. In Handbook of cardiac electrophysiology (vol. 1, pp. 176–179). London: Remedica; 2002.

9 Haines DE, Verow AF. Observations on electrode-tissue interface temperature and effect on electrical impedance during radiofrequency ablation of ventricular myocardium. Circulation. 1990;82:1034–1038.

10 Müssigbrodt A, Grothoff M, Dinov B, Kosiuk J, Richter S, Sommer P, *et al*. Irrigated tip catheters for radiofrequency ablation in ventricular tachycardia. Biomed Res Int. 2015;2015:389294–6.

11 Ramoul K, Wright M, Sohal M, Shah A, Castro-Rodriguez J, Verbeet T, *et al*. Does diffuse irrigation result in improved radiofrequency catheter ablation? A prospective randomized study of right atrial typical flutter ablation. Europace. 2015;17:295–299.

12 Nguyen DT, Olson M, Zheng L, Barham W, Moss JD, Sauer WH. Effect of irrigant characteristics on lesion formation after radiofrequency energy delivery using

ablation catheters with actively cooled tips. J Cardio Electrophysiol. 2015;26:792–798.

13 Doshi SK, Reddy VY. In Catheter ablation of cardiac arrhythmias (eds. Huang SKS, Miller JM, vol. 1, pp. 69–84). Amsterdam: Elsevier Saunders; 2015.

14 Yamada T, Kay GN. In Catheter ablation of cardiac arrhythmias (eds. Huang SKS, Miller JM, pp. 685–701). Amsterdam: Elsevier Saunders; 2015.

15 Bohnen M, Stevenson WG, Tedrow UB, Michaud GF, John RM, Epstein LM, *et al*. Incidence and predictors of major complications from contemporary catheter ablation to treat cardiac arrhythmias. Heart Rhythm. 2011;8:1661–1666.

16 Manolis AS, Vassilikos V, Maounis TN, Chiladakis J, Cokkinos DV. Radiofrequency ablation in pediatric and adult patients: comparative results. J Interv Card Electrophysiol. 2001;5:443–453.

17 Hindricks G. The Multicentre European Radiofrequency Survey (MERFS): complications of radiofrequency catheter ablation of arrhythmias. The Multicentre European Radiofrequency Survey (MERFS) investigators of the Working Group on Arrhythmias of the European Society of Cardiology. Eur Heart J. 1993;14:1644–1653.

18 Santilli R, Perego M. In Veterinary image-guided interventions (eds. Weisse C, Berent A, pp. 531–540). Hoboken: John Wiley & Sons, Inc.; 2015.

19 Shepard RK, Wood MA. In Catheter ablation of cardiac arrhythmias (eds. Huang SKS, Miller JM, pp. 421–446). Amsterdam: Elsevier Saunders; 2015.

20 Kalahasty G, Wood MA. In Catheter ablation of cardiac arrhythmias (eds. Huang SKS, Miller JM, pp. 447–460). Amsterdam: Elsevier Saunders; 2015.

21 Miller JM, Das MK, Jain R, Bhakta D. In Catheter ablation of cardiac arrhythmias (eds. Huang SKS, Miller JM, pp. 461–473). Amsterdam: Elsevier Saunders; 2015.

22 Kalman JM, Nisbet AM, Teh AW, Roberts-Thomson KC. In Catheter ablation of cardiac arrhythmias (eds. Huang SKS, Miller JM, pp. 183–202). Amsterdam: Elsevier Saunders; 2015.

23 Feld GK, McGarry T, Olson N, Lalani G, Schricker A. In Catheter ablation of cardiac arrhythmias (eds. Huang SKS, Miller JM, pp. 203–231). Amsterdam: Elsevier Saunders; 2015.

24 Pérez FJ, Schubert CM, Parvez B, Pathak V, Ellenbogen KA, Wood MA. Long-term outcomes after catheter ablation of cavo-tricuspid isthmus dependent atrial flutter: a meta-analysis. Circ Arrhythm Electrophysiol. 2009;2:393–401.

20

Arrhythmias in Canine Cardiomyopathies and Valvular Heart Disease

Gerhard Wess and Marin Torti

Introduction

Dilated cardiomyopathy (DCM) is an important cause of cardiac morbidity and mortality in dogs and is the most commonly acquired cardiac disorder in medium-sized, large and giant-breed dogs. In most cases, DCM is a genetic disease, even if the disease has a slow onset and is usually detected later in life, in middle-aged or older dogs. DCM is the most common cause of congestive heart failure (CHF) and sudden cardiac death (SCD) in medium-sized and large-breed dogs.[1]

Both European and North American studies have shown that Doberman Pinschers are one of the most commonly affected breeds with DCM, and in this breed DCM is an inherited, slowly progressive primary myocardial disease.[2] Furthermore, DCM has been described in other dog breeds as well, namely in Boxers, Newfoundland Dogs, Airedale Terriers, Portuguese Water Dogs, Great Danes, Saint Bernard Dogs, Cocker Spaniels and Irish Wolfhounds.[3]

The natural progression of DCM can be described by three distinct stages:[2]

- *Stage I* is characterised by a morphologically and electrically normal heart; there is no evidence or clinical signs of heart disease in a predisposed breed, but the disease is already present at a cellular or genetic level. Currently, this stage cannot be detected.
- *Stage II* is characterised by evidence of cardiac remodelling or arrhythmias but without clinical signs of heart disease. This stage is known as the *occult, preclinical* or *silent* stage of disease. These terms refer to the owner's perspective that the dog appears normal despite evidence of cardiac abnormalities on further testing. The morphological changes consist of left ventricular (LV) enlargement in systole, diastole or both.[3] Arrhythmias such as ventricular premature contractions or complexes (VPCs) or atrial fibrillation may be documented during this phase. The cardiac remodelling and arrhythmias may coexist or be of

predominantly one form at any time during the pre-clinical stage.[1,2]

- *Stage III* is characterised by the presence of clinical signs of heart failure and is referred to as the *overt* or *clinical* stage of DCM. Whereas the first and second stages can persist for years, stage III has often a comparatively short duration of several months, after the development of CHF.[4,5]

Detection of early stages of the disease is important for each specific dog as well as for all dogs of a particular breed, given the desire to perpetuate breeding programs that result in healthy dogs. Whilst detecting the clinical stage of the disease when the dogs develop clinical signs of left or right heart failure (consisting of pulmonary oedema or ascites and pleural effusion, respectively) is comparatively easy, this is only the tip of an iceberg, as recognition of the pre-clinical phase of the disease is much more challenging.

For breeding purposes as well as for initiating drug therapy to delay the progression of the disease,[5] it is mandatory to detect and identify the early stages of the disease. To diagnose pre-clinical disease in an individual dog, it is necessary to know the prevalence of DCM and early clinical signs for specific dog breeds in the pre-clinical phase of DCM.

Arrhythmias accompanying canine DCM are wide-ranging: from atrial premature contractions and paroxysmal supraventricular tachycardia to atrial fibrillation, VPCs and ventricular tachyarrhythmia.[2,3]

Arrhythmias in Breed-specific Cardiomyopathies

Doberman Pinscher Cardiomyopathy

Doberman Pinschers are one of the most commonly affected breeds, and DCM in this breed is an inherited, slowly progressive primary myocardial disease.[1,6–9]

Guide to Canine and Feline Electrocardiography, First Edition. Ruth Willis, Pedro Oliveira and Antonia Mavropoulou.
Companion website: www.wiley.com/go/willis/electrocardiography

The pre-clinical stage of the disease is characterised by evidence of cardiac remodelling and/or arrhythmias in the absence of clinical signs of heart disease.[1,10–13] The echocardiographic changes include left ventricular (LV) enlargement in systole and later in diastole. VPCs are a common finding in the pre-clinical phase of DCM in Doberman Pinschers.[14] SCD, caused by ventricular tachycardia (VT) or ventricular fibrillation, occurs during the pre-clinical phase in at least 25 to 30% of affected dogs (see Figure 20.1).[8,12,14] These echocardiographic changes and arrhythmias can coexist or one form may predominate at any time during this pre-clinical stage.[1,4]

Existing prevalence information on cardiomyopathy in Doberman Pinschers is from dogs in the United States or Canada, where prevalence ranges between 45 and 63%.[1] A study from Europe showed a similar prevalence with 58% of the dogs being affected.[4] This European study showed that 37% of the dogs had only VPCs without echocardiographic changes and that arrhythmias often were the first abnormality detected. Only a small proportion of dogs (13%) presented with only echocardiographic changes and no arrhythmias on 24 h ambulatory ECG (Holter) examination. Another interesting finding was that although there was no overall difference in the occurrence of cardiomyopathy between male and female dogs, there was a difference between sex concerning disease manifestation.[4,11] Female dogs had significantly more VPCs without echocardiographic changes than male dogs, and this difference became more apparent with increasing age. On the other hand, male dogs developed earlier echocardiographic changes than did female dogs. Some older studies concerning Doberman Pinscher

cardiomyopathy (DoCM) found a higher prevalence of the disease in male dogs. However, the prevalence study from Europe found an equal sex distribution, which supports the suspected autosomal dominant mode of inheritance.[1,4,11] The different findings concerning the sex distribution may be explained by the results of the study that showed an equal sex distribution but different disease progression between male and female dogs. Female dogs seem to experience a slower progression of disease, with VPCs as the only abnormality found even in the older age groups. Male dogs, on the contrary, showed echocardiographic changes earlier than female dogs. These changes are easier to detect because no 24 h ambulatory ECG (Holter) examination is necessary, and male dogs therefore are also more likely to develop CHF at an earlier age than female dogs and also die earlier from their disease.[4]

The average age of detection of pre-clinical DoCM is between 5 and 7 years, but some dogs are affected as young as 2 years of age. Therefore, screening for pre-clinical DoCM should be started in Doberman Pinschers at 2–3 years of age and should include 24 h ambulatory ECG (Holter) and echocardiography. A one-time screening is not sufficient to rule out future development of DoCM, because the disease is acquired and may develop with increasing age. Given that the disease can develop over time coupled with the known rate of progression, screening should ideally be repeated on a yearly basis.[4,12]

5-minute in-house ECG

Sometimes, 24 h ambulatory ECG (Holter) is not readily available to the veterinarian, and therefore a study that evaluated the use of an in-house ECG and compared the

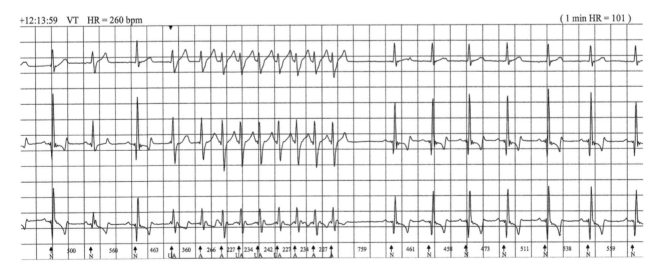

Figure 20.1 Ventricular arrhythmias in pre-clinical DoCM. An asymptomatic, 5-year-old, female, entire Doberman presented for screening for dilated cardiomyopathy. The 24 h ambulatory ECG trace revealed 398 ventricular beats during the recording period, including examples of complex ventricular ectopy such as the short paroxysm of rapid (260 bpm) monomorphic ventricular tachycardia. On Doberman Pinscher ambulatory ECG traces, the QRS complexes of the ventricular beats are often narrower than seen in other breeds, which sometimes makes analysis technically challenging. [5-year-old, female, Doberman Pinscher with DCM at stage II]

results to those of 24 h ambulatory ECG (Holter) recordings, the gold standard for detection of arrhythmias in Doberman Pinschers, was conducted.[12,15] This study showed that a 5 min in-house ECG had low sensitivity but a high specificity for predicting more than 100 VPCs in 24 h, if at least one VPC was detected within 5 min.[12,15] The absence of VPCs in the 5 min in-house ECG should not lead to the assumption that the dog is healthy, because false negative cases were found in 35.8% of the examinations. We can therefore conclude that the finding of at least one VPC in a 5 min in-house ECG strongly warrants further examination, because of the high specificity (96.7%) and positive predictive value (85.6%).[12,15]

24-hour Ambulatory ECG (Holter)

Fewer than 50 single VPCs in 24 h is considered to be normal in Dobermans, although detection of any number of VPCs is cause for concern.[6,16] Greater than 300 VPCs in 24 h, or two subsequent recordings within a year showing 50 to 300 VPCs in 24 h, is considered diagnostic of pre-clinical DCM in Doberman Pinschers regardless of the concurrent echocardiographic findings.[11,17] Many studies have used >100 VPCs in 24 h as the cut-off value for establishing a diagnosis of DoCM, but the authors believe that the results of the recent study cited above should be the basis of current recommendations.

Comments on special situations:

1) *24 h ambulatory ECG (Holter) examination shows 1–50 VPCs/24 h:* In Doberman Pinschers, detection of any number of VPCs is cause for concern, even if only a few VPCs are detected in 24 h (<50 VPC/24 h). In these cases, VPCs that have a short coupling interval (Vmax >250/min) and complexity should also be

considered as a diagnostic criterion, as couplets, triplets or single short runs of VPCs with a fast rate (instantaneous heart rate >260/min) are potentially dangerous and are less likely caused by systemic diseases (Figure 20.2). In these cases, DoCM cannot be ruled out, and a follow-up 24 h ambulatory ECG (Holter) examination should be performed within 3–6 months.

2) *24 h ambulatory ECG (Holter) examination shows 50–300 VPCs/24 h, and a follow-up 24 h ambulatory ECG (Holter) within 12 months shows <50 VPCs/24 h.* Dogs in this category remain a challenge as DoCM cannot be definitively ruled out; therefore, ongoing screening is strongly recommended.

3) It is also important to acknowledge that some dogs will have normal echocardiograms but still have pre-clinical DoCM diagnosed based on the 24 h ambulatory ECG (Holter) examination results. Systemic diseases that could potentially cause VPCs should always be excluded. Ventricular escape beats and accelerated idioventricular rhythms are not considered to be diagnostic for DoCM (Figure 20.3). The role of atrial premature contractions and atrial tachycardia in the diagnosis of DoCM in Doberman Pinschers is currently unknown. Atrial fibrillation is an exception and may be seen, particularly in dogs at stage 3 of the disease (figure 20.4).

Screening for DoCM should be started at 2–3 years of age (ideally at 2 years of age) and should include 24 h ambulatory ECG (Holter) monitoring as well as echocardiography. Annual screening examinations should be performed, ideally in both genders; however, if for financial reasons this is not possible, at least male

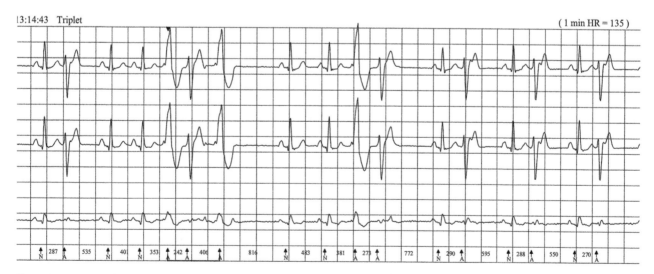

Figure 20.2 Ventricular triplet, couplet and bigeminy in a Doberman Pinscher with DoCM. In this trace, an isolated VPC (beat 2), a triplet (beats 5–7), a couplet (beats 10 and 11) and ventricular bigeminy (from beat 12 onwards) can be seen. The triplet and couplet are composed of ectopic beats with different origins (multifocal). The maximum instantaneous rate on this trace is between the first two beats of the triplet and is 248 bpm. [Unknown age, male Doberman Pinscher dog with DoCM]

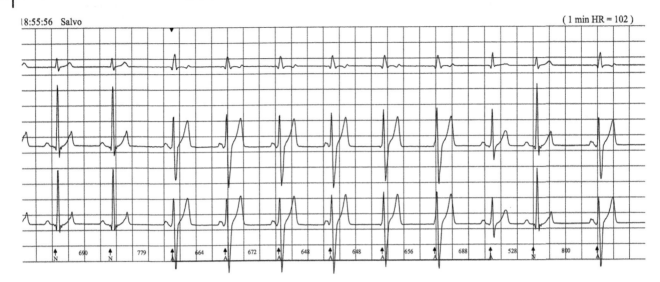

Figure 20.3 Idioventricular rhythm in a Doberman Pinscher. A ventricular rhythm is seen with an instantaneous rate of approximately 92 bpm during a 24 h Holter. This is not diagnostic of DoCM, and an extracardiac cause should be investigated. [5-year-old, female, Doberman Pinscher dog]

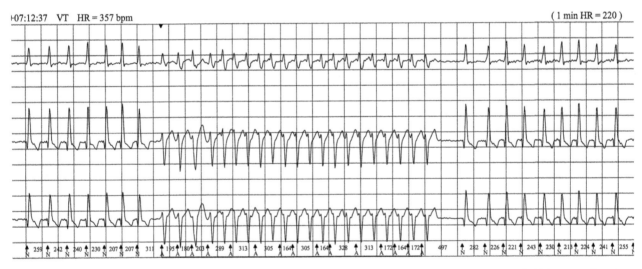

Figure 20.4 Atrial fibrillation and ventricular tachycardia in a Doberman Pinscher with DoCM. This is an extract of a Holter recording from a Doberman Pinscher at the overt stage of DoCM with a history of syncope and signs of congestive heart failure at presentation. The underlying rhythm is atrial fibrillation with a rate of approximately 200 bpm and is interrupted by an episode of monomorphic ventricular tachycardia with an instantaneous rate of 357 bpm. [7-year-old, female, Doberman Pinscher with DoCM]

Doberman Pinschers should be screened annually due to their higher impact on the dog population and female dogs every 2 years.

Sudden Cardiac Death

In Doberman Pinschers suffering from DoCM, only limited research has been devoted to evaluating risk factors that can be helpful to predict SCD.

Historically, in Doberman Pinschers with DoCM, risk factors proposed were VT,[12] ventricular late potentials detected by signal-averaged electrocardiography,[13,18,19] and echocardiographic evidence of heart enlargement.[12]

More recently, several echocardiographic, 24 h ambulatory ECG (Holter) variables, and cardiac troponin I (cTnI) and N-terminal prohormone of B-type natriuretic peptide (NT-proBNP) concentrations, were evaluated as possible predictors of SCD in Doberman Pinschers. An enlarged heart, represented by a left ventricular end-diastolic volume/body surface area (LVEDV/BSA) score of >91.3 mL/m^2, was found to be the most important and single statistically significant variable to identify Doberman Pinschers with DCM carrying a high risk to die of SCD. The probability of SCD occurrence increases 8.5-fold for each 50 mL/m^2 unit increment of LVEDV/

BSA. However, cardiac enlargement alone is insufficient to predict SCD in Dobermans, because many dogs who die of SCD have no echocardiographic changes.[9,11] Other variables of importance were VT, an elevated cTnI concentration and VPC with a beat-to-beat rate of >260 bpm, which might be additional prognostic markers for SCD risk assessment. The total number of VPCs, however, was not a predictor of SCD.[20]

In human medicine, left ventricular dysfunction measured by ejection fraction (EF) ≤30% is the most important measurement used for risk stratification to identify patients at high risk of SCD.[21–23] Additional variables for risk evaluation of SCD in humans include electrophysiology testing,[24] signal-averaged electrocardiography,[25,26] cardiac magnetic resonance imaging[22,23,27] and measurement of cardiac biomarker concentrations.[28,29] Currently, there is no consensus, but a combination of cardiac magnetic resonance imaging and electrophysiology testing appears to be promising in the human medical field.

Treatment of DoCM

Stage I
At stage 1, there are no detectable signs of disease, and treatment is not warranted.

Stage II
In asymptomatic Doberman Pinschers with echocardiographic evidence of cardiac enlargement and/or ventricular arrhythmias, there is evidence that treatment with pimobendan may prolong the pre-clinical period.[30]

Many anti-arrhythmic drugs have been used for treatment of ventricular arrhythmias in Dobermans, with several studies investigating the efficacy and toxicity of amiodarone. The rationale for use of this medication includes the multiple mechanisms of anti-arrhythmic action and the fact that amiodarone has less effect on systolic function than other anti-arrhythmic drugs, which may be advantageous in DoCM.

When considering the use of amiodarone in Dobermans, it is worthwhile noting that this breed is predisposed to hepatopathy[31] and hypothyroidism,[32] and therefore haematology and serum biochemistry, including bile acids, should be carefully monitored in view of the tendency of amiodarone to raise hepatic enzyme levels and lower total thyroid hormone concentration.[33] Hepatopathy associated with amiodarone administration has been reported 1.5–8 months after starting treatment; and haematological abnormalities such as neutropenia and a positive Coombs' test have also been associated with amiodarone administration.[34,35] Because of the side effects, the authors of this book recommend that amiodarone should be used only by specialists or after consulting with a specialist in dogs with very malignant arrhythmias, as other drugs (such as sotalol, mexiletine or a combination of both) are alternatives with fewer side effects.

In one study of stage 2 Dobermans, amiodarone was used for treatment of ventricular arrhythmias that persisted or relapsed after use of mexiletine, tocainide, atenolol, quinidine, procainamide, carvedilol or sotalol. In some cases, amiodarone was administered concurrently with tocainide or mexiletine. In this group of dogs, signs of amiodarone toxicity were seen in 10 of the 22 dogs (45%) at both loading and maintenance doses, with signs including anorexia, vomiting and diarrhoea, and there were corresponding increases in hepatic enzyme concentrations. These changes were reversible after discontinuation of drug in the majority of cases (9/10) or use of a lower dose in one case.[36] In this study, the authors state that whether amiodarone had any influence on survival time or the severity of arrhythmias could not be evaluated from this study due to small patient numbers and the absence of a control group.[36]

In stage 2 cases with arrhythmias and normal echocardiographic examination, anti-arrhythmic treatment is administered, especially to those dogs with malignancy criteria (couplets, triplets, VT and fast instantaneous rate of the VPCs). Prospective studies are not yet available, and therefore the actual risks and benefits of this approach in Dobermans are unclear.

Stage III
In symptomatic patients, treatment is warranted and will consist of CHF and/or anti-arrhythmic treatment.

Congestive Heart Failure Treatment

In dogs at risk of or already in CHF, treatment with a diuretic and an ACE inhibitor is warranted. Additionally, the benefit of treatment with pimobendan is well established[37] and is normally started when a systolic dysfunction is detected on ultrasound.

Anti-arrhythmic Treatment

> In a recent study, the following criteria were used when deciding to start treatment:
>
> - History of collapse
> - Malignant ventricular ectopy on 24 h ambulatory ECG (Holter) – couplets, triplets or VT with instantaneous rate >280 bpm.[20]

Assessing the Risks Versus Benefits of Anti-arrhythmic Treatment
The evidence for anti-arrhythmic drug efficacy has not been fully established. Whilst there is an understandable desire to suppress ventricular ectopy, studies in human

medicine have shown that whilst some drugs are very effective in reducing the frequency and severity of ventricular ectopy, their use does not reduce the risk of sudden death.[38] It is important to remember that whilst sudden death in DoCM is assumed to be associated with ventricular tachyarrhythmias, collapse associated with bradyarrhythmia also has been documented.[39] This is clinically relevant because whilst medical suppression of VT may reduce the risk of sudden death, in some patients it may not reduce (and could increase) the frequency of syncope, which may be understandably distressing for owners.

In a recent European study, Dobermans with stage II or III DoCM were treated with anti-arrhythmic drugs if they fulfilled the criteria stated in this chapter.[20] These dogs were treated with several anti-arrhythmics, including sotalol in 15 (28%) of the control group dogs and 15 (37%) of the SCD group, and amiodarone in eight control group dogs (15%) and eight (20%) SCD group dogs. Whilst this study suggested that Dobermanns receiving anti-arrhythmic therapy were at higher risk of SCD, this was attributed to a pre-selection bias in that dogs with the most severe ventricular arrhythmias received anti-arrhythmic therapy.[20]

A retrospective study on the use of amiodarone included two Dobermans with DCM who were treated for a short period (27 and 136 days) and tolerated this drug without evidence of hepatopathy until death.[40]

An earlier study recruited 19 Dobermans with abnormal echocardiographic findings, and it documented VT and 1–2 episodes of collapse or syncope.[16] Sixteen of these dogs were treated with ACE inhibitors and furosemide as required. Anti-arrhythmic treatment included tocainide (six dogs) and mexiletine (seven dogs), whilst another six dogs did not receive any anti-arrhythmic therapy. The median survival time of dogs treated with anti-arrhythmic drugs was significantly longer (198 days [78–345]) than that of untreated dogs (11 days [3–38]). When arrhythmias worsened (typically after 2–6 months), further medications such as procainamide, quinidine, amiodarone or a β-blocker were added sequentially or in combination with the original anti-arrhythmic. β-blockers were commonly combined with tocainide and mexiletine. Subsequent 24 h ambulatory ECG (Holter) recordings confirmed a reduction in the frequency of ventricular ectopy and suppression of sustained (>30 s) VT in all 13 treated dogs. All 19 dogs in this study died suddenly without overt evidence of worsening CHF, and this occurred during periods of both rest and exercise.[16]

Anti-arrhythmic drugs were prescribed only if several malignancy criteria were fulfilled, such as having >50 couplets, triplets, VT or a fastest instantaneous rate (FR) of VPC >280 bpm.

Arrhythmogenic Right Ventricular Cardiomyopathy (ARVC)

ARVC is a well-described form of cardiomyopathy in humans that has also been described in dogs and more recently in cats.[41,42] This is particularly true for Boxer dogs, in whom this disease was also known as Boxer cardiomyopathy or arrhythmogenic right ventricular dysplasia. Additionally, there have been isolated reports of ARVC in other breeds, including English Bulldogs,[43] Dachshunds,[44] Labrador Retrievers,[45] Bullmastiffs,[46] Siberian Huskies,[47] Weimaraners,[48] Shetland Sheepdogs[49] and Dalmatians.[49] In Boxer dogs, ARVC is an adult-onset, familial primary myocardial disease characterised by the progressive replacement of ventricular myocardium (primarily right ventricular myocardium) with fatty or fibro-fatty tissue which leads to arrhythmias, SCD and right ventricular failure. ARVC is primarily an electrical disease.[50]

Three stages of ARVC in Boxer dogs have been described:

- *Stage I*: Asymptomatic dogs with VPCs
- *Stage II*: Dogs with syncope due to VTs
- *Stage III*: Development of systolic dysfunction.[51]

The disease therefore shows a variable clinical picture with a long pre-clinical phase, in which the dogs appear to be unremarkable to their owners but, despite this, usually have ventricular arrhythmias, which can lead to syncope or SCD. However, bradycardia at the time of collapse has also been documented in Boxers with frequent and/or complex ventricular ectopy.[52] Although ARVC in Boxer dogs is a familial cardiomyopathy, with many dogs having the genetic mutation, it appears that most dogs do not develop the phenotype until middle age.[53–55] In a recent study looking at the natural progression of ARVC in Boxer dogs, it was found that the detection of more than 300 VPCs in 24 h was generally not apparent before 6 years of age.[53] It was also shown that the development of arrhythmias in Boxer dogs might be fairly abrupt.[55,56] In Boxers with ARVC, multivariate analysis showed that in Boxers without left ventricular enlargement (left ventricular diastolic diameter in diastole <35 mm), the presence of VT, male sex and age >4.5 years were independent predictors of cardiac mortality.[57]

ARVC is a cardiomyopathy that is characterised by ventricular arrhythmias that originate in the right ventricle (see chapter 11), and they typically manifest as VPCs with left bundle branch block morphology with varying degrees of complexity – occurring as single VPCs, couplets, triplets or runs of VT (Figure 20.5).[55,58] In some affected dogs, the morphology of the VPCs can be different. However, if a Boxer shows multifocal VPCs or VPCs not typical for ARVC (without the LBBB appearance), a different cause from ARVC should be considered.

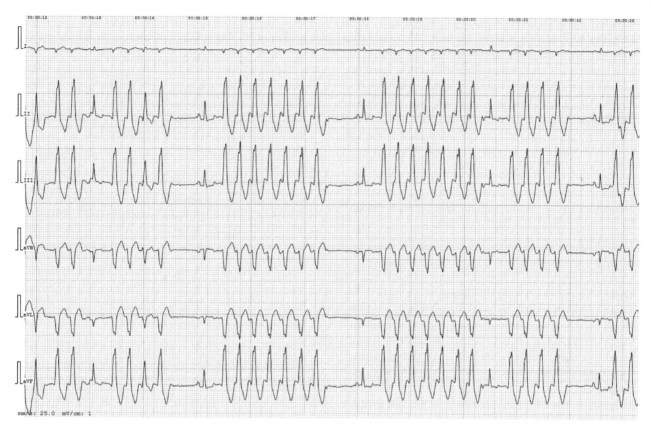

Figure 20.5 Ventricular arrhythmias in a Boxer with ARVC. An underlying sinus rhythm is seen frequently interrupted by repetitive brief periods of ventricular tachycardia with a rate of approximately 240 bpm. The ventricular ectopic beats display a left bundle branch block morphology (main positive deflection in leads II, III and aVF; main negative deflection in leads aVR and aVL), suggestive of an origin in the right ventricle. An isolated beat (beat 8) and a couplet (beats 5 and 6) are also seen. [10-year-old, male neutered Boxer dog with ARVC] (25 mm/s; 10 mm/mV)

Atrial fibrillation and other supraventricular arrhythmias have also been described in ARVC.[59]

As ARVC is an adult-onset disease and can occur at varying ages, it is currently recommended that the first 24 h ambulatory ECG (Holter) be performed at 3 years of age and repeated on an annual basis.[54,59] The reason to perform screening examinations in young dogs is to detect early-affected dogs, who have a risk to die suddenly, and to exclude these dogs from breeding. A 24 h ambulatory ECG (Holter) recording should be evaluated for the number of VPCs and their complexity, as already described in this chapter.

In-house ECG

Brief (2–5 min in duration) in-house ECG is a convenient way to assess heart rhythm and screen for arrhythmias. However, it is insensitive for detection of intermittent ventricular arrhythmias, and it is further confounded by the fact that the number of VPCs varies significantly on a day-to-day basis in dogs (by as much as 83% in Boxers).[60,61] A study comparing in-house ECG and 24 h ambulatory ECG (Holter) for detection of VPCs in mature Boxer dogs

has shown that the in-house ECG is highly specific (93%) for detection of at least 50 VPCs during a 24 h period.[61] However, in-house ECG is insensitive, and a lack of VPCs does not preclude clinically significant ventricular ectopy. Sensitivity of the in-house ECG does increase as the prevalence of VPCs increases or when symptomatic dogs were evaluated (e.g. dogs with syncope).[60,61]

> *To summarise*: If VPCs are present on brief in-house ECG, further evaluation is strongly warranted; also, normal in-house ECG findings do not rule out ARVC.

24-hour Ambulatory ECG (Holter)

24 h ambulatory ECG (Holter) is typically the diagnostic test of choice, and is generally recommended as it allows better assessment of the overall frequency and complexity of the rhythm disturbances; it also serves as an important guide in monitoring the success of anti-arrhythmic therapy.[57] 24 h ambulatory ECG (Holter) is an important part of the diagnostic workup, screening and management of ARVC in dogs. Multiple-day recordings may

ultimately prove to be even more valuable than a single 24 h ambulatory ECG (Holter) recording.[60] Interpretation of the 24 h ambulatory ECG (Holter) recording can sometimes pose a challenge, primarily because strict criteria for ARVC diagnosis do not exist. However, it is unusual for adult, mature dogs to have ventricular arrhythmias, as it was found that the median number of VPCs detected in mature, asymptomatic Boxer dogs was 10 VPCs in 24 h; the 25 and 75% confidence intervals were 2 and 110 VPCs, respectively.

> The following classification system has been developed for screening asymptomatic Boxer dogs:[62]
>
> *Grade 1 – within normal limits*: 0 to 50 single VPCs per 24 h
>
> *Grade 2 – repeat testing in 6 to 12 months*: 51 to 100 VPCs in 24 h
>
> *Grade 3 – suspicious*: 100 to 300 single VPCs in 24 h
>
> *Grade 4 – the dog is likely affected*: 100 to 300 VPCs in 24 h with increased complexity (i.e. occurrence of frequent couplets, triplets or runs of VT), or 300 to 1000 VPCs in 24 h
>
> *Grade 5 – the dog is affected*: More than 1000 VPCs in 24 h. Start anti-arrhythmic therapy – discussed in the remainder of this section.

These criteria are based on evaluation of a single 24 h ambulatory ECG (Holter) recording in adult, mature Boxer dogs with no clinical signs, and they represent a starting point for making screening recommendations. As mentioned, ARVC represents primarily an electrical abnormality rather than myocardial dysfunction, so screening efforts should be based on repeated, annual 24 h ambulatory ECG (Holter) monitoring.

In patients with a history of collapse, an ambulatory ECG (Holter) is often very useful to document the underlying rhythm during such an episode should it occur whilst wearing the monitor. This is particularly important to distinguish episodes of collapse due to ventricular tachyarrhythmias (Figure 20.6) from those associated with a bradyarrhythmia such as vasovagal syncope (Figure 20.7).

Treatment of Asymptomatic Boxers

When a ventricular arrhythmia is detected in an asymptomatic Boxer, this presents a challenge on how best to advise the owner. As discussed in this chapter, reducing the frequency of ventricular ectopy does not automatically

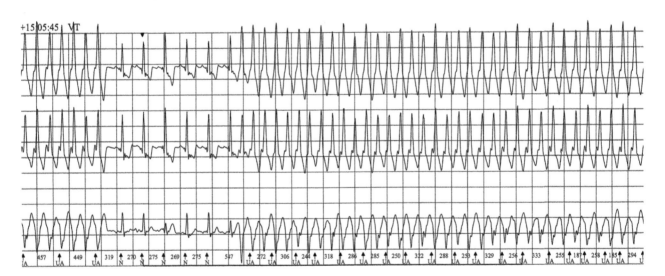

Figure 20.6 Ventricular tachycardia causing collapse in a Boxer with ARVC. Ambulatory ECG trace showing rapid monomorphic ventricular tachycardia (≈330 bpm) at the time of collapse in a Boxer dog with ARVC. [5-year-old, female, Boxer with ARVC]

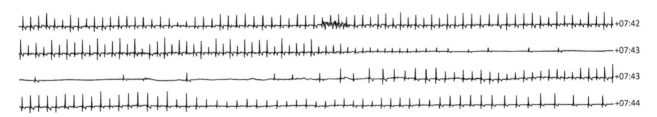

Figure 20.7 Bradyarrhythmia causing collapse in a Boxer with suspicion of vasovagal syncope. Ambulatory ECG trace showing an episode of pronounced sinus bradycardia with sudden onset following a period of sinus tachycardia during exercise. This lasted for several seconds and resulted in a syncopal episode. Evidence of structural heart disease or ventricular arrhythmias was not found in this case. [2-year-old, female, Boxer]

reduce the risk of sudden death.[38] Additionally, although anti-arrhythmic administration can reduce frequency of syncope in human patients,[63] this may not be the case in all canine patients, and there is always a risk of pro-arrhythmia. Owners also need to be counselled about the potential costs of anti-arrhythmic therapy, including the costs of medication, blood samples to monitor for signs of toxicity, and also subsequent 24 h ambulatory ECG (Holter) recordings to ensure a significant reduction in the frequency or complexity of ventricular ectopy. In light of the marked day-to-day variability in the frequency of ventricular ectopy, marked reductions (e.g. >80%) are required before any change can be attributed to drug administration.[60]

---

24 h ambulatory criteria that might prompt treatment in an asymptomatic dog include:

- Sustained (>30 s) VT
- The ventricular beats occur very early in diastole, resulting in R-on-T phenomena and an instantaneous heart rate >260 bpm.

There is limited evidence that omega-3 fatty acid supplementation (fish oil) administration can reduce the frequency of ventricular ectopy in Boxers.[64] Whilst efficacy of fish oils may be limited, fish oil administration carries the advantage of low toxicity.

Treatment of Boxers with Syncope or Exercise Intolerance

Treatment is recommended in Boxers with ARVC that present with complex or frequent ventricular arrhythmias and clinical signs such as syncope and/or exercise intolerance. A study assessing the efficacy of four anti-arrhythmic treatment protocols in Boxers with VTs and syncope has shown that treatment with sotalol (1.5–2 mg/kg PO q12h) *OR* a combination of mexiletine (5–8 mg/kg PO q8h) and atenolol (12.5 mg/dog PO q12h) was efficacious and well tolerated.[65] Treatment with procainamide or atenolol monotherapy was not effective. As mexiletine may sometimes result in gastrointestinal signs such as anorexia, vomiting or diarrhoea, the addition of atenolol is advantageous as it allows a lower dose of mexiletine to be used and minimises these side effects. Potential adverse effects of sotalol include hypotension and pro-arrhythmia. The combination of mexiletine and sotalol is also used by many cardiologists with good results, as illustrated in Figure 20.8.

Treatment of Boxers with Ventricular Arrhythmias and Systolic Dysfunction

In this group, signs of CHF are managed using standard therapy (diuretics, ACE inhibitors, spironolactone and pimobendan), and lower doses of drugs such as sotalol may be gradually up-titrated to effect. L-carnitine supplementation (50 mg/kg PO q8h) has been used in a family of Boxers with cardiac enlargement, systolic dysfunction and arrhythmias, and it did result in some improvement.[66] However, although myocardial carnitine levels are difficult to assess (as endomyocardial biopsy is required), carnitine deficiency is not thought to be a cause of ARVC in Boxers.

Irish Wolfhound Cardiomyopathy

In Irish wolfhounds (IWHs), the reported prevalence of DCM is around 30%. The mean age of onset has been estimated at 4.5 years; female dogs are less frequently affected and develop the disease at an older age than males.[67] IWHs often develop atrial fibrillation, which is frequently detected years before the dogs develop DCM. However, not all dogs with atrial fibrillation will develop the classical DCM.[68,69] Often, the dogs present with lone atrial fibrillation, although VPCs may also be found (Figure 20.9). The progression of IWH cardiomyopathy is poorly understood but appears to be slow, with the development of atrial fibrillation preceding the development of DCM by approximately 24 months.[70,71] In a small number of IWHs, additional electrocardiographic abnormalities have been described. They include VPCs, atrial premature contractions (APCs), right bundle branch block and left anterior fascicular block.[72] A recent North American study[73] has shown that IWHs diagnosed with a single APC did trend towards development of atrial fibrillation. Furthermore, the sensitivity of atrial fibrillation as a diagnostic marker of DCM was 40% and had a sensitivity of 89% for identifying left atrial enlargement (measured as the left atrial to aortic root ratio from two dimensions).[73] Also, significant ventricular arrhythmias were noted in several IWHs in the same study, which warranted anti-arrhythmic therapy and in which sudden death was attributable to severe ventricular arrhythmias.[73] The results of a recent European study looking at the long-term outcome of IWHs with atrial fibrillation showed that atrial fibrillation (lone atrial fibrillation) is associated with increased mortality and development of DCM in IWHs, and that it represents a strong predictor of cardiac death.[72] Furthermore, when comparing the ECG findings of IWHs with DCM to those without, atrial fibrillation was the most common ECG abnormality detected. Additionally, VPCs were detected both in healthy IWHs and in IWHs with DCM.[72,74] Multifocal VPCs and VPCs of increased complexity were mainly found in IWHs with DCM. In a proportion of IWHs with sudden death, ventricular arrhythmias were recorded before sudden death occurred.[70,75]

In summary, in-house ECG is an acceptable diagnostic screening tool for detection of IWH cardiomyopathy, and it should be done annually, ideally together with echocardiography.[73]

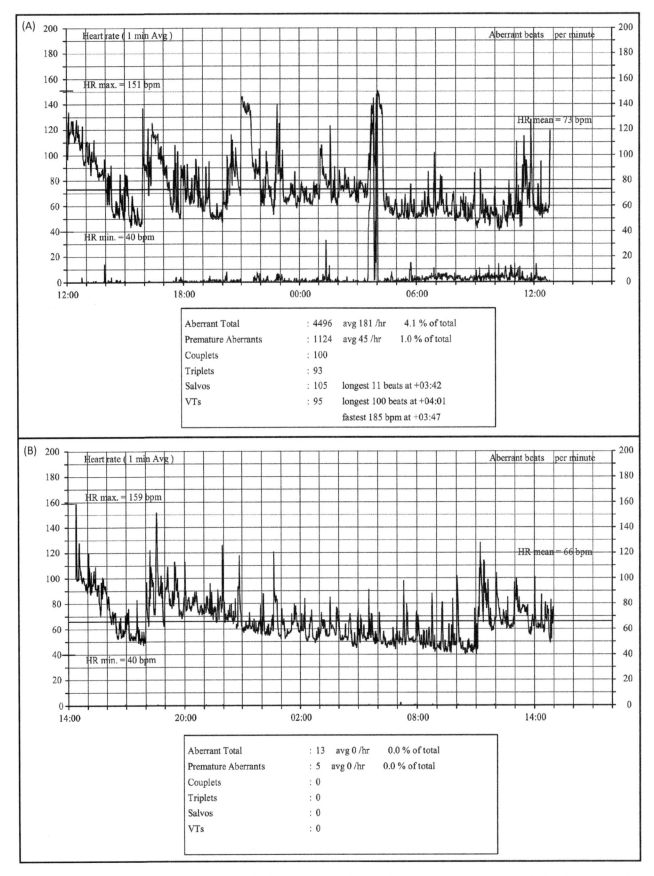

Figure 20.8 Anti-arrhythmic treatment in a Boxer with ARVC. (A) The total count of ventricular ectopic beats and 24 h tachogram may be seen in a Boxer with ARVC that had been stable on treatment on sotalol and an ACE inhibitor for many months. At the time of this recording, the owner reported that the dog had recently become more lethargic and exercise intolerant. The echocardiographic findings were normal. An elevated number of ventricular beats (4496/24 h) may be seen with more complex ventricular arrhythmias, including 95 episodes of ventricular tachycardia. This is also obvious from analysis of the tachogram. (B) Addition of mexiletine to the existing treatment plan resulted in marked improvement with a significant reduction in the number of ventricular arrhythmias, and this was accompanied by clinical improvement. [11-year-old, male neutered Boxer dog with ARVC]

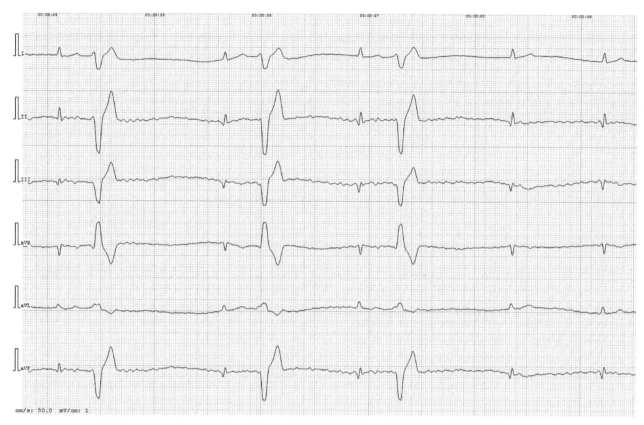

Figure 20.9 Lone atrial fibrillation and ventricular premature complexes in an Irish Wolfhound with DCM. The underlying rhythm is an irregular narrow-QRS rhythm without visible P waves and undulations of the baseline, consistent with lone atrial fibrillation with a rate of 90–100 bpm. Additionally, isolated ventricular premature complexes may be seen with a right bundle branch block morphology suggestive of a left ventricular origin. Atrial fibrillation is the most common electrocardiographic finding in IWH and appears to precede the development of DCM by approximately 24 months. The concurrent presence of ventricular arrhythmias originating in the left ventricle increases suspicion of DCM. [7-year-old, male neutered Irish Wolfhound with electrocardiographic and echocardiographic evidence of DCM] (50 mm/s, 10 mm/mV)

Treatment of Irish Wolfhound Cardiomyopathy

The results of 24 h ambulatory ECG (Holter) recordings will determine whether ventricular rate control is required for dogs with atrial fibrillation, as discussed in chapter 9. In dogs with systolic dysfunction, complex ventricular ectopy and atrial fibrillation, class III anti-arrhythmic drugs such as amiodarone may merit consideration.[76]

Dilated Cardiomyopathy in Great Danes and Newfoundlands

Great Danes (GDs) are known to be predisposed to DCM, and this is one of the most common breeds identified in retrospective analyses.[1,77] A recent study reported a prevalence of 35.9% for DCM and suspects an autosomal dominant mode of inheritance.[78] In the pre-clinical phase, GDs can have ventricular arrhythmias, which are a potential cause of sudden death in this dog breed.[79] Similar to IWHs, some GDs develop atrial fibrillation before they develop the classical DCM type, but this appears less common compared to ventricular arrhythmias.[53,78]

Familial adult-onset DCM without a gender predisposition has been reported in Newfoundland dogs.[80,81] The most common electrocardiographic abnormality was atrial fibrillation, but isolated VPCs also occur.[81] Annual screening evaluations are warranted and should include an ambulatory ECG and ideally echocardiography.

Arrhythmias Associated with Chronic Valvular Degenerative Disease (CVDD)

Arrhythmias are a common finding in dogs affected by CVDD, and, as might be expected, the frequency and severity of arrhythmias are reported to be higher in dogs with clinical disease. A longitudinal study of 257 dogs with degenerative atrioventricular valve disease showed that the heart rate increases and heart rate variability decreases in the year prior to death, and therefore careful monitoring of heart rate is a useful non-invasive indicator of advancing disease.[82] In another study, 50% of dogs ($n = 7$) with pre-clinical CVDD were reported to have supraventricular arrhythmias, 57% ($n = 8$) had ventricular arrhythmias and 21% ($n = 3$) had both ventricular and supraventricular arrhythmias. In the group of dogs with clinical disease, 72% of dogs ($n = 16$) had supraventricular arrhythmias, 86% ($n = 19$) had ventricular arrhythmias and 68% ($n = 15$) had both ventricular and supraventricular arrhythmias.[83]

24 h ambulatory ECG (Holter) findings in dogs with advanced degenerative mitral valve disease and syncope have also been described.[84] Sinus arrhythmia was seen less frequently in dogs with a history of syncope, as these dogs tended to have more advanced heart disease. A syncopal episode was observed during 24 h ambulatory ECG (Holter) monitoring in four dogs in this study – three dogs had sinus rhythm, and one dog had sinus arrest followed by escape rhythm.[84]

Atrial fibrillation requires a critical mass of atrial tissue to be sustained; therefore, it tends to be seen in small-breed dogs with CVDD, resulting in severe atrial enlargement and, more commonly, in medium-sized breeds such as Border collies.

References

1 O'Grady, M. R. & O'Sullivan, M. L. Dilated cardiomyopathy: an update. *Vet. Clin. North Am. Small Anim. Pract.* **34**, 1187–1207 (2004).

2 Tidholm, A., Häggström, J., Borgarelli, M. & Tarducci, A. Canine idiopathic dilated cardiomyopathy. Part I: Aetiology, clinical characteristics, epidemiology and pathology. *Vet J* **162**, 92–107 (2001).

3 Tidholm, A. & Jonsson, L. A retrospective study of canine dilated cardiomyopathy (189 cases). *J Am Anim Hosp Assoc* **33**, 544–550 (1997).

4 Wess, G., Schulze, A., Butz, V., Simak, J., Killich, M., Keller, L. J. M., Maeurer, J. & Hartmann, K. Prevalence of dilated cardiomyopathy in Doberman Pinschers in various age groups. *J. Vet. Intern. Med.* **24**, 533–538 (2010).

5 O'Grady, M. R. & Horne, R. The prevalence of dilated cardiomyopathy in Doberman Pinschers: a 4.5 year follow up. *Journal of Veterinary Internal Medicine* **12**, 199

6 Calvert, C. A., Chapman, W. L. J. & Toal, R. L. Congestive cardiomyopathy in Doberman pinscher dogs. *J. Am. Vet. Med. Assoc.* **181**, 598–602 (1982).

7 Petric, A. D., Stabej, P. & Zemva, A. Dilated cardiomyopathy in Doberman Pinschers: Survival, *Causes of Death and a Pedigree Review in a Related Line. J Vet Cardiol* **4**, 17–24 (2002).

8 Calvert, C. A., Pickus, C. W., Jacobs, G. J. & Brown, J. Signalment, survival, and prognostic factors in Doberman pinschers with end-stage cardiomyopathy. *J. Vet. Intern. Med.* **11**, 323–326 (1997).

9 Calvert, C. A., Hall, G., Jacobs, G. & Pickus, C. Clinical and pathologic findings in Doberman pinschers with occult cardiomyopathy that died suddenly or developed congestive heart failure: 54 cases (1984-1991). *J. Am. Vet. Med. Assoc.* **210**, 505–511 (1997).

10 O'Grady, M. R., O'Sullivan, M. L., Minors, S. L. & Horne, R. Efficacy of benazepril hydrochloride to delay the progression of occult dilated cardiomyopathy in Doberman Pinschers. *J. Vet. Intern. Med.* **23**, 977–983 (2009).

11 Calvert, C. A., Jacobs, G., Pickus, C. W. & Smith, D. D. Results of ambulatory electrocardiography in overtly healthy Doberman Pinschers with echocardiographic abnormalities. *J. Am. Vet. Med. Assoc.* **217**, 1328–1332 (2000).

12 Calvert, C. A., Jacobs, G. J., Smith, D. D., Rathbun, S. L. & Pickus, C. W. Association between results of ambulatory electrocardiography and development of cardiomyopathy during long-term follow-up of Doberman pinschers. *J. Am. Vet. Med. Assoc.* **216**, 34–39 (2000).

13 Hazlett, M. J., Maxie, M. G., Allen, D. G. & Wilcock, B. P. A retrospective study of heart disease in doberman pinscher dogs. *Can Vet J* **24**, 205–210 (1983).

14 Martin, M. W. S., Stafford Johnson, M. J. & Celona, B. Canine dilated cardiomyopathy: a retrospective study of signalment, presentation and clinical findings in 369 cases. *J Small Anim Pract* **50**, 23–29 (2009).

15 Wess, G., Schulze, A., Geraghty, N. & Hartmann, K. Ability of a 5-minute electrocardiography (ECG) for predicting arrhythmias in Doberman Pinschers with cardiomyopathy in comparison with a 24-hour ambulatory ECG. *J. Vet. Intern. Med.* **24**, 367–371 (2010).

16 Calvert, C. A. & Brown, J. Influence of antiarrhythmia therapy on survival times of 19 clinically healthy Doberman pinschers with dilated cardiomyopathy that experienced syncope, ventricular tachycardia, and sudden death (1985-1998). *J Am Anim Hosp Assoc* **40**, 24–28 (2004).

17 Geraghty, N. & Wess, G. Vergleich verschiedener Holterkriterien zur Diagnose des arrhythmischen Stadiums der dilatativen Kardiomyopathie beim Dobermann. 1–107 (2011).

18 Calvert, C. A., Kraus, M., Jacobs, G. & Kushner, L. Possible late potentials in 4 dogs with sustained ventricular tachycardia. *J. Vet. Intern. Med.* **12**, 96–102 (1998).

19 Calvert, C. A., Jacobs, G. J., Kraus, M. & Brown, J. Signal-averaged electrocardiograms in normal

Doberman pinschers. *J. Vet. Intern. Med.* **12**, 355–364 (1998).

20 Klüser, L., Holler, P. J., Simak, J., Tater, G., Smets, P., Rügamer, D., Küchenhoff, H. & Wess, G. Predictors of Sudden Cardiac Death in Doberman Pinschers with Dilated Cardiomyopathy. *Journal of Veterinary Internal Medicine* **30**, 722–732 (2016).

21 Manolis, A. S. Sudden death risk stratification in non-ischemic dilated cardiomyopathy using old and new tools: a clinical challenge. *Expert Rev Cardiovasc Ther* **15**, 315–325 (2017).

22 Grimm, W., Christ, M., Bach, J., Muller, H.-H. & Maisch, B. Noninvasive arrhythmia risk stratification in idiopathic dilated cardiomyopathy: results of the Marburg Cardiomyopathy Study. *Circulation* **108**, 2883–2891 (2003).

23 Solomon, S. D., Zelenkofske, S., McMurray, J. J. V., Finn, P. V., Velazquez, E., Ertl, G., Harsanyi, A., Rouleau, J. L., Maggioni, A., Kober, L., White, H., Van de Werf, F., Pieper, K., Califf, R. M. & Pfeffer, M. A. Sudden death in patients with myocardial infarction and left ventricular dysfunction, heart failure, or both. *N Engl J Med* **352**, 2581–2588 (2005).

24 Zaman, S. & Kovoor, P. Sudden cardiac death early after myocardial infarction: pathogenesis, risk stratification, and primary prevention. *Circulation* **129**, 2426–2435 (2014).

25 Pandey, A. K., Das, A., Singwala, A. K. & Bhatt, K. N. Prediction and stratification of the future cardiovascular arrhythmic events: signal averaged electrocardiography versus ejection fraction. *Indian J Physiol Pharmacol* **54**, 123–132 (2010).

26 Gomes, J. A., Cain, M. E., Buxton, A. E., Josephson, M. E., Lee, K. L. & Hafley, G. E. Prediction of long-term outcomes by signal-averaged electrocardiography in patients with unsustained ventricular tachycardia, coronary artery disease, and left ventricular dysfunction. *Circulation* **104**, 436–441 (2001).

27 Chugh, S. S. Early identification of risk factors for sudden cardiac death. *Nat Rev Cardiol* **7**, 318–326 (2010).

28 Berger, R., Huelsman, M., Strecker, K., Bojic, A., Moser, P., Stanek, B. & Pacher, R. B-type natriuretic peptide predicts sudden death in patients with chronic heart failure. *Circulation* **105**, 2392–2397 (2002).

29 Galante, O., Amit, G., Zahger, D., Wagshal, A., Ilia, R. & Katz, A. B-type natriuretic peptide levels stratify the risk for arrhythmia among implantable cardioverter defibrillator patients. *Clin Cardiol* **31**, 586–589 (2008).

30 Summerfield, N. J., Boswood, A., O'Grady, M. R., Gordon, S. G., Dukes McEwan, J., Oyama, M. A., Smith, S., Patteson, M., French, A. T., Culshaw, G. J., Braz Ruivo, L., Estrada, A., O'Sullivan, M. L., Loureiro, J., Willis, R. & Watson, P. Efficacy of pimobendan in the prevention of congestive heart failure or sudden death in Doberman Pinschers with preclinical dilated cardiomyopathy (the PROTECT Study). *Journal of Veterinary Internal Medicine* **26**, 1337–1349 (2012).

31 Mandigers, P. J. J., van den Ingh, T. S. G. A. M., Spee, B., Penning, L. C., Bode, P. & Rothuizen, J. Chronic hepatitis in Doberman pinschers. A review. *Vet Q* **26**, 98–106 (2004).

32 Beier, P., Reese, S., Holler, P. J., Simak, J., Tater, G. & Wess, G. The role of hypothyroidism in the etiology and progression of dilated cardiomyopathy in Doberman Pinschers. *J. Vet. Intern. Med.* **29**, 141–149 (2015).

33 Bicer, S., Nakayama, T. & Hamlin, R. L. Effects of chronic oral amiodarone on left ventricular function, ECGs, serum chemistries, and exercise tolerance in healthy dogs. *J. Vet. Intern. Med.* **16**, 247–254 (2002).

34 Jacobs, G., Calvert, C. & Kraus, M. Hepatopathy in 4 dogs treated with amiodarone. *J. Vet. Intern. Med.* **14**, 96–99 (2000).

35 Calvert, C. A., Sammarco, C. & Pickus, C. Positive Coombs' test results in two dogs treated with amiodarone. *J. Am. Vet. Med. Assoc.* **216**, 1933–6– 1926 (2000).

36 Kraus, M. S., Thomason, J. D., Fallaw, T. L. & Calvert, C. A. Toxicity in Doberman Pinchers with ventricular arrhythmias treated with amiodarone (1996–2005). *J. Vet. Intern. Med.* **23**, 1–6 (2009).

37 Fuentes, V. L., Corcoran, B., French, A., Schober, K. E., Kleemann, R. & Justus, C. A double-blind, randomized, placebo-controlled study of pimobendan in dogs with dilated cardiomyopathy. *J. Vet. Intern. Med.* **16**, 255–261 (2002).

38 Echt, D. S., Liebson, P. R., Mitchell, L. B., Peters, R. W., Obias-Manno, D., Barker, A. H., Arensberg, D., Baker, A., Friedman, L. & Greene, H. L. Mortality and morbidity in patients receiving encainide, flecainide, or placebo. The Cardiac Arrhythmia Suppression Trial. *N Engl J Med* **324**, 781–788 (1991).

39 Calvert, C. A., Jacobs, G. J. & Pickus, C. W. Bradycardia-associated episodic weakness, syncope, and aborted sudden death in cardiomyopathic Doberman Pinschers. *J. Vet. Intern. Med.* **10**, 88–93 (1996).

40 Pedro, B., Lopez-Alvarez, J., Fonfara, S., Stephenson, H. & Dukes McEwan, J. Retrospective evaluation of the use of amiodarone in dogs with arrhythmias (from 2003 to 2010). *J Small Anim Pract* **53**, 19–26 (2012).

41 Fox, P. R., Maron, B. J., Basso, C., Liu, S. K. & Thiene, G. Spontaneously occurring arrhythmogenic right ventricular cardiomyopathy in the domestic cat: A new animal model similar to the human disease. *Circulation* **102**, 1863–1870 (2000).

42 Harvey, A. M., Battersby, I. A., Faena, M., Fews, D., Darke, P. G. G. & Ferasin, L. Arrhythmogenic right ventricular cardiomyopathy in two cats. *J Small Anim Pract* **46**, 151–156 (2005).

43 Santilli, R. A., Bontempi, L. V., Perego, M., Fornai, L. & Basso, C. Outflow tract segmental arrhythmogenic right ventricular cardiomyopathy in an English Bulldog. *Journal of Veterinary Cardiology* **11**, 47–51 (2009).

44 Bright, J. M. & McEntee, M. Isolated right ventricular cardiomyopathy in a dog. *J. Am. Vet. Med. Assoc.* **207**, 64–66 (1995).

45 Mohr, A. J. & Kirberger, R. M. Arrhythmogenic right ventricular cardiomyopathy in a dog. *J S Afr Vet Assoc* **71**, 125–130 (2000).

46 Simpson, K. W., Bonagura, J. D. & Eaton, K. A. Right ventricular cardiomyopathy in a dog. *J. Vet. Intern. Med.* **8**, 306–309 (1994).

47 Fernandez del Palacio, M. J., Bernal, L. J., Bayon, A., Bernabe, A., Montes de Oca, R. & Seva, J. Arrhythmogenic right ventricular dysplasia/cardiomyopathy in a Siberian husky. *J Small Anim Pract* **42**, 137–142 (2001).

48 Eason, B. D., Leach, S. B. & Kuroki, K. Arrhythmogenic right ventricular cardiomyopathy in a weimaraner. *Can Vet J* **56**, 1035–1039 (2015).

49 Nakao, S., Hirakawa, A., Yamamoto, S., Kobayashi, M. & Machida, N. Pathological features of arrhythmogenic right ventricular cardiomyopathy in middle-aged dogs. *J Vet Med Sci* **73**, 1031–1036 (2011).

50 Basso, C., Fox, P. R., Meurs, K. M., Towbin, J. A., Spier, A. W., Calabrese, F., Maron, B. J. & Thiene, G. Arrhythmogenic right ventricular cardiomyopathy causing sudden cardiac death in boxer dogs: a new animal model of human disease. *Circulation* **109**, 1180–1185 (2004).

51 Harpster, N. K. in *Current Veterinary Therapy* (ed. Kirk, R.) **VIII**, 329–337 (1983).

52 Thomason, J. D., Kraus, M. S., Surdyk, K. K., Fallaw, T. & Calvert, C. A. Bradycardia-associated syncope in 7 Boxers with ventricular tachycardia (2002-2005). *J. Vet. Intern. Med.* **22**, 931–936 (2008).

53 Meurs, K. M., Stern, J. A., Reina-Doreste, Y., Spier, A. W., Koplitz, S. L. & Baumwart, R. D. Natural history of arrhythmogenic right ventricular cardiomyopathy in the boxer dog: a prospective study. *J. Vet. Intern. Med.* **28**, 1214–1220 (2014).

54 Caro-Vadillo, A., Garcia-Guasch, L., Carreton, E., Montoya-Alonso, J. A. & Manubens, J. Arrhythmogenic right ventricular cardiomyopathy in boxer dogs: a retrospective study of survival. *Vet. Rec.* **172**, 268–268 (2013).

55 Harpster, N. K. Boxer cardiomyopathy. A review of the long-term benefits of antiarrhythmic therapy. *Vet. Clin. North Am. Small Anim. Pract.* **21**, 989–1004 (1991).

56 Meurs, K. M., Spier, A. W., Miller, M. W., Lehmkuhl, L. & Towbin, J. A. Familial ventricular arrhythmias in boxers. *J. Vet. Intern. Med.* **13**, 437–439 (1999).

57 Mõtsküla, P. F., Linney, C., Palermo, V., Connolly, D. J., French, A., Dukes McEwan, J. & Luis-Fuentes, V. Prognostic Value of 24-Hour Ambulatory ECG (Holter) Monitoring in Boxer Dogs. *Journal of Veterinary Internal Medicine* **27**, 904–912 (2013).

58 Kraus, M. S., Moïse, N. S., Rishniw, M., Dykes, N. & Erb, H. N. *Morphology of Ventricular Arrhythmias in the Boxer as Measured by 12-Lead Electrocardiography with Pace-Mapping Comparison.* **16**, 153–158 (2002).

59 Baumwart, R. D., Meurs, K. M., Atkins, C. E., Bonagura, J. D., DeFrancesco, T. C., Keene, B. W., Koplitz, S., Luis Fuentes, V., Miller, M. W., Rausch, W. & Spier, A. W. Clinical, echocardiographic, and electrocardiographic abnormalities in Boxers with cardiomyopathy and left ventricular systolic dysfunction: 48 cases (1985-2003). *J. Am. Vet. Med. Assoc.* **226**, 1102–1104 (2005).

60 Spier, A. W. & Meurs, K. M. Evaluation of spontaneous variability in the frequency of ventricular arrhythmias in Boxers with arrhythmogenic right ventricular cardiomyopathy. *J. Am. Vet. Med. Assoc.* **224**, 538–541 (2004).

61 Meurs, K. M., Spier, A. W., Wright, N. A. & Hamlin, R. L. Comparison of in-hospital versus 24-hour ambulatory electrocardiography for detection of ventricular premature complexes in mature Boxers. *J. Am. Vet. Med. Assoc.* **218**, 222–224 (2001).

62 Meurs, K. M. Boxer dog cardiomyopathy: an update. *Vet. Clin. North Am. Small Anim. Pract.* **34**, 1235–44– viii (2004).

63 Priori, S. G., Aliot, E., Blomstrom-Lundqvist, C., Bossaert, L., Breithardt, G., Brugada, P., Camm, A. J., Cappato, R., Cobbe, S. M., Di Mario, C., Maron, B. J., McKenna, W. J., Pedersen, A. K., Ravens, U., Schwartz, P. J., Trusz-Gluza, M., Vardas, P., Wellens, H. J. & Zipes, D. P. Task Force on Sudden Cardiac Death of the European Society of Cardiology. *Eur Heart J* **22**, 1374–1450 (2001).

64 Smith, C. E., Freeman, L. M., Rush, J. E., Cunningham, S. M. & Biourge, V. Omega-3 fatty acids in Boxer dogs with arrhythmogenic right ventricular cardiomyopathy. *J. Vet. Intern. Med.* **21**, 265–273 (2007).

65 Meurs, K. M., Spier, A. W., Wright, N. A., Atkins, C. E., DeFrancesco, T. C., Gordon, S. G., Hamlin, R. L., Keene, B. W., Miller, M. W. & Moïse, N. S. Comparison of the effects of four antiarrhythmic treatments for familial ventricular arrhythmias in Boxers. *J. Am. Vet. Med. Assoc.* **221**, 522–527 (2002).

66 Keene, B. W., Panciera, D. P., Atkins, C. E., Regitz, V., Schmidt, M. J. & Shug, A. L. Myocardial L-carnitine deficiency in a family of dogs with dilated cardiomyopathy. *J. Am. Vet. Med. Assoc.* **198**, 647–650 (1991).

67 Vollmar, A. C. The prevalence of cardiomyopathy in the Irish wolfhound: a clinical study of 500 dogs. *J Am Anim Hosp Assoc* **36**, 125–132 (2000).

68 Vollmar, A. C. & Fox, P. R. Long-term Outcome of Irish Wolfhound Dogs with Preclinical Cardiomyopathy, Atrial Fibrillation, or Both Treated with Pimobendan, Benazepril Hydrochloride, or Methyldigoxin Monotherapy. *Journal of Veterinary Internal Medicine* **30**, 553–559 (2016).

69 Vollmar, A. C., C, T., R, K. & al, E. Cardiomyopathy in Irish Wolfhounds. in *ACVIM Forum Proceedings*

70 C, V., Keene, B. W., B, K. & al, E. Long term outcome of Irish Wolfhounds with lone atrial fibrillation. in *ACVIM Forum Proceedings, Indianapolis, -June*

71 Brownlie, S. E. & Cobb, M. A. Observations on the development of congestive heart failure in Irish wolfhounds with dilated cardiomyopathy. *J Small Anim Pract* **40**, 371–377 (1999).

72 C, V. & Vollmar, A. C. Findings from electrocardiography in Irish Wolfhounds with and without cardiomyopathy. in *th ECVIM-CA Congress Proceedings, Goteborg, - September*

73 WD, T., Abbott, J., H, G. & al, E. An Update on cardiac disease in the Irish Wolfhound: The North American Experience. in *ACVIM Forum Proceedings, Indianapolis, -June*

74 Schmitt, K. E., WD, T. & G, P. Characterization and clinical significance of ventricular premature complexes in Irish Wolfhounds. in *ACVIM Forum Proceedings Seattle, June -,*

75 Bulmer, B. J., Oyama, M. A., Lamont, L. A. & Sisson, D. D. Implantation of a Single-Lead Atrioventricular Synchronous (VDD) Pacemaker in a Dog with Naturally Occurring 3rd-Degree Atrioventricular Block. *Journal of Veterinary Internal Medicine* **16**, 197–200 (2002).

76 Saunders, A. B., Miller, M. W., Gordon, S. G. & Van De Wiele, C. M. Oral amiodarone therapy in dogs with atrial fibrillation. *J. Vet. Intern. Med.* **20**, 921–926 (2006).

77 Borgarelli, M., Santilli, R. A., Chiavegato, D., D'Agnolo, G., Zanatta, R., Mannelli, A. & Tarducci, A. Prognostic indicators for dogs with dilated cardiomyopathy. *J. Vet. Intern. Med.* **20**, 104–110 (2006).

78 Stephenson, H. M., Fonfara, S., Lopez-Alvarez, J., Cripps, P. & Dukes McEwan, J. Screening for dilated cardiomyopathy in Great Danes in the United Kingdom. *J. Vet. Intern. Med.* **26**, 1140–1147 (2012).

79 Martin, M. W. S., Stafford Johnson, M. J., Strehlau, G. & King, J. N. Canine dilated cardiomyopathy: a retrospective study of prognostic findings in 367 clinical cases. *J Small Anim Pract* **51**, 428–436 (2010).

80 Lee, B.-H., Dukes-McEwan, J., French, A. T. & Corcoran, B. M. Evaluation of a novel doppler index of combined systolic and diastolic myocardial performance in Newfoundland dogs with familial prevalence of dilated cardiomyopathy. *Vet Radiol Ultrasound* **43**, 154–165 (2002).

81 Tidholm, A. & Jonsson, L. Dilated cardiomyopathy in the Newfoundland: a study of 37 cases (1983–1994). *J Am Anim Hosp Assoc* **32**, 465–470 (1996).

82 Lopez-Alvarez, J., Boswood, A., Moonarmart, W., Hezzell, M. J., Lotter, N. & Elliott, J. Longitudinal electrocardiographic evaluation of dogs with degenerative mitral valve disease. *Journal of Veterinary Internal Medicine* **28**, 393–400 (2014).

83 Crosara, S., Borgarelli, M., Perego, M., Häggström, J., La Rosa, G., Tarducci, A. & Santilli, R. A. Holter monitoring in 36 dogs with myxomatous mitral valve disease. *Aust. Vet. J.* **88**, 386–392 (2010).

84 Rasmussen, C. E., Falk, T., Domanjko Petric, A., Schaldemose, M., Zois, N. E., Moesgaard, S. G., Åblad, B., Nilsen, H. Y., Ljungvall, I., Hoglund, K., Häggström, J., Pedersen, H. D., Bland, J. M. & Olsen, L. H. Holter monitoring of small breed dogs with advanced myxomatous mitral valve disease with and without a history of syncope. *Journal of Veterinary Internal Medicine* **28**, 363–370 (2014).

21

Arrhythmias in Feline Cardiomyopathies
Erin L. Anderson

Hypertrophic Cardiomyopathy

Hypertrophic cardiomyopathy (HCM) is the most common acquired cardiomyopathy of domestic cats with prevalence as high as 14–15% in the asymptomatic population.[1] The disease is characterized by spontaneous and unnecessary hypertrophy (thickening) of the myocardium, most commonly in the left ventricle (LV) in the absence of primary causes of compensatory concentric hypertrophy (e.g. aortic stenosis, systemic hypertension and hyperthyroidism).[1,5–9] Genetic mutations encoding proteins of the sarcomere (specifically, beta-myosin heavy chain [β-MHC] and myosin-binding protein C [MBPC]) have been implicated in the development of HCM in humans as well as the Ragdoll and Maine Coon breeds.[10–15] These mutations interrupt the normal structure and function of the sarcomere and result in decreased force production.[5,11,13,16,17] Stress-responsive growth factors are thus stimulated, causing myocyte hypertrophy and fibroblast proliferation.[11,17] Hallmark histopathological findings in HCM include myocardial hypertrophy, myocyte disarray, interstitial and replacement fibrosis, and microvascular remodelling/coronary arteriosclerosis.[16–21]

Hypertrophy and fibrosis of the LV impose diastolic dysfunction and variable ventricular outflow tract obstruction and myocardial ischaemia.[11,16,18,22] Coronary atherosclerosis contributes to altered myocardial perfusion and ischaemia, leading to myocardial cell death. Cellular repair mechanisms result in replacement fibrosis. Both myocardial ischaemia and fibrosis impose viscoelastic burdens on the myocardium that further impede diastolic filling and likely interrupt transmission of normal electrical impulses, creating a substrate for cardiac arrhythmias.[11,22,23]

The presence and extent of hypertrophy, myocyte disarray and cardiac fibrosis have all been implicated in the origin of ventricular arrhythmias and increased risk for sudden death in people with HCM.[24–26]

Ventricular Arrhythmias

Ventricular arrhythmias can be an indicator of the presence of underlying structural heart disease in cats. Only 4/106 cats with ventricular tachyarrhythmias on in-hospital electrocardiogram (ECG) tracings had normal echocardiographic exams in one retrospective study.[2] The abnormal echocardiographic findings included 66 cats with HCM, 17 with restrictive or unclassified cardiomyopathy (RCM/UCM) and six with dilated cardiomyopathy (DCM), and the remaining had either valvular or congenital lesions. In comparison, the authors described statistically significantly fewer dogs (95/138) over the same study period, with abnormal echocardiograms associated with ventricular arrhythmias, suggesting a greater specificity of ventricular tachyarrhythmias for indicating underlying structural heart disease in cats compared to dogs.[2]

Ventricular arrhythmias are common in cats with HCM and, as in people, may increase the risk of syncope and sudden death.[3–6] A 2014 study described that 17/17 cats with HCM had ventricular arrhythmias on 24h Holter monitoring and that these arrhythmias occurred with greater frequency and complexity than ventricular arrhythmias recorded on 24h Holter monitors in normal cats.[28] Ventricular arrhythmias in cats with HCM may be characterized by single premature ventricular complexes/contractions (VPCs, also called ventricular premature complexes/contractions, depolarisations or extrasystoles), couplets, triplets or runs of ventricular tachycardia (see Figure 21.1). Rapid or sustained ventricular ectopy can be haemodynamically significant because it decreases diastolic filling time (which is particularly detrimental in HCM wherein diastolic function is already impaired) and decreases myocardial perfusion, which can propagate electrical instability. The overall heart rate at which these risks become more likely has not been definitively determined.

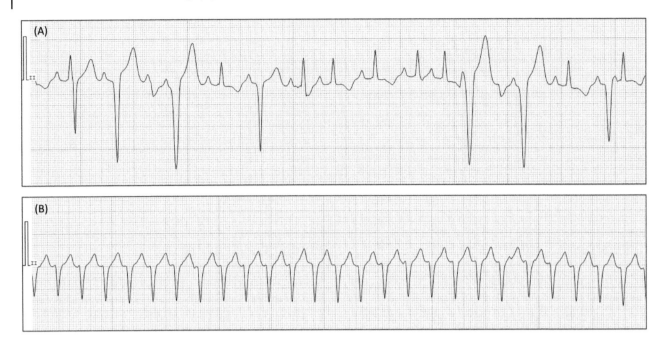

Figure 21.1 Electrocardiographic manifestations of ventricular arrhythmias in cats with hypertrophic cardiomyopathy (HCM). (A) Several ventricular ectopic beats (beats 1, 2, 3, 5, 11, 12 and 14) in a cat with HCM with a right bundle branch morphology suggestive of a left ventricular origin. The remaining beats are sinus with normal P-QRS and a first-degree atrioventricular block (PR, 100–120 ms; normal, 60–90). [7-year-old, female, neutered Domestic Shorthair cat with HCM] (lead II, 50 mm/sec, 20 mm/mV) (B) Ventricular tachycardia with a right bundle branch morphology at a rate of approximately 240 bpm. [14-year-old, male neutered, Persian cat with HCM and congestive heart failure] (lead II, 50 mm/sec, 20 mm/mV)

Mechanisms of Ventricular Arrhythmias in HCM

The most commonly proposed mechanisms of ventricular ectopy in HCM include triggered activity and re-entry.[7-9] Experimental models of LV hypertrophy provide evidence of prolonged transmembrane action potential duration (APD).[7] Patch-clamp studies on myocytes from human HCM patients undergoing surgical myectomy provide more specific evidence that the APD prolongation results from increased late inward sodium and calcium currents and decreased repolarising potassium currents.[8,9] Interrupted repolarisation allows for oscillations in membrane potential that can reach threshold and depolarise the cell again (e.g. an early afterdepolarisation).[7,8,10,11] Prolonged transient calcium currents also increase intracellular diastolic calcium concentrations, which provoke delayed afterdepolarisations, oscillations in resting membrane that produce VPCs when they are sufficiently large to reach threshold.

Re-entry can result from early afterdepolarisations or from conduction delay or blocks attributable to myocardial ischaemia and intracellular fibrosis.[7] In re-entry, hypertrophied or otherwise compromised regions of myocardium fail to conduct depolarisations fully or rapidly, while these depolarisations disperse normally through adjacent tissue. By the time a slowed depolarisation reaches normal tissue, the normal tissue may

have repolarised and be susceptible to stimulation again. Alternatively, if the diseased tissue blocks conduction altogether, then the depolarisation that was conducted through normal tissue can 're-enter' the diseased tissue in a retrograde fashion and depolarise normal tissue again.

In humans, the presence and extent of myocardial fibrosis as detected by late gadolinium enhancement on cardiac magnetic resonance imaging (cMRI) are associated with a higher rate of ventricular tachycardia and sudden cardiac death.[12,13] While cMRI is accurate for measuring LV mass in cats with HCM, a study of 26 affected Maine Coon cats and 10 normal controls revealed contrast enhancement in only one affected cat, suggesting low utility of cMRI for identifying myocardial fibrosis in cats.[14]

Clinical Approach to Ventricular Arrhythmias

Auscultation of a cat with ventricular arrhythmias may reveal either sustained tachycardia and/or an irregular rhythm characterized by premature beats. Clinicians often describe auditory findings by the 'pause' following the ectopic beat since the prematurity can be difficult to identify amid the frequently rapid heart rate of cats. A compensatory pause occurs after a VPC when the subsequent sinus depolarisation reaches the ventricles and finds them still refractory from the preceding VPC. Audible heart murmurs are neither specific nor particularly sensitive for identifying cats with acquired cardiomyopathy, so the identification of an arrhythmia warrants pursuit of a diagnostic ECG as well as an echocardiogram. Notably, Jackson *et al.* provided Holter evidence that low-grade ventricular arrhythmias occurred commonly in cats even in the absence of structural heart disease, so ventricular arrhythmias should not be considered specific for HCM.[28]

Rapid, sustained ventricular tachyarrhythmias can promote clinical signs of exercise intolerance (which, admittedly, may be difficult for owners to identify in cats with largely sedentary lifestyles), syncope, worsening congestive heart failure (CHF) or sudden death. Sudden death was less common than aortic thromboembolism or CHF in two reports of cats with HCM.[6,15] The overall heart rate at which these risks become more likely has not been definitively determined.

When rapid arrhythmias result in clinical signs or the perceived imminent risk of such, anti-arrhythmic therapy may be necessary. To avoid the risk of pro-arrhythmic potential with many anti-arrhythmics, their use requires discriminate consideration of any contributing arrhythmogenic factors that are controllable without pharmacotherapy. Factors like hypoxia, which can occur in fulminant CHF; hyperthyroidism, which may cause cardiac hypertrophy that is echocardiographically indistinct from HCM; anaemia; hypokalaemia or extracardiac morbidity can all cause ventricular arrhythmias that require specific treatment other than, or in addition to, anti-arrhythmic drugs. When these factors have been adequately controlled and ventricular tachyarrhythmias remain at rates that threaten normal cardiac output (>250 beats/min), then anti-arrhythmic treatment to suppress the frequency and severity of ventricular arrhythmias may be considered with one of several different anti-arrhythmic drugs.

Lidocaine is a class 1b sodium channel blocker that decreases the APD, increases the refractory period, decreases the dispersion of refractoriness and reduces the rate of phase 4 depolarisation.[16–18] It is delivered intravenously (because high first-pass metabolism precludes enteral absorption) at doses of 0.25–0.5 mg/kg and may be repeated up to a total of three times if ineffective but well tolerated.[16] Lidocaine has the potential for adverse neurologic and gastrointestinal effects and may be particularly cardiovascularly depressing in cats, causing significant bradycardia and decreased measures of cardiac output.[17–19] Most cats with HCM have preserved systolic function, so this effect may not have overt clinical consequences, but slow, vigilantly monitored administration to effect is still an appropriate precaution.

Ventricular tachycardia unresponsive to lidocaine may require consideration of an intravenous (IV) β-blocker.

Esmolol is a short-acting β-1 adrenoreceptor antagonist which can reduce catecholamine-induced ventricular arrhythmias when delivered as an IV bolus of 50–500 mcg/kg and followed with a continuous rate infusion at 25–200 mcg/kg/min.[17,19] Alternatively, propranolol is a relatively longer acting non-selective adrenoreceptor antagonist that can be dosed at 0.05–4 mg/cat or 0.02–0.06 mg/kg IV slowly and to effect.

Less commonly used acute treatments for ventricular tachycardia include amiodarone, a class III anti-arrhythmic that is generally avoided in cats due to known thyrotoxic and hepatotoxic effects, and magnesium sulphate. Although not thoroughly evaluated in cats, canine doses of 30 mg/kg magnesium sulphate by slow IV injection may successfully control ventricular tachycardia by reversing hypomagnesaemia-induced prolongation of repolarising potassium currents.[1]

Chronic oral anti-arrhythmic options include atenolol (6.25–12.5 mg PO q12–24h), propranolol (2–5 mg/kg PO q12h), sotalol (2 mg/kg or 10–20 mg PO q12h) and procainamide (3–5 mg/kg PO q8–12h). Pure β-blockers like atenolol and propranolol and partial β-blockers like sotalol should be used with caution, at initially low doses, or avoided entirely in acute CHF as β-blockade can exacerbate cardiac decompensation. In patients receiving chronic treatment with atenolol prior to the onset of acute CHF, the dose is often halved until resolution of the acute crisis.

Supraventricular Tachyarrhythmias

Supraventricular arrhythmias have been reported in cats with structurally normal hearts, but cats with HCM appear to have a higher incidence of such arrhythmias.[4,20,21] Jackson *et al.*[4] reported supraventricular arrhythmias on 24h Holter monitors in 88% of cats with HCM compared to 60% of normal controls.

Atrial premature complexes (APCs) arise from supraventricular sites outside the sinus node and above the ventricles at rates faster than the sinus node. They may occur as single depolarisations or as sustained tachyarrhythmias (supraventricular tachycardia [SVT], atrial flutter and atrial fibrillation [AF]) (see Figure 21.2). Atrial fibrillation is the most commonly occurring arrhythmia in humans with HCM, affecting up to 20% of patients.[26] The most commonly proposed mechanism for atrial tachyarrhythmias in HCM is thought to be re-entry, although abnormal automaticity and triggered activity also occur.[11,22] These mechanisms are enabled by the ultrastructural abnormalities that occur with HCM; specifically, interstitial fibrosis, cellular hypertrophy and degeneration, and thickened myocardial basement membranes were observed in cats with cardiomyopathy and were worse in cats with more severe enlargement of the

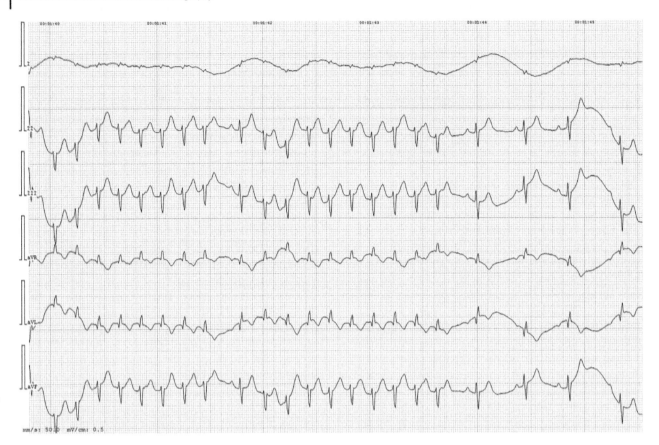

Figure 21.2 Supraventricular tachycardia in a cat with hypertrophic cardiomyopathy (HCM). Brief episodes of narrow-QRS tachycardia (beats 1–8 and 10–18) with a rate of approximately 300 bpm. The remaining beats are sinus with a rate of approximately 160–180 bpm. The QRS morphology (left anterior fascicular block) and duration (40 ms) are the same during tachycardia and sinus rhythm, indicating a supraventricular origin for the episodes of tachycardia. [7-year-old, female neutered, Domestic Shorthair cat with HCM] (50 mm/sec, 20 mm/mV)

left atrium.[23] These changes are associated with reduced resting membrane potentials and reduced action potential amplitudes, particularly in association with atrial enlargement.[22]

SVT can be more specifically described, based on the mechanism and site of origin, as sinus node or atrioventricular (AV) node re-entrant tachycardia, automatic atrial or junctional tachycardia, or orthodromic AV nodal re-entrant tachycardia.[24,25] These distinctions are paramount in treatment decisions in arrhythmic humans, in regard to both medical therapy and the potential success of catheter-based ablation therapy, but given the limitations of ablation therapy in cats, SVT is often a clinically acceptable general grouping.

Atrial Fibrillation

Perhaps the most common supraventricular tachyarrhythmia encountered in feline cardiomyopathic patients is AF. AF is characterized by rapid and chaotic atrial depolarisations with variable and unpredictable conduction through the AV node. The resulting arrhythmia is irregular and often rapid, depending on the inherent discretion of an individual AV node. The haemodynamic consequences of AF are twofold: (1) since the atria are fibrillating and not properly, uniformly contracting, ventricular filling – and ultimately cardiac output – are decreased by as much as 20%; and (2) the rapid ventricular response rate also reduces cardiac output.[26]

In a retrospective study of 50 cats with AF, all 50 cats had echocardiographic evidence of structural heart disease. Restrictive/unclassified cardiomyopathy was present in 19/50 cats (38%), while HCM (18/50 [36%]) and DCM (6/50 [12%]) were less common.[27] Other reported forms of structural heart disease included AV valve dysplasia (2/50 [4%]), mitral stenosis, cor pulmonale, arrhythmogenic right ventricular cardiomyopathy (ARVC), primary mitral regurgitation with systolic dysfunction, and RCM/UCM with LV adenocarcinoma.[27] Of 39 cats that had echocardiographic measurements of the left atrium, 35 were reported to have atrial enlargement, providing clinical support to the findings of electrophysiological alterations in cats with atrial enlargement.[23,27] Atrial enlargement/ remodelling and tissue fibrosis can lead to abnormal expression and function of ion channels, paving the way for abnormal automaticity, triggered activity, or one or multiple re-entrant circuits.[28] Competing hypotheses regarding the origin and maintenance of AF are discussed in chapter 9.

Clinical Approach to Atrial Fibrillation

AF is most often diagnosed in cats when they present with clinical signs of decompensated heart disease – dyspnoea associated with CHF, paresis or paralysis secondary to thromboembolism, or non-specific signs of lethargy, inappetence or general malaise. In the previously cited retrospective publication of 50 affected cats, AF was an incidental finding in the minority (22%) of patients.[27]

Salient physical exam findings in cats with AF include an irregular tachyarrhythmia accompanied by femoral pulse deficits which reflect the beat-by-beat variability in diastolic filling time and subsequent cardiac output. Accompanying findings relating to CHF or thromboembolism are variably present. Electrocardiographic findings include an irregularly irregular rhythm, a complete and convincing absence of P waves in all leads, and possibly a coarse, 'fibrillatory' baseline (see Figure 21.3). Because AV conduction necessarily varies in AF and the

instantaneous heart rates as calculated on ECG are so variable, ventricular rate should be measured over a period of time on the ECG (usually at least 1 min).

Treatment is indicated when the ventricular rate is inappropriately high (>250 beats/min in the hospital setting, or greater than an average of 160 bpm/24 h Holter). Electrocardioversion, which is a major treatment consideration in people and sometimes in dogs, has not been reported in cats.[26,28,29] Medical therapy is used to slow AV nodal conduction, thus controlling the ventricular response rate, and is not expected to convert the rhythm to sinus. The most commonly used drugs include diltiazem (1–2.5 mg/kg PO q8h or 7.5–15 mg/cat PO q8h) and atenolol (6.25–12.5 mg/cat PO q12h). Extended-release formulations of diltiazem should be avoided due to variable absorption and a seemingly high risk of gastrointestinal adverse effects and lethargy.[29] Initiation of atenolol should be avoided in acute CHF as β-blockade can exacerbate decompensated heart disease. The oral solution of atenolol can facilitate gradual uptitration of the dose. Some authors use sotalol (2 mg/kg q12h) as an alternative to diltiazem or atenolol. Digoxin has a long half-life in cats which increases the risk of toxicity, and therefore its use is not recommended.

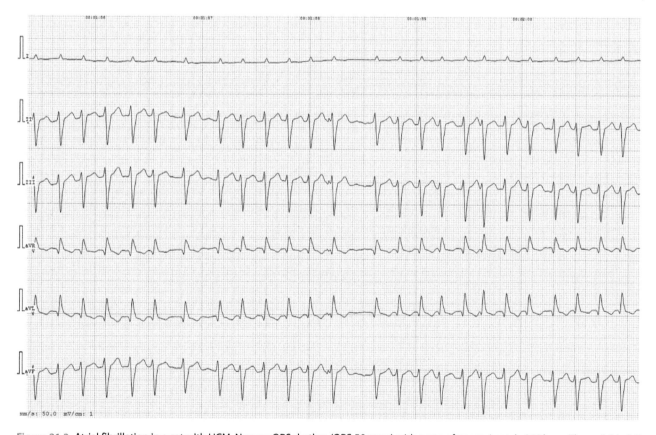

Figure 21.3 Atrial fibrillation in a cat with HCM. Narrow-QRS rhythm (QRS 50 msec) with a rate of approximately 240 bpm. The variable R-R interval and absence of P waves are consistent with atrial fibrillation. There is also left anterior fascicular block, which is characterized by negatively deflected QRS complexes in leads II, III and aVF and positively deflected QRS complexes in leads I, aVL and aVR. [5-year-old, male neutered, Domestic Shorthair cat with HCM and congestive heart failure] (50 mm/s, 10 mm/mV)

Bradyarrhythmias: Atrioventricular block

Atrioventricular block (AVB) occurs when conduction through the AV node is slowed or entirely inhibited. In cats with HCM, this is attributed to degeneration and fibrous replacement of the AV conductive fibres, specifically of the central fibrous body and endocardial and myocardial portions of the proximal interventricular septum.[30,31]

In first-degree AVB, conduction through the AV node is slowed but still complete, such that the atria and ventricles maintain normal synchrony. This can occur with structural heart disease or with any factor that increases vagal tone, specifically diseases of the gastrointestinal, respiratory or central nervous systems, or with drugs like calcium channel blockers, β-blockers or digoxin. Pharmacotherapy is an important consideration since first-degree AVB, although uncommon in cats, may appear in patients receiving atenolol or diltiazem. Clinical signs are not expected with first-degree AVB.

In second-degree AVB, conduction through the AV node occurs but not consistently so. Type I second-degree AVB is also called the Wenckebach phenomenon and is described as a gradually increasing PR interval in the complexes preceding the blocked P wave. In Type II second-degree AVB, there is a fixed PR interval in all conducted complexes with no change before or after blocked P waves. The higher the grade/severity of type II second-degree AVB, the more frequently transmission through the AV node is incomplete, and the more lone P waves (without a subsequent QRS complex) appear on an ECG tracing.

Type I second-degree AVB may be mechanistically more similar to first-degree AVB (i.e. it may occur in cats with abnormally high vagal tone or with β-blockade or calcium channel blockade), while type II second-degree AVB is more commonly thought to represent conduction tissue disease.

In third-degree AVB, the AV node fails to transmit any impulses whatsoever, and AV synchrony is entirely lost. The absence of a ventricular stimulus prompts subsidiary pacemakers in the AV junction or ventricles to assume pacing function of the heart at rates (60–140 beats/min) that are substantially lower than the inherent sinus rate (Figure 21.4). Bradycardic cats are at risk for clinical signs of exercise intolerance or collapse. They may also develop bradycardia-induced volume overload and secondary CHF. In a 2008 report of 21 cats with third-degree AVB, 6/21 cases were diagnosed incidentally,

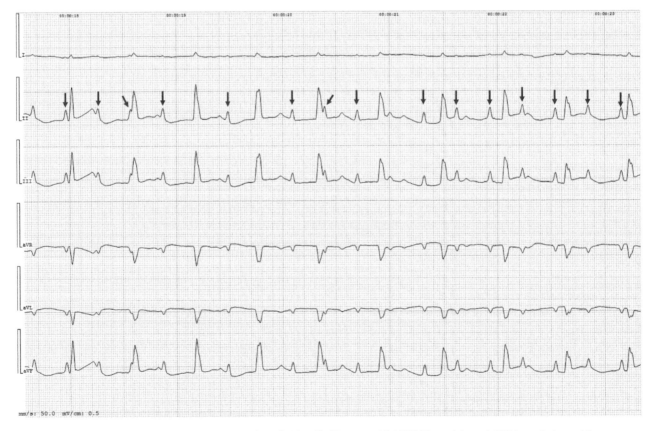

Figure 21.4 Third-degree atrioventricular block incidentally identified in a cat with HCM. The atrial rate is 200 beats/min, and P waves are indicated by arrows. The QRS complexes, which have no consistent relation to the P waves, occur as a ventricular escape rhythm with a rate of approximately 120 bpm. [15-year-old, male neutered, Domestic Shorthair cat with HCM and CHF] (50 mm/sec, 20 mm/mV)

while the others presented with syncope or in respiratory distress secondary to CHF.[32] Eleven of 18 cats undergoing echocardiographic evaluation had evidence of structural heart disease, and seven of those were primary cardiomyopathies (HCM, UCM/RCM or DCM).[32] No AV nodal lesions were identified echocardiographically.[32] Interestingly, only 1/21 cats received a surgically placed pacemaker, the treatment of choice in symptomatic third-degree AVB, and yet the median survival time was respectably long (median, 386 days; range, 1–2013 days), even given the advanced median age of 14 years in the reported cats.[32] Survival time was not influenced by the presence or absence of either structural heart disease or CHF, and no cats were reported to have died suddenly.[32] This suggests that, depending on the ventricular rate, third-degree AVB may be relatively well tolerated in cats.

Bradyarrhythmias: Sinus Bradycardia

Inappropriate sinus bradycardia may occur with severe, acute CHF or cardiogenic shock in cats. This is an important and species-specific distinction, since both conditions would more commonly be expected to produce sinus tachycardia (see Figure 21.5).

Other ECG Findings

Left anterior fascicular block is not an arrhythmia as it does not interrupt the underlying cardiac rhythm, but it does constitute a common ECG finding in cats with HCM. Termination of an electrical impulse through the left anterior (or dorsal) arm of the bundle branch penetrating the LV may occur as a result of fibrosis or degeneration in the His–Purkinje fibres.[19,30,31] The ECG appearance of LAFB includes a left axis deviation between –30 and –90°, characterized by negative QRS complexes in leads II, III and aVF (rS morphology), and positive QRS complexes in leads I and aVL (qR morphology) (see Figures 21.3 and 21.6). It is particularly important not to misinterpret this appearance of the QRS complexes for ventricular ectopic beats.

ST segment elevation or depression may also be found in cases with myocardial infarction (see Figure 21.7).

Restrictive and Unclassified Cardiomyopathy

Restrictive cardiomyopathy (RCM) is an acquired cardiomyopathy in domestic cats of largely unidentified aetiology. Reported hypotheses include infectious or

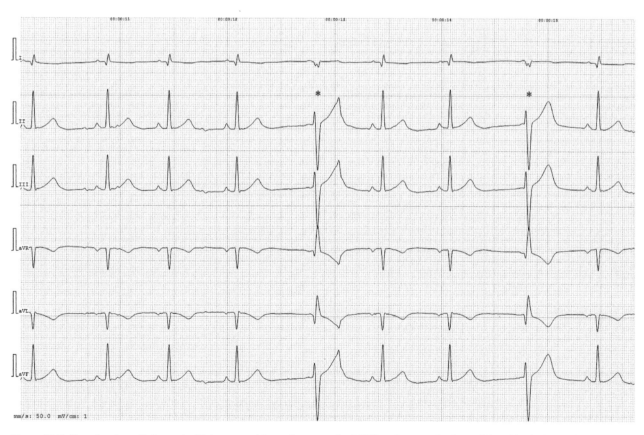

Figure 21.5 Sinus bradycardia in a cat with hypertrophic cardiomyopathy (HCM) and congestive heart failure (CHF). The underlying rhythm is sinus with a rate of approximately 90–120 bpm. Occasional ventricular escape beats (*) are also present. [2-year-old, male neutered, Domestic Shorthair cat with HCM and CHF] (50 mm/sec, 10 mm/mV)

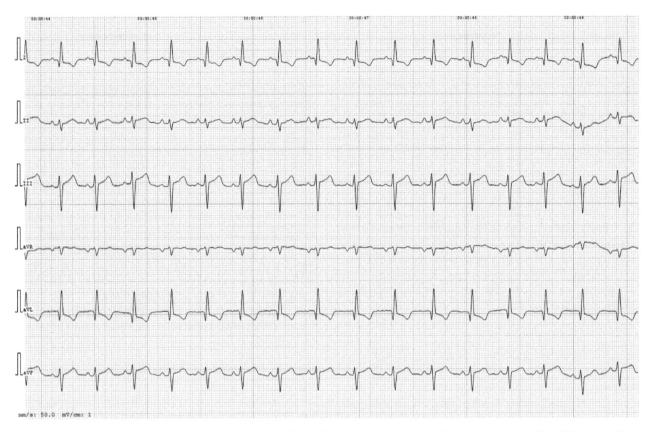

Figure 21.6 Sinus rhythm with left anterior fascicular block. The underlying rhythm is sinus with a rate of 170 bpm. The QRS is normal in duration (40 ms), and the MEA is deviated to the left at approximately −60° (−30 to −90°). The QRS has a rS morphology in leads II, III and aVF, and qR morphology in leads I and aVL. [3-year-old, male neutered, Domestic Shorthair cat with HCM] (50 mm/s; 10 mm/mV).

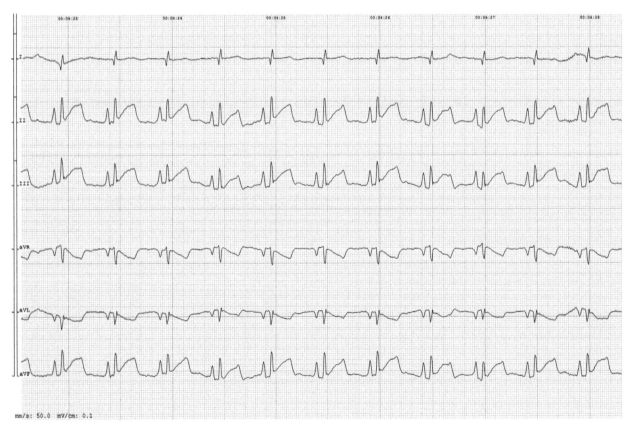

Figure 21.7 ST elevation due to myocardial infarction in a cat with HCM. The underlying rhythm is sinus bradycardia with a rate of 135 bpm. The ST segment is elevated due to myocardial infarction visible on echocardiography. [5-year-old, male neutered, Domestic Shorthair cat with HCM] (50 mm/sec, 20 mm/mV)

immune-mediated endo- or myocarditis, end-stage ('burn-out') HCM complicated by myocardial failure, or eosinophilia-induced cardiac damage.[19,33–37] Commonly implicated genetic mutations in humans with RCM have not been identified in cats.[38] The disease is characterized by diastolic dysfunction despite normal (or variably hypertrophied) myocardial wall diameters and subsequently increased ventricular filling pressures. Fibrosis variably occurs and, depending on its location, can result in distinction between endomyocardial and myocardial forms of RCM.[34,36,38] The decreased compliance of the LV ultimately leads to elevated atrial pressures, which can result in clinical complications of CHF, thrombus formation and thromboembolic events, or arrhythmias. Because auscultable abnormalities such as audible murmurs, gallop sounds or arrhythmias occur in a minority of patients (36% in one report), patients with RCM are often not identified until after severe disease results in the onset of these complications.[1] Physical exam findings may include tachypnoea or dyspnoea associated with CHF, an audible arrhythmia, or hindlimb paresis associated with thromboembolism.

Echocardiographic findings in RCM may include normal or variably hypertrophied LV wall diameters with or without subendocardial hyperechogenicity (indicating fibrosis), normal to variably increased or decreased LV chamber size with frequently preserved systolic function, biatrial enlargement with or without spontaneous echo contrast or a formed thrombus, and criteria of diastolic dysfunction.[39]

Although less well defined, clinicians generally accept that the term *unclassified* (or *undetermined*) *cardiomyopathy* (UCM) is used to describe cases with similar echocardiographic findings but without documented restrictive physiology.[19,33,39] Alternatively, UCM may be used to describe findings when other defined criteria of HCM, RCM, DCM or ARVC are not met in a cat with clear echocardiographic diastolic/systolic dysfunction and atrial enlargement.[19,33]

Arrhythmias in RCM and UCM

Arrhythmias in cats with RCM likely arise from similar mechanisms as in HCM. The predominant atrial enlargement is a logical source for commonly reported atrial tachyarrhythmias like AF. In 50 cats with AF, the most common echocardiographic diagnosis was RCM or UCM, occurring in 19 cats (38%) at a mean ventricular response rate of 223 ± 36 beats/min.[27] A retrospective study by Kimura *et al.* reported pathologic arrhythmias in 19/34 cats with RCM, including APCs (9/34; 26%), AF (5/34; 15%), VPCs (5/34; 15%) and third-degree AV block (1/34).[40] An additional report documented non-sustained SVT in 8/35 cats and VPCs in 10/35 cats presenting with RCM, with one additional cat developing AF 10 months after diagnosis.[38] Haemodynamically significant tachyarrhythmias portend a risk for CHF, syncope or near syncope, or sudden death in patients with RCM. The cause of sudden death in humans with RCM has not been unequivocally associated with arrhythmias; a study of 18 paediatric human patients with RCM documented rate-dependent ST segment depression on Holter monitoring (consistent with myocardial ischaemia) in all five patients suffering sudden cardiac death, but rhythm derangements were not reported.[41]

The prognosis for RCM is generally guarded given the often late diagnosis and high risk of complications associated with severe disease. Reported survival times vary greatly from 3 to 1560 days (median, 102 days) in one study[38] and 1–977 days (median, 30) in another.[40]

Arrhythmogenic Right Ventricular Cardiomyopathy

ARVC is an uncommon primary myocardial disease of cats, accounting for 2–4% of all feline cardiomyopathies.[33,42,43] Paige *et al.*[44] documented ARVC in 1 of 103 apparently healthy cats, while Wilkie *et al.*[45] made a post-mortem diagnosis of ARVC in 4/87 cats suffering sudden or unexpected deaths. As in Boxer dogs and humans, ARVC in cats is characterized by myocyte death and replacement with fibrous or fibrofatty tissue, predominantly within the right ventricle.[42,46,47] Genetic mutations have been reported in people and Boxers with ARVC but have not been described in cats.[46–50]

In a case series of 12 cats with ARVC, the median age was 7.3 ± 5.2 years, and no sex or breed predilections were identified.[42] Common presenting complaints may include dyspnoea associated with pulmonary oedema or pleural effusion, ascites, lethargy, anorexia or collapse. Most cats are diagnosed once they develop signs referable to right-sided CHF.[42] Physical exam may reveal an audible murmur secondary to tricuspid valve regurgitation, a gallop sound or arrhythmia, muffled lung sounds secondary to pleural effusion, jugular distension or pulsation, and/or abdominal distension with or without a palpable fluid wave.

In cats as opposed to dogs, ARVC is an echocardiographic diagnosis. Findings include right ventricular and right atrial dilation with a normal tricuspid valve. Tricuspid dysplasia is the major differential for right heart enlargement in cats. Other variable abnormalities include paradoxical motion of the interventricular septum, tricuspid regurgitation, abnormal trabeculations, regional dyskinesis or akinesis associated with localized aneurysms, and variable left heart enlargement.[39,42]

Arrhythmias in ARVC

The arrhythmias occurring in cats with ARVC vary widely and can include any combination of ventricular or

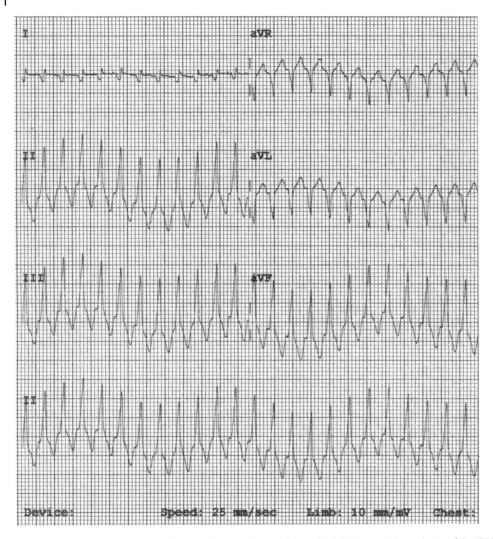

Figure 21.8 Rapid ventricular tachycardia in a cat with suspicion of ARVC. The positive polarity of the QRS complexes in lead II, referred to as *left bundle branch block morphology*, suggests an origin within the right ventricle. [11-year-old, male neutered, Domestic Shorthair cat with suspicion of ARVC] (25 mm/msec, 10 mm/mV)

supraventricular tachyarrhythmias and variable degrees of AV block (see Figure 21.8).[33,42] Although not strictly an arrhythmia, right bundle branch block may also occur with right ventricular enlargement. Treatment is aimed at controlling rapid arrhythmias as needed and as described previously. Additional treatment may be indicated to treat or prevent CHF or thromboembolism.

Dilated Cardiomyopathy

Diseases of systolic dysfunction are uncommon in cats, specifically since taurine deficiency was associated with reversible myocardial failure in 1987, prompting reformulation of many commercial feline diets to include supplemental taurine.[1,33,51–54] Since that time, systolic dysfunction in cats is more commonly linked to idiopathic DCM, tachycardia-induced cardiomyopathy, end-stage/ burn-out HCM or doxorubicin cardiotoxicosis.[33,55] In Ferasin's[1] retrospective report of 106 cats with cardiomyopathy, DCM was the third most common diagnosis, occurring in 11 cats (10.4% of cases), with HCM and RCM occurring more commonly. A causative genetic mutation has not been identified in cats as it has in Doberman Pinschers with DCM, but genetics may still play a factor in disease.[56,57]

Cats with DCM may present asymptomatically and may or may not have an audible heart murmur, gallop sound or arrhythmia. More commonly, they are diagnosed after the onset of clinical signs, particularly tachypnoea or dyspnoea associated with CHF, syncope related to arrhythmias, lethargy or anorexia. Audible arrhythmias and gallop sounds were previously reported in 79% of cats with DCM, and murmurs of mitral regurgitation were less common.[58] Additional physical exam findings may include muffled or abnormal lung sounds secondary to pleural effusion or pulmonary oedema, abdominal distension secondary to right-sided CHF, pulse deficits associated with arrhythmias, hypodynamic pulses secondary to poor cardiac output, and central retinal lesions.[19,33,52]

A diagnosis of DCM in cats is based on echocardiographic identification of ventricular dilation (increased end-systolic LV diameter, increased E-point to septal separation), normal to thin myocardial wall diameters, low fractional shortening or other measures of impaired systolic function (reduced velocity of circumferential fibre shortening, increased pre-ejection period, decreased LV ejection time), focal or global hypokinesis, and atrial dilation.[39,58,59] Additional features may include reduced systolic myocardial velocity on Tissue Doppler, spontaneous echo contrast or thrombus within an enlarged atrium, or AV valve regurgitation secondary to annular dilation.[39,59]

Taurine levels should be measured in cats with echocardiographic findings suggestive of DCM, particularly in cats receiving a diet other than a complete and balanced, commercially available cat food. While endomyocardial samples are most reflective of intracellular myocardial taurine, the need for general anaesthesia and the impracticality of endomyocardial biopsy often preclude its use.[33] Instead, taurine concentrations are measured in plasma or whole blood; whole blood concentrations are preferred, as these are more likely to include taurine concentrated in platelets and granulocytes and less likely to be affected by the patient's fed or fasted state.[19,33,51,52] Whole blood concentrations <250 nmol/L are considered deficient and require dietary taurine supplementation (250 mg/cat PO q12h).

Arrhythmias in DCM

Arrhythmias appear to be both common and variable in cats with DCM and may include atrial or ventricular tachyarrhythmias or pathologic bradycardia.[58] In cats receiving treatment with pimobendan, a positive inotrope commonly indicated for dogs with DCM, 7/32 had ECG evidence of arrhythmias, including VPCs ($n=3$), ventricular tachycardia ($n=1$), APCs ($n=1$) and SVT ($n=2$).[60] In canine DCM, particularly in Doberman Pinschers, ventricular arrhythmias are common and rep-

resent a substantial risk factor for sudden death.[61,62] Whether or not this is similarly true in cats with DCM is not clear, at least in part because of the currently low incidence of the disease. Six of 106 cats (5.7%) with ventricular arrhythmias described by Côté et al.[2] had an echocardiographic diagnosis of DCM.

Treating ventricular arrhythmias in cats with DCM may present a formidable challenge since β-blockers like sotalol and atenolol have the potential to exacerbate systolic dysfunction, particularly if gradual up-titration of the dose over several days or weeks is not possible. In such cases, it is imperative to keep in mind the extraneous factors that may exacerbate arrhythmias. Addressing such factors may make specific anti-arrhythmic therapy less essential. A common example of this principle is the occurrence of ventricular arrhythmias in patients with acute CHF and associated hypoxia. Appropriate treatment would prioritise supplemental oxygen, diuretics and/or therapeutic thoracocentesis to improve oxygenation, which often stabilises arrhythmias without the need for anti-arrhythmic drugs. When these factors have been eliminated or controlled and ventricular tachyarrhythmias persist at rates that threaten normal cardiac output (approximately >250 bpm), then anti-arrhythmic drugs may be necessary. Options include lidocaine 0.25–2 mg/kg by slow IV injection and only to effect, with the potential option of a continuous rate at 10–40 mcg/kg/min; mexiletine 5 mg/kg PO q8h; or sotalol 2 mg/kg PO q8h.[16,17,19,33,63] Another important treatment consideration in feline DCM is use of a positive inotrope such as digoxin 0.007 mg/kg PO q48h (approximately 1/8 to 1/4 of a 0.125 mg tablet PO q48h) or pimobendan 0.25 mg/kg PO q12h, both of which require informed owner consent as their use in cats is off-label.[19]

Supraventricular arrhythmias, including atrial fibrillation, may require rate-control treatment with diltiazem 1–2.5 mg/kg PO q8h if the ventricular response rate is fast enough to threaten normal cardiac output.

In several countries, diltiazem is licensed in cats for the treatment of primary hypertrophic cardiomyopathy, but it is important to note that no anti-arrhythmic drugs are licensed for treatment of arrhythmias in cats. Therefore, informed owner consent should be obtained prior to administration of anti-arrhythmic drugs, especially in the settings of CHF and concurrent disease.

References

1 Ferasin L, Sturgess CP, Cannon MJ, Caney SMA, Gruffydd-Jones TJ, Wotton PR. Feline idiopathic cardiomyopathy: a retrospective study of 106 cats (1994–2001). J Feline Med Surg. 2003;5:151–159.

2 Cote E, Jaeger R. Ventricular tachyarrhythmias in 106 cats: associated structural cardiac disorders. J Vet Intern Med. 2008;22:1444–1446.

3 Maron BJ. Hypertrophic cardiomyopathy and other causes of sudden cardiac death in young competitive athletes, with considerations for preparticipation screening and criteria for disqualification. Cardiol Clin. 2007;25:399–414–vi.

4 Jackson BL, Lehmkuhl LB, Adin DB. Heart rate and arrhythmia frequency of normal cats compared to cats

with asymptomatic hypertrophic cardiomyopathy. J Vet Cardiol. 2014;16:215–225.

5 Payne JR, Borgeat K, Connolly DJ, Boswood A, Dennis S, Wagner T, *et al*. Prognostic indicators in cats with hypertrophic cardiomyopathy. J Vet Intern Med. 2013;27:1427–1436.

6 Payne JR, Borgeat K, Brodbelt DC, Connolly DJ, Luis Fuentes V. Risk factors associated with sudden death vs. congestive heart failure or arterial thromboembolism in cats with hypertrophic cardiomyopathy. J Vet Cardiol. 2015;17(Suppl. 1):S318–S328.

7 Aronson RS. Mechanisms of arrhythmias in ventricular hypertrophy. J Cardio Electrophysiol. 1991;2:249–261.

8 Rials SJ, Wu Y, Ford N, Pauletto FJ, Abramson SV, Rubin AM, *et al*. Effect of left ventricular hypertrophy and its regression on ventricular electrophysiology and vulnerability to inducible arrhythmia in the feline heart. Circulation. 1995;91:426–430.

9 Coppini R, Ferrantini C, Yao L, Fan P, Del Lungo M, Stillitano F, *et al*. Late sodium current inhibition reverses electromechanical dysfunction in human hypertrophic cardiomyopathy. Circulation. 2013;127:575–584.

10 Passini E, Mincholé A, Coppini R, Cerbai E, Rodriguez B, Severi S, *et al*. Mechanisms of pro-arrhythmic abnormalities in ventricular repolarisation and anti-arrhythmic therapies in human hypertrophic cardiomyopathy. J Mol Cell Cardiol. 2016;96:72–81.

11 Heller LJ, Stauffer EK, Fox WD. Electrical and mechanical properties of cardiac muscles from spontaneously hypertensive rats (SHR). Fed Proc. 1978;37:349.

12 Adabag AS, Maron BJ, Appelbaum E, Harrigan CJ, Buros JL, Gibson CM, *et al*. Occurrence and frequency of arrhythmias in hypertrophic cardiomyopathy in relation to delayed enhancement on cardiovascular magnetic resonance. J Am Coll Cardiol. 2008;51:1369–1374.

13 O'Hanlon R, Grasso A, Roughton M, Moon JC, Clark S, Wage R, *et al*. Prognostic significance of myocardial fibrosis in hypertrophic cardiomyopathy. J Am Coll Cardiol. 2010;56:867–874.

14 MacDonald KA, Wisner ER, Larson RF, Klose T, Kass PH, Kittleson MD. Comparison of myocardial contrast enhancement via cardiac magnetic resonance imaging in healthy cats and cats with hypertrophic cardiomyopathy. Am J Vet Res. 2005;66:1891–1894.

15 Rush JE, Freeman LM, Fenollosa NK, Brown DJ. Population and survival characteristics of cats with hypertrophic cardiomyopathy: 260 cases (1990–1999). J Am Vet Med Assoc. 2002;220:202–207.

16 Muir WM III, Sams RA, Moise SN. In Textbook of canine and feline cardiology (eds. Fox PR, Sisson D, Moise SN, pp. 307–330). Philadelphia: Saunders; 1999.

17 Fox PR, Harpster NK. In Textbook of canine and feline cardiology (eds. Fox PR, Sisson D, Moise SN, pp. 386–399). Philadelphia: Saunders; 1999.

18 Pypendop BH, Ilkiw JE. Assessment of the hemodynamic effects of lidocaine administered IV in isoflurane-anesthetized cats. Am J Vet Res. 2005;66:661–668.

19 Côté E, MacDonald KA, Meurs KM, Sleeper MM. Feline cardiology. Hoboken: John Wiley & Sons, Inc.; 2011. doi:10.1002/9781118785782

20 Ware WA. Twenty-four-hour ambulatory electrocardiography in normal cats. J Vet Intern Med. 1999;13:175–180.

21 Abbott JA. Heart rate and heart rate variability of healthy cats in home and hospital environments. J Feline Med Surg. 2005;7:195–202.

22 Boyden PA, Tilley LP, Albala A, Liu SK, Fenoglio JJ, Wit AL. Mechanisms for atrial arrhythmias associated with cardiomyopathy: a study of feline hearts with primary myocardial disease. Circulation. 1984;69:1036–1047.

23 Boyden PA, Tilley LP, Albala A, Liu SK, Fenoglio JJ, Wit AL. Mechanisms for atrial arrhythmias associated with cardiomyopathy: a study of feline hearts with primary myocardial disease. Circulation. 1984;69:1036–1047.

24 Wright KN. In Kirks current veterinary therapy (eds. Bonagura JD, Twedt DC). Amsterdam: Elsevier; 2014.

25 Cote E. In Textbook of veterinary internal medicine (ed. Ettinger S, pp. 1159–1187). Amsterdam: Elsevier; 2010.

26 Nattel S. New ideas about atrial fibrillation 50 years on. Nature. 2002;415:219–226.

27 Cote E, Harpster NK, Laste NJ, MacDonald KA, Kittleson MD, Bond BR, *et al*. Atrial fibrillation in cats: 50 cases (1979–2002). J Am Vet Med Assoc. 2004;225:256–260.

28 Bright JM, Martin JM, Mama K. A retrospective evaluation of transthoracic biphasic electrical cardioversion for atrial fibrillation in dogs. J Vet Cardiol. 2005;7:85–96.

29 Wall M, Calvert CA, Sanderson SL, Leonhardt A, Barker C, Fallaw TK. Evaluation of extended-release diltiazem once daily for cats with hypertrophic cardiomyopathy. J Am Anim Hosp Assoc. 2005;41:98–103.

30 Liu SK, Tilley LP, Tashjian RJ. Lesions of the conduction system in the cat with cardiomyopathy. Recent Adv Stud Cardiac Struct Metab. 1975;10:681–693.

31 Kaneshige T, Machida N, Itoh H, Yamane Y. The anatomical basis of complete atrioventricular block in cats with hypertrophic cardiomyopathy. J Comp Pathol. 2006;135:25–31.

32 Kellum HB, Stepien RL. Third-degree atrioventricular block in 21 cats (1997–2004). J Vet Intern Med. 2006;20:97–103.

33 MacDonald KA. In Textbook of veterinary internal medicine (eds. Ettinger SJ, Feldman EC, pp. 1328–1431). Hoboken: John Wiley & Sons, Inc.; 2010.

34 Liu SK. Pathology of feline heart diseases. Vet Clin North Am. 1977;7:323–339.

35 Meurs KM, Fox PR, Magnon AL, Liu S, Towbin JA. Molecular screening by polymerase chain reaction detects panleukopenia virus DNA in formalin-fixed hearts from cats with idiopathic cardiomyopathy and myocarditis. Cardiovasc Pathol. 2000;9:119–126.

36 Fox PR. Endomyocardial fibrosis and restrictive cardiomyopathy: pathologic and clinical features. J Vet Cardiol. 2004;6:25–31.

37 Stalis IH, Bossbaly MJ, Van Winkle TJ. Feline endomyocarditis and left ventricular endocardial fibrosis. Vet Pathol. 1995;32:122–126.

38 Fox PR, Basso C, Thiene G, Maron BJ. Spontaneously occurring restrictive nonhypertrophied cardiomyopathy in domestic cats: a new animal model of human disease. Cardiovasc Pathol. 2014;23:28–34.

39 De Madron E. In Clinical echocardiography of the dog and cat (ed. De Madron E, pp. 207–228). Amsterdam: Elsevier; 2016.

40 Kimura Y, Fukushima R, Hirakawa A, Kobayashi M, Machida N. Epidemiological and clinical features of the endomyocardial form of restrictive cardiomyopathy in cats: a review of 41 cases. J Vet Med Sci. 2016;78:781–784.

41 Rivenes SM, Kearney DL, Smith EO, Towbin JA, Denfield SW. Sudden death and cardiovascular collapse in children with restrictive cardiomyopathy. Circulation. 2000;102:876–882.

42 Fox PR, Maron BJ, Basso C, Liu SK, Thiene G. Spontaneously occurring arrhythmogenic right ventricular cardiomyopathy in the domestic cat: a new animal model similar to the human disease. Circulation. 2000;102:1863–1870.

43 Fox PR. In Textbook of canine and feline cardiology (eds. Fox PR, Sisson D, Moise SN, pp. 621–678). Philadelphia: Saunders; 1999.

44 Paige CF, Abbott JA, Elvinger F, Pyle RL. Prevalence of cardiomyopathy in apparently healthy cats. J Am Vet Med Assoc. 2009;234:1398–1403.

45 Wilkie LJ, Smith K, Luis Fuentes V. Cardiac pathology findings in 252 cats presented for necropsy; a comparison of cats with unexpected death versus other deaths. J Vet Cardiol. 2015;17(Suppl. 1):S329–S340.

46 Basso C, Fox PR, Meurs KM, Towbin JA, Spier AW, Calabrese F, et al. Arrhythmogenic right ventricular cardiomyopathy causing sudden cardiac death in boxer dogs: a new animal model of human disease. Circulation. 2004;109:1180–1185.

47 Basso C, Corrado D, Marcus FI, Nava A, Thiene G. Arrhythmogenic right ventricular cardiomyopathy. Lancet. 2009;373:1289–1300.

48 Oyama MA, Reiken S, Lehnart SE, Chittur SV, Meurs KM, Stern J, et al. Arrhythmogenic right ventricular cardiomyopathy in Boxer dogs is associated with calstabin2 deficiency. J Vet Cardiol. 2008;10:1–10.

49 Meurs KM, Mauceli E, Lahmers S, Acland GM, White SN, Lindblad-Toh K. Genome-wide association identifies a deletion in the 3′ untranslated region of striatin in a canine model of arrhythmogenic right ventricular cardiomyopathy. Human Genet. 2010;128:315–324.

50 Meurs KM, Stern JA, Sisson DD, Kittleson MD, Cunningham SM, Ames MK, et al. Association of dilated cardiomyopathy with the striatin mutation genotype in boxer dogs. J Vet Intern Med. 2013;27:1437–1440.

51 Pion PD, Kittleson MD, Rogers QR, Morris JG. Myocardial failure in cats associated with low plasma taurine: a reversible cardiomyopathy. Science. 1987;237:764–768.

52 Pion PD, Kittleson MD, Thomas WP, Skiles ML, Rogers QR. Clinical findings in cats with dilated cardiomyopathy and relationship of findings to taurine deficiency. J Am Vet Med Assoc. 1992;201:267–274.

53 Pion PD, Kittleson MD, Thomas WP, Delellis LA, Rogers QR. Response of cats with dilated cardiomyopathy to taurine supplementation. J Am Vet Med Assoc. 1992;201:275–284.

54 Fox PR, Sturman JA. Myocardial taurine concentrations in cats with cardiac disease and in healthy cats fed taurine-modified diets. Am J Vet Res. 1992;53:237–241.

55 Cesta MF, Baty CJ, Keene BW, Smoak IW, Malarkey DE. Pathology of end-stage remodeling in a family of cats with hypertrophic cardiomyopathy. Vet Pathol. 2005;42:458–467.

56 Meurs KM, Lahmers S, Keene BW, White SN, Oyama MA, Mauceli E, et al. A splice site mutation in a gene encoding for PDK4, a mitochondrial protein, is associated with the development of dilated cardiomyopathy in the Doberman pinscher. Human Genet. 2012;131:1319–1325.

57 Lawler DF, Templeton AJ, Monti KL. Evidence for genetic involvement in feline dilated cardiomyopathy. J Vet Intern Med. 1993;7:383–387.

58 Sisson DD, Knight DH, Helinski C, Fox PR, Bond BR, Harpster NK, et al. Plasma taurine concentrations and M-mode echocardiographic measures in healthy cats and in cats with dilated cardiomyopathy. J Vet Intern Med. 1991;5:232–238.

59 Novotny MJ, Hogan PM, Flannigan G. Echocardiographic evidence for myocardial failure induced by taurine deficiency in domestic cats. Can J Vet Res. 1994;58:6–12.

60 Hambrook LE, Bennett PF. Effect of pimobendan on the clinical outcome and survival of cats with

non-taurine responsive dilated cardiomyopathy. J Feline Med Surg. 2012;14:233–239.

61 Petric AD, Stabej P, Zemva A. Dilated cardiomyopathy in Doberman Pinschers: survival, causes of death and a pedigree review in a related line. J Vet Cardiol. 2002;4:17–24.

62 Calvert CA, Jacobs G, Pickus CW, Smith DD. Results of ambulatory electrocardiography in overtly healthy Doberman Pinschers with echocardiographic abnormalities. J Am Vet Med Assoc. 2000;217:1328–1332.

63 Kittleson MD. In Small animal cardiovascular medicine (eds. Kittleson MD, Kienle RD, pp. 469–493). St. Louis: Mosby; 1998.

22

Inherited Ventricular Arrhythmias in German Shepherd Dogs
Thibault Ribas and Romain Pariaut

Introduction

Inherited ventricular arrhythmias (VA) in the German Shepherd dog (GSD) is a primary electric disorder first described by N.S. Moïse and colleagues in 1994.[1] Their investigations followed reports of sudden cardiac death in puppies. These animals had severe VAs, and a significant number of them died suddenly without prodromes. A research colony of affected dogs was established at Cornell University to study the pathophysiology and genetic inheritance of this condition.

Epidemiology

This inherited arrhythmia seems to be specific to the GSD, although VAs with similar electrocardiographic characteristics are occasionally detected in young dogs from other breeds. It is likely to be a trait with simple autosomal dominant transmission and incomplete penetrance or a polygenic trait.[2] So far, detailed genetic analyses have failed to identify one or several specific mutations, but studies have pointed to locations on chromosome 6 and chromosome 11.[3]

Although VA can be triggered experimentally in affected dogs as young as 7 weeks of age with intravenous administration of phenylephrine (10 µg/kg), puppies usually spontaneously develop arrhythmias after 12 weeks of age.[2] An age dependence of the arrhythmia has been demonstrated.[4] Indeed, the incidence and severity of VA increase between 7 and 28 weeks and then decrease from 28 to 44 weeks. The VA severity, based on the number of ectopic beats and the complexity of the rhythm (couplets, triplets and runs of ventricular tachycardia), peaks between 20 and 28 weeks. Therefore, young GSDs between the ages of 12 and 50 weeks are considered to be in the vulnerable period which carries the highest risk of sudden cardiac death from ventricular tachycardia degenerating into ventricular fibrillation.

Whenever dogs survive beyond the age of 2 years, the arrhythmia progressively regresses, which eliminates the risk of arrhythmic death. However, in rare cases, dogs up to 30 months of age have died suddenly. The incidence of sudden death has been estimated to be between 15 and 20% in families of affected dogs.[5]

Clinical Presentation

The distinctive feature of this inherited arrhythmia is that it is not associated with the typical clinical signs (exercise intolerance, lethargy or syncope) reported with tachyarrhythmias. Therefore, it is more common to suspect the disease in apparently healthy dogs during cardiac auscultation or on an electrocardiogram (ECG). In the severe form of the disease, sudden cardiac death is the only clinical manifestation. Death occurs most frequently during sleep, especially during phases of rapid eye movement (REM) sleep, but also during rest, recovery after periods of exercise or excitement, and the early morning hours.[2] The risk of sudden death is higher in dogs that have more than 10 short runs of rapid (frequently >450 beats/min) and polymorphic ventricular tachycardia per 24h.[1,2]

Diagnosis

Detection of inherited VAs in GSDs is challenging because the disease is occult until the arrhythmia resolves spontaneously or the animal dies suddenly. In addition, the prevalence of this condition is low, which explains why systematic screening by 24h Holter monitoring is not routinely performed, although it remains the best method to identify affected dogs. Considering that the propensity for VA is higher during periods of bradycardia, ventricular ectopies might be rare or absent during physical examination or routine electrocardiographic

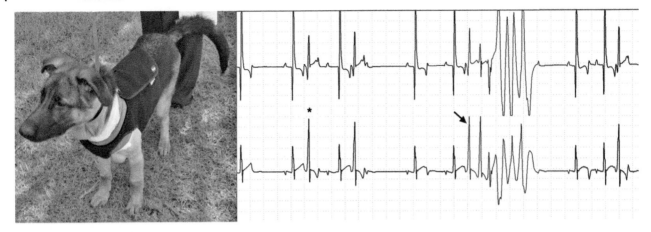

Figure 22.1 Representative sample of a 24 h Holter recording from a 5-month-old German Shepherd dog with inherited ventricular arrhythmia. The underlying rhythm is respiratory sinus arrhythmia. Most sinus beats are followed by a ventricular premature beat (*), and occasional rapid runs of polymorphic ventricular tachycardia (arrow) occur during periods of slow heart rate.

recording in the stressful environment of a veterinary hospital. Twenty-four-hour Holter monitoring in a familiar environment provides a much better assessment of the arrhythmia during periods of exercise, rest and sleep.[2,6] Screening with a Holter should be strongly recommended in young GSDs whenever:

- There is a history of unexplained or cardiac-related sudden death in the dog's family.
- An arrhythmia is suspected or confirmed during physical examination.
- VAs are detected on an ECG. It is not unusual that the arrhythmia is first detected when young GSDs are anaesthetized to be neutered, and their heart rate decreases secondary to the action of sedatives and anaesthetic agents.

The diagnosis is solely based on the presence of VAs, as affected dogs do not have obvious abnormalities on routine haematology, serum biochemistry, thoracic radiographs and transthoracic echocardiogram. However, those tests may be necessary to rule out other causes of VAs. Circulating cardiac troponin I levels measured in a limited number of suspected cases were within the reference interval or mildly increased (unpublished observations).

Subtle electrocardiographic changes have been reported during sinus rhythm in affected GSDs: prolongation of the PR interval by 18%;[7] a notching of the T wave is present during sinus rhythm in some dogs that have frequent ventricular tachycardia;[2] and ST segment elevation is more important in affected than healthy dogs.[8] There is no prolongation of the QT interval. Moreover, this disease is not associated with structural cardiac abnormalities in the young affected dogs and in the adults after resolution of VA. Finally, there are no lesions on gross examination of the heart.[1]

Although the arrhythmia burden can be as low as 10 to 100 ventricular ectopies per hour, VA can represent up to

60% of the heart beats over 24 h in the most severe cases. Ventricular premature complexes usually have a right bundle branch morphology,[9] and they occur as rapid non-sustained runs of polymorphic ventricular tachycardia during periods of sinus bradycardia, often after a pause of the sinus rhythm. During those runs of ventricular tachycardia, the heart rate is frequently over 400 bpm (see Figure 22.1).[4] A young GSD is considered affected if the number of ventricular premature beats exceeds 10 per hour on a 24 h Holter. In addition, these ectopic beats have to be pause-dependent and more frequent during periods of slower sinus rhythm. Finally, it is important to rule out a structural cardiac disease or systemic condition. However, the diagnosis remains challenging because on occasion, the electrocardiographic manifestation of the disease is a monomorphic sustained ventricular tachycardia with a slower rate (200–250 bpm).[2] A few dogs also have occasional supraventricular arrhythmias, including atrial premature beats and short runs of tachycardia. It must, however, be emphasized that it is common to misdiagnose ventricular premature beats as supraventricular beats if examined from a single-lead electrocardiographic recording, and therefore a 6 or 12-lead ECG is strongly recommended to confirm the origin of the ectopic beats.

An increase in heart rate using artificial pacing or drugs (e.g. atropine, glycopyrrolate or isoproterenol) suppresses VA. Usually, arrhythmias disappear if the heart rate exceeds 130 beats per minute.[2] Conversely, phenylephrine, bradycardia and pronounced sinus arrhythmia exacerbate VA. In young GSDs that do not spontaneously have arrhythmias during physical examination, baroreflex-mediated slowing of the heart rate may reveal VAs.[4] However, because of the risk of sudden death, vagal manoeuvres to trigger the arrhythmia are not recommended.

It remains challenging to predict which dogs have a higher risk of sudden cardiac death. Rather than the total number of ventricular ectopic beats, it is the presence of frequent (more than 10 per hour) runs of polymorphic ventricular tachycardia that may identify individuals at higher risk of sudden death.

Mechanism of Arrhythmias

The typical form of VA is described as pause-dependent because most ventricular ectopic beats during sinus rhythm follow long R-R intervals, and they are less frequent when the sinus rate increases.[1] Experimental studies have associated the arrhythmia trigger to early afterdepolarisations (EADs) originating in the Purkinje fibres of the left ventricle.[2,10] EADs increase in frequency when repolarisation of myocytes is prolonged, for example during reflex bradycardia mediated by systemic vasoconstriction following the intravenous injection of the alpha-1 agonist phenylephrine. Phenylephrine also directly promotes abnormal automaticity and EADs in the left ventricular Purkinje fibres by altering the potassium channel currents I_{K1} and I_{Ks}.[11]

The substrate for the arrhythmia is created by abnormalities of cardiac repolarisation in various regions of the left ventricle. Action potential duration measured in the anteroseptal region is significantly longer in affected GSDs, particularly at cycle lengths exceeding 1000 ms (heart rates below 60 bpm).[12] This delay in repolarisation has been attributed to alterations in transmembrane potassium (I_{to}, I_{Kr} and I_{Ks}) and calcium (I_{Ca-L}) currents.[2,8,13,14] In addition to electrophysiologic changes, abnormal sympathetic innervation of the left ventricle is present in affected dogs, specifically in the anterior interventricular septum and portions of left ventricular free wall, and response to adrenergic stimulation is altered.[2,11,12,15–17] It is likely that the lack of sympathetic innervation impacts normal cardiac ion channel development. While EADs trigger the arrhythmia, runs of tachycardia could result from re-entries as a result of an heterogeneity of left ventricular repolarisation, which is reflected by T wave changes on the surface ECT at baseline.[18]

Approximately 17% of afflicted dogs also show monomorphic ventricular tachycardia with slower rate. This type of VA is secondary to triggered activity attributable to delayed afterdepolarisations (DADs).[12] DADs are induced by beta-1-adrenergic receptor stimulation, which is consistent with the higher frequency of this type of arrhythmia during sinus tachycardia.[12]

Treatment

Medical Therapy

One strategy to limit the occurrence of ventricular ectopies is to prevent bradycardia, which can be achieved short term by increasing the heart rate with atropine,

glycopyrrolate or isoproterenol.[2] Lidocaine (2 mg/kg intravenously), a sodium channel blocker which also shortens action potential duration, is very effective at suppressing the arrhythmia,[2] for example during anaesthesia. Conversely, bradycardia should be avoided, and therefore the use of beta-adrenergic antagonist medications is likely to be contraindicated.

Long-term management with oral medications is challenging. Sotalol, as monotherapy, exacerbates VA in GSDs. Experimentally, it prolongs action potential duration in isolated Purkinje fibres and increases the number of EADs.[7,19,20] Despite the real efficacy of lidocaine, mexiletine, used alone, does not significantly decrease VA.[19] However, a synergic effect seems to exist when mexiletine is combined with sotalol, causing a reduction in the number of ventricular premature beats but not the number of runs of VT.[19] Based on current data that suggest a small beneficial effect of this treatment protocol, the combination therapy of mexiletine (8 mg/kg PO q8h) and sotalol (2.5 mg/kg PO q12h) is used for arrhythmia management during the vulnerable period of the disease. Unfortunately, no published study has clearly investigated the effect of medical treatment on the risk of sudden death. Therefore, even a significant reduction in VA with treatment does not necessarily imply a reduction in the risk of sudden cardiac death.

Implantable Cardioverter-Defibrillator (ICD)

The feasibility of ICDs has been tested experimentally in a few dogs, and one report has been published on the use of an ICD in a client-owned dog with inherited VAs considered to be at high risk for sudden death.[21] This dog had severe VAs that showed poor response to medical treatment with mexiletine and sotalol. After implantation of the device, the dog initially received several inappropriate shocks during periods of rapid sinus tachycardia that was erroneously identified as ventricular tachycardia by the device, and subsequently the ICD became infected. Ultimately, the dog survived the vulnerable period, and the device was removed 6 months after implantation. The use of ICDs to terminate ventricular fibrillation in the most severely affected dogs requires further work.

Prognosis

The risk of sudden death correlates with severity of arrhythmias.[2] 15 to 20% of affected dogs die suddenly, most frequently during their first year of life.[2] In dogs that survive beyond the age of 2 years, the frequency of VA remains stable throughout the animal's life or completely resolves in some dogs.[2]

References

1 Moise NS, Meyers-Wallen V, Flahive WJ, Valentine BA, Scarlett JM, Brown CA, *et al.* Inherited VAs and sudden death in German shepherd dogs. J Am Coll Cardiol. 1994;24:233–243.

2 Moise NS, Gilmour RFJ, Riccio ML. An animal model of spontaneous arrhythmic death. J Cardiovasc Electrophysiol. 1997;8:98–103.

3 Brisbin A, Cruickshank J, Moïse NS, Gunn T, Bustamante CD, Mezey JG. Fast, exact linkage analysis for categorical traits on arbitrary pedigree designs. Genet Epidemiol. 2011;35:371–380.

4 Moise NS, Riccio ML, Kornreich B, Flahive WJJ, Gilmour RFJ. Age dependence of the development of VAs in a canine model of sudden cardiac death. Cardiovasc Res. 1997;34:483–492.

5 Moise NS, Gilmour RF, Riccio ML, Flahive WF. Diagnosis of inherited ventricular tachycardia in German shepherd dogs. J Am Vet Med Assoc. 1997;210:403–410.

6 Moise NS, Brittain DD, Flahive WJJ, Riccio ML, Ernst RS, Scarlett J, *et al.* Relationship of ventricular tachycardia to sleep/wakefulness in a model of sudden cardiac death. Pediatr Res. 1996;40:344–350.

7 Merot J, Probst V, Debailleul M, Gerlach U, Moise NS, Le Marec H, *et al.* Electropharmacological characterization of cardiac repolarization in German shepherd dogs with an inherited syndrome of sudden death: abnormal response to potassium channel blockers. J Am Coll Cardiol. 2000;36:939–947.

8 Protas L, Sosunov EA, Anyukhovsky EP, Moïse NS, Rosen MR, Robinson RB. Regional dispersion of L-type calcium current in ventricular myocytes of German shepherd dogs with lethal cardiac arrhythmias. Heart Rhythm. 2005;2:172–176.

9 Hamlin RL. Animal models of VAs. Pharmacol Ther. 2007;113:276–295.

10 Gilmour RFJ, Moise NS. Triggered activity as a mechanism for inherited VAs in German shepherd dogs. J Am Coll Cardiol. 1996;27:1526–1533.

11 Sosunov EA, Obreztchikova MN, Anyukhovsky EP, Moïse NS, Danilo PJ, Robinson RB, *et al.* Mechanisms of alpha-adrenergic potentiation of VAs in dogs with inherited arrhythmic sudden death. Cardiovasc Res. 2004;61:715–723.

12 Sosunov EA, Gainullin RZ, Moise NS, Steinberg SF, Danilo P, Rosen MR. Beta(1) and beta(2)-adrenergic receptor subtype effects in German shepherd dogs with inherited lethal VAs. Cardiovasc Res. 2000;48:211–219.

13 Freeman LC, Pacioretty LM, Moise NS, Kass RS, Gilmour RFJ. Decreased density of Ito in left ventricular myocytes from German shepherd dogs with inherited arrhythmias. J Cardiovasc Electrophysiol. 1997;8:872–883.

14 Jesty SA, Jung SW, Cordeiro JM, Gunn TM, Di Diego JM, Hemsley S, *et al.* Cardiomyocyte calcium cycling in a naturally occurring German shepherd dog model of inherited VA and sudden cardiac death. J Vet Cardio. 2013;15:5–14.

15 Dae MW, Lee RJ, Ursell PC, Chin MC, Stillson CA, Moise NS. Heterogeneous sympathetic innervation in German shepherd dogs with inherited VA and sudden cardiac death. Circulation. 1997;96:1337–1342.

16 Sosunov EA, Anyukhovsky EP, Shvilkin A, Hara M, Steinberg SF, Danilo PJ, *et al.* Abnormal cardiac repolarization and impulse initiation in German shepherd dogs with inherited VAs and sudden death. Cardiovasc Res. 1999;42:65–79.

17 Sosunov EA, Anyukhovsky EP, Gainullin RZ, Plotnikov A, Danilo PJ, Rosen MR. Long-term electrophysiological effects of regional cardiac sympathetic denervation of the neonatal dog. Cardiovasc Res. 2001;51;659–669.

18 Obreztchikova MN, Sosunov EA, Anyukhovsky EP, Moïse NS, Robinson RB, Rosen MR. Heterogeneous ventricular repolarization provides a substrate for arrhythmias in a German shepherd model of spontaneous arrhythmic death. Circulation. 2003;108:1389–1394.

19 Gelzer ARM, Kraus MS, Rishniw M, Hemsley SA, Moïse NS. Combination therapy with mexiletine and sotalol suppresses inherited ventricular arrhythmias in German shepherd dogs better than mexiletine or sotalol monotherapy: a randomized cross-over study. J Vet Cardiol. 2010;12:93–106.

20 Moise NS. From cell to cageside: autonomic influences on cardiac rhythms in the dog. J Small Anim Pract. 1998;39:460–468.

21 Pariaut R, Saelinger C, Queiroz-Williams P, Strickland KN, Marshall HC. Implantable cardioverter-defibrillator in a German shepherd dog with ventricular arrhythmias. J Vet Cardiol. 2011;13:203–210.

23

Systemic Disease and Arrhythmias, Including Selected Non-cardiogenic Causes of Collapse

Jon Wray

Introduction

A large number of extra-cardiac disorders may provoke cardiac rhythm disturbances in dogs and cats. Therefore, it is important to interpret the electrocardiogram (ECG) in the context of the patient's clinical presentation and history, results of physical examination findings, known comorbidities and current drug therapy. This chapter is not intended to be an exhaustive, comprehensive review, but it does include clinically important and well-recognised disorders, including:

- Autonomic disturbances
- Hypoxia
- Electrolyte and acid–base disturbances
- Endocrinopathies
- Abdominal disease
- Trauma
- Drugs and intoxications
- Non-cardiac causes of collapse and episodic weakness.

Autonomic

The anatomy and physiological role of the autonomic nervous system in heart rate and rhythm control are described in chapters 1 and 2.

Vagotonia in Respiratory and Gastrointestinal Disease

In dogs, increased vagal tone may produce bradyarrhythmias such as sinus bradycardia, sinus block, sinus arrest and first and second-degree (usually Mobitz type I) atrioventricular block. These abnormalities are rarely reported in cats due to the inherent sympathetic dominance in this species. Increased vagal tone is seen in patients with respiratory disease, including after lung surgery,[1] and with severe gastrointestinal disorders. Breeds affected by components of brachycephalic obstructive airway syndrome will often display periods of sinus node block, sinus node arrest and first and second-degree atrioventricular block.

Vagotonia in Central Nervous System (CNS) and Ocular Disorders

Animals with severe CNS disorders may develop bradyarrhythmias through a variety of causes, including:

- Direct stimulation of vagal efferent pathways in some brainstem and cranial cervical spinal cord lesions[2]
- Development of vagal afferent hypersensitivity with cervical spinal disorders
- Cushing's reflex – hypertension and concurrent bradycardia as a result of increased vagal tone secondary to increased intracranial pressure.

The oculocardiac reflex resulting in raised vagal tone may be stimulated by:

- Manipulation of the ophthalmic, maxillary or mandibular branches of the trigeminal nerve
- Space-occupying ocular or peri-ocular lesions causing ocular compression
- During ophthalmic surgery.[3]

Dysautonomia

Dysautonomia is an uncommon syndrome affecting both cats and dogs in which degeneration of autonomic ganglia of unknown aetiology produces dysfunction of both sympathetic and parasympathetic nervous systems. Sinus bradycardia and failure to elevate heart rate in response to stimulation are reported in both cats and dogs and are assumed to be due to loss of sympathetic function.[4]

Myocardial Hypoxia

Ischaemic heart disease has been reported commonly at necropsy in cats with left ventricular hypertrophy, and in dogs with heart failure.[5,6] Atherosclerosis has been reported predominantly in dogs with hyperlipidaemia secondary to hypothyroidism and diabetes mellitus.[7–9] The ECG findings associated with infarction include ventricular tachycardia, atrial fibrillation and ventricular premature complexes (VPCs), intraventricular conduction abnormalities, deviation of the ST segment, tall, peaked T-waves, change in T-wave polarity, development of Q-waves and slurring of the R-wave descent (see Figure 23.1).[5,10]

Electrolyte Abnormalities

Common electrolyte changes that may affect the ECG include changes in potassium (K^+), calcium (Ca^{2+}) and magnesium (Mg^{2+}). As described in chapter 2, transmembrane shifts of ions are key to the normal action potential. ECG changes associated with hyperkalaemia have been studied extensively and therefore are presented in more detail followed by other electrolytes in Table 23.3.

Hyperkalaemia

In dogs and cats, hyperkalaemia may be associated with a number of conditions, including urethral obstruction, hypoadrenocorticism, acute oliguric or anuric renal failure, acidosis, acute tumour lysis or reperfusion injury.[11–15] Traditionally, the ECG changes with hyperkalaemia were investigated by administering potassium to healthy dogs, and the changes were described as occurring in a linear fashion proportional to the amount of potassium administered, as shown in Table 23.1.[11,13,14]

However, whilst these changes are reproducible in experimental situations, in clinical cases these characteristic ECG changes may not occur. In a study of 40 dogs and cats with hyperkalaemia, only 12 ECGs showed changes typical of those described in Table 23.1. In this

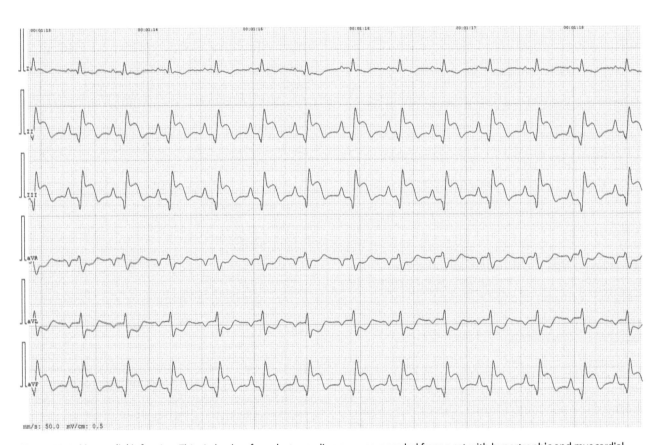

Figure 23.1 Myocardial infarction. This six-lead surface electrocardiogram was recorded from a cat with hypertrophic and myocardial infarction. The suspected area of infarction was visible on echocardiography as a large aneurysmal area on the left ventricular free wall with a very thin and hypomotile myocardium. The electrocardiogram shows a sinus rhythm with an obvious ST elevation visible in all leads except lead I. The increased duration of the P wave (50 ms) and QRS (50 ms) was attributed to significant chamber enlargement. Underlying electrolyte abnormalities were not present in this patient. The PR interval was at the higher end of normal (90 ms). Q waves, another possible finding with myocardial infarction, may be seen in leads I, II, III and aVF. [5-year-old, male neutered, Domestic Shorthair cat with hypertrophic cardiomyopathy and myocardial infarction] (50 mm/s; 20 mm/mV)

Table 23.1 ECG changes seen after administering potassium-containing solution to healthy dogs

Serum potassium concentration	ECG change
5.5–6.5 mEq/L	Tall, peaked T waves
6.6–7 mEq/L	Decrease in R wave amplitude, prolonged QRS and PR intervals, and ST segment depression
7.1–8.5 mEq/L	Decreased P wave amplitude, increased P wave duration and prolongation of QT interval
8.6–10 mEq/L	Lack of P waves (atrial standstill) and sinoventricular rhythm
>10.1 mEq/L	Widening of QRS complex and eventual replacement of the QRS complex with a smooth biphasic waveform; ventricular fibrillation, flutter or asystole

Note: For univalent ions like potassium, 1 mEq/L equals 1 mmol/L.

Table 23.2 ECG changes observed at different serum potassium concentrations in clinical cases

Serum potassium concentration	Number of dogs and cats	ECG changes observed that differed from the expected pattern
5.5–6.5 mEq/L	4 cats, 1 dog	Normal sinus rhythm (2 cats, 1 dog) Sinus bradycardia (1 cat) Sinoventricular rhythm (1 cat)
6.6–7 mEq/L	0 cats, 2 dogs	Normal sinus rhythm
7.1–8.5 mEq/L	6 cats, 6 dogs	Normal sinus rhythm (5 cats, 3 dogs) Sinus tachycardia (1 cat) Tall T waves (1 dog)
8.6–10 mEq/L	5 cats, 2 dogs	Normal sinus rhythm (1 cat, 1 dog) Ventricular tachycardia (1 cat) Tall T waves, atrial standstill, bradycardia (1 cat)
>10.1 mEq/L	7 cats, 4 dogs	Normal sinus rhythm (1 dog) Sinus tachycardia (1 cat) Atrioventricular dissociation with second-degree atrioventricular block (1 dog) Sinoventricular rhythm (1 cat)

ATP-ase, Enzymes that catalyse the decomposition of adenosine triphosphate into adenosine diphosphate.

study, total magnesium, calcium and venous blood gases were also measured, and hypocalcaemia was observed in the cases with the most severe hyperkalaemia.[16]

In a later publication, the same authors described the ECG changes at specific potassium concentrations in more detail, and their findings are summarised in Table 23.2.[15] Other concurrent electrolyte abnormalities documented in this study included hyponatraemia (7/35), hypochloridaemia (15/35), hypermagnesaemia (12/18), hypocalcaemia (6/30) and venous acidaemia (17/18), and it is logical to conclude that the complex interactions between electrolytes in different disease states explain the differences between the changes observed in clinical and experimental situations.

The ECG changes seen with hyperkalaemia are attributed to inactivation of Na-K channels in the cell membrane; reduced potassium efflux during the resting stage, so cells reach threshold potential more slowly; and also prolongation of phase 3 (repolarisation), thereby increasing action potential duration – see Figures 23.2 and 23.3 for ECG changes associated with hyperkalaemia.[11,13,14] The cardiotoxicity of potassium is increased by simultaneous hypocalcaemia, hyponatraemia and acidaemia.

It is important to note that some of the changes seen with hyperkalaemia (e.g. peaked T waves and wide-QRS complexes) are non-specific, and other causes are described in chapter 4.

Endocrinopathies

Thyroid Hormones and Arrhythmias

The heart is sensitive to the effects of thyroid hormone. The thyroid gland produces both triiodothyronine (T_3)

and thyroxine (T_4), with T_3 being the more metabolically active molecule and T_4 acting as a circulating reservoir for conversion to T_3. The effects of T_3 include acting within the cell nucleus stimulating changes in protein synthesis, changes in the activity of sarcolemmal $3Na^+/2K^+$ and $3Na^+/1Ca^{2+}$ channels (see chapter 2) and altered responsiveness to adrenergic stimulation, and it is likely to be the latter actions which can potentially result in arrhythmias.

Increases in sarcolemmal Na^+/K^+ pump activity result in increased myocardial oxygen consumption that is required to fuel the changes in protein synthesis with increased myosin synthesis and also a change in myosin isoenzyme to the fast type.[40,41] Increases in sarcolemmal $3Na^+/1Ca^{2+}$ pump number increase the efficiency of calcium uptake and release that results in an increase in contractility.[41]

This explains why increased levels of thyroid hormone result in myocardial hypertrophy and an increased inotropic state.[42]

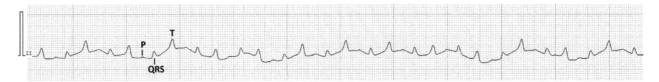

Figure 23.2 Sinus bradycardia and other ECG changes attributed to hyperkalaemia. This electrocardiogram was recorded from a cat with hyperkalaemia (8.3 mEq/L) due to urethral obstruction. Sinus bradycardia (140 bpm) is seen with low-amplitude P waves (0.05 mV; normal <0.2), QRS complexes (0.15 mV; normal <0.9) and tall T waves (0.2 mV; normal <0.3). The duration of the P waves (45 ms; normal <35) and QRS complexes (55 ms; normal <40) are increased, as is the PR interval (110 ms; normal 50–90). [6-year-old, male neutered, Domestic Shorthair cat with urethral obstruction] (50 mm/s; 20 mm/mV)

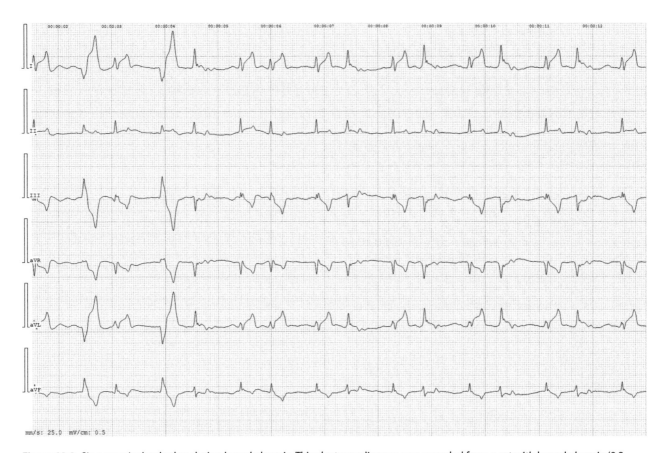

Figure 23.3 Sino-ventricular rhythm during hyperkalaemia. This electrocardiogram was recorded from a cat with hyperkalaemia (9.2 mEq/L) due to acute renal injury. Significant bradycardia (80 bpm) is seen, without visible P waves, wide QRS (90–140 ms; normal <40) and a significantly prolonged QT interval (330 ms; normal 70–200). Additionally, the RR intervals are irregular. These findings are suggestive of a sino-ventricular rhythm in which the sinus node is still able to depolarise, albeit more slowly, and the conduction system still conducts the impulses to the ventricles causing ventricular depolarisation. The atrial myocytes, however, remain in a permanent state of depolarisation due to the high potassium levels, effectively causing atrial standstill. Beats 1 and 3 show a wide, bizarre QRS complex morphology and may be ventricular in origin. [6-year-old, male neutered, Domestic Shorthair cat with acute renal injury] (25 mm/s; 20 mm/mV)

The relationship between thyroid hormones and the sympathetic nervous system is complicated – it has been shown that administration of thyroid hormone can increase the number of β-adrenergic receptors, making the myocardium more sensitive to the effects of circulating catecholamines.[43,44] This is supported by the observation that the administration of β-adrenergic blockade attenuates the effects of thyroid hormone on the heart.[45]

Canine Hypothyroidism

The most common ECG changes reported with hypothyroidism in dogs are sinus bradycardia, low-amplitude P and R waves and inverted T waves.[46–48] In a study

Table 23.3 Electrophysiological alterations, causes and ECG changes associated with electrolyte abnormalities

Electrolyte abnormality	Cardiac electrophysiological effect	Causes	Effect on ECG
Hypokalaemia	• Resting membrane potential more negative (hyperpolarised) • Rapid phase 0 • Delayed ventricular repolarisation • Prolonged action potential duration • Enhanced automaticity	• Increased loss through the gastrointestinal tract (e.g. vomiting and diarrhoea) • Increased urinary loss (e.g. renal failure) • Prolonged decreased intake • Alkalosis or insulin therapy • Iatrogenic (e.g. after furosemide or albuterol administration)[17]	• Supraventricular and ventricular arrhythmias • Prolongation of the QT interval • Prominent U waves • Low-amplitude T waves • ST segment changes[18,19]
Hypercalcaemia	• Impaired conduction through AVN • Raises threshold potential of cardiomyocytes, thereby hindering depolarisation • Shortens early ventricular repolarisation	• Hypercalcaemia of malignancy • Primary hyperparathyroidism • Vitamin D excess • Chronic renal failure • Granulomatous disease • Idiopathic hypercalcaemia in cats	• Long PR • Short QT • Ventricular arrhythmias[20,21] • In humans, an Osborn wave occurs (notching of the terminal section of the QRS complex); however, this has not been reported in hypercalcaemic dogs[22]
Hypocalcaemia	• Prolonged phase 2 of action potential • Threshold potential closer to the resting membrane potential, which results in hyperexcitability[13]	• Hypoparathyroidism (both primary and iatrogenic after bilateral thyroidectomy surgery) • Puerperal tetany (eclampsia) • Intoxication with ethylene glycol • Intestinal hypovitaminosis D • Cats with urethral obstruction may be hypocalcaemic and hyperkalaemic[23]	• Prolonged ST segment and QT interval[13,21] occurred in 4 of 17 dogs with naturally occurring hypoparathyroidism[24] • Tachycardia • Deep wide T waves • Bradycardia[25]
Hypermagnesaemia	• Mg is a co-factor for both sodium–potassium–ATPase and calcium–ATPase[26] • Faster cardiomyocyte repolarisation • Delayed atrioventricular node and intraventricular conduction	• Renal failure • Iatrogenic over-dosage • Endocrinopathies (e.g. hyperparathyroidism, hypothyroidism, hypoadrenocorticism)[26] • Critical illness[27]	• Prolongation of the QRS complex • Shortened QT interval • Prolonged PR interval[13,28] • Increases in potassium and magnesium have opposite effects on the QT interval, and therefore hypomagnesaemia may at least partially negate the effects of hyperkalaemia[29]

(Continued)

Table 23.3 (Continued)

Electrolyte abnormality	Cardiac electrophysiological effect	Causes	Effect on ECG
Hypomagnesaemia	• Decreased intracellular potassium concentration and increased intracellular sodium • Increase in cell resting membrane potential closer to the threshold potential • Increased intracellular sodium, activates $3Na^+/1Ca^{2+}$ counter-transport (see chapter 2) mechanisms resulting in slowed calcium flux which may cause cell injury • Blockage of the voltage-dependent potassium channels resulting in prolonged repolarisation[30] • Lowered threshold for catecholamine-induced ventricular arrhythmias	• Decreased oral intake • Decreased intestinal absorption • Excessive loss via the gastrointestinal or urinary tracts • Endocrine disorders (hyperadrenocorticism, hyperthyroidism, hyperaldosteronism and diabetes mellitus)[26] • Hypomagnesaemia and hypocalcaemia have been associated with protein-losing enteropathy in dogs, especially Yorkshire terriers[31] • Critical illness[27,30]	• Atrial fibrillation • Narrow-QRS complex tachyarrhythmias • Ventricular premature beats • Ventricular tachycardia[9,32]
Acidaemia	• Decreased β-adrenergic receptors available in cardiac nodal tissue[33–35] • Increasing ionised and total serum calcium[14] • Functional impairment of transient outward K^+ current $I_{(to)}$[36] • Electrophysiological effects of acidosis in dogs are known to differ in neonates versus adults[37] and between different myocardial sites[38]	• Respiratory acidosis • Metabolic acidosis	• Ventricular arrhythmias, including ventricular fibrillation and asystole[39]

involving 38 dogs, ECG changes associated with hypothyroidism (in addition to sinus bradycardia) were prolongation of the P wave, PR interval, QRS complex and QT interval.[49] These changes are reversible after adequate thyroid hormone supplementation.[46] Atherosclerosis of coronary vessels is associated with hypothyroidism in dogs and may result in arrhythmias.[9]

Hypothyroidism has been postulated to play a role in development of dilated cardiomyopathy (DCM) in dogs; however, other studies have not supported this theory.[50–52] Dobermans diagnosed with hypothyroidism have a 1.76-fold increased risk of developing DCM, and a dog suffering from DCM has a 2.26-fold increased risk of developing hypothyroidism.[47] However, in this same study, the presence of hypothyroidism in Dobermans did not appear to result in a significant difference in the frequency of VPCs.[47] Human patients with hypothyroidism may show increased frequency of ventricular ectopy, but this has not been observed in Dobermans.[47]

Two Great Danes with hypothyroidism and myocardial failure also had atrial fibrillation.[53] There is a case report of a dog with hypothyroidism and atrial fibrillation that converted back to sinus rhythm after 2 weeks of levothyroxine supplementation.[54] However, in this case, the development of atrial fibrillation was attributed to medetomidine sedation and altered autonomic tone rather than hypothyroidism. A study of large and giant breeds with atrial fibrillation showed that the frequency of primary hypothyroidism in dogs with atrial fibrillation is higher than in the control dogs without atrial fibrillation.[55] Amiodarone administration is contraindicated in hypothyroid dogs due to the effects of this drug on thyroid function.[56]

Feline Hyperthyroidism

As mentioned in this chapter, there is interaction between thyroid hormones and the sympathetic nervous system, and therefore common ECG findings in hyperthyroid cats include sinus tachycardia and increased QRS complex voltage in leads II, III and aVF.[57–59] In another larger study population, low frequencies of atrial and ventricular arrhythmias and intraventricular conduction abnormalities such as left axis deviation and increased QRS complex duration were also recorded.[57,60]

These arrhythmias may resolve once a euthyroid state is re-established. β-adrenergic antagonists help to restore normal heart rates in hyperthyroid cats, providing indirect evidence of the role of the sympathetic nervous system in the genesis of arrhythmias seen in this condition.[61]

Unusual arrhythmias reported in cats with hyperthyroidism include:

- Escape-capture-bigeminy, although whether the hyperthyroidism was the cause of the arrhythmia was not established[62]
- Advanced second-degree atrioventricular block with ventricular escape beats and ventricular tachycardia which persisted after 4 weeks of treatment of hyperthyroidism[63]
- Ventricular pre-excitation[57,64]
- In a retrospective review of cats with third-degree atrioventricular block, three individuals had a palpable goitre, thereby raising suspicion of concurrent hyperthyroidism.[65]

Canine Hyperthyroidism

Hyperthyroidism occurs in dogs due to functional thyroid tumours, excessive supplementation and also feeding of raw diets containing poultry necks.[66,67] The electrocardiographic changes reported associated with hyperthyroidism in dogs include sinus tachycardia, supraventricular ectopy and atrial flutter and increased T wave amplitude.[68,69]

Parathyroid Disease

Parathyroid disease can potentially result in hypo- or hypercalcaemia, and the associated ECG changes have been described previously in Table 23.3.

Adrenal Dysfunction

Hypoadrenocorticism

This condition is caused by a deficiency of either cortisol or mineralocorticoid secretion from the adrenal gland.[70] The mineralocorticoid effects are mediated by aldosterone that controls extracellular fluid balance by modulating sodium excretion and potassium absorption in the renal collecting ducts. Aldosterone deficiency results in profound hypovolaemia, hyponatraemia, hypochloraemia and hyperkalaemia that may result in ECG abnormalities described earlier in this chapter. In a study involving 225 dogs with hypoadrenocorticism, atrial standstill was detected in 47%, bradycardia in 29%, atrial or ventricular extrasystoles in 6% and second or third-degree atrioventricular block in 5%.[71]

There is also a report of a single case that developed atrial fibrillation 40 h after initial evaluation and 30 h after hyperkalaemia had resolved.[72]

Hyperadrenocorticism

Cases with hyperadrenocorticism are considered to be hypercoagulable and therefore at risk of pulmonary thromboembolic disease which could result in pulmonary hypertension. The ECG is an insensitive means of detecting pulmonary hypertension, but, in patients with severe and chronic pulmonary hypertension, there may be ECG changes seen with right heart enlargement such as tall, peaked P waves in lead II, a right ventricular enlargement pattern and a right axis deviation. Left

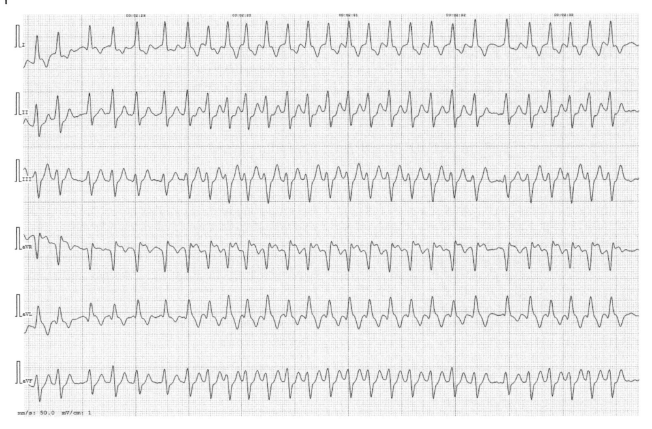

Figure 23.4 Electrocardiographic findings in a dog with pheochromocytoma. This electrocardiogram was recorded from a dog with a pheochromocytoma. An irregular wide-QRS (80 ms) rhythm is seen, with a rate of approximately 230 bpm, and without obvious P waves. These findings were suggestive of ventricular tachycardia, although the possibility of atrial fibrillation with concomitant aberrant ventricular conduction was also considered given the irregularity of the rhythm. Treatment with oral sotalol was successful in converting this rhythm to a regular sinus rhythm. [11-year-old, female neutered, Crossbreed dog with pheochromocytoma] (50 mm/s; 10 mm/mV)

ventricular hypertrophy has been reported in dogs with hyperadrenocorticism and may result in ECG changes (see chapter 4).[73]

Pheochromocytoma

Pheochromocytomas are rare neuroendocrine tumours originating from the medulla of the adrenal glands. They may be functionally active or inactive. Functionally active tumours secrete catecholamines, most commonly norepinephrine, that can lead to systemic effects. As expected, sinus tachycardia was the most common arrhythmia reported in 15% (4 of 26) of cases in one study,[74] and in the same study ventricular ectopy was noted in 24% (5 of 21) of dogs. In another study, unspecified tachyarrhythmias were noted in 43% (9 of 21) of dogs. See Figure 23.4 for an example of an arrhythmia in a dog with pheochromocytoma.[75]

However, other arrhythmias have been reported. In a retrospective study of nine dogs, ECGs were obtained from five – one case showed third-degree atrioventricular block, one case showed atrial premature beats and an idioventicular rhythm, and one case showed ventricular premature beats.[76] Third-degree atrioventricular block and phaechromocytoma in two dogs has also been reported.[77]

Primary Hyperaldosteronism (Conn's syndrome)

This is a rare endocrinopathy in cats and seen even less frequently in dogs. The associated excessive aldosterone secretion results in systemic arterial hypertension, hypernatraemia and hypokalaemia. In cats, severe hypokalaemia was associated with atrioventricular conduction abnormalities with increased PR, QRS and QT intervals. Prominent U waves, atrioventricular dissociation, paroxysmal ventricular tachycardia and reduced T wave amplitude have also been reported with this condition in cats.[78,79] A dog with this condition showed sinus tachycardia, ST segment depression and a slightly increased P wave amplitude on the resting ECG.[80]

Abdominal and Systemic Disease States

Gastric Dilation and Volvulus

Gastric dilation and torsion is a disease most commonly seen in large and giant-breed dogs, and the mechanical distension and twisting of the stomach may result in a large number of metabolic derangements. These include hypovolaemic shock, acidosis, myocardial ischaemia, increased circulating levels of catecholamines and pro-inflammatory cytokines, and pancreatic ischaemia which may lead to production of myocardial depressant factor (MDF).[81–84]

Cardiac arrhythmias are usually reported to be ventricular in origin (VPCs, accelerated idioventricular rhythm, paroxysmal and sustained ventricular tachycardia, and multiform ventricular tachycardia), and they are usually seen 12–36 h after onset of clinical signs.[85,86] Supraventricular rhythm disturbances, including atrial fibrillation, have also been reported.[85]

Cardiac arrhythmia has been reported in 40% (78/193) of dogs with gastric dilation volvulus (GDV) in one study[87] and 42% (48/115) of dogs in another[88] with preoperative arrhythmias being associated with significantly higher mortality than non-arrhythmogenic dogs in some studies[89,90] but not in another.[87] Dogs with GDV often have increased circulating troponin levels, and the magnitude of this increase is correlated to the severity of arrhythmias and also patient outcome.[91]

Whilst these ventricular arrhythmias may be self-limiting within 2–4 days, treatment with lidocaine was successful at re-establishing sinus rhythm in 9 of 11 dogs.[92]

More recently, a prospective non-controlled study was used to compare historical controls with the effect of lidocaine administration to suppress ventricular arrhythmias in cases with gastric dilation and torsion. It showed that early treatment with a lidocaine bolus followed by a continuous rate infusion significantly reduced hospitalisation time and improved outcome.[93] The lidocaine infusion was continued until arrhythmias had improved and then slowly decreased (e.g. by halving the rate every 6 h over a 12 h period).[90]

The role of intracellular magnesium in arrhythmias in GDV patients has been investigated and suggests that intracellular hypomagnesaemia is not a significant contributor to the arrhythmias observed in these patients.[94] Other forms of supportive care to improve outcome for patients with GDV is described elsewhere.[95]

Splenic Disease and Ventricular Arrhythmias

When 24 h ambulatory ECG (Holter) was used to monitor dogs in the 48 h post splenectomy (due to neoplasia, torsion or immune-mediated disease), rapid ventricular tachycardia was detected in 22 of 50 dogs.[96] See Figure 23.5 for an example of an arrhythmia in a dog post

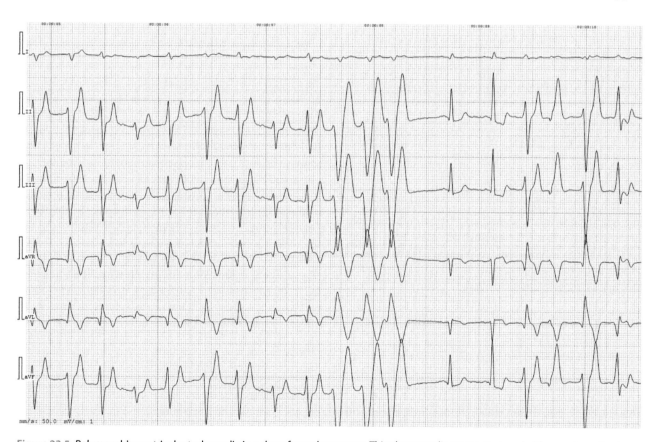

Figure 23.5 Polymorphic ventricular tachycardia in a dog after splenectomy. This electrocardiogram was recorded from a dog a few hours after splenectomy. A wide-QRS rhythm is seen with a rate of approximately 180–200 bpm, consistent with ventricular tachycardia. Beats 13 and 14 are sinus beats with normal P-QRS-T. The ventricular ectopic beats display varying morphology, suggesting more than one ectopic foci. [7-year-old, male Rhodesian Ridgeback post splenectomy] (50 mm/s; 10 mm/mV)

splenectomy. In this study, postoperative ventricular tachycardia was more common in dogs with ruptured splenic masses. Similar results were obtained in a more recent retrospective study of 60 dogs with non-traumatic haemoabdomen, where 11/25 with haemangiosarcoma had ventricular arrhythmias in the postoperative period.[97]

The mechanisms causing the ventricular arrhythmias with splenic disease are thought to be:

- Myocardial ischaemia and hypoxia secondary to reduced venous return and/or anaemia
- Hypovolaemic shock from mass rupture and blood loss
- Acid–base and electrolyte imbalance
- Microemboli
- Pancreatic hypoperfusion or ischaemia, resulting in myocardial depressant factor (MDF) release[53,98]
- Myocardial metastases
- Local or systemic catecholamine release.

As a result of the high frequency of ventricular arrhythmias post splenectomy, continuous ECG monitoring is advised. Although these ventricular arrhythmias will generally resolve spontaneously within 5 days postoperatively, treatment would be indicated if there was haemodynamic instability associated with rapid ventricular tachycardia or frequent/complex ventricular ectopy. Treatment for ventricular arrhythmias post splenectomy generally involves bolus(es) of lidocaine followed by a continuous rate infusion, oxygen supplementation and, in rare cases, short-term treatment with oral sotalol.

Pancreatitis

Although cardiac arrhythmias are anecdotally reported in association with pancreatitis, objective descriptions of specific rhythm disturbances are lacking. It has been postulated that release of MDF secondary to pancreatic ischaemia, or due to haemorrhagic pancreatic necrosis, may contribute to the genesis of arrhythmias, as may electrolyte disturbances resulting from pancreatitis, with both supraventricular and ventricular rhythm disturbances, interventricular conduction disturbances and ST segment changes being described.

Miscellaneous Systemic Disease States Associated with Arrhythmias

Heat Stroke

Sinus tachycardia, T wave and ST segment alterations and ventricular extrasystoles have been reported in association with heat stroke in dogs. Sinus tachycardia appears common, and ventricular arrhythmias are rare but associated with worse outcome in affected dogs.[99]

Electrocution

Electrocution may induce ventricular fibrillation with exposure to low-voltage sources, and higher voltage exposure may induce asystole, ventricular arrhythmias (including ventricular tachycardia) or sinus tachycardia.

Myasthenia Gravis

Third-degree atrioventricular block was reported in association with acquired myasthenia gravis in four dogs, although the mechanism responsible was unclear.[100]

Arrhythmias in Association with Systemic Infectious Diseases

Bradyarrhythmias associated with borreliosis and trypanosomiasis are discussed in more detail in chapter 7.

- *Borrelia burgdorferi*: Complete heart block[101]
- *Clostridium tetani*: bradycardia, sinus arrest and second-degree atrioventricular block[102]
- *Trypanosoma cruzi* infections in dogs may result in ECG changes and arrhythmias, including prolonged PR interval, atrioventricular block, decreased R-wave amplitude with progression to VPCs, and multiform ventricular tachycardia.[103–105]

Trauma

Several published studies report the incidence of cardiac abnormalities presumed to be due to traumatic myocardial injury in dogs who have sustained a blunt chest injury (BCI).[106–108] Increased automaticity, conduction block and triggered activity may all contribute to arrhythmias in BCI patients. Additionally, concurrent hypoxia, acidosis, electrolyte disturbances, enhanced sympathetic tone and catecholamine release may contribute to loss of organised depolarisation. A prospective study of 30 dogs which had presented with motor vehicle trauma occurring in the previous 24 h and in which 24 h ambulatory ECG monitoring was performed revealed ventricular ectopy in 29 dogs (97%) at a rate ranging from <100 VPCs/24 h to 191,953 VPCs/24 h.[108]

Arrhythmias reported in dogs with BCI have included:

- Ventricular premature depolarisations and ventricular tachycardia[108,109]
- Third-degree atrioventricular block[110]
- Paroxysmal atrial fibrillation[111]
- Second-degree atrioventricular block[108]
- Supraventricular tachycardia[108,112]
- Sinus arrest with ventricular or junctional escape[108]
- Abnormal ST elevation or depression.[112]

An early priority in veterinary patients with arrhythmia secondary to BCI should be to establish (1) whether the arrhythmia is haemodynamically significant and (2) whether identification and correction of concurrent pathological states (especially correction of electrolyte disturbances, provision of fluid and oxygen therapy to counter acid–base disturbances and hypoxia, provision of adequate analgesia and correction of blood loss) would result in correction of the arrhythmia.

Toxicity and Arrhythmias

Methylxanthines

Methylxanthines are plant-derived alkaloids such as caffeine, theobromine and theophylline that are commonly found in human foodstuffs. Caffeine is found in coffee, tea and other soft drinks, especially energy drinks. Theobromine is found in cacao seeds and in products manufactured from these seeds, such as chocolate. Methylxanthine toxicity as a result of chocolate ingestion is one of the most common toxicities encountered in dogs and may result in arrhythmias.[113,114]

Theophylline is found in tea and is also used as a bronchodilator.

The effects of methylxanthines include:

- Increased cyclic adenosine monophosphate (cAMP)
- Enhanced release of catecholamines
- Increased intracellular calcium whilst inhibiting sequestration of calcium in the sarcoplasmic reticulum.

The result of methylxanthine ingestion is stimulation of the CNS and cardiac muscle, bronchodilation and diuresis.

Methylxanthine toxicity is more common in dogs than cats and is usually caused by chocolate ingestion. The concentration of theobromine varies according to the type of chocolate, with dark chocolate and cocoa powder containing the highest concentrations (e.g. 4.4–8.8 mg theobromine/g) and milk or white chocolate containing lower concentrations (e.g. 1–2 mg/g). Clinical signs are likely in dogs ingesting >20 mg/kg of theobromine, with signs occurring 2–4 h post ingestion and peak levels reached around 10 h after ingestion. Signs observed include hypertension, ventricular arrhythmias, muscle rigidity, ataxia, seizures and coma. Death secondary to cardiac arrhythmias or respiratory failure has been seen at doses >200 mg/kg, although clinical reports exist of case fatalities with doses lower than this and as low as 80 mg/kg.[115] However, if emesis and gastric decontamination are undertaken promptly, then the prognosis may be good.[114]

Oleander Toxicity

Oleander (*Nerium oleander*) is an ornamental shrub found principally in the southeastern United States. It contains cardenolides which are cardiac glycosides acting in a similar fashion to digoxin (inhibition of sarcomlemmal $3Na^+/2K^+$ exchange), and toxicity may result in digoxin-like arrhythmogenic effects along with acute vomiting and diarrhoea. Sporadic cases of small animal oleander toxicity are reported with arrhythmias, including ventricular extrasystoles, bradycardia, sinus pauses and second-degree atrioventricular block.[116] Diagnosis of oleander toxicity can be confirmed using a digoxin radio-immunoassay, as there is cross-reactivity with this assay.[116]

Cocaine

Arrhythmias have been reported in 10/19 dogs after cocaine toxicosis. Sinus tachycardia was reported in all cases.[117]

Cyclic Antidepressants

Intoxication with cyclic antidepressants (agents containing aromatic nuclei and an aliphatic aminopropyl side chain) can result in central anticholinergic effects and α1-adrenergic blockade. At high doses, toxicity may be seen with repolarisation abnormalities and afterdepolarisations.[118] Common cyclic antidepressant drugs in use include amitriptyline, imipramine and clomipramine. Reported arrhythmias with cyclic antidepressant toxicity include sinus tachycardia, ventricular tachycardia, ventricular fibrillation, prolongation of QRS complexes and PR and QT intervals.[118–120]

Anticholinergics

Many plants and prescription medications have anticholinergic properties, as summarised in Table 23.4.

Anticholinesterases

Anticholinesterases are usually found in organophosphate and carbamate insecticidal/parasiticidal compounds, and also in some industrial flame-retardant preparations. Cardiovascular signs of anticholinesterase toxicity largely result from muscarinic effects, including sinus bradycardia. However, other pro-arrhythmogenic effects which have been attributed to nicotinic stimulation include multiform VPCs which were reported in a cat with organophosphate toxicity,[121] and tachycardia was reported in a dog with acetylcholinesterase inhibitor toxicosis.[122]

Table 23.4 Examples of plants and medications with anticholinergic properties

Plants	Medications
Deadly nightshade (*Atropa belladonna*)	Belladonna alkaloids, including atropine, scopolamine, tropicamide and propantheline
Angel's trumpet (*Brugmansia candida*)	Anti-parkinsonian drugs including benztropine, trihexyphenidyl, procyclidine and biperiden
Night-blooming jessamine (*Cestrum diurnum*)	H1 anti-histaminergic drugs, such as diphenhydramine, chlorpheniramine, clemastine, meclizine and hydroxyzine
Trumpet lily (*Datura arborea*)	Phenothiazines
Jimson weed (*Datura stramonium*)	
Henbane (*Hyocyamus niger*)	
Mandrake (*Mandragora officinarum*)	
Matrimony vine (*Lycium halmifolium*)	
Chalice vine / cup-of-gold (*Solandra* spp.)	

Envenomation

Most envenomations reported to be associated with arrhythmias have occurred with snake or spider bites, or scorpion stings, and are reported in dogs. Arrhythmias induced by envenomation by the European adder (*Vipera berus*) have been studied in 17 dogs prospectively using 24 h ambulatory ECG analysis, and 47% of these demonstrated ventricular arrhythmias.[123] Similar ECG changes were documented in another study of European adder bites.[124] The degree of myocardial damage is likely to be proportional to the degree of troponin elevation.[125]

Envenomation by eastern diamondback rattlesnakes (*Crotalus adamanteus*) resulted in cardiac arrhythmias, predominantly VPCs, in 13/31 (42%) of dogs.[126] Ventricular arrhythmias have also been reported after envenomation of dogs by the Palestinian viper (*Vipera palaestinae*).[127,128]

A variety of arrhythmias were noted after envenomation by Indian red scorpions.[129] This study reported conduction defects (similar to those seen in human patients with myocardial infarction) that were attributed to catecholamine release and autonomic storm. The arrhythmias seen in these cases resolved after administration of insulin. Excessive catecholamine release is also a feature of Sydney funnel web spider envenomation, and tachyarrhythmias have been noted.[130,131]

Approximately 2% of dogs treated with tick antitoxin serum for tick paralysis caused by the Australian paralysis tick (*Ixodes holocyclus*) exhibited a Bezold Jarisch reflex, a vagally mediated cholinergic response typified by bradycardia in combination with systemic vasodilation and mild reduction in myocardial contractility. This is thought to be caused by chemical stimulation of cardiac receptors in the posterior wall of the left ventricle.[132] This reflex is attenuated by atropine administration.

Selected Non-cardiac causes of Episodic Weakness and Collapse

Whilst the following conditions are non-cardiac, the presenting signs are often mistaken for cardiac disease, and therefore awareness of these conditions can be useful in directing appropriate further investigation.

Duchenne Muscular Dystrophy (DMD)

DMD is a rare condition caused by an X-linked mutation on the DMD gene resulting in loss of the protein dystrophin. The absence of dystrophin leads to myofibre membrane fragility and necrosis, with eventual muscle atrophy and contractures ultimately resulting in death due to respiratory failure or cardiomyopathy.[133] ECG changes associated with this condition in Golden Retrievers have been described, including a short PR interval, deep Q waves and ventricular arrhythmias.[134] The deep Q waves have been attributed to changes in the Purkinje fibres.[135]

Autosomal Recessive Centronuclear Myopathy (CNM) in Labrador Retrievers

CNM in Labrador Retrievers is a hereditary myopathy characterised by skeletal muscle problems such as muscle weakness and exercise intolerance. It is also known as hereditary myopathy of the Labrador Retriever (HMLR) with an autosomal recessive pattern of inheritance. Clinical signs in affected dogs develop within the first 1–7 months of life and include gait abnormalities, generalised weakness, exercise intolerance, absence of patellar reflexes, and generalised muscle atrophy prominently affecting limb, cervical and temporal muscles.[136,137]

L-2-Hydroxyglutaric Aciduria (L-2-HGA) in Staffordshire Bull Terriers

L-2-HGA in Staffordshire Bull Terriers is a neurometabolic disorder characterised by elevated levels of L-2-hydroxyglutaric acid in urine, plasma and cerebrospinal fluid. L-2-HGA affects the CNS, with clinical signs usually apparent between 6 months and 1 year (although they can appear later). Symptoms include epileptic seizures, 'wobbly' gait, tremors, muscle stiffness as a result of exercise or excitement and altered behaviour. The mutation probably occurred spontaneously in a single dog but, once in the population, has been inherited from generation to generation like any other gene. The disorder shows an autosomal recessive mode of inheritance.[138]

Canine Epileptoid Cramping Syndrome (CECS or Spike's disease)

CECS, also known as Spike's disease, is a hereditary canine disease with similarities to canine epilepsy, and Border Terriers are reported to be predisposed. This disease is characterised by paroxysms of involuntary movements that occur at rest with no loss of consciousness. Episodes last from minutes to hours, and dogs are completely normal between episodes. Some affected individuals appear to respond favourably to a gluten-free diet.[139]

Border Collie Collapse (BCC)

BCC is a recognised condition in Border Collies in the United States, Europe and Australia. These dogs are normal at rest but intermittently exhibit signs after 5–15 min of strenuous exercise. Abnormalities observed after exercise include upper motor neuron paresis and general proprioceptive ataxia in all four limbs, increased extensor tone and scuffing/knuckling of the pelvic limbs, crossing of the pelvic limbs, and exaggerated stepping or 'stomping' with the thoracic limbs. Many affected dogs are described as having truncal swaying and as staggering or falling to the side, suggesting a balance problem, although none developed a head tilt or abnormal nystagmus. Most of the dogs evaluated were mentally abnormal during BCC episodes, with mentation described by their owners and investigators as dull, disoriented or distracted.[140] Curiously, some dogs can be roused from this dazed state by voice commands or familiar actions, such as putting the dog on the lead. Episodes are unpredictable, and dogs will recover spontaneously. Investigation using standardised exercise tests showed no consistent significant differences in exercising body temperature, heart rate or rhythm (sinus tachycardia), blood gas analysis, serum biochemistry and muscle biopsy findings between normal and affected dogs performing a standardised exercise protocol.[140]

There has been speculation that this condition is a form of generalised non-convulsive seizure. Whilst hot environmental temperature has been proposed as a trigger, DNA from the dogs with BCC did not contain the ryanodine receptor mutation on chromosome 1 which is associated with malignant hyperthermia. Additionally, creatine kinase activity and rectal temperature during collapse and recovery were similar to those of normal dogs performing the same exercise, making malignant hyperthermia very unlikely. Borders Collies with this condition test negative for the dynamin-1 (DNM1) muta-

tion – see the 'Exercise-induced collapse in Labradors' section for more information about this mutation.

Exercise-induced Collapse in Labradors

Exercise-induced collapse (EIC) is a recognised problem in Labradors; it tends to affect athletic young adult dogs often with excitable temperament, and working dogs with high drive. The condition is characterised by episodic weakness at exercise with ataxia and weakness affecting the hindlimbs, then forelimbs, recumbency without loss of consciousness, panting, followed by gradual but complete recovery. Owners report that events are more likely in warm weather.

In 2008, a mutation in the gene encoding the DNM1 protein was reported as being associated with this condition.[141] The frequency of DNM1 mutant allele carriers in Labrador Retrievers from conformation show, field trial/hunt test, pet or service lines ranged from 17.9 to 38.0%, and the frequency of homozygous mutant (EE genotype) individuals ranged from 1.8 to 13.6%; 83.6% of these EE Labradors were reported to have collapsed by 4 years of age.[142] DNM1 is found at synaptic membranes in the CNS and is required for normal neural function, especially during sustained stimulation as occurs during exercise. Although collapse in Labradors has been attributed to dogs who are homozygous for the DNM1 mutation, there are reported cases in dogs heterozygous for this gene mutation and also dogs without the gene mutation who exhibit clinical signs.

In a review of 109 Labrador Retrievers suspected of having EIC, 74 of dogs (68%) were homozygous for the DNM1 mutation, and the remaining 32% were heterozygous or did not have the mutation. A study from Japan showed similar results, with only 4.5% of dogs (6 of 133) being homozygous for the DNM1 mutation.[143] As a significant number of affected dogs do not have the DMN1 mutation, it seems likely that this condition is either multifactorial or not associated with the DMN1 mutation.

The features of collapse in the DNM1 mutation homozygous dogs were:

- First episode of collapse when dogs were <2 years old
- Collapse originating in hindlimbs with or without progression to forelimbs. Collapse predominantly affecting the hindlimbs without progression to the forelimbs showed poor sensitivity (42%) but high specificity (94%) for identification of dogs with EIC.
- Low muscle tone in the affected limbs during collapse
- Clinically normal mentation during collapse
- Rapid recovery (<60 min) from collapse episodes.[144]

As a result of the variation in genotype and phenotype, the authors concluded that there are likely to be other causes of episodic collapse in otherwise healthy Labradors. Labrador Retrievers are predisposed to idiopathic epilepsy,[145] and exercise, excitement and hyperventilation can trigger seizures in epileptic humans.

Dogs heterozygous for the DNM1 mutation and dogs homozygous for the mutation with a collapse phenotype were also detected in Chesapeake Bay Retrievers, Curly-coated Retrievers, Boykin Spaniels, Pembroke Welsh Corgis and mixed-breed dogs thought to be Labrador Retriever crosses. The DNM1 mutation was not identified in Golden, Flat-coated, or Nova Scotia Duck Tolling Retrievers, or 15 other non-retrieving breeds.[142]

Differences between Exercise-induced Collapse and Border Collie Collapse

While Labradors with EIC remain alert and have relatively flaccid but uncoordinated pelvic limbs during an episode, dogs with BCC are mentally abnormal during episodes, are ataxic in all four limbs and have increased extensor tone in the rear limbs with scuffing and knuckling during walking. Labradors with EIC usually try to continue to run and retrieve while dragging their flexed and flaccid rear legs, while dogs with BCC tend to wander aimlessly or stagger and fall.[140]

Conclusion

Systemic disease is a common cause of arrhythmias in small animal patients, and this chapter emphasises the importance of interpreting ECG changes in light of the patient's history, the physical examination and the results of other tests.

References

1 Kocaturk M, Salci H, Yilmaz Z, Bayram AS, Koch J. Pre- and post-operative cardiac evaluation of dogs undergoing lobectomy and pneumonectomy. J Vet Sci. 2010;11257–264.

2 Kube S, Owen T, Hanson S. Severe respiratory compromise secondary to cervical disk herniation in two dogs. J Am Anim Hosp Assoc. 2003;39:513–517.

3 Selk Ghaffari M, Marjani M, Masoudifard M. Oculocardiac reflex induced by zygomatic arch fracture in a crossbreed dog. J Vet Cardiol. 2009;11:67–69.

4 Harkin KR, Andrews GA, Nietfeld JC. Dysautonomia in dogs: 65 cases (1993–2000). J Am Vet Med Assoc. 2002;220:633–639.

5 Driehuys S, Van Winkle TJ, Sammarco CD, Drobatz KJ. Myocardial infarction in dogs and cats: 37 cases (1985–1994). J Am Vet Med Assoc. 1998;213:1444–1448.

6 Kidd L, Stepien RL, Amrheiw DP. Clinical findings and coronary artery disease in dogs and cats with acute and subacute myocardial necrosis: 28 cases. J Am Anim Hosp Assoc. 2000;36:199–208.

7 Hess RS, Kass PH, Van Winkle TJ. Association between diabetes mellitus, hypothyroidism or hyperadrenocorticism, and atherosclerosis in dogs. J Vet Intern Med. 2003;17:489–494.

8 Kagawa Y, Hirayama K, Uchida E, Izumisawa Y, Yamaguchi M, Kotani T, *et al.* Systemic atherosclerosis in dogs: histopathological and immunohistochemical studies of atherosclerotic lesions. J Comp Pathol. 1998;118:195–206.

9 Liu SK, Tilley LP, Tappe JP, Fox PR. Clinical and pathologic findings in dogs with atherosclerosis: 21 cases (1970–1983). J Am Vet Med Assoc. 1986;189:227–232.

10 Patterson DF, Detweiler DK, Hubben K, Botts RP. Spontaneous abnormal cardiac arrhythmias and conduction disturbances in the dog: a clinical and pathologic study of 3,000 dogs. Am J Vet Res. 1961;22:355–369.

11 Ettinger PO, Regan TJ, Oldewurtel HA. Hyperkalemia, cardiac conduction, and the electrocardiogram: a review. Am Heart J. 1974;88:360–371.

12 Norman BC, Cote E, Barrett KA. Wide-complex tachycardia associated with severe hyperkalemia in three cats. J Feline Med Surg. 2006;8:372–378.

13 Surawicz B. Relationship between electrocardiogram and electrolytes. Am Heart J. 1967;73:814–834.

14 Surawicz B. Electrolytes and the electrocardiograim. Postgrad Med. 1974;55:123–129.

15 Tag TL, Day TK. Electrocardiographic assessment of hyperkalemia in dogs and cats. J Vet Emerg Crit Care. 2008;18:61–67.

16 Tag TL, Day TK. Electrocardiographic assessment of hyperkalaemia in dogs and cats. J Vet Emerg Crit Care. 2004;14:S1–S17.

17 Romito G, Cote E, Domenech O. ECG of the month: sinus tachycardia due to albuterol-induced hypokalemia. J Am Vet Med Assoc. 2013;243:1108–1110.

18 Bahler RC, Rakita L. Cardiovascular function in potassium-depleted dogs. Am Heart J. 1971;81:650–657.

19 Felkai F. Electrocardiographic signs in ventricular repolarisation of experimentally induced hypokalaemia and appearance of the U-wave in dogs. Acta Vet Hung. 1985;33:221–228.

20 Surawicz B. Effect of Ca on duration of QT interval and ventricular systole in dog. Am J Physiol. 1963;205:785–789.

21 Feldman EC, Ettinger SJ. Electrocardiographic changes associated with electrolyte disturbances. Vet Clin North Am. 1977;7:487–496.

22 Otero J, Lenihan DJ. The 'normothermic' Osborn wave induced by severe hypercalcemia. Tex Heart Inst J. 2000;27:316–317.

23 Drobatz KJ, Hughes D. Concentration of ionized calcium in plasma from cats with urethral obstruction. J Am Vet Med Assoc. 1997;211:1392–1395.

24 Russell NJ, Bond KA, Robertson ID, Parry BW, Irwin PJ. Primary hypoparathyroidism in dogs: a retrospective study of 17 cases. Aust Vet J. 2006;84:285–290.

25 Sherding RG, Meuten DJ, Chew DJ, Knaack KE, Haupt KH. Primary hypoparathyroidism in the dog. J Am Vet Med Assoc. 1980;176:439–444.

26 Humphrey S, Kirby R, Rudloff E. Magnesium physiology and clinical therapy in veterinary critical care. J Vet Emerg Crit Care. 2015;25:210–225.

27 Toll J, Erb H, Birnbaum N, Schermerhorn T. Prevalence and incidence of serum magnesium abnormalities in hospitalized cats. J Vet Intern Med. 2002;16:217–221.

28 Nakayama T, Nakayama H, Miyamoto M, Hamlin RL. Hemodynamic and electrocardiographic effects of magnesium sulfate in healthy dogs. J Vet Intern Med. 1999;13:485–490.

29 Martin LG. Hypercalcemia and hypermagnesemia. Vet Clin North Am Small Anim Pract. 1998;28:565–585.

30 Khanna C, Lund EM, Raffe M, Armstrong PJ. Hypomagnesemia in 188 dogs: a hospital population-based prevalence study. J Vet Intern Med. 1998;12:304–309.

31 Kimmel SE, Waddell LS, Michel KE. Hypomagnesemia and hypocalcemia associated with protein-losing enteropathy in Yorkshire terriers: five cases (1992–1998). J Am Vet Med Assoc. 2000;217:703–706.

32 Dhupa N, Proulx J. Hypocalcemia and hypomagnesemia. Vet Clin North Am Small Anim Pract. 1998;28:587–608.

33 Marsh JD, Margolis TI, Kim D. Mechanism of diminished contractile response to catecholamines during acidosis. Am J Physiol. 1988;254:H20–H27.

34 Orchard CH, Kentish JC. Effects of changes of pH on the contractile function of cardiac muscle. Am J Physiol. 1990;258:C967–C981.

35 Mitchell JH, Wildenthal K, Johnson RLJ. The effects of acid-base disturbances on cardiovascular and pulmonary function. Kidney Int. 1972;1:375–389.

36 Du Z, Chaoqian X, Shan H, Lu Y, Ren N. Functional impairment of cardiac transient outward K+ current as a result of abnormally altered cellular environment. Clin Exp Pharmacol Physiol. 2007;34:148–152.

37 Geller JC, Rosen MR. Age related differences in the response to acidosis, hypoxia, and hyperkalaemia in canine cardiac Purkinje fibers. Cardiovasc Res. 1994;28:125–128.

38 Gilmour RFJ, Zipes DP. Different electrophysiological responses of canine endocardium and epicardium to combined hyperkalemia, hypoxia, and acidosis. Circ Res. 1980;46:814–825.

39 Calvert MH. The effect of acute acidosis and its correction on the heart of the conscious dog. Br J Surg. 1971;58:308.

40 Dillmann WH. Hormonal influences on cardiac myosin ATPase activity and myosin isoenzyme distribution. Mol Cell Endocrinol. 1984;34:169–181.

41 Dillmann WH. Biochemical basis of thyroid hormone action in the heart. Am J Med. 1990;88:626–630.

42 Buccino RA, Spann JFJ, Pool PE, Sonnenblick EH, Braunwald E. Influence of the thyroid state on the intrinsic contractile properties and energy stores of the myocardium. J Clin Invest. 1967;46:1669–1682.

43 Dillmann WH. Cellular action of thyroid hormone on the heart. Thyroid. 2002;12:447–452.

44 Ojamaa K, Klein I, Sabet A, Steinberg SF. Changes in adenylyl cyclase isoforms as a mechanism for thyroid hormone modulation of cardiac beta-adrenergic receptor responsiveness. Metabolism. 2000;49:275–279.

45 Kupfer LE, Bilezikian JP, Robinson RB. Regulation of alpha and beta adrenergic receptors by triiodothyronine in cultured rat myocardial cells. Naunyn Schmiedebergs Arch Pharmacol. 1986;334:275–281.

46 Panciera DL. An echocardiographic and electrocardiographic study of cardiovascular function in hypothyroid dogs. J Am Vet Med Assoc. 1994;205:996–1000.

47 Beier P, Reese S, Holler PJ, Simak J, Tater G, Wess G. The role of hypothyroidism in the etiology and progression of dilated cardiomyopathy in Doberman Pinschers. J Vet Intern Med. 2015;29:141–149.

48 Nijhuis AH, Stokhof AA, Huisman GH, Rijnberk A. ECG changes in dogs with hypothyroidism. Tijdschr Diergeneeskd. 1978;103:736–741.

49 Pasławska U, Noszczyk-Nowak A, Kungl K, Bioły K, Popiel J, Nicpon J. Thyroid hormones concentrations and ECG picture in the dog. Pol J Vet Sci. 2006;9:253–257.

50 Scott-Moncrieff JC. Clinical signs and concurrent diseases of hypothyroidism in dogs and cats. Vet Clin North Am Small Anim Pract. 2007;37:709–722.

51 Calvert CA, Jacobs GJ, Medleau L, Pickus CW, Brown J, McDermott M. Thyroid-stimulating hormone stimulation tests in cardiomyopathic Doberman pinschers: a retrospective study. J Vet Intern Med. 1998;12:343–348.

52 Tidholm A, Jonsson L. A retrospective study of canine dilated cardiomyopathy (189 cases). J Am Anim Hosp Assoc. 1997;33:544–550.

53 Phillips DE, Harkin KR. Hypothyroidism and myocardial failure in two Great Danes. J Am Anim Hosp Assoc. 2003;39:133–137.

54 Chow B, French A. Conversion of atrial fibrillation after levothyroxine in a dog with hypothyroidism and arterial thromboembolism. J Small Anim Pract. 2014;55:278–282.

55 Gerritsen RJ, van den Brom WE, Stokhof AA. Relationship between atrial fibrillation and primary hypothyroidism in the dog. Vet Q. 1996;18:49–51.

56 Bicer S, Nakayama T, Hamlin RL. Effects of chronic oral amiodarone on left ventricular function, ECGs, serum chemistries, and exercise tolerance in healthy dogs. J Vet Intern Med. 2002;16:247–254.

57 Peterson ME, Keene B, Ferguson DC, Pipers FS. Electrocardiographic findings in 45 cats with hyperthyroidism. J Am Vet Med Assoc. 1982;180:934–937.

58 Moise NS, Dietze AE, Mezza LE, Strickland D, Erb HN, Edwards NJ. Echocardiography, electrocardiography, and radiography of cats with dilatation cardiomyopathy, hypertrophic cardiomyopathy, and hyperthyroidism. Am J Vet Res. 1986;47:1476–1486.

59 Broussard JD, Peterson ME, Fox PR. Changes in clinical and laboratory findings in cats with hyperthyroidism from 1983 to 1993. J Am Vet Med Assoc. 1995;206:302–305.

60 Fox PR, Peterson ME, Broussard JD. Electrocardiographic and radiographic changes in cats with hyperthyroidism: comparison of populations evaluated during 1992–1993 vs. 1979–1982. J Am Anim Hosp Assoc. 1999;35:27–31.

61 Klein I, Levey GS. New perspectives on thyroid hormone, catecholamines, and the heart. Am J Med. 1984;76:167–172.

62 Visser LC, Scansen BA, Bonagura JD. ECG of the month: escape-capture bigeminy in a cat. J Am Vet Med Assoc. 2014;245:52–54.

63 Martinelli E, Spalla I, Quintavalla C, Brambilla P, Riscazzi G, Locatelli C. ECG of the month. Arrhythmia due to hyperthyroidism in a cat. J Am Vet Med Assoc. 2013;243:787–789.

64 Riesen SC, Lombard CW. ECG of the month. Pleural effusion with hyperthyroidism. J Am Vet Med Assoc. 2005;227:556–558.

65 Kellum HB, Stepien RL. Third-degree atrioventricular block in 21 cats (1997–2004). J Vet Intern Med. 2006;20:97–103.

66 Broome MR, Peterson ME, Kemppainen RJ, Parker VJ, Richter KP. Exogenous thyrotoxicosis in dogs attributable to consumption of all-meat commercial dog food or treats containing excessive thyroid hormone: 14 cases (2008–2013). J Am Vet Med Assoc. 2015;246:105–111.

67 Kohler B, Stengel C, Neiger R. Dietary hyperthyroidism in dogs. J Small Anim Pract. 2012;53:182–184.

68 Fine DM, Tobias AH, Bonagura JD. Cardiovascular manifestations of iatrogenic hyperthyroidism in two dogs. J Vet Cardiol. 2010;12:141–146.

69 Hoey A, Page A, Brown L, Atwell RB. Cardiac changes in experimental hyperthyroidism in dogs. Aust Vet J. 1991;68:352–355.

70 Klein SC, Peterson ME. Canine hypoadrenocorticism: part I. Can Vet J. 2010;51:63–69.

71 Peterson ME, Kintzer PP, Kass PH. Pretreatment clinical and laboratory findings in dogs with hypoadrenocorticism: 225 cases (1979–1993). J Am Vet Med Assoc. 1996;208:85–91.

72 Riesen SC, Lombard CW. ECG of the month: atrial fibrillation secondary to hypoadrenocorticism. J Am Vet Med Assoc. 2006;229:1890–1892.

73 Takano H, Kokubu A, Sugimoto K, Sunahara H, Aoki T, Fijii Y. Left ventricular structural and functional abnormalities in dogs with hyperadrenocorticism. J Vet Cardiol. 2015;17:173–181.

74 Gilson SD, Withrow SJ, Wheeler SL, Twedt DC. Pheochromocytoma in 50 dogs. J Vet Intern Med. 1994;8:228–232.

75 Barthez PY, Marks SL, Woo J, Feldman EC, Matteucci M. Pheochromocytoma in dogs: 61 cases (1984–1995). J Vet Intern Med. 1997;11:272–278.

76 Edmondson EF, Bright JM, Halsey CH, Ehrhart EJ. Pathologic and cardiovascular characterization of pheochromocytoma-associated cardiomyopathy in dogs. Vet Pathol. 2015;52:338–343.

77 Mak G, Allen J. Simultaneous pheochromocytoma and third-degree atrioventricular block in 2 dogs. J Vet Emerg Crit Care. 2013;23:610–614.

78 Atkins CE. The role of noncardiac disease in the development and precipitation of heart failure. Vet Clin North Am Small Anim Pract. 1991;21:1035–1080.

79 Flood SM, Randolph JF, Gelzer AR, Refsal K. Primary hyperaldosteronism in two cats. J Am Anim Hosp Assoc. 1999;35:411–416.

80 Breitschwerdt EB, Meuten DJ, Greenfield CL, Anson LW, Cook CS, Fulghum RE. Idiopathic hyperaldosteronism in a dog. J Am Vet Med Assoc. 1985;187:841–845.

81 Sharp CR, Rozanski EA. Cardiovascular and systemic effects of gastric dilatation and volvulus in dogs. Top Companion Anim Med. 2014;29:67–70.

82 Muir WW, Weisbrode SE. Myocardial ischemia in dogs with gastric dilatation-volvulus. J Am Vet Med Assoc. 1982;181:363–366.

83 Orton EC, Muir WW. 3. Isovolumetric indices and humoral cardioactive substance bioassay during clinical and experimentally induced gastric dilatation-volvulus in dogs. Am J Vet Res. 1983;44:1516–1520.

84 Prabhu SD. Cytokine-induced modulation of cardiac function. Circ Res. 2004;95:1140–1153.

85 Muir WW, Bonagura JD. Treatment of cardiac arrhythmias in dogs with gastric distention-volvulus. J Am Vet Med Assoc. 1984;184:1366–1371.

86 Horne WA, Gilmore DR, Dietze AE, Freden GO, Short CE. Effects of gastric distention-volvulus on coronary blood flow and myocardial oxygen consumption in the dog. Am J Vet Res. 1985;46:98–104.

87 Brockman DJ, Washabau RJ, Drobatz KJ. Canine gastric dilatation/volvulus syndrome in a veterinary critical care unit: 295 cases (1986–1992). J Am Vet Med Assoc. 1995;207:460–464.

88 Muir WW. Gastric dilatation-volvulus in the dog, with emphasis on cardiac arrhythmias. J Am Vet Med Assoc. 1982;180:739–742.

89 Brourman JD, Schertel ER, Allen DA, Birchard SJ, DeHoff WD. Factors associated with perioperative mortality in dogs with surgically managed gastric dilatation-volvulus: 137 cases (1988–1993). J Am Vet Med Assoc. 1996;208:1855–1858.

90 Mackenzie G, Barnhart M, Kennedy S, DeHoff W, Schertel E. A retrospective study of factors influencing survival following surgery for gastric dilatation-volvulus syndrome in 306 dogs. J Am Anim Hosp Assoc. 2010;46:97–102.

91 Schober KE, Cornand C, Kirbach B, Aupperle H, Oechtering, G. Serum cardiac troponin I and cardiac troponin T concentrations in dogs with gastric dilatation-volvulus. J Am Vet Med Assoc. 2002;221:381–388.

92 Muir WW, Lipowitz AJ. Cardiac dysrhythmias associated with gastric dilatation-volvulus in the dog. J Am Vet Med Assoc. 1978;172:683–689.

93 Bruchim Y, Itay S, Shira B-H, Kelmer E, Sigal Y, Itamar A, *et al*. Evaluation of lidocaine treatment on frequency of cardiac arrhythmias, acute kidney injury, and hospitalization time in dogs with gastric dilatation volvulus. J Vet Emerg Crit Care. 2012;22:419–427.

94 Bebchuk TN, Hauptman JG, Braselton WE, Walshaw R. Intracellular magnesium concentrations in dogs with gastric dilatation-volvulus. Am J Vet Res. 2000;61:1415–1417.

95 Bruchim Y, Kelmer E. Postoperative management of dogs with gastric dilatation and volvulus. Top Companion Anim Med. 2014;29:81–85.

96 Marino DJ, Matthiesen DT, Fox PR, Lesser MB, Stamoulis ME. Ventricular arrhythmias in dogs undergoing splenectomy: a prospective study. Vet Surg.1994;23:101–106.

97 Aronsohn MG, Dubiel B, Roberts B, Powers BE. Prognosis for acute nontraumatic hemoperitoneum in the dog: a retrospective analysis of 60 cases (2003–2006). J Am Anim Hosp Assoc. 2009;45:72–77.

98 Knapp DW, Aronsohn MG, Harpster NK. Cardiac arrhythmias associated with mass lesions of the canine spleen. J Am Anim Hosp Assoc. 1993;122.

99 Drobatz KJ, Macintire DK. Heat-induced illness in dogs: 42 cases (1976–1993). J Am Vet Med Assoc. 1996;209:1894–1899.

100 Hackett TB, Van Pelt DR, Willard MD, Martin LG, Shelton GD, Wingfield WE. Third degree atrioventricular block and acquired myasthenia gravis in four dogs. J Am Vet Med Assoc. 1995;206:1173–1176.

101 Levy SA, Duray PH. Complete heart block in a dog seropositive for Borrelia burgdorferi. Similarity to human Lyme carditis. J Vet Intern Med. 1988;2:138–144.

102 Panciera DL, Baldwin CJ, Keene BW. Electrocardiographic abnormalities associated with

tetanus in two dogs. J Am Vet Med Assoc. 1988;192:225–227.

103 Barr SC, Simpson RM, Schmidt SP, Bunge MM, Authement JM, Lozano F. Chronic dilatative myocarditis caused by *Trypanosoma cruzi* in two dogs. J Am Vet Med Assoc. 1989;195:1237–1241.

104 Barr SC, Holmes RA, Klei TR. Electrocardiographic and echocardiographic features of trypanosomiasis in dogs inoculated with North American *Trypanosoma cruzi* isolates. Am J Vet Res. 1992;53:521–527.

105 Meurs KM, Anthony MA, Slater M, Miller MW. Chronic *Trypanosoma cruzi* infection in dogs: 11 cases (1987–1996). J Am Vet Med Assoc. 1998;213:497–500.

106 Schober KE, Kirbach B, Oechtering G. Noninvasive assessment of myocardial cell injury in dogs with suspected cardiac contusion. J Vet Cardiol. 1999;1:17–25.

107 Campbell VL, King LG. Pulmonary function, ventilator management, and outcome of dogs with thoracic trauma and pulmonary contusions: 10 cases (1994–1998). J Am Vet Med Assoc. 2000;217:1505–1509.

108 Snyder PS, Cooke KL, Murphy ST, Shaw NG, Lewis DD, Lanz OI. Electrocardiographic findings in dogs with motor vehicle-related trauma. J Am Anim Hosp Assoc. 2001;37:55–63.

109 Macintire DK, Snider TG. 3. Cardiac arrhythmias associated with multiple trauma in dogs. J Am Vet Med Assoc. 1984;184:541–545.

110 Nicholls PK, Watson PJ. Cardiac trauma and third degree AV block in a dog following a road accident. J Small Anim Pract. 1995;36:411–415.

111 Madewell BR, Nelson DT, Hill K. Paroxysmal atrial fibrillation associated with trauma in a dog. J Am Vet Med Assoc. 1977;71:273–275.

112 Harpster NK, VanZwieten MJ, Bernstein M. Traumatic papillary muscle rupture in a dog. J Am Vet Med Assoc. 1974;165:1074–1079.

113 Bates N, Rawson-Harris P, Edwards N. Common questions in veterinary toxicology. J Small Anim Pract. 2015;56:298–306.

114 Cortinovis C, Caloni F. Household food items toxic to dogs and cats. Front Vet Sci. 2016;3:26.

115 Bates N, Rawson-Harris P, Edwards N. Common questions in veterinary toxicology. J Small Anim Pract. 2015;56:298–306.

116 Page C, Murtaugh RJ. Hypoglycemia associated with oleander toxicity in a dog. J Med Toxicol. 2015;11:141–143.

117 Thomas EK, Drobatz KJ, Mandell DC. Presumptive cocaine toxicosis in 19 dogs: 2004–2012. J Vet Emerg Crit Care. 2014;24:201–207.

118 Ansel GM, Coyne K, Arnold S, Nelson SD. Mechanisms of ventricular arrhythmia during

amitriptyline toxicity. J Cardiovasc Pharmacol. 1993;22:798–803.

119 Lheureux P, Vranckx M, Leduc D, Askenasi R. Flumazenil in mixed benzodiazepine/tricyclic antidepressant overdose: a placebo-controlled study in the dog. Am J Emerg Med. 1992;10:184–188.

120 Mitsumori Y, Nakamura Y, Hoshiai K, Nagayama Y, Adachi-Akahane S, Koizumi S, et al. In vivo canine model comparison of cardiovascular effects of antidepressants milnacipran and imipramine. Cardiovasc Toxicol. 2010;10:275–282.

121 Price PM. ECG of the month: organophosphate intoxication in a cat. J Am Vet Med Assoc. 1989;195:325.

122 Tse YC, Sharp CR, Evans T. Mechanical ventilation in a dog with acetylcholinesterase inhibitor toxicosis. J Vet Emerg Crit Care. 2013;23:442–446.

123 Vestberg AR, Tidholm A, Ljungvall I. Twenty-four-hour ambulatory electrocardiography characterization of heart rhythm in *Vipera berus*–envenomed dogs. Acta Vet Scand. 2017;59:28.

124 Pelander L, Ljungvall I, Häggström J. Myocardial cell damage in 24 dogs bitten by the common European viper (*Vipera berus*). Vet Rec. 2010;166:687–690.

125 Segev G, Ohad DG, Shipov A, Kass PH, Aroch I. Cardiac arrhythmias and serum cardiac troponins in *Vipera palaestinae* envenomation in dogs. J Vet Intern Med. 2008;22:106–113.

126 Willey JR, Schaer M. Eastern Diamondback Rattlesnake (*Crotalus adamanteus*) envenomation of dogs: 31 cases (1982–2002). J Am Anim Hosp Assoc. 2005;41:22–33.

127 Aroch I, Segev G, Klement E, Shipov A, Harrus S. Fatal *Vipera xanthina palestinae* envenomation in 16 dogs. Vet Hum Toxicol. 2004;46:268–272.

128 Segev G, Ohad DG, Shipov A, Kass PH, Aroch I. Cardiac arrhythmias and serum cardiac troponins in *Vipera palaestinae* envenomation in dogs. J Vet Intern Med. 2008;22:106–113.

129 Murthy RR, Vakil AE, Yeolekar KE. Insulin administration reverses the metabolic and electrocardiographic changes in acute myocarditis induced by Indian red scorpion (*Buthus tamulus*) venom in experimental dogs. Indian Heart J. 1990;42:35–42.

130 Duncan AW, Tibballs J, Sutherland SK. Effects of Sydney funnel-web spider envenomation in monkeys, and their clinical implications. Med J Aust. 1980;2:429–435.

131 Tibballs J, Sutherland SK, Duncan AW. Effects of male Sydney funnel-web spider venom in a dog and a cat. Aust Vet J. 1987;64:63–64.

132 Atwell RB, Campbell FE. Reactions to tick antitoxin serum and the role of atropine in treatment of dogs and cats with tick paralysis caused by Ixodes holocyclus: a pilot survey. Aust Vet J. 2001;79:394–397.

133 Kornegay JN. The golden retriever model of Duchenne muscular dystrophy. Skelet Muscle. 2017;7:9.

134 Moise NS, Valentine BA, Brown CA, Erb HN, Beck KA, Cooper BJ, et al. Duchenne's cardiomyopathy in a canine model: electrocardiographic and echocardiographic studies. J Am Coll Cardiol. 1991;17:812–820.

135 Urasawa N, Wada MR, Machida N, Yuasa K, Shimatsu Y, Wakao Y, et al. Selective vacuolar degeneration in dystrophin-deficient canine Purkinje fibers despite preservation of dystrophin-associated proteins with overexpression of Dp71. Circulation. 2008;117:2437–2448.

136 Maurer M, Mary J, Guillaud L, Fender M, Pele M, Bilzer T, et al. Centronuclear myopathy in Labrador retrievers: a recent founder mutation in the PTPLA gene has rapidly disseminated worldwide. PLoS ONE. 2012;7:e46408.

137 Gortel K, Houston DM, Kuiken T, Fries CL, Boisvert B. Inherited myopathy in a litter of Labrador retrievers. Can Vet J. 1996;37:108–110.

138 Shea A, De Risio L, Carruthers H, Ekiri A, Beltran E. Clinical features and disease progression of L-2-hydroxyglutaric aciduria in 27 Staffordshire bull terriers. Vet Rec. 2016. Nov 26;179(21):545.

139 Lowrie M, Garden OA, Hadjivassiliou M, Harvey RJ, Sanders DS, Powell R, et al. The clinical and serological effect of a gluten-free diet in Border Terriers with epileptoid cramping syndrome. J Vet Intern Med. 2014;29:1564–1568.

140 Taylor S, Shmon C, Su L, Epp T, Minor K, Mickelson J, et al. Evaluation of dogs with Border Collie collapse, including response to two standardized strenuous exercise protocols. J Am Anim Hosp Assoc. 2016;52:281–290.

141 Patterson EE, Minor KM, Tchernatynskaia AV, Taylor SM, Shelton GD, Ekenstedt KJ, et al. A canine DNM1 mutation is highly associated with the syndrome of exercise-induced collapse. Nat Genet. 2008;40:1235–1239.

142 Minor KM, Patterson EE, Keating MK, Gross SD, Ekenstedt KJ, Taylor SM, et al. Presence and impact of the exercise-induced collapse associated DNM1 mutation in Labrador retrievers and other breeds. Vet J. 2011;189:214–219.

143 Takanosu M, Mori H, Suzuki H, Suzuki K. Genotyping of exercise-induced collapse in Labrador retrievers using an allele-specific PCR. Vet J. 2012;193:293–295.

144 Furrow E, Minor KM, Taylor SM, Mickelson JR, Patterson EE. Relationship between dynamin 1 mutation status and characteristics of recurrent episodes of exercise-induced collapse in Labrador Retrievers. J Am Vet Med Assoc. 2013;242:786–791.

145 Jaggy A, Faissler D, Gaillard C, Srenk P, Graber H. Genetic aspects of idiopathic epilepsy in Labrador retrievers. J Small Anim Pract. 1998;39:275–280.

24

Cardiac Arrhythmias and Anaesthesia
Frances Downing and Louise Clark

Introduction

Arrhythmias represent an important cause of perioperative complications. A number of clinical situations may trigger changes in cardiac rhythm.[1] These rhythm changes may be due to a primary aetiology, or to reversible causes related to anaesthesia or surgery. While the incidence of perioperative arrhythmias in people is extremely high (the Multicenter Study of General Anaesthesia reported a 70.2% incidence of tachycardia, bradycardia or arrhythmias in 17,201 patients having general anaesthesia), only 1.6% of these will require clinically significant management.[2,3] Whilst comparable information is not currently available in veterinary species, Redondo *et al.* reported an incidence of bradycardia in 36.3% of anaesthetised dogs.[4]

Vital organs such as the brain, heart and kidneys must be adequately perfused during general anaesthesia and surgery. Physiological alterations during anaesthesia and the effects of pharmacological agents are the major causes of autonomic changes resulting in perioperative arrhythmia production. Many anaesthetic agents have direct myocardial depressant effects, resulting in reduced contractility as well as reduced sympathetic stimulation of the peripheral vasculature. The net effect is a fall in cardiac output with concomitant vasodilation and hypotension, which may result in organ hypo-perfusion. When this is coupled with hypovolaemia (e.g. in septic shock), the risk of arrhythmia increases; this can decrease cardiac output and organ perfusion further.

Patients with underlying structural heart disease are at greatest risk for developing either supraventricular or ventricular arrhythmias during the induction of anaesthesia secondary to hypotension, autonomic imbalance or airway manipulation. In addition, during cardiac or major vascular surgery, patients may experience arrhythmia during dissection of the pericardium, placement of atrial sutures[5] or cardiac manipulation. Other factors such as electrolyte abnormalities, co-morbidity, hormone mediators or direct physical stimulation by either the surgeon or anaesthetist can precipitate arrhythmia.

Some of the most common conditions in the perioperative environment that predispose patients to arrhythmias are listed in Table 24.1. These conditions are usually reversible, and they should be treated before considering use of pharmacological anti-arrhythmic therapies.

The clinician should be aware that anti-arrhythmic drugs can also be pro-arrhythmic, and this may occur more readily under conditions of general anaesthesia in the presence of other drugs. In an attempt to treat a perioperative arrhythmia, there is a risk of iatrogenic deterioration, and therefore knowing the physiology of the cardiac rhythm, knowing anaesthetic pharmacology and weighing the risks and benefits of anti-arrhythmic drug administration are necessary. Most perioperative arrhythmias are benign, without significant haemodynamic consequences. In symptomatic cases where the arrhythmia can evolve into a life-threatening malignant arrhythmia, timely treatment should be provided.

Perioperative Cardiac Arrhythmias

Clinical Approach to the Patient

ABC Patient Assessment
Determine if the arrhythmia is causing serious cardiovascular compromise with altered heart rate, cardiac output, organ perfusion and blood pressure (see Figure 24.1).
Obtain help if needed
Assess the anaesthetic. Check:

- Oxygenation (peripheral blood oxygen saturation $[SpO_2] > 90\%$ and/or partial pressure of arterial oxygen $[P_aO_2] > 60$ mmHg)
- Ventilation and end tidal carbon dioxide ($ETCO_2 < 55$ mmHg and/or $P_aCO_2 < 60$ mmHg)
- Is the depth of anaesthesia inadequate for surgery?
- Drug error or interaction?

Guide to Canine and Feline Electrocardiography, First Edition. Ruth Willis, Pedro Oliveira and Antonia Mavropoulou.
© 2018 John Wiley & Sons Ltd. Published 2018 by John Wiley & Sons Ltd.
Companion website: www.wiley.com/go/willis/electrocardiography

Assess the surgery. Check for:

- Vagal stimulation (e.g. because of organ traction)
- Sympathetic stimulation due to surgical dissection and manipulation
- Possible air or fat embolism
- Unexpected haemorrhage and hypovolaemia
- Mediastinal or intrathoracic manipulation
- Adrenaline injection (including sub-conjunctival or intra-cameral).

Record a six-lead electrocardiogram (ECG) where possible, and correct the underlying cause.

Table 24.1 Common conditions in the perioperative environment that predispose patients to arrhythmias[6]

- Hypoxaemia – $SpO_2 < 90\%$ or $P_aO_2 < 60$ mmHg
- Hypercapnia
- Metabolic acidosis
- Hypotension – MAP < 60 mmHg or Doppler BP < 90 mmHg (dogs)
- Electrolyte abnormalities
- Mechanical irritation, including;
  - Surgery
  - Chest drain
- Hypothermia – temperature <37 °C
- Adrenergic stimulation (light anaesthesia, inadequate analgesia)
- Pro-arrhythmic drugs
- Micro or macro shock
- Cardiac ischaemia

MAP, Mean arterial blood pressure.

Common Anaesthetic Drugs and Arrhythmias

A number of drugs commonly used as part of balanced anaesthesia have the potential to cause cardiac arrhythmias, through both direct and indirect mechanisms. This section aims to briefly summarise the most common anaesthetic drug-induced arrhythmias, the underlying mechanisms behind them and potential treatment options where appropriate risk factors for anaesthetic-induced arrhythmias and interactions between anaesthetic agents and common anti-arrhythmic drugs (see Tables 24.3 and 24.4).

α2-Adrenoreceptor Agonists

The use of the α2-adrenoreceptor agonists medetomidine and dexmedetomidine as sedative and analgesic agents has now become commonplace in companion animal medicine. The clinical effects of these drugs are mediated through the activation of α-adrenoreceptors within a number of target organs, including the brain, heart and peripheral vasculature. The predominant effects of stimulation of these receptors are summarised in Table 24.2. Medetomidine and dexmedetomidine have a greater selectivity for α2-receptors over α1-receptors (1620:1); conversely, xylazine, which is used less frequently, has a α2:α1 selectivity of only 160:1. Medetomidine is a racemic mix of two optical enantiomers, dexmedetomidine and levomedetomidine, with the latter being believed to contribute minimally towards the observed clinical effect of the mixture.[7,8] Dexmedetomidine is the clinically active

Table 24.2 Summary of the predominant effects of α-adrenoreceptor stimulation

	α1-receptor stimulation	α2-receptor stimulation
CNS	Increased alertness Increased sympathetic tone	Sedation Anxiolysis Decreased NE release
Kidneys	Anti-diuresis Anti-natriuresis Increased renal vascular resistance Decreased GFR	Increased diuresis Inhibited renin release
Myocardium	Positive inotropy Hypertrophy Decreased conduction speed and automaticity of Purkinje fibres Prolong AP duration and refractory period	
Coronary circulation	Vasoconstriction	Vasoconstriction
Peripheral vasculature	Vasoconstriction	Vasoconstriction
Pancreas		Decreased insulin secretion
Liver	Glycogenolysis	

AP, Action potential; CNS, central nervous system; GFR, glomerular filtration rate; NE, norepinephrine.[10,11]

isomer, with effects at both α2-adrenoreceptors and imidazoline receptors; activity at imidazoline receptors may be responsible for some of the centrally mediated hypotensive and anti-arrhythmogenic effects observed.[9]

In addition to their sedative and analgesic properties, medetomidine and dexmedetomidine can have marked effects on cardiovascular function; most commonly, they are associated with a decrease in cardiac output, a reduction in heart rate and alterations in blood pressure.[12] The haemodynamic effects of these drugs are minimally dose-dependent, with doses of medetomidine as low as 5 mcg/kg intravenously (IV) having been shown to produce a near-maximal effect in dogs.[8,12,13] Currently, the doses of medetomidine recommended by manufacturers in the UK for sedation in dogs prior to induction of anaesthesia with propofol range from 10 to 40 mcg/kg when administered intramuscularly (IM) or IV.[14]

The cardiovascular effects of medetomidine are often described as biphasic:

1) Initial peripheral vasoconstriction, due to stimulation of α2-adrenoreceptors within vascular smooth muscle, causes an increase in blood pressure (hypertension) and systemic vascular resistance (SVR). The increase in blood pressure causes a baroreceptor-mediated decrease in heart rate. The duration of this phase depends on the dose of drug given and the route of administration, with high IV doses tending to have the greatest effect.

2) After the initial vasoconstrictive phase has passed, blood pressure tends to return to normal but bradycardia persists. The bradycardia is thought to be due to a centrally mediated reduction in sympathetic tone, although the exact mechanism for this is still unclear.

Cardiac arrhythmias attributed to the administration of medetomidine and dexmedetomidine are most often secondary to baroreceptor reflex triggered by peripheral vasoconstriction and increase in blood pressure (Phase 1). The most common cardiac arrhythmias observed in dogs following the administration of these drugs are bradyarrhythmias,[15] particularly first- and second-degree atrioventricular (AV) block. In cats, AV block is observed less commonly, whilst sinus bradycardia and idioventricular rhythm can be seen (see Figure 24.2). Dexmedetomidine is also reported to have anti-arrhythmic properties; the

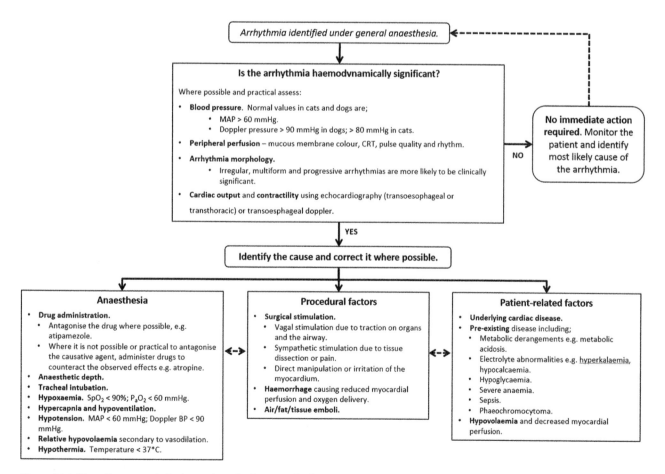

Figure 24.1 Flow diagram to help determine whether an arrhythmia occurring in a patient under general anaesthesia is clinically significant and likely to require treatment, and what the most likely cause of the arrhythmia is. Once the likely cause of the arrhythmia has been identified, the clinician is then more able to decide on an appropriate treatment protocol. In cases of clinically insignificant arrhythmias, the likely cause should ideally still be identified, and the patient monitored for signs of deterioration.

exact mechanism for this is still unclear but is proposed to be related to activity at imidazoline receptors and/or vagal stimulation.[9]

The need to treat the bradyarrhythmias caused by α2 agonists should be decided based on the individual patient. In general, bradycardia should be treated if it is causing a clinically significant decrease in cardiac output, blood pressure, tissue perfusion and oxygen delivery or if it precipitates ventricular arrhythmias (escape beats or ventricular premature complexes). Atipamezole, an α2-adrenoreceptor receptor antagonist, can be administered to counteract the cardiovascular effects of medetomidine and dexmedetomidine.[16] It is important to note that the sedative and analgesic effects of the drugs will also be antagonised. It is always important to rule out other causes of bradycardia, such as hypothermia and the administration of other drugs, before antagonising α2-receptor agonists.

Anticholinergic drugs, such as atropine and glycopyrrolate, can be used to increase the heart rate in patients with a persistently low heart rate and hypotension. Their use is not advisable in the presence of vasoconstriction and hypertension (Phase 1); this can increase myocardial work and can precipitate further arrhythmias. The pre-emptive use of atropine has been shown to reduce the occurrence of bradycardia following medetomidine and dexmedetomidine administration in dogs, but it can exacerbate and prolong hypertension, induce tachycardia, precipitate ventricular arrhythmias and cause pulsus alternans;[17–19] it is therefore not advisable. Additionally, it is important to note that an increase in the patient's heart rate does not necessarily equate to an increase in cardiac output.[20] It is also worth noting that the administration of anticholinergic drugs can themselves induce arrhythmias. Whilst their administration is most commonly associated with tachycardia, they can induce bradyarrhythmias, including second-degree AV block (see Figure 24.3); this is particularly notable when low doses are used.[21]

The administration of sympathomimetic drugs, including a low dose of ketamine (0.1–0.2 mg/kg IV), has been

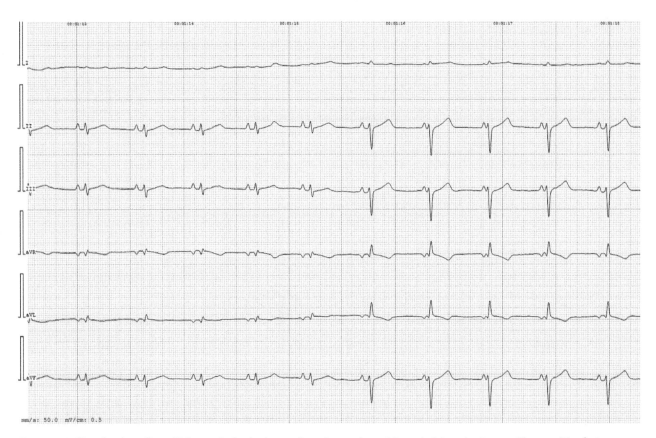

Figure 24.2 Sinus bradycardia and idioventricular rhythm attributed to medetomidine administration in a cat. The transition between sinus bradycardia with a rate of ≈115 bpm (first five beats) to a wide-QRS rhythm (last five beats) can be seen. The QRS of the sinus beats has a normal duration (40 ms) and is preceded by a normal-looking P wave with a constant PR interval within normal limits (75 ms); the abnormal appearance of the QRS was attributed to dorsal recumbency, as there was no evidence of structural heart disease in this case on echocardiography. The last five beats display a wide QRS (80 ms), and even though normal-looking P waves may be seen preceding each QRS, the PR interval is variable (45 to 70 ms), suggesting atrioventricular dissociation. This was an idioventricular rhythm with a rate of ≈110–115 bpm that became apparent as the sinus rate lowered. On an anaesthesia monitor, the variable PR interval could be difficult to distinguish, and this could have been confused with right bundle branch block. It should not be confused with ventricular tachycardia. This electrocardiographic trace was recorded during sedation with methadone (0.2 mg/kg) and medetomidine (10 mcg/kg) for an abdominal ultrasound. [6-year-old, male, neutered Domestic Shorthair cat with lower urinary tract disease] (50 mm/s; 20 mm/mV)

suggested as an alternative to anticholinergics as a means of increasing the heart rate when the bradycardia is centrally mediated (Phase 2).[15] It has also been proposed that lidocaine could be used to treat dexmedetomidine-mediated bradycardia due to a vagolytic effect seen in conditions of high vagal tone, resulting in an increase in the rate of sinoatrial (SA) activity.[22] This is not a widely used treatment and is not currently recommended by the authors.

Acepromazine

Acepromazine (ACP) is a phenothiazine drug with sedative and anxiolytic properties. Its cardiovascular effects are due to its antagonistic effects on α1-adrenoreceptors, causing peripheral vasodilation and a fall in blood pressure. ACP has been reported to have anti-arrhythmic properties, reducing the occurrence of catecholamine-induced arrhythmias in halothane-anaesthetised dogs[23] but not in cats.[24] A number of mechanisms for this have been proposed, including direct effects on α1-adrenoreceptors in the heart, a reduction in sympathetic tone and a decrease in conduction velocity within cardiac myocytes and increased refractory period. The clinical significance of this effect is not known.

Ketamine

Ketamine is a phencyclidine derivative capable of inducing analgesia and anaesthesia. Ketamine's primary mechanism of action is mediated by non-competitive antagonism at N-methyl-D-aspartate (NMDA) receptor Ca^{2+} channels.[25] Other reported mechanisms of action include an interaction with opioid receptors; antagonistic actions at monoamine oxidase, muscarinic and nictotinic receptors; and inhibitory effects at neuronal Na^+ channels.[25]

The administration of ketamine is most commonly associated with an increase in heart rate, blood pressure and cardiac output due to stimulation of the sympathetic nervous system. Tachycardia can have detrimental effects in patients susceptible to ischaemia due to reduced myocardial filling, increased myocardial work and oxygen requirement. Ketamine itself is a direct myocardial depressant; however, this action is usually counteracted by the systemic increase in sympathetic activity. Arrhythmias associated with the administration of ketamine usually do not require specific treatment; careful monitoring of cardiovascular variables, supportive treatment and discontinuation of ketamine administration may be required.

Propofol

Propofol, (2,6-diisopropylpenol) is a commonly used intravenous induction agent in humans and companion animals. The administration of propofol is associated with a dose-dependent decrease in SVR, cardiac output and blood pressure, with little or no associated change in heart rate; it can cause mild bradycardia and have a direct negative inotropic effect.[26] These effects are generally considered to be mild in healthy patients at clinically relevant doses and do not require treatment.

Alfaxalone

Alfaxalone is a neuroactive steroid that can be used for induction and maintenance of anaesthesia in dogs and cats.[27,28] The administration of alfaxalone IV can cause a dose-dependent decrease in SVR, blood pressure and cardiac output and may reduce myocardial contractility.[27,29,30] This can be accompanied by a transient baroreceptor-mediated tachycardia, in response to the decrease in blood pressure. It is also reported that alfaxalone can cause a dose-dependent decrease in heart rate in cats.[29] These effects are generally considered to be mild at clinically relevant doses and do not require treatment.

Volatile Agents

This group contains the inhalational gases isoflurane, sevoflurane, desflurane and halothane, which are used for maintenance of anaesthesia in companion animals and humans. The most common cardiovascular effect is hypotension secondary to dose-dependent vasodilation and decreases in SVR, cardiac output and myocardial contractility. If hypotension results in decreased myocardial perfusion and oxygen delivery, this may precipitate cardiac arrhythmias. Desflurane can also cause an increase in heart rate.[31] In addition, the use of halothane can increase myocardial sensitivity to catecholamine-induced arrhythmias. In humans, these agents have been found to delay ventricular repolarisation and prolong the QT interval, with isoflurane causing ventricular dysrhythmias in 2.5% of human patients.[31,32] Currently, similar information is not available in veterinary species. The most effective way of reducing the cardiovascular side effects of the volatile agents is to reduce the dose required to maintain anaesthesia by using a balanced, multimodal approach. Diligent haemodynamic monitoring is recommended during anaesthesia, and if hypotension persists further supportive treatment, including intravenous fluid therapy, may be required.

Risk Factors for Anaesthetic Agent–induced Arrhythmias

Risk factors for the development of anaesthetic-induced arrhythmias can be classified as modifiable and non-modifiable. Underlying cardiac disease is an important non-modifiable risk factor. Cardiac dilation can result in abnormal automaticity, whereas anaerobic metabolism in ischaemic myocardial tissues can raise the resting membrane potential which may result in abnormal impulse conduction.[32]

It is important to identify patients who might be at risk for developing drug-induced arrhythmias, so measures can be taken to minimize the modifiable factors. Given that electrolytes are integral in the generation and propagation of electrical depolarisations within the heart, it is important to ensure that electrolytes are within physiological range. Where there is a history of arrhythmias, there is increased risk of recurrence when certain medications are administered (e.g. skeletal muscle myopathies with succinylcholine administration).

Systemic disease may produce metabolic conditions that can alter the pharmacokinetics of drugs, potentially increasing the risk of medication-induced arrhythmias. A decrease in renal or hepatic drug clearance can increase plasma concentration levels of certain medications or their metabolites. This is particularly important in medications with a narrow therapeutic index. Such patients often have complex medical regimens, with multiple potential pharmacokinetic or pharmacodynamic interactions.[32]

Intra-operative Arrhythmias: Specific Considerations in the Anaesthetised Patient

Whilst the general principles of arrhythmia management have been extensively covered elsewhere, it is important to remember that when under the influence of anaesthetic drugs that have significant cardiovascular side effects themselves, there is the potential for more severe effects on cardiovascular function than might be expected with any specific arrhythmia in the conscious patient. The arrhythmogenic potential of anaesthesia drugs is discussed elsewhere in this chapter. Anaesthesia can also 'uncover' latent arrhythmia, particularly sick sinus syndrome.

Sinus Bradycardia

Sinus bradycardia is generally only a problem if the heart rate falls to a point that affects cardiac output. In a healthy heart during anaesthesia, the fall in heart rate will tend to allow an increase in pre-load and a subsequent increase in stroke volume, thus maintaining an adequate cardiac output. Whilst we are limited in our

Table 24.3 Interactions between anaesthetic agents and anti-arrhythmic drugs (from human data)[31]

Cardiac drug	Potential anaesthetic interactions
General	• General anaesthesia may 'uncover' sick sinus syndrome.
Adenosine	• Vasodilation with isoflurane and neuraxial blockade • Bronchoconstriction with neostigmine • Asystole with neostigmine/edrophonium/α2-adrenergic agonists and opioids
Amiodarone	• Myocardial depression and vasodilation with anaesthetic agents • Several studies suggest increased risk of severe intra-operative complications; dysrhythmias and bradycardias were particularly evident. • Any drugs that cause bradycardia may be potentiated: β-blockers, calcium channel blockers.
β-blockers	• Marked hypotensive effect due to negative inotropic effect • Myocardial depression potentiated by halothane • Bronchoconstriction with atracurium and neostigmine • Bronchoconstriction in asthmatics
Calcium channel blockers	• Bradycardia and myocardial depression with halogenated agents • Bradycardia and myocardial depression with dantrolene • Potentiates neuromuscular blockade • The effects of verapamil on the SA and AV nodes are additive with β-blocking drugs. The use of these two together can give rise to catastrophic bradycardia.
Digoxin	• Bradycardia potentiated by halothane and succinyl choline • Care with calcium and diuretics (hypokalaemia)
Dobutamine	• Dobutamine is directly arrhythmogenic, causing dose-dependent tachycardia; doses higher than 5 µg/kg/min are prone to cause arrhythmia and generate little benefit in oxygen transportation.
Lidocaine	• May potentiate opioid-induced bradyarrhythmia
Magnesium	• Potentiates and prolongs action of neuromuscular blockade
Procainamide	• Antagonises neostigmine • May cause ventricular arrhythmias in the presence of phenothiazines (ACP)
Quinidine	• Prolongs the action of neuromuscular blockade

Table 24.4 The most frequently reported arrhythmias in dogs and cats associated with the use of commonly used anaesthetic drugs, their underlying causes and a practical approach to managing them where necessary

Drug	Most common arrhythmias observed after administration	Cause of the arrhythmia	Treatment (if required)
Acepromazine (ACP)	• None likely	• Arrhythmias may be seen as a result of hypotension and hypoperfusion caused by ACP.	• Supportive treatment to correct hypotension, including: – IV fluid administration – Vasopressor administration in severe cases only, for example norepinephrine, phenylephrine or ephedrine. (*These drugs can cause arrhythmias. Concurrent invasive blood pressure monitoring is recommended during use.*)
Medetomidine/ dexmedetomidine	• Sinus bradycardia • First and second-degree AV block (dogs) • Idioventricular rhythm (cats)	• Initial α2-adrenoreceptor mediated peripheral vasoconstriction, hypertension and reflex bradycardia • Subsequent centrally mediated bradycardia	• Atipamezole (*Note: Will also reverse sedative and analgesic effects.*) • Anticholinergic drugs, such as atropine and glycopyrrolate, should not be used if hypertension is present.
Ketamine	• Sinus tachycardia and occasional ventricular arrhythmias reported	• Sympathetic stimulation and subsequent increase in myocardial work and oxygen requirement • Ketamine is a direct myocardial depressant; this generally masks its systemic autonomic effects.	• Discontinuation of ketamine administration may be required if tachycardia is clinically significant. • Further supportive treatment may include: – Supplemental oxygen administration – Drugs to reduce heart rate and sympathetic tone, including low doses of pure or partial mu agonists (e.g. 0.1–0.2 mg/kg methadone slow IV).
Benzodiazepines (e.g. midazolam, diazepam)	• None likely	N/A	N/A
Methadone, morphine and fentanyl	• Sinus bradycardia • First and second-degree AV block (dogs) • Idioventricular rhythm (cats)	• Vagally mediated bradycardia	• Anticholinergic drugs: – Atropine: 0.01–0.04 mg/kg IV or IM – Glycopyrrolate: 0.005–0.01 mg/kg IV or IM. • If effects are prolonged or severe, antagonise using naloxone. (*Note: Will also reverse analgesic effects.*)
Propofol	• None likely – bradycardia has been reported.	• Exact mechanism of bradycardia is unclear.	• Usually transient and no treatment required
Alfaxalone	• Tachycardia	• Baroreceptor-mediated response to a decrease in SVR and hypotension	• Usually transient and no treatment required
Volatile gases – isoflurane, sevoflurane and desflurane	• None likely	• Arrhythmias may be a result of hypotension and hypoperfusion due to dose-dependent vasodilation and myocardial depression.	• Reduce volatile administration where possible. • Further supportive treatment to correct hypotension if needed, including: – IV fluid administration – Vasopressor administration in severe cases only, for example norepinephrine, phenylephrine or ephedrine. (*These drugs can cause arrhythmias, and concurrent invasive blood pressure monitoring is recommended during use.*)
Nitrous oxide (N_2O)	• None likely – tachycardia and ectopic beats have been reported.	• Sympathetic stimulation • N_2O can cause direct myocardial depression; this generally masks its systemic autonomic effects.	• Switch off the flow of N_2O.

Note: Arrhythmias may be multifactorial and not the result of the administration of a single drug; therefore, it is essential to consider all potential factors that may be contributing to an observed arrhythmia before deciding upon treatment. AV block, Atrioventricular block.

ability to measure cardiac output in the clinical situation (trans-oesophageal Doppler and echocardiography are available in some institutions), we tend to use blood pressure as a surrogate, although with limitations. Thus, if sinus bradycardia is associated with hypotension, the use of anticholinergics can be considered. Opioids, widely used in the perioperative situation, are parasympathomimetic drugs and tend to potentiate bradycardia, especially at high doses. Potent, short-acting opioids such as fentanyl and alfentanil have relatively short half-lives, and therefore reducing the rate of infusion is often the treatment of choice. There are specific considerations relating to pharmacologically induced bradycardia and α2-adrenoceptor agonists (see Table 24.4).

Sinus Tachycardia

Tachycardia increases myocardial oxygen consumption, and whilst this is associated with increased mortality in people, its significance in domestic species is unknown. One assumes that it will have detrimental effects in patients susceptible to ischaemia due to reduced myocardial filling and increased myocardial work and oxygen requirement. Extreme tachycardia can result in decreased ventricular filling time and hence decreased cardiac output; therefore, it should be treated.

The aetiology should be considered. Sinus tachycardia can, for example, be a response to hypotension (e.g. from haemorrhage or vasodilation), and an effort to maintain cardiac output and, in this situation, address the cause of the hypotension is paramount. No attempt should be made to reduce heart rate until cardiac output (if possible), blood pressure and perfusion have been assessed and managed.

Where sinus tachycardia is a result of sympathetic stimulation from nociception, improving intra-operative analgesia should be the first objective. Short-acting opioids (e.g. fentanyl) are routinely used for this purpose, but side effects such as respiratory depression should be considered. Very low doses of α2-adrenoceptor agonists can also be used for this purpose, but their cardiovascular effects should be considered.

When other therapies has been ineffective, β-blockers can be used for this purpose, and during anaesthesia drugs with a short half-life such as esmolol are appropriate. Extreme care should be taken where the presence of a catecholamine-secreting tumour is suspected.

Supraventricular Tachycardia (SVT)

Perioperative SVTs should be considered as a sign of a potentially life-threatening underlying clinical condition. The initial approach is, as noted previously, to look for an underlying cause, usually pathology or procedure-related, and possible repercussions. Many of these conditions are reversible with appropriate management (see Figure 24.1), and anti-arrhythmic drugs should be considered only after these potential aetiologies have been eliminated.

Furthermore, the effect of the arrhythmia on haemodynamic stability (e.g. hypotension) should be assessed. Where profound haemodynamic instability is present, electrical cardioversion (when available) may be the appropriate initial response. Perioperative cardioversion may not be completely effective or even may not be able to maintain an organized rhythm for an adequate period. This is because cardioversion itself does not reverse the baseline cause of the arrhythmia. The process of cardioversion is described in chapter 9.

Most patients with perioperative SVTs maintain moderate haemodynamic stability; therefore, they do not need immediate electrical cardioversion. For this reason, heart rate control is the most important objective to prevent hypotension, rate-related myocardial ischaemia, heart failure and pulmonary oedema.

There are no clear guidelines as to which pharmacological agent is preferred, but treatment options are discussed in chapters 8, 10 and 17. All anti-arrhythmic drugs should be titrated to effect, and they have the common side effect of exacerbating hypotension.

Opioids may also be used for rate control; short and ultra-short-acting opioids such as fentanyl and alfentanil are para-sympathomimetic and thus will tend to reduce heart rate. They can be very useful in that they also provide profound analgesia; nociception may be a cause of intra-operative SVT. These drugs are not without side effects: they can cause profound bradycardia and hypoventilation, and this must be addressed promptly.

Atrial Fibrillation

Initial Management
Ensure correction of any pre-existing metabolic disturbances, including hypoxaemia and acidosis. Calcium channel antagonists verapamil or diltiazem are preferred agents for rate control.

Intra-operative Management
Where AF occurs in the presence of normal systolic function and with a normal ventricular rate, it is usually asymptomatic and does not cause any major anaesthetic problems. AF with a rapid ventricular response can cause significant cardiovascular complications, including hypotension, rate-related myocardial ischaemia and heart failure.

Normal atrial activity accounts for at least 10% of ventricular filling, which can increase up to 40% at higher heart rates. Where pathology is present that reduces systolic function and particularly ventricular elastance, the patient is more dependent on atrial filling to contribute to cardiac output. Thus, the adverse effects of AF with a

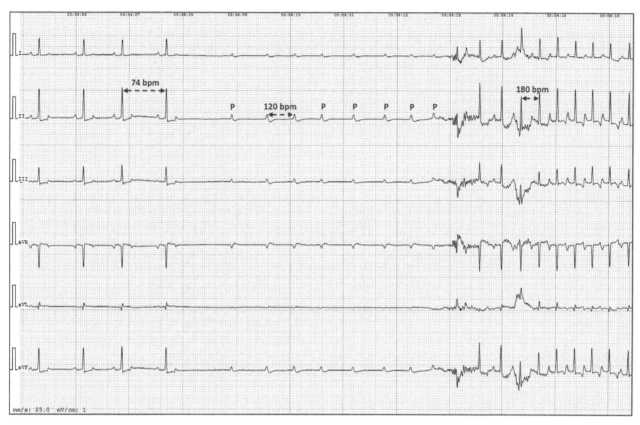

Figure 24.3 Second-degree atrioventricular block following IV administration of atropine. This electrocardiographic trace was recorded from a dog with gastrointestinal disease and bradycardia despite hypotension. Atropine was administered at a dose of 0.02 mg/kg intravenously in an attempt to increase heart rate, as it was suspected to be due to elevated vagal tone. The first four beats are sinus beats with a rate of 70–80 bpm, followed by eight non-conducted P waves (second-degree atrioventricular block), despite an increase in sinus rate to 120 bpm; then, it is followed by sinus tachycardia at ≈ 180 bpm for the last nine beats. [9-year-old, male, entire Bull Terrier with inflammatory bowel disease] (25 mm/s; 10 mm/mV)

rapid ventricular response rate are more profound in cases with underlying cardiac disease. The first step in managing these patients is to identify any precipitating causes and attempt to correct these.

Specific treatment should be commenced when adverse signs develop, such as hypotension secondary to the tachycardia. The evidence regarding the specificity of ST segment changes relating to cardiac ischaemia in domestic species is limited. There are no clear guidelines as to which pharmacological agent is preferred, but treatment options are discussed in chapters 9 and 17. All anti-arrhythmic drugs should be titrated to effect, and they have the common side effect of exacerbating hypotension. Opioids may also be used for rate control, as described in this chapter.

Multiple risk factors have been identified for the development of atrial fibrillation in human patients undergoing surgery. Some of these may be relevant in domestic species, and consideration should be taken of the following.

System aetiology assessment
- *Cardiac disease*: Valvular heart disease, cardiomyopathy, pre-existing excitatory syndromes and sinus node disease

- *Respiratory dysfunction*: Hypoxaemia and its pathophysiology, including pneumonia, pleural effusion and thromboembolic disease
- Metabolic acidosis, diabetes mellitus and other endocrine dysfunctions
- Hypovolaemia

Ventricular Tachycardia

Paroxysmal Ventricular Tachycardia
This is a common perioperative occurrence, especially during thoracic or cardiac surgery, and in the absence of cardiac disease it does not require treatment. In patients with cardiomyopathies, this non-sustained rhythm can predict malignant ventricular arrhythmias. The main strategy in paroxysmal VT would be prevention, instituting immediate treatment when possible risk factors arise.

Sustained Ventricular Tachycardia
An accelerated idioventricular rhythm becomes VT when heart rate is ≥180 bpm in the dog. VT is associated with a large decrease in cardiac output, hypotension and reduced tissue perfusion. It may also be self-reinforcing

due to a precipitous fall in coronary perfusion which may occur earlier when there is a pre-existing influence of anaesthetic drugs. The treatments detailed in chapters 8–11 are relevant to anaesthetised cases and should be instigated immediately. Where risk factors for deterioration of this arrhythmia are present, communication with the surgeon is paramount, and abandoning the procedure may be necessary. Equipment preparation (staff and defibrillator) in case of deterioration is mandatory.

Unstable VT, Pulseless VT and Ventricular Fibrillation (VF)

The management strategies for patients with perioperative unstable VT, pulseless VT or VF are not pharmacological. They are immediate defibrillation, cardiopulmonary resuscitation (CPR) in case of cardiorespiratory arrest, and correction of reversible causes (see chapter 11).

Summary

The distinction between a benign arrhythmia and those that carry the risk of sudden death is fundamental. Prevention is as important as treatment: the most important steps in prevention are recognition of risk factors, including pre-existing pathology and procedure factors; appropriate anaesthetic technique for each patient; and

monitoring. The management in perioperative arrhythmia does not always include the use of anti-arrhythmic agents, although they should not be delayed when indicated.

Key Points

- Cardiac arrhythmias can be a significant cause of perioperative complications. Before treating an arrhythmia under anaesthesia, it is important to establish whether it is clinically significant (and therefore whether treatment is needed) and, where possible, identify the underlying cause. **The treatment of life-threatening arrhythmias under anaesthesia should never be delayed.**
- Causes of arrhythmias under anaesthesia can be broadly categorised as anaesthesia, procedural and patient-related factors.
- A comprehensive patient history and thorough clinical examination will help identify factors that may increase the risk of arrhythmia under general anaesthesia. This information should then be incorporated into the patient's anaesthetic plan.
- The clinician should be aware of the arrhythmogenic potential of the anaesthetic drugs they use regularly, how and when to treat these arrhythmias and the potential for interaction between these drugs and other commonly used medications.

References

1 Fisher MD. Perioperative cardiac dysrhythmias. Anaesthesiology. 1997;86:1397–1424.

2 Forrest JB, Cahalan MK, Rehder K, Goldsmith CH, Levy WJ, Strunin L, *et al.* Multicenter study of general anesthesia. II. Results. Anesthesiology. 1990;72:262–268.

3 Forrest JB, Rehder K, Cahalan MK, Goldsmith CH. Multicenter study of general anesthesia. III. Predictors of severe perioperative adverse outcomes. Anesthesiology. 1992;76:3–15.

4 Redondo JI, Rubio M, Soler G, Serra I, Soler C, Gómez-Villamandos RJ. Normal values and incidence of cardiorespiratory complications in dogs during general anaesthesia: a review of 1281 cases. J Vet Med A Physiol Pathol Clin Med. 2007;54;470–477.

5 Waldo AL, Henthorn RW, Epstein AE, Plumb VJ. Diagnosis and treatment of arrhythmias during and following open heart surgery. Med Clin North Am. 1984;68:1153–1169.

6 Thompson A, Balser JR. Perioperative cardiac arrhythmias. Br J Anaesth. 2004;93:86–94.

7 MacDonald E, Scheinin M, Scheinin H, Virtanen R. Comparison of the behavioral and neurochemical effects of the two optical enantiomers of medetomidine, a

selective alpha-2-adrenoceptor agonist. J Pharm Exper Therap. 1991;259:848–854.

8 Kuusela E, Raekallio M, Anttila M, Falck I, Mölsä S, Vainio O. Clinical effects and pharmacokinetics of medetomidine and its enantiomers in dogs. J Vet Pharmacol Therap. 2000;23:15–20.

9 Kamibayashi, T, Mammoto, T, Hayashi, Y, Yamatodani, A, Takada, K, Sasaki, S, *et al.* Further characterization of the receptor mechanism involved in the antidysrhythmic effect of dexmedetomidine on halothane/epinephrine dysrhythmias in dogs. Anesthesiology. 1995;83: 1082–1089.

10 Rang HP, Dale MM, Ritter JM. In Pharmacology (eds. Rang HP, Dale MM, Ritter JM, Hunter MG, Simmons B, pp. 139–163). Edinburgh: Churchill Livingstone; 2001.

11 Long KM, Kirby R. An update on cardiovascular adrenergic receptor physiology and potential pharmacological applications in veterinary critical care. J Vet Emerg Crit Care. 2008;18:2–25.

12 Murrell JC, Hellebrekers LJ. Medetomidine and dexmedetomidine: a review of cardiovascular effects and antinociceptive properties in the dog. Vet Anaesth Analg. 2005;32:117–127.

13 Pypendop BH, Verstegen JP. Hemodynamic effects of medetomidine in the dog: a dose titration study. Vet Surg. 1998;27:612–622.

14 NOAH. Noah Compendium: domitor 1 mg/ml solution for injection: dosage and administration. Enfield: NOAH; 2017.

15 Murrell J. In BSAVA manual of canine and feline anaesthesia and analgesia (eds. Duke-Novakovski T, De Vries M, Seymour C, pp. 170–189). Gloucester: BSAVA; 2016.

16 Vähä-Vahe AT. The clinical effectiveness of atipamezole as a medetomidine antagonist in the dog. J Vet Pharmacol Therap. 1990;13:198–205.

17 Alibhai HI, Clarke KW, Lee YH, Thompson J. Cardiopulmonary effects of combinations of medetomidine hydrochloride and atropine sulphate in dogs. Vet Rec. 1996;138:11–13.

18 Ko JC, Fox SM, Mandsager RE. Effects of preemptive atropine administration on incidence of medetomidine-induced bradycardia in dogs. J Am Vet Med Assoc. 2001;218:52–58.

19 Congdon JM, Marquez M, Niyom S, Boscan P. Evaluation of the sedative and cardiovascular effects of intramuscular administration of dexmedetomidine with and without concurrent atropine administration in dogs. J Am Vet Med Assoc. 2011;239:81–89.

20 Ko JC, Barletta M, Sen I, Weil AB, Krimins RA, Payton ME, *et al*. Influence of ketamine on the cardiopulmonary effects of intramuscular administration of dexmedetomidine-buprenorphine with subsequent reversal with atipamezole in dogs. J Am Vet Med Assoc. 2013;242:339–345.

21 Richards DLS, Clutton RE, Boyd C. Electrocardiographic findings following intravenous glycopyrrolate to sedated dogs: a comparison with atropine. Vet Anaesth Analg. 1989;16:46–50.

22 Lieberman NA, Harris RS, Katz RI, Lipschutz HM, Dolgin M, Fisher VJ. The effects of lidocaine on the electrical and mechanical activity of the heart. Am J Cardiol. 1968;22:375–380.

23 Muir WW, Werner LL, Hamlin RL. Effects of xylazine and acetylpromazine upon induced ventricular fibrillation in dogs anesthetized with thiamylal and halothane. Am J Vet Res. 1975;36:1299–1303.

24 Walsh KP, Brearley JC, Cullum-Hanshaw KS. The effect of pre-anaesthetic medication on the incidence of cardiac arrhythmias during halothane anaesthesia in cats. Vet Anaesth Analg. 2000;27:45–49.

25 Pai A, Heining M. Ketamine. Cont Ed Anaesth. 2007;7(2):59–63.

26 Tramèr MR, Moore RA, McQuay HJ. Propofol and bradycardia: causation, frequency and severity. Br J Anaesth. 1997;78:642–651.

27 Ambros B, Duke-Novakovski T, Pasloske KS. Comparison of the anesthetic efficacy and cardiopulmonary effects of continuous rate infusions of alfaxalone-2-hydroxypropyl-β-cyclodextrin and propofol in dogs. J Am Vet Med Assoc. 2008;233:1590–1590.

28 Warne LN, Beths T, Whittem T, Carter JE, Bauquier SH. A review of the pharmacology and clinical application of alfaxalone in cats. Vet J. 2015;203:141–148.

29 Muir W, Lerche P, Wiese A, Nelson L, Pasloske K, Whittem T. The cardiorespiratory and anesthetic effects of clinical and supraclinical doses of alfaxalone in cats. Vet Anaesth Analg. 2009;36:42–54.

30 Taboada FM, Murison PJ. Induction of anaesthesia with alfaxalone or propofol before isoflurane maintenance in cats. Vet Rec. 2010;167:85–89.

31 Lorentz MN, Vianna BSB. Cardiac dysrhythmias and anesthesia. Rev Bras Anestesiol. 2011;61:798–813.

32 Barnes BJ, Hollands JM. Drug-induced arrhythmias. Crit Care Med. 2010;38:S188–S197.

Appendix 1

Normal ECG Measurements for Cats and Dogs

Measurements are taken from lead II, with a paper speed of 50 mm/s.

Parameter	Dog	Cat
Heart rate (bpm)	Adult: 70–160 Puppy: 70–200	Adult: 140–220
P wave amplitude (mV)	<0.4	<0.2
P wave width (ms)	Adult: <40 Giant breed: <50	<40
PR interval (ms)	60–130*	50–90
QRS amplitude (mV)	>0.5 and <3	<0.9
QRS width (ms)	<70	<40
QT duration (ms)	150–250**	120–180
QTc (ms)	150–240	70–200
ST segment	Elevation/depression: <0.2 mV	
T wave amplitude	Positive, negative or biphasic. No more than 25% of height of R wave.	Positive, negative or biphasic

Source: Adapted from Tilley[1].
*The PR interval is inversely correlated to heart rate.[2]
**The QT interval also decreases at high heart rates.

Guide to Canine and Feline Electrocardiography, First Edition. Ruth Willis, Pedro Oliveira and Antonia Mavropoulou.
© 2018 John Wiley & Sons Ltd. Published 2018 by John Wiley & Sons Ltd.
Companion website: www.wiley.com/go/willis/electrocardiography

Corrected QT Interval (QTc)

Measure the QT interval on the electrocardiogram and the RR interval of the preceding beat. The corresponding QTc (calculated using a logarithmic formula) may be found on the following table with prolonged QTc denoted by pink font:

Table showing QTc calculated using a logarithmic formula[3] for calculating QTc

					Measured QT (ms)							
	160	**170**	**180**	**190**	**200**	**210**	**220**	**230**	**240**	**250**	**260**	**270**
200	193	205	217	229	241	254	266	278	290	302	314	326
250	185	197	209	220	232	243	255	266	278	290	301	313
300	179	191	202	213	224	236	247	258	269	280	292	303
350	175	186	197	207	218	229	240	251	262	273	284	295
400	171	182	192	203	214	224	235	246	256	267	278	288
450	168	178	188	199	209	220	230	241	251	262	272	283
500	165	175	185	196	206	216	226	237	247	257	268	278
550	162	172	182	193	203	213	223	233	243	253	264	274
600	160	170	180	190	200	210	220	230	240	250	260	270
650	158	168	178	188	198	207	217	227	237	247	257	267
700	156	166	176	186	195	205	215	225	234	244	254	264
800	153	163	172	182	191	201	211	220	230	239	249	258
900	150	160	169	179	188	197	207	216	226	235	245	254
1000	148	157	167	176	185	194	204	213	222	232	241	250
1200	144	153	162	171	180	189	198	208	217	226	235	244

Preceding RR (ms)

References

1 Tilley LP. Essentials of canine and feline electrocardiography. St. Louis: Mosby; 1995.

2 Osborne BE, Leach GD. The beagle electrocardiogram. Food Cosmet Toxicol. 1971;9:857–864.

3 Matsunaga T, Mitsui T, Harada T, Inokuma M, Murano H, Shibutani Y. QT corrected for heart rate and relation between QT and RR intervals in beagle dogs. J Pharmacol Toxicol Meth. 1997;38:201–209.

Appendix 2

Arrhythmias – A Brief Review

This chapter aims to illustrate common and abnormal rhythms in a standardised format to encourage a logical and systematic approach to ECG interpretation. To do this, we are going to use the following ten concepts:

General

1) Is the rhythm fast or slow?
2) Is the rhythm regular or irregular? If irregular, is it regularly irregular or irregularly irregular?

P waves

3) Are any P waves present?
4) Is the P wave morphology consistent?
5) Is there a P for every QRS, and vice versa?
6) Is the PR interval constant?

QRS

7) Are the P waves and QRS complexes coupled together?
8) Are the QRS complexes narrow or wide?
9) Are matching QRS complexes grouped or not grouped?
10) Are there any dropped beats?

The next three sections develop these concepts with brief explanatory notes. More detailed information can be found in the associated chapters.

General

Is the rhythm fast or slow? Many rhythms are defined by their rate – for example, bradycardia in dogs is defined as heart rates ≤60 bpm and tachycardia as ≥180 bpm; and in cats, bradycardia is ≤100 bpm and tachycardia ≥220 bpm.

Is the rhythm regular or irregular? A ruler or callipers can be useful to determine if P-P and R-R intervals are regular. The next question is whether the rhythm is regularly irregularly or irregularly irregular; this may initially sound confusing but refers to whether there is an underlying pattern or if the rhythm is chaotic.

P waves

Are any P waves present? The presence of P waves implies that the rhythm has some atrial or supraventricular component.

Is the P wave morphology consistent? P waves which all appear identical imply that they are all being generated by the same pacemaker site. If there is variation in P wave morphology, then this could suggest that there is >1 pacemaker site or that some other component of the ECG complex is superimposed on the P wave.

Is there a P for every QRS, and vice versa? If the ratio is not 1:1, then this implies either atrioventricular block or an ectopic focus.

Is the PR interval constant? This is useful in the identification of atrial premature beats, and also when determining whether a wide-QRS complex is due to a supraventricular beat with aberrant ventricular conduction or a ventricular beat.

QRS Complexes

Are the P waves and QRS complexes coupled together? If P waves and QRS complexes are coupled, then the resulting complex may be a normal beat, an atrial premature beat or low-grade (first-degree) atrioventricular block. During ventricular tachycardia, there may be fusion or capture beats which are preceded by a P wave.

Guide to Canine and Feline Electrocardiography, First Edition. Ruth Willis, Pedro Oliveira and Antonia Mavropoulou.
© 2018 John Wiley & Sons Ltd. Published 2018 by John Wiley & Sons Ltd.
Companion website: www.wiley.com/go/willis/electrocardiography

Are the QRS complexes wide or narrow? Narrow-QRS complexes are conducted through the ventricles via the normal conduction pathways and typically are associated with supraventricular and junctional rhythms. Wide-QRS complexes are most commonly ventricular in origin but can also be seen with supraventricular beats that are conducted aberrantly through the ventricles.

Are matching QRS complexes grouped or not grouped? This can be useful in determining if atrioventricular block is present or if there is a pattern of recurring premature beats. In ventricular bigeminy, sinus beats alternate with ventricular beats; and in ventricular trigeminy, there is one sinus beat followed by two ventricular beats or two sinus beats followed by a single ventricular beat.

Are there any dropped beats? Dropped beats occur in sinus or atrioventricular node dysfunction.

Sinus Rhythms

Sinus Rhythm

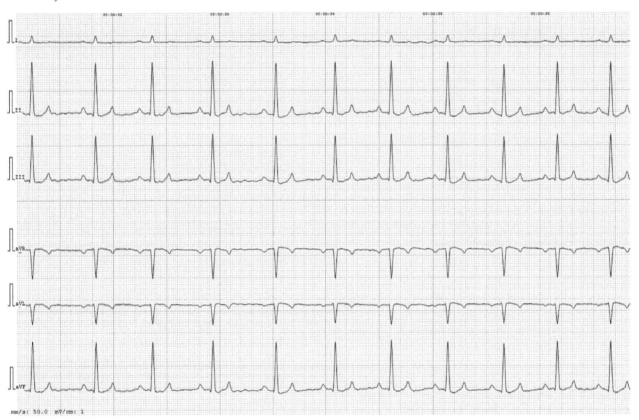

[9-year-old, male Lurcher dog] (50 mm/s; 10 mm/mV)

Rate	Dog 60–180 bpm Cat 100–220 bpm	PR interval	Dog 60–130 ms Cat 50–90 ms
Rhythm	Regular	QRS	Dog <70 ms (+40° to +100°) Cat <40 ms (0° to +160°)
P wave	Present Positive in leads II, III and aVF; positive or biphasic in lead I; negative in aVR and aVL. Dog (−18° to +90°) Cat (−0° to +90°)	Grouping	None
P:QRS	1:1	Dropped beats	None

Sinus rhythm is the normal rhythm seen in cats and dogs. In this rhythm, the sinoatrial node is the dominant pacemaker, and all measurements are within their respective reference ranges unless there is concomitant atrioventricular block or aberrant intraventricular conduction.

Respiratory Sinus Arrhythmia

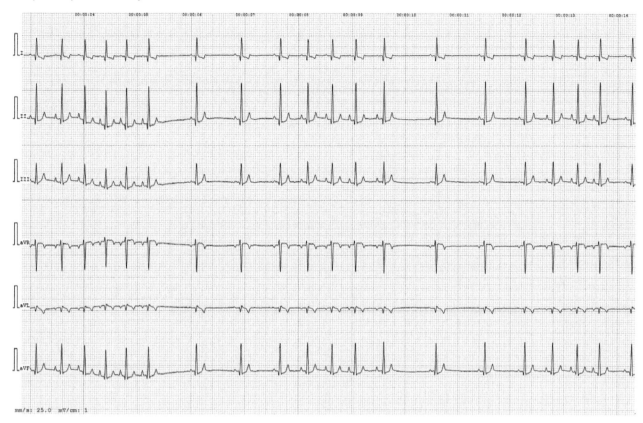

[3-year-old, male neutered, Staffordshire Bull Terrier dog] (25 mm/s; 10 mm/mV)

Rate (approx.)	Dog 60–120 bpm Cat 100–130 bpm	PR interval	Dog 60–130 ms Cat 50–90 ms
Rhythm	Regularly irregular	QRS	Normal
P wave	Present	Grouping	None
P:QRS	1:1	Dropped beats	Only if sinus arrhythmia is very marked
Respiratory sinus arrhythmia is a cyclical variation of the heart rate related to autonomic tone variations during the respiratory phases. It is very common in dogs but rarely seen in the clinical setting in cats. As may be seen in the example given here, the P-QRS-T complexes are normal, but there is a cyclical increase and decrease of the heart rate during inspiration and expiration, respectively.			

Wandering Pacemaker

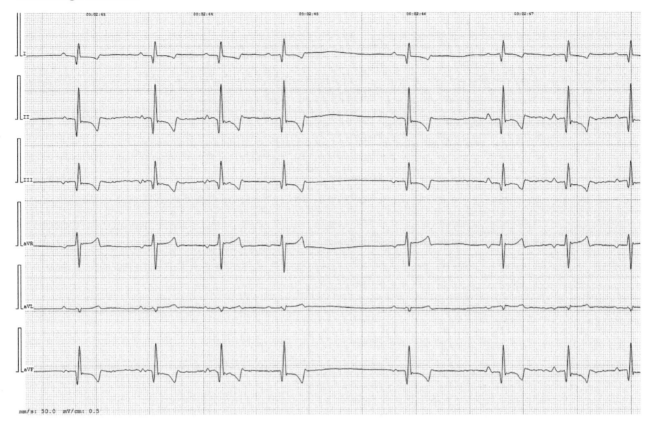

[6-year-old, female neutered, Boxer dog] (50 mm/s; 20 mm/mV)

Rate (approx.)	Dog 60–120 bpm	PR interval	Normal to prolonged
Rhythm	Regularly irregular	QRS	Normal
P wave	Present with variable morphology	Grouping	None
P:QRS	1:1	Dropped beats	None
Wandering pacemaker is a regular variation in P wave morphology presumed to occur as a result of fluctuations in autonomic tone influencing the point of impulse generation within the sinoatrial node. It is frequently seen in dogs but is rare in cats.			

Sinus Bradycardia

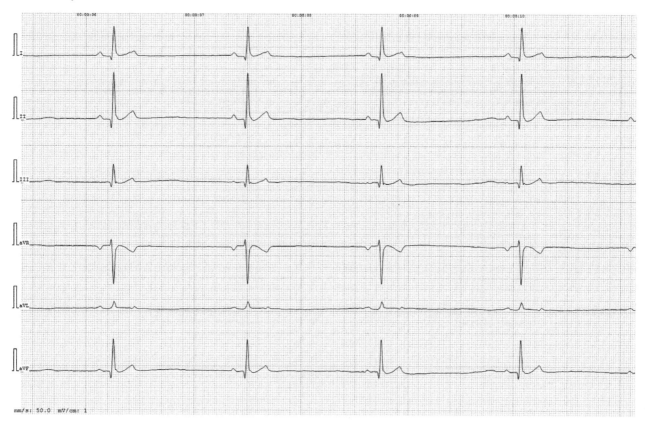

[6-year-old, female neutered, Labrador Retriever dog] (50 mm/s; 10 mm/mV)

Rate (approx.)	Dog <60 bpm Cat <100 bpm	PR interval	Normal to slightly prolonged
Rhythm	Regular	QRS	Normal
P wave	Present	Grouping	None
P:QRS	1:1	Dropped beats	None

Sinus bradycardia is a slow, regular heart rhythm commonly seen in resting dogs or cats. As this rhythm is associated with high resting vagal tone, it is sometimes seen in conjunction with sinus arrhythmia, wandering pacemaker and first-degree atrioventricular block. In the example here, a regular sinus rhythm is seen (normal P-QRS-T) with a heart rate of 60 bpm in a dog. The PR interval is at the higher end of the normal range or slightly prolonged (130–140 ms).

Sinus Tachycardia

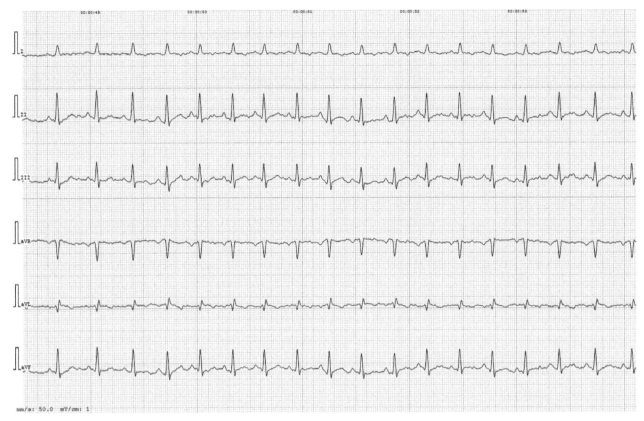

[2-year-old, male neutered, Staffordshire Bull Terrier dog] (50 mm/s; 10 mm/mV)

Rate (approx.)	Dog >180 bpm Cat >220 bpm	PR interval	Normal to slightly shortened
Rhythm	Regular	QRS	Normal to slightly shortened
P wave	Present	Grouping	None
P:QRS	1:1	Dropped beats	None
Sinus tachycardia is a rapid regular rhythm caused by conditions that require increased cardiac output that may be physiological (such as exercise, pain or fear) or pathological (such as hypovolaemia, hypoxia or haemorrhage). Sinus tachycardia has gradual onset and offset. In the example here, a regular sinus rhythm is seen (normal P-QRS-T) with a heart rate of approximately 200 bpm in a dog. The PR interval is at the lower end of the normal range (70 ms).			

Ectopic Foci

Atrial Premature Complex or Beat (APC or APB)

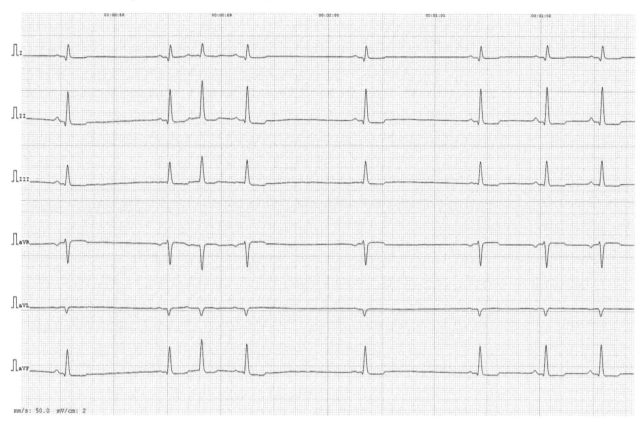

[9-year-old, male neutered, Cavalier King Charles Spaniel dog] (50 mm/s; 5 mm/mV)

Rate	Depends on underlying rhythm	PR interval	Variable in the APC
Rhythm	Irregular	QRS	Normal Dog <70 ms (+40° to +100°) Cat <40 ms (0° to +160°)
P wave	Present, but P wave of atrial premature beat may show different morphology from the sinus beats	Grouping	Sometimes – in the example shown, the rhythm alternates between sinus beats and APCs
P:QRS	1:1	Dropped beats	None

An atrial ectopic beat is a beat originating in the atrial tissue outside the sinus node. It is often premature (it occurs before the next sinus beat is due) and followed by a pause. If it does not depolarise the sinus node, the next sinus beat will occur after a normal P-P interval, and the sum of P-P' and P'-P will be twice the sinus P-P – this is termed a *compensatory pause*. If the APC is able to depolarise the sinus node and reset it, the next sinus beat will occur sooner, and the sum of P-P' and P'-P will be less than twice the sinus P-P – this is termed a *non-compensatory pause*. If a pause is not seen after the premature, it is termed an interpolated beat, as seen in the example here, where the third beat is an interpolated APC.

Ventricular Premature Beat or Contraction (VPB or VPC)

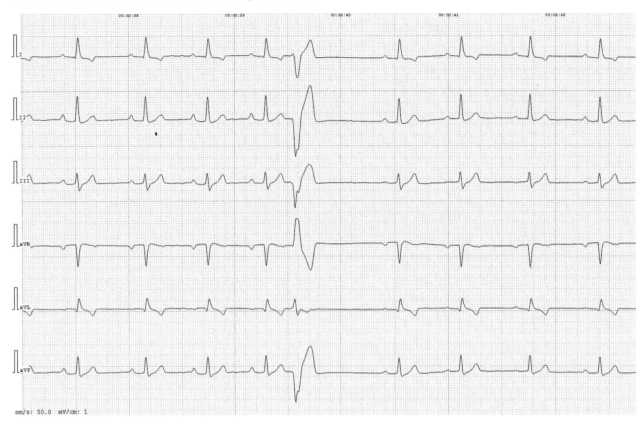

[9-year-old, male neutered, Irish Terrier dog] (50 mm/s; 10 mm/mV)

Rate	Depends on underlying rhythm	PR interval	Normal
Rhythm	Irregular	QRS	Premature beat has wide QRS and different T wave morphology
P wave	None associated with premature beat	Grouping	None
P:QRS	P < QRS	Dropped beats	None

A ventricular ectopic beat is a beat originating in any structure located below the atrioventricular junction. It is often premature (it occurs before the next sinus beat is due) and may be followed by a pause or may be interpolated. In the example here, the fifth beat is a VPC followed by a compensatory pause. The QRS is wide and abnormal and is not preceded by a P wave.

Ventricular Bigeminy

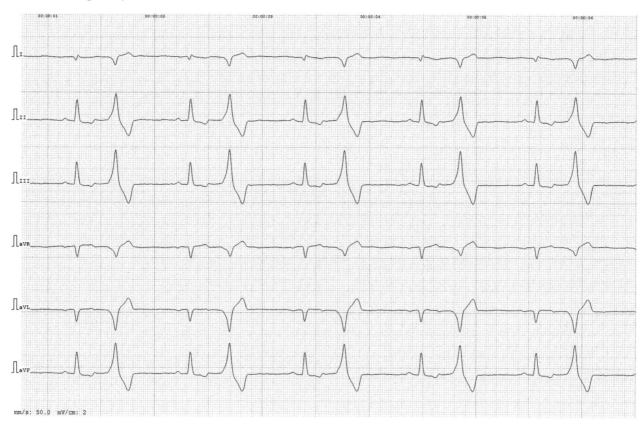

[14-year-old, male neutered, Border Collie dog] (50 mm/s; 5 mm/mV)

Rate	Variable	PR interval	Normal on sinus beats; no P wave coupled to the ventricular beats
Regularity	Irregular	QRS	Ventricular beats are wide with different morphology to the sinus beats
P wave	None with the premature beats	Grouping	Alternating sinus and ventricular beats
P:QRS	P < QRS	Dropped beats	None
Ventricular bigeminy is the term used to describe a rhythm where ventricular ectopic beats alternate with sinus beats in a 1:1 arrangement.			

Ventricular Trigeminy

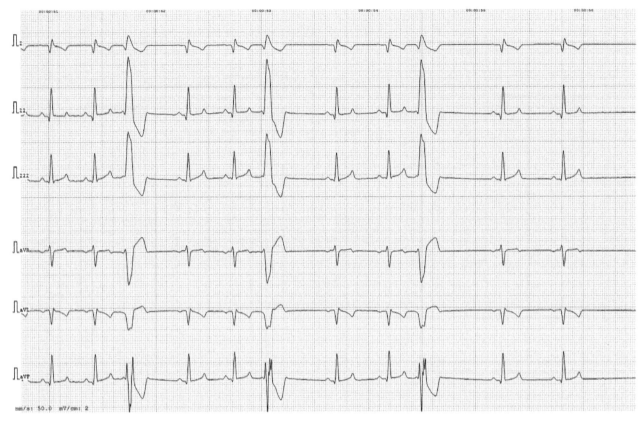

[8-year-old, female neutered, Labrador Retriever dog] (50 mm/s; 5 mm/mV)

Rate	Variable	PR interval	Normal on sinus beats; no P wave coupled to the ventricular beats
Rhythm	Irregular	QRS	Ventricular beats are wide with different morphology from the sinus beats
P wave	None with the premature beats	Grouping	Regular repeating pattern of two sinus beats followed by a ventricular beat, or two ventricular beats followed by a sinus beat
P:QRS	P < QRS	Dropped beats	None
Ventricular trigeminy is the term used to describe a rhythm where two ventricular ectopic beats alternate with one sinus beat, or two sinus beats alternate with one ventricular ectopic beat.			

Ventricular Escape Beat

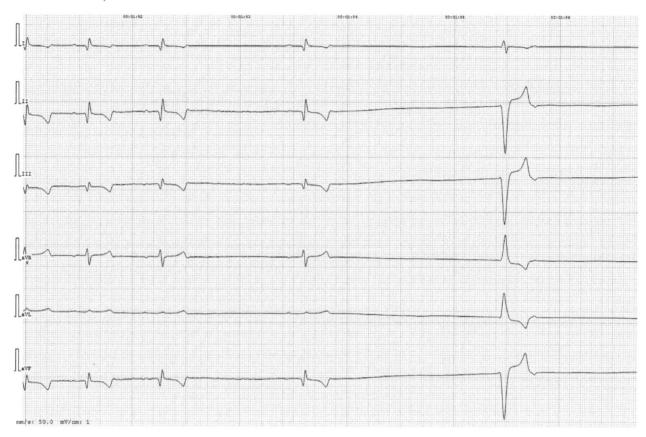

[14-year-old, male neutered, Border Collie dog] (50 mm/ms; 10 mm/mV)

Rate	Depends on underlying rhythm	PR interval	None
Rhythm	Irregular	QRS	Wide and different QRS morphology from the sinus beats
P wave	None associated with escape beat	Grouping	None
P:QRS	None associated with escape beat	Dropped beats	Yes – pause prior to the escape beat
A ventricular escape beat is a ventricular ectopic beat that occurs after a pause caused by a period of sinus node inactivity or block. It is the result of spontaneous depolarisation of a subsidiary pacemaker located in the ventricular tissue. In the example here, the last beat is a ventricular escape beat.			

Junctional Escape Beat

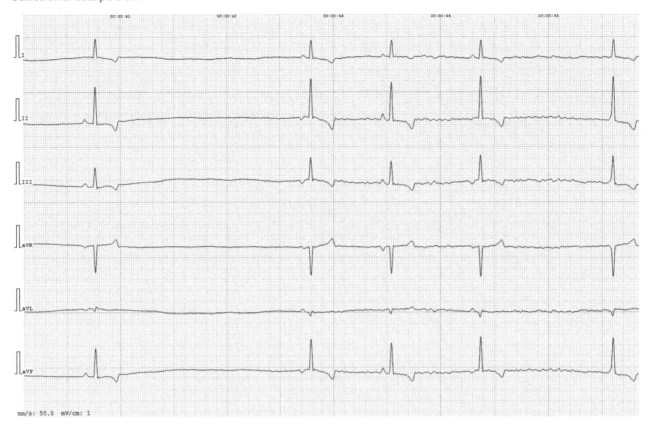

[11-year-old, female neutered, West Highland White Terrier dog] (50.mm/s; 10mm/mV)

Rate	Depends on underlying rhythm	PR interval	None, short or P after QRS
Rhythm	Irregular	QRS	Normal Dog <70 ms (+40° to +100°) Cat <40 ms (0° to +160°)
P wave	Variable (none, antegrade or retrograde after QRS)	Grouping	None
P:QRS	None or 1:1 if P is present	Dropped beats	Yes – pause prior to the junctional escape beat
A junctional escape beat is an ectopic beat that occurs after a pause caused by a period of sinus node inactivity or block. It is the result of spontaneous depolarisation of a subsidiary pacemaker located in the atrioventricular junction; and, as such, the QRS is similar to the sinus beats in terms of duration and appearance. In the example here, the second, fourth and fifth beats are junctional escape beats.			

Junctional Escape Rhythm

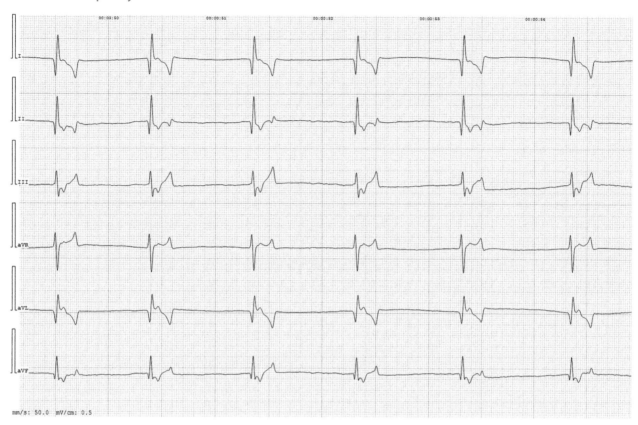

[12-year-old, male neutered, Staffordshire Bull Terrier dog] (50 mm/s; 20 mm/mV)

Rate	Slow	PR interval	None, short or P after QRS
Rhythm	Regular	QRS	Normal Dog <70 ms (+40° to +100°) Cat <40 ms (0° to +160°)
P wave	Variable	Grouping	None
P:QRS	None or 1:1 If P is present	Dropped beats	None

A junctional escape rhythm is a rhythm originating from the atrioventricular junction as the result of the depolarisation of a subsidiary pacemaker. It occurs when the rate of the sinus rhythm falls below the intrinsic rate of the subsidiary pacemaker. Depending on the origin of the impulse, a retroconducted P wave (negative in leads II, III and aVF) may be seen before or after the QRS; or may not be seen if it occurs at the same time as the QRS. In the example here, a retroconducted P may be seen following the QRS in the ST segment. The QRS is normal in duration and appearance, and a sinus P is not seen before the QRS. The heart rate is 60 bpm.

Ventricular Escape Rhythm

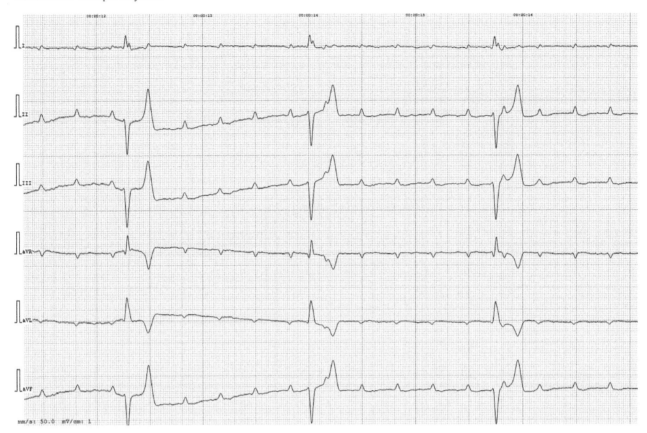

[8-year-old, male neutered, Dogue de Bordeaux dog] (50 mm/s; 10 mm/mV)

Rate	Slow <60 bpm	PR interval	None
Rhythm	Regular	QRS	Abnormal; wide Dogs >70 ms Cats >40 ms
P wave	None	Grouping	None
P:QRS	None	Dropped beats	None
A ventricular escape rhythm is a rhythm originating from the ventricles as the result of depolarisation of a subsidiary pacemaker. It occurs when the rate of the sinus rhythm falls below the intrinsic rate of the subsidiary pacemaker or in case of third degree atrioventricular block, as in the example given here.				

Conduction Abnormalities

Sinus Pause

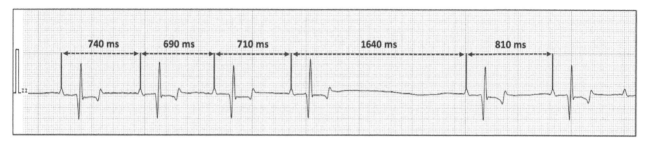

[4-year-old, male neutered, Boxer dog] (50 mm/s, 20 mm/mV)

Rate	Variable	PR interval	Normal
Rhythm	Irregular	QRS	Normal
P wave	Present except during the dropped beats	Grouping	None
P:QRS	1:1	Dropped beats	Yes – pause is not a multiple of the normal P-P interval

A sinus pause corresponds to a period of sinus inactivity. On the electrocardiogram, it is seen as a pause between two beats. This may be due to either a lack of sinus node depolarisation or the inability of the impulse to exit the sinus node and depolarise the atrial tissue (sinoatrial block). This is not possible to distinguish on the surface electrocardiogram unless the pause is an exact multiple of the normal P-P interval, suggesting a second-degree sinoatrial block (as shown next).

Second-degree Sinoatrial Block

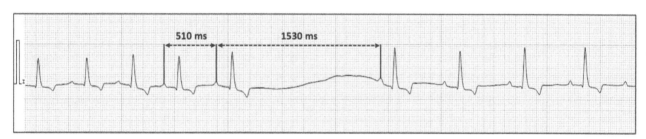

[9-year-old, male neutered, Boxer dog] (50 mm/s, 20 mm/mV)

Rate	Variable	PR interval	Normal
Rhythm	Irregular	QRS	Normal
P wave	Present except during the dropped beats	Grouping	None
P:QRS	1:1	Dropped beats	Yes – pause is a multiple of the normal P-P interval

In sinoatrial block (SAB), the sinus impulse is unable to exit the sinus node to depolarise the atrial tissue and initiate a beat. There are three degrees of SAB: (1) there is a delay in conduction through the sinus node; (2) occasional beats are blocked; and (3) none of the sinus depolarisations manage to reach the atrial tissue. It is not possible to identify first- and third-degree SAB on the surface electrocardiogram; however, a sinus pause that is an exact multiple of the normal P-P interval is highly suggestive of a second-degree SAB. In the example here, a sinus pause that is exactly three times longer than the preceding P-P is suggestive of second-degree SAB.

Sinus Node Arrest

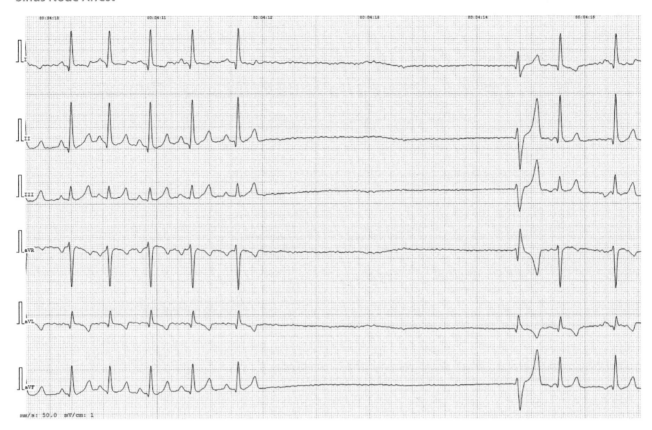

[11-year-old, female neutered, Staffordshire Bull Terrier] (50 mm/s, 10 mm/mV)

Rate	Variable, generally slow	PR interval	Normal
Rhythm	Irregular	QRS	Normal
P wave	Present except during the periods of asystole	Grouping	None
P:QRS	1:1	Dropped beats	Yes

Sinus pauses and sinus node arrest describe periods of sinus node inactivity or block. Sinus pauses are commonly seen in resting dogs, whereas sinus arrest describes a longer interruption of normal sinus node activity. In the example here, a long pause is seen without P-QRS-T complexes until a ventricular escape beat occurs.

First-degree Atrioventricular Block

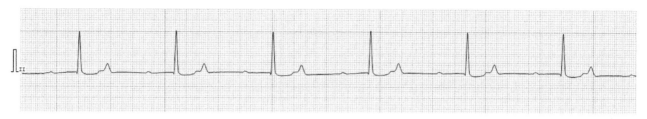

[9-year-old, male English Bulldog] (50 mm/s, 10 mm/mV)

Rate	Depends on underlying rhythm	PR interval	Constant but prolonged
Rhythm	Regular or regularly irregular if sinus arrhythmia is also present	QRS	Normal
P wave	Normal	Grouping	None
P:QRS	1:1	Dropped beats	None

With first-degree atrioventricular block, there is a delay in conduction through the atrioventricular node, resulting in a longer than normal PR interval. All P waves are followed by a QRS unless there is concomitant second-degree atrioventricular block. In the example here, the PR interval is constant but prolonged (260 ms).

Second-degree Atrioventricular Block Mobitz Type I

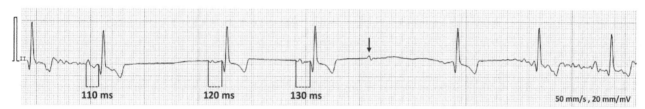

[10-year-old, male Boxer dog] (50 mm/s, 20 mm/mV)

Rate	Depends on underlying rhythm	PR interval	Variable – lengthens prior to block
Rhythm	Regularly irregular	QRS	Normal
P wave	Present	Grouping	Present and variable
P:QRS	P > QRS	Dropped beats	Yes

With second-degree atrioventricular block (2AVB), there is intermittent block of the impulse in the atrioventricular node. On the surface ECG, one or more P waves are not followed by a QRS. In 2AVB Mobitz type I, there is a progressive prolongation of the PR interval until the impulse is blocked, as illustrated in the example given here. Normally, only one P wave is not followed by a QRS.

Second-degree Atrioventricular Block Mobitz type II

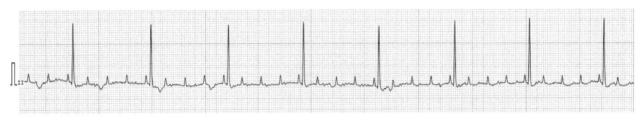

[10-year-old, male neutered, Cavalier King Charles Spaniel dog] (50 mm/s, 10 mm/mV)

Rate	Depends on underlying rhythm	PR interval	Variable due to intermittent block; constant PR on conducted P waves
Rhythm	Regularly irregular	QRS	Normal
P wave	Present	Grouping	Present and variable
P:QRS	P > QRS, 4:1 in this example	Dropped beats	Yes

With second-degree atrioventricular block (2AVB), there is intermittent block of the impulse in the atrioventricular node. On the surface ECG, one or more P waves are not followed by a QRS. In 2AVB Mobitz type II, one or more P waves are not followed by a QRS with a constant PR interval before the impulse is blocked.

Third-degree Atrioventricular Block

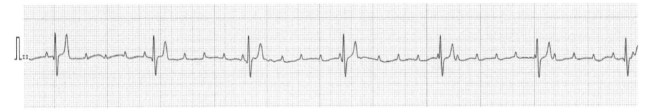

[10-year-old, male neutered, Boxer dog] (25 mm/s, 10 mm/mV)

Rate	Slow with separate atrial (P waves) and ventricular (QRS) rates	PR interval	No coupling between P waves and QRS complexes
Rhythm	Regular but different P and QRS rates	QRS	Normal or wide, depending on the origin of the underlying escape rhythm
P wave	Present	Grouping	None
P:QRS	P > > QRS	Dropped beats	None

With third-degree atrioventricular block (3AVB), all atrial impulses are blocked in the atrioventricular node (complete block). The P waves are not associated with the QRS, and the ventricular rate and QRS appearance will depend on the underlying escape rhythm (junctional vs. ventricular). In the example here, sinus P waves may be seen with a rate of approximately 140 bpm and are not associated with the QRS (there is no constant PR). The QRS are wide (80–90 ms), and the ventricular rate is approximately 30 bpm, consistent with a ventricular escape rhythm.

Left Bundle Branch Block

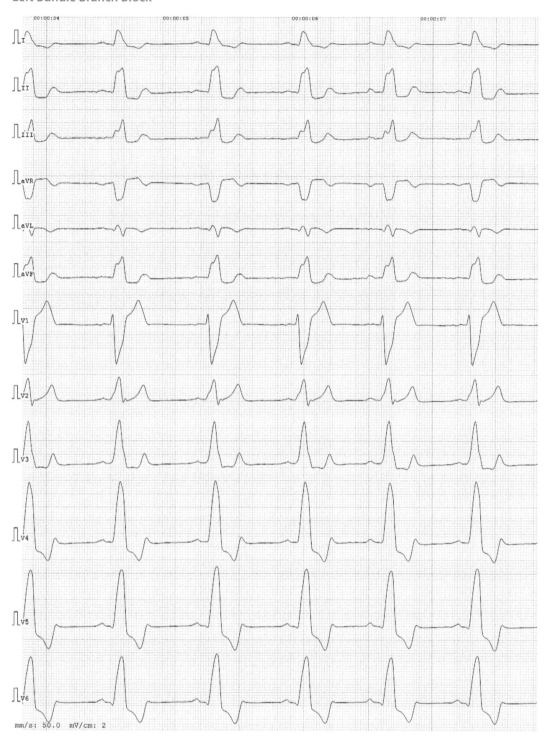

[8-year-old, male, Gordon Setter dog] (50 mm/s, 5 mm/mV)

Rate	Depends on underlying rhythm	PR interval	Normal
Rhythm	Regular or irregular	QRS	Wide
P wave	Present	Grouping	Sometimes
P:QRS	1:1	Dropped beats	None

With left bundle branch block, ventricular depolarisation occurs via the right bundle branch towards the right ventricle, and then slowly via the working myocardium to the left ventricle. This results in a wide QRS (>80 ms) with a normal mean electrical axis. The QRS is prevalently positive in leads I, II, III, aVF and V2 to V6. A normal P wave is seen before each QRS with a normal PR interval (unless there is concomitant atrioventricular block).

Right Bundle Branch Block

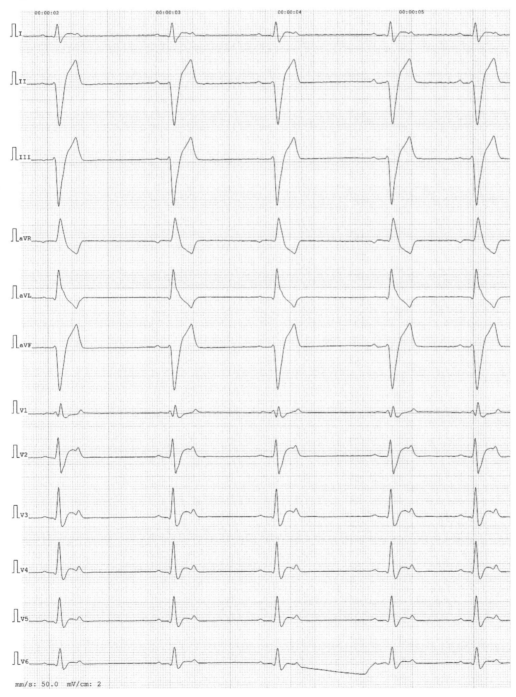

mm/s: 50.0 mV/cm: 2

[10-year-old, male neutered, Cairn Terrier dog] (50 mm/s, 5 mm/mV)

Rate	Depends on underlying rhythm	PR interval	Normal
Rhythm	Regular or irregular	QRS	Wide
P wave	Present	Grouping	Sometimes
P:QRS	1:1	Dropped beats	None

With right bundle branch block, ventricular depolarisation occurs via the left bundle branch to the left ventricle, and then slowly via the working myocardium towards the right ventricle. This results in a wide QRS (>80 ms) with a right deviation of the MEA (up to –110°). Large wide S waves are seen in leads II, III and aVL; a positive R wave is seen in lead aVR; and an r' or R' wave may be seen in V1. A normal P wave is seen before each QRS with a normal PR interval (unless there is concomitant atrioventricular block).

Sinus Rhythm With Ventricular Pre-excitation Via an Accessory Pathway

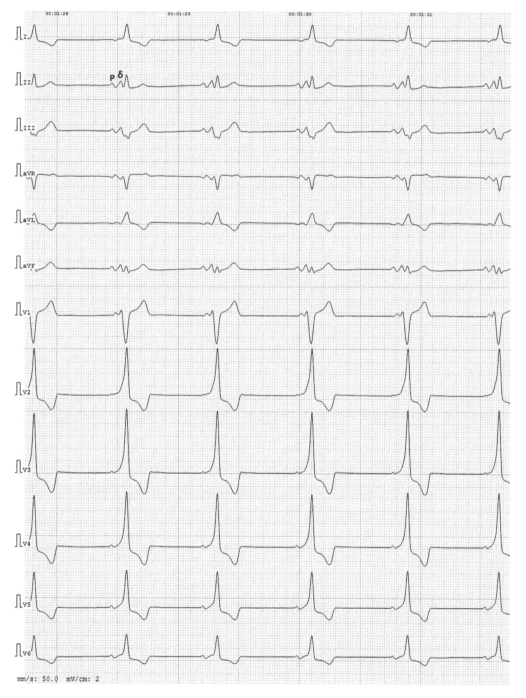

[8-year-old, female neutered, Labrador Retriever] (50 mm/s; 5 mm/mV)

Rate	Depends on underlying rhythm	PR interval	Short
Rhythm	Regular or irregular	QRS	Wide
P wave	Present	Grouping	None
P:QRS	1:1	Dropped beats	None

With ventricular pre-excitation, atrioventricular conduction occurs via both the atrioventricular node (AVN) and an accessory pathway. The impulse travelling through the accessory pathway reaches the ventricles before the normally conducted impulse via the AVN–His–Purkinje, causing early excitation of that area of ventricle. On the surface electrocardiogram, this is seen as a short PR interval and a QRS that is wider than normal. The initial part of the QRS may appear as a slope or a distinct wave termed the delta wave (δ) that reflects early ventricular depolarisation.

Tachycardias

Atrial Fibrillation

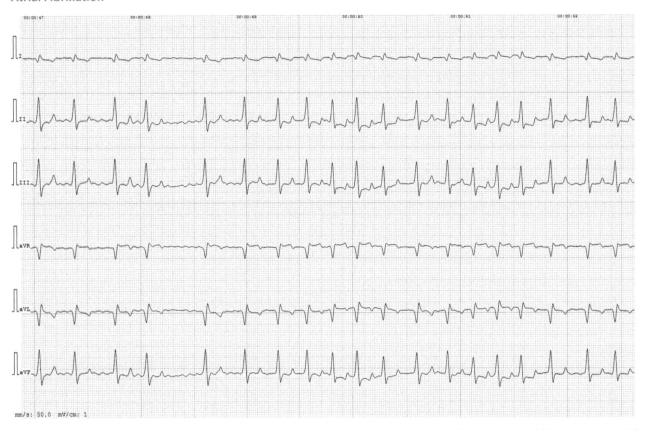

[2-year-old, male Saint Bernard dog] (50 mm/s; 10 mm/mV)

Rate	Variable	PR interval	None
Rhythm	Irregularly irregular	QRS	Normal
P wave	None – chaotic atrial activity, f waves	Grouping	None
P:QRS	None	Dropped beats	None

Atrial fibrillation is a chaotic atrial rhythm with simultaneous depolarisation of multiple areas of the atrial tissue that may be seen on the surface electrocardiogram as small undulations of baseline (f waves), as seen on the example given here. The resulting rhythm is irregular, as many atrial depolarisations reach the atrioventricular node but only a fraction actually reach the ventricles. On the surface electrocardiogram, atrial fibrillation is characterised by an irregular rhythm without visible P waves, and possible visible f waves. The heart rate is often elevated but may also be normal (lone atrial fibrillation).

Atrial Flutter

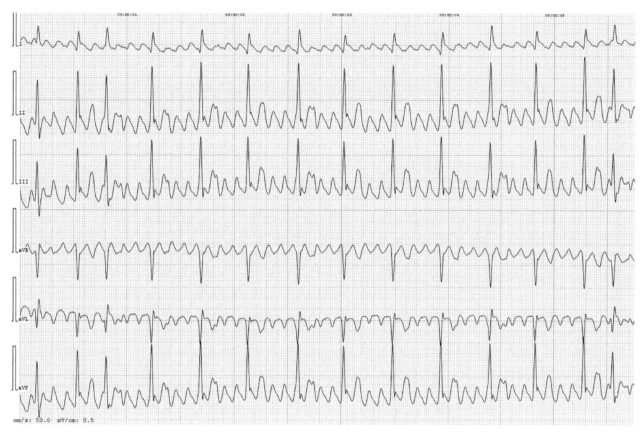

[13-year-old, male neutered, Crossbreed dog] (50 mm/s; 20 mm/mV)

Rate	Atrial rate >300 bpm Ventricular rate variable	FR interval	Variable
Rhythm	Irregular or less commonly regular depending on A:V conduction ratio	QRS	Normal
P wave	Saw-tooth appearance F waves	Grouping	None
F:QRS	F>>QRS	Dropped beats	None

Atrial flutter is a rapid atrial tachycardia caused by the presence of a macro re-entrant circuit in the atrial wall. On the surface ECG, P waves are replaced by flutter (F) waves that represent the cyclic atrial activation loop with an atrial rate between 300 to 600 bpm. The F waves often have a typical saw-tooth appearance as seen in the example here between each QRS. The QRS is normal in appearance (unless there is concomitant bundle branch block), and the rhythm may be regular or irregular depending on conduction of atrial impulses through the atrioventricular node.

Focal Atrial Tachycardia

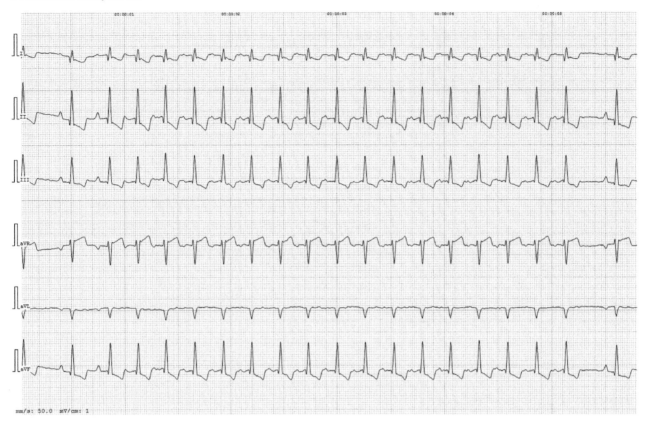

[11-year-old, male Border Terrier dog] (50 mm/s; 10 mm/mV)

Rate	Variable		PR interval	Normal or slightly different
Rhythm	Irregular		QRS	Normal
P wave	Present but morphology of ectopic P' is different from the sinus P which may be visible or superimposed on ST segment of preceding beat		Grouping	Short paroxysms of tachycardia interrupt sinus rhythm
P:QRS	1:1 unless there is second-degree atrioventricular block at offset		Dropped beats	Short pause after offset due to overdrive suppression of sinus node
Focal atrial tachycardia (FAT) is the result of depolarisation of an ectopic focus in the atria. One (focal) or more (multifocal) foci may be present, generating ectopic P' waves with varying morphology depending on their origin, and different from the sinus P. They may be difficult to identify at higher rates, as they may appear superimposed on the T wave or ST segment of the previous beat. In the example here, an episode of FAT may be seen (beats 3 to 18) where the ectopic P' is seen superimposed on the T wave and is only discernible in some of the beats. The QRS is normal unless there is concomitant bundle branch block.				

Isorhythmic Atrioventricular Dissociation Type I

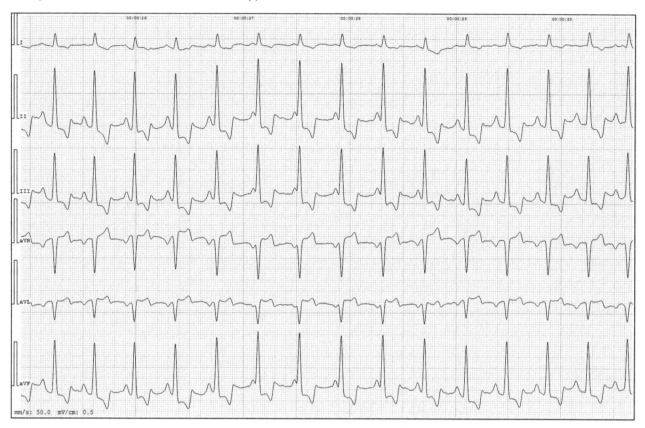

[12-year-old, male Labrador Retriever dog] (50 mm/s; 20 mm/mV)

Rate	Variable	PR interval	Variable with rhythmic fluctuation
Rhythm	Slightly irregular	QRS	Normal
P wave	Present	Grouping	None
P:QRS	1:1	Dropped beats	None

The term *isorhythmic AV dissociation* (IAVD) indicates the presence of two rhythms (a sinus and an ectopic junctional rhythm) that coexist and show some degree of synchronisation (have similar discharge rates). On the electrocardiogram, this is seen as normal P waves that are not associated with the QRS; the P-P and R-R intervals are similar, but the PR interval varies. With IAVD type I, a rhythmic variation of the sinus P wave position is seen in relation to the QRS. It is often seen moving closer to and then away from the QRS, as in the example here. Occasionally, the P wave might move into and get buried within the QRS complex, only to move back out again in front of the QRS in the subsequent beats.

Isorhythmic Atrioventricular Dissociation Type II

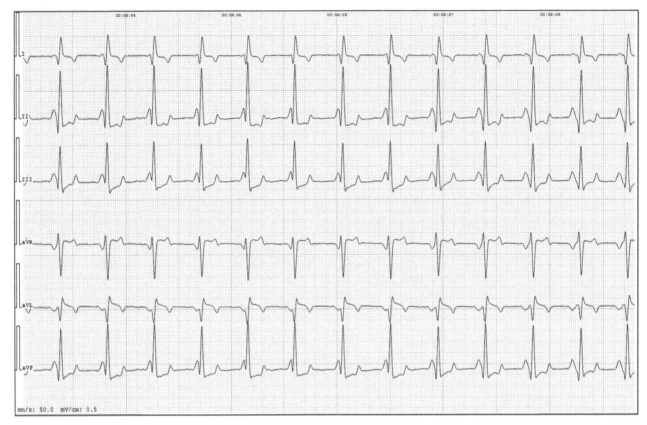

[13-year-old, male neutered, Labrador Retriever dog] (50 mm/s; 20 mm/mV)

Rate	Variable	PR interval	Fixed but P may be before or after QRS.
Rhythm	Slightly irregular	QRS	Normal
P wave	Present	Grouping	None
P:QRS	1:1	Dropped beats	None

The term *isorhythmic AV dissociation* (IAVD) indicates the presence of two rhythms (a sinus and an ectopic junctional rhythm) that coexist and show some degree of synchronisation (have similar discharge rates). On the electrocardiogram, this is seen as normal P waves that are not associated with the QRS; the P-P and R-R intervals are similar, but the PR interval varies. With IAVD type II, the relationship between P and QRS is fixed, and the rhythmic fluctuation seen in type 1 synchronisation does not occur. The P wave may precede the QRS complex, may coincide with it being hidden or may be superimposed on the ST segment or the first half of the T wave. In the example here, the P is seen in a fixed position just before the ascending R wave.

Junctional Tachycardia

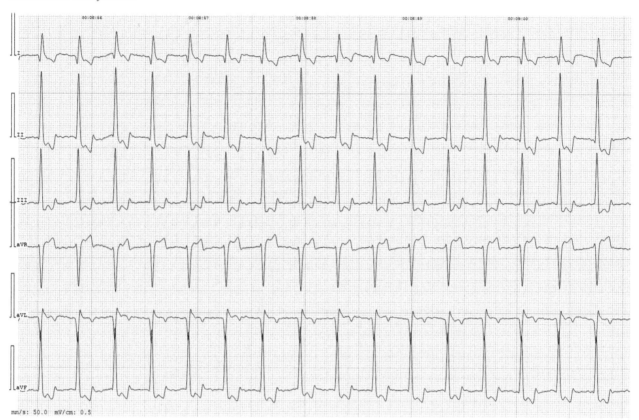

[12-year-old, female neutered, Labrador Retriever dog] (50 mm/s; 20 mm/mV)

Rate	>100 bpm	PR interval	No coupling between P waves and QRS complexes
Rhythm	Regular	QRS	Normal
P wave	Present with isorhythmic atrioventricular dissociation; may be retrograde in ST segment if ventriculoatrial depolarisation	Grouping	None
P:QRS	P waves do not consistently precede QRS complex	Dropped beats	None
Junctional tachycardia is the result of depolarisation of an ectopic focus located within or in the area immediately adjacent to the atrioventricular junction. Depending on the origin of the impulse, a retroconducted P' wave (negative in leads II, III and aVF) may be seen before or after the QRS; or may not be seen if it occurs at the same time as the QRS. In the example here, a retroconducted P' may be seen in the descending R/initial part of the ST segment. The QRS is normal in duration unless there is concomitant bundle branch block.			

Orthodromic Atrioventricular Reciprocating Tachycardia

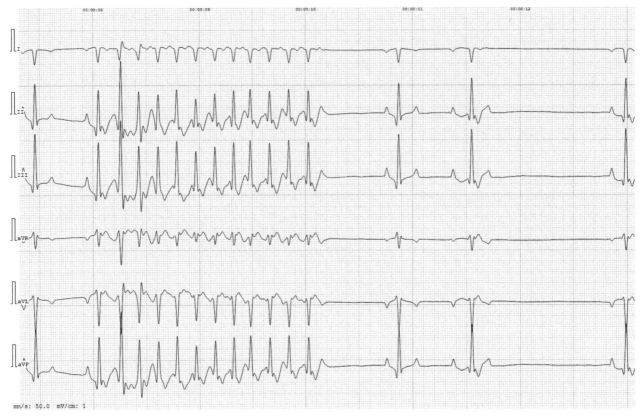

[4-month-old, male Staffordshire Bull Terrier dog] (50 mm/s; 10 mm/mV)

Rate	>180 bpm	PR interval	RP′ < P′R
Rhythm	Regular	QRS	Normal unless concomitant bundle branch block
P wave	Retrograde P (negative in leads II, III and aVF) visible on the ST segment	Grouping	None
P:QRS	P = QRS	Dropped beats	None
Orthodromic atrioventricular reciprocating tachycardia is the result of a macro re-entrant rhythm where the impulse travels down the atrioventricular node and normal conduction pathways from the atria to the ventricles and up to the atria again via an accessory pathway. Episodes of tachycardia are seen with sudden onset and offset, such as in the example here (beats 3 to 13). The QRS during tachycardia is similar in appearance to the sinus beats, and a retrograde P (negative in leads II, III and aVF) may be seen on the ST segment.			

Ventricular Tachycardia

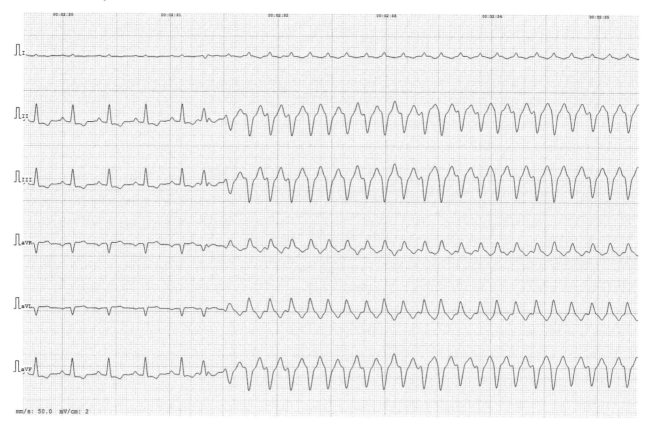

[8-year-old, male Siberian Husky dog] (50 mm/s; 5 mm/mV)

Rate	>180 bpm	PR interval	No coupling
Rhythm	Regular	QRS	Wide with different morphology from the sinus beats
P wave	Often superimposed on ventricular beats but occasionally visible	Grouping	Clusters of ventricular beats
P:QRS	P < QRS	Dropped beats	May be short pause after offset

Ventricular tachycardia (VT) is the result of depolarisation of an ectopic focus in the tissues below the atrioventricular junction with a rate above 180 bpm. One (unifocal) or more (multifocal) foci may be present, generating wide QRS with abnormal morphology depending on their origin. In the example given here, an episode of VT is seen from beat 7 onwards with a rate of approximately 340 bpm. The QRS is wide with a morphology similar to a right bundle branch block, suggesting an origin in the left ventricle.

Appendix 3

Mean Electrical Axis

The mean electrical axis (MEA) is the net vector of depolarisation of a current moving across the myocardium, and further information on this concept is presented in chapters 3 and 4. Additionally, the electrical axis of the P or P' waves is described in chapter 8. The electrocardiographic (ECG) lead systems used in dogs and cats are derived from those used in human patients; obviously, the shape of the thorax is quite different in veterinary patients and can even vary dramatically between different breeds. In light of these anatomical variations, care should be taken to not over-interpret the accuracy of the MEA value obtained – perhaps considering it as an estimate rather than a true value. As further clinical electrophysiological studies are performed, we will glean further information about the accuracy of MEA estimations in veterinary patients.

Various ways of estimating the MEA were described in chapter 4. As the graphical method (see Figure 4.24) follows a mathematical formula, tables have been derived to facilitate rapid estimation of the MEA, and these are presented in this appendix as a guide for clinicians.[1,2]

Directions for Using Tables to Determine the Mean Electrical Axis

1) Using the amplitudes of the deflections, calculate the algebraic sum of the positive and negative waves in lead I (see Figure 4.24 for an example).
   If the sum is positive, use Table A3.1 or A3.2; if negative, use Table A3.3 or A3.4.
2) Determine the algebraic sum of the positive and negative waves in lead III (see Figure 4.24 for an example).
   If negative, use Table A3.2 or A3.3; if positive, use Table A3.1 or A3.4.
3) Plot the values obtained on the appropriate table. The intersection of the lead I column with the lead III row shows the MEA in degrees.

Guide to Canine and Feline Electrocardiography, First Edition. Ruth Willis, Pedro Oliveira and Antonia Mavropoulou.
© 2018 John Wiley & Sons Ltd. Published 2018 by John Wiley & Sons Ltd.
Companion website: www.wiley.com/go/willis/electrocardiography

Table A3.1

	Lead I positive																					
Lead III positive	0.0	0.5	1.0	1.5	2.0	2.5	3.0	3.5	4.0	4.5	5.0	6.0	7.0	8.0	9.0	10.0	11.0	12.0	13.0	14.0	15.0	20.0
0	90	30	30	30	30	30	30	30	30	30	30	30	30	30	30	30	30	30	30	30	30	30
0.5	90	60	49	44	41	39	38	37	36	35	35	34	33	33	33	32	32	32	32	32	32	31
1.0	90	71	60	53	49	46	44	42	41	40	39	38	37	36	35	35	34	34	34	33	33	32
1.5	90	76	67	60	55	52	49	47	45	44	43	41	39	38	38	37	36	36	36	35	35	33
2.0	90	79	71	65	60	56	53	51	49	47	46	44	42	41	40	39	38	38	37	37	36	35
2.5	90	81	74	68	64	60	57	54	52	51	49	47	45	43	42	41	40	39	39	38	38	36
3.0	90	82	76	71	67	63	60	57	55	53	52	49	47	45	44	43	42	41	40	39	39	37
3.5	90	83	78	73	69	66	63	60	58	56	54	51	49	47	46	44	43	42	42	41	40	38
4.0	90	84	79	75	71	68	65	62	60	58	56	53	51	49	47	46	45	44	43	42	42	39
4.5	90	85	80	76	73	69	67	64	62	60	58	55	53	51	49	48	47	45	44	43	43	40
5.0	90	85	81	77	74	71	68	66	64	62	60	57	55	52	51	49	48	47	46	45	44	41
6.0	90	86	82	79	76	73	71	69	67	65	63	60	57	55	53	52	50	49	48	47	46	43
7.0	90	87	83	81	78	75	73	71	69	67	65	63	60	58	56	54	53	51	50	49	48	44
8.0	90	87	84	82	79	77	75	73	71	69	68	65	62	60	58	56	55	53	52	51	50	46
9.0	90	87	85	82	80	78	76	74	73	71	69	67	64	62	60	58	57	55	54	53	52	48
10.0	90	88	85	83	81	79	77	76	74	72	71	68	66	64	62	60	58	57	56	54	53	49
11.0	90	88	86	84	82	80	78	77	75	73	72	70	67	65	63	62	60	59	57	56	55	50
12.0	90	88	86	84	82	81	79	78	76	75	73	71	69	67	65	63	61	60	59	57	56	52
13.0	90	88	86	84	83	81	80	78	77	76	74	72	70	68	66	64	63	61	60	59	58	53
14.0	90	88	87	85	83	82	80	79	78	77	75	73	71	69	67	66	64	63	61	60	59	55
15.0	90	88	87	85	84	82	81	80	78	77	76	74	72	70	68	67	65	64	62	61	60	55
20.0	90	89	88	87	85	84	83	82	81	80	79	77	76	74	72	71	70	68	67	65	65	60

Table A3.2

Lead III negative \ Lead I positive	0.0	0.5	1.0	1.5	2.0	2.5	3.0	3.5	4.0	4.5	5.0	6.0	7.0	8.0	9.0	10.0	11.0	12.0	13.0	14.0	15.0	20.0
0	-90	30	30	30	30	30	30	30	30	30	30	30	30	30	30	30	30	30	30	30	30	30
0.5	-90	-30	0	11	16	19	21	22	23	24	25	26	26	27	27	27	28	28	28	28	28	29
1.0	-90	-60	-30	-11	0	7	11	14	16	18	19	21	22	23	24	25	25	26	26	26	27	27
1.5	-90	-71	-49	-30	-16	-7	0	5	7	11	13	16	18	20	21	22	23	23	24	24	25	26
2.0	-90	-76	-60	-44	-30	-19	-11	-5	0	4	7	11	14	16	18	19	20	21	22	22	23	25
2.5	-90	-79	-67	-53	-41	-30	-21	-14	-8	-4	0	6	9	12	14	16	17	19	20	20	21	23
3.0	-90	-81	-71	-60	-49	-39	-30	-22	-16	-11	-7	0	5	8	11	13	15	16	17	18	19	22
3.5	-90	-82	-74	-65	-55	-46	-38	-30	-23	-18	-13	-6	0	4	7	10	12	14	15	16	17	21
4.0	-90	-83	-76	-68	-60	-52	-44	-37	-30	-24	-19	-11	-5	0	4	7	9	11	13	14	15	19
4.5	-90	-84	-78	-71	-64	-56	-49	-42	-36	-30	-25	-16	-9	-4	0	3	6	8	10	12	13	18
5.0	-90	-85	-79	-73	-67	-60	-53	-47	-41	-35	-30	-21	-14	-8	-4	0	3	6	8	9	11	16
6.0	-90	-86	-81	-76	-71	-66	-60	-54	-49	-44	-39	-30	-22	-16	-11	-7	-3	0	3	5	7	13
7.0	-90	-86	-82	-78	-74	-69	-65	-60	-55	-51	-46	-38	-30	-23	-18	-13	-9	-6	-3	0	2	10
8.0	-90	-87	-83	-80	-76	-72	-68	-64	-60	-56	-52	-44	-37	-30	-24	-19	-15	-11	-8	-5	-2	7
9.0	-90	-87	-84	-81	-78	-74	-71	-67	-64	-60	-56	-49	-42	-36	-30	-25	-20	-16	-13	-9	-7	3
10.0	-90	-87	-85	-82	-79	-76	-73	-70	-67	-63	-60	-53	-47	-41	-35	-30	-25	-21	-17	-14	-11	0
11.0	-90	-88	-85	-83	-80	-77	-75	-72	-69	-66	-63	-57	-51	-45	-40	-35	-30	-26	-22	-18	-15	-3
12.0	-90	-88	-86	-83	-81	-79	-76	-74	-71	-68	-66	-60	-54	-49	-44	-39	-34	-30	-26	-22	-19	-7
13.0	-90	-88	-86	-84	-82	-80	-77	-75	-73	-70	-68	-63	-57	-52	-47	-43	-38	-34	-30	-26	-23	-10
14.0	-90	-88	-86	-84	-82	-80	-78	-76	-74	-72	-69	-65	-60	-55	-51	-46	-42	-38	-34	-30	-27	-13
15.0	-90	-88	-87	-85	-83	-81	-79	-77	-75	-73	-71	-67	-62	-58	-53	-49	-45	-41	-37	-33	-30	-16
20.0	-90	-89	-87	-86	-85	-83	-82	-81	-79	-78	-76	-73	-70	-67	-63	-60	-57	-53	-50	-47	-44	-30

Lead I negative

Lead III positive	0.0	0.5	1.0	1.5	2.0	2.5	3.0	3.5	4.0	4.5	5.0	6.0	7.0	8.0	9.0	10.0	11.0	12.0	13.0	14.0	15.0	20.0
0		−150	−150	−150	−150	−150	−150	−150	−150	−150	−150	−150	−150	−150	−150	−150	−150	−150	−150	−150	−150	−150
0.5	90	150	180	−169	−164	−161	−159	−158	−157	−156	−155	−154	−154	−153	−153	−153	−152	−152	−152	−152	−152	−151
1.0	90	120	150	169	180	−173	−169	−166	−164	−162	−161	−159	−158	−157	−156	−155	−155	−154	−154	−154	−153	−153
1.5	90	109	131	150	164	173	180	−175	−172	−169	−167	−164	−162	−160	−159	−158	−157	−157	−156	−156	−155	−154
2.0	90	104	120	136	150	161	169	175	180	−176	−173	−169	−166	−164	−162	−161	−160	−159	−158	−158	−157	−155
2.5	90	101	113	127	139	150	159	166	172	176	180	−174	−171	−168	−166	−164	−163	−161	−160	−160	−159	−157
3.0	90	99	109	120	131	141	150	158	164	169	173	180	−175	−172	−169	−167	−165	−164	−163	−162	−161	−158
3.5	90	98	106	115	125	134	142	150	157	162	167	174	180	−176	−173	−170	−168	−166	−165	−164	−163	−159
4.0	90	97	104	112	120	128	136	143	150	156	161	169	175	180	−176	−173	−171	−169	−167	−166	−165	−161
4.5	90	96	102	109	116	124	131	138	144	150	155	164	171	176	180	−177	−174	−172	−170	−168	−167	−162
5.0	90	95	101	107	113	120	127	133	139	145	150	159	166	172	176	180	−177	−174	−172	−171	−169	−164
6.0	90	94	99	104	109	114	120	126	131	136	141	150	158	164	169	173	177	180	−177	−175	−173	−167
7.0	90	94	98	102	106	111	115	120	125	129	134	142	150	157	162	167	171	174	177	180	−178	−170
8.0	90	93	97	100	104	108	112	116	120	124	128	136	143	150	156	161	165	169	172	175	178	−173
9.0	90	93	96	99	102	106	109	113	116	120	124	131	138	144	150	155	160	164	167	171	173	−177
10.0	90	93	95	98	101	104	107	110	113	117	120	127	133	139	145	150	155	159	163	166	169	180
11.0	90	92	95	97	100	103	105	108	111	114	117	123	129	135	140	145	150	154	158	162	165	177
12.0	90	92	94	97	99	101	104	106	109	112	114	120	126	131	136	141	146	150	154	158	161	173
13.0	90	92	94	96	98	100	103	105	107	110	112	117	123	128	133	137	142	146	150	154	157	170
14.0	90	92	94	96	98	100	102	104	106	108	111	115	120	125	129	134	138	142	146	150	153	167
15.0	90	92	93	95	97	99	101	103	105	107	109	113	118	122	127	131	135	139	143	147	150	164
20.0	90	91	93	94	95	97	98	99	101	102	104	107	110	113	117	120	123	127	130	133	136	150

Lead I negative

Lead III negative	0.0	0.5	1.0	1.5	2.0	2.5	3.0	3.5	4.0	4.5	5.0	6.0	7.0	8.0	9.0	10.0	11.0	12.0	13.0	14.0	15.0	20.0
0	-150	-150	-150	-150	-150	-150	-150	-150	-150	-150	-150	-150	-150	-150	-150	-150	-150	-150	-150	-150	-150	-150
0.5	-90	-120	-131	-136	-139	-141	-142	-143	-144	-145	-145	-146	-147	-147	-147	-148	-148	-148	-148	-148	-148	-149
1.0	-90	-109	-120	-127	-131	-134	-136	-138	-139	-140	-141	-142	-143	-144	-145	-145	-146	-146	-146	-147	-147	-148
1.5	-90	-104	-113	-120	-125	-128	-131	-133	-135	-136	-137	-139	-141	-142	-142	-143	-144	-144	-144	-145	-145	-147
2.0	-90	-101	-109	-115	-120	-124	-127	-129	-131	-133	-134	-136	-138	-139	-140	-141	-142	-142	-143	-143	-144	-145
2.5	-90	-99	-106	-112	-116	-120	-123	-126	-128	-129	-131	-133	-135	-137	-138	-139	-140	-141	-141	-142	-142	-144
3.0	-90	-98	-104	-109	-113	-117	-120	-123	-125	-127	-128	-131	-133	-135	-136	-137	-138	-139	-140	-141	-141	-143
3.5	-90	-97	-102	-107	-111	-114	-117	-120	-122	-124	-126	-129	-131	-133	-134	-136	-137	-138	-138	-139	-140	-142
4.0	-90	-96	-101	-105	-109	-112	-115	-118	-120	-122	-124	-127	-129	-131	-133	-134	-135	-136	-137	-138	-138	-141
4.5	-90	-95	-100	-104	-107	-111	-113	-116	-118	-120	-122	-125	-127	-129	-131	-132	-133	-135	-136	-137	-137	-140
5.0	-90	-95	-99	-103	-106	-109	-112	-114	-116	-118	-120	-123	-125	-128	-129	-131	-132	-133	-134	-135	-136	-139
6.0	-90	-94	-98	-101	-104	-107	-109	-111	-113	-115	-117	-120	-123	-125	-127	-128	-130	-131	-132	-133	-134	-137
7.0	-90	-93	-97	-99	-102	-105	-107	-109	-111	-113	-115	-117	-120	-122	-124	-126	-127	-129	-130	-131	-132	-136
8.0	-90	-93	-96	-98	-101	-103	-105	-107	-109	-111	-112	-115	-118	-120	-122	-124	-125	-127	-128	-129	-130	-134
9.0	-90	-93	-95	-98	-100	-102	-104	-106	-107	-109	-111	-113	-116	-118	-120	-122	-123	-125	-126	-127	-128	-132
10.0	-90	-92	-95	-97	-99	-101	-103	-104	-106	-108	-109	-112	-114	-116	-118	-120	-122	-123	-124	-126	-127	-131
11.0	-90	-92	-94	-96	-98	-100	-102	-103	-105	-107	-108	-110	-113	-115	-117	-118	-120	-121	-123	-124	-125	-130
12.0	-90	-92	-94	-96	-98	-99	-101	-102	-104	-105	-107	-109	-111	-113	-115	-117	-119	-120	-121	-123	-124	-128
13.0	-90	-92	-94	-96	-97	-99	-100	-102	-103	-104	-106	-108	-110	-112	-114	-116	-117	-119	-120	-121	-122	-127
14.0	-90	-92	-93	-95	-97	-98	-100	-101	-102	-103	-105	-107	-109	-111	-113	-114	-116	-117	-119	-120	-121	-125
15.0	-90	-92	-93	-95	-96	-98	-99	-100	-102	-103	-104	-106	-108	-110	-112	-113	-115	-116	-118	-119	-120	-125
20.0	-90	-91	-92	-93	-95	-96	-97	-98	-99	-100	-101	-103	-104	-106	-108	-109	-110	-112	-113	-115	-115	-102

References

1 Jackson GE, Winsor T. Aids for determining magnitude and direction of electric axes of the electrocardiogram. Circulation. 1950;1;975–981.

2 Singh PN, Athar MS. Simplified [correction of Simlified] calculation of mean QRS vector (mean electrical axis of heart) of electrocardiogram. Indian J Physiol Pharmacol. 2003;47:212–216.

Appendix 4

Anti-Arrhythmic Drugs and Dosages*

> *Disclaimer:* The doses listed in this document are published recommendations available at the time when this document was prepared. Primary responsibility for all decisions regarding treatment remains with the primary clinician. All patients should be carefully monitored for adverse effects and idiosyncratic reactions regularly during therapy.
>
> Drugs are listed in alphabetical order; the order in no way reflects a recommendation or preference. More detailed discussion of drug properties can be found in chapter 17. Knowledge of specific indications and contraindications is the responsibility of the attending clinician.

---

* Refer to main text for detailed information and references.

Guide to Canine and Feline Electrocardiography, First Edition. Ruth Willis, Pedro Oliveira and Antonia Mavropoulou.
© 2018 John Wiley & Sons Ltd. Published 2018 by John Wiley & Sons Ltd.
Companion website: www.wiley.com/go/willis/electrocardiography

Adverse effects

Drug	Dose	Cardiovascular	Other	Comments
Amiodarone	*Dogs*: 8–10 mg/kg q12h for 1 week followed by 5–10 mg/kg q24h PO **OR** 10–15 mg/kg PO q12h for 7 days followed by 7.5 mg/kg PO q12h for 14 days and then 5–7.5 mg PO q24h 2 mg/kg IV in 10 min, followed by CRI of 0.8 mg/kg/h for 6 h, then 0.4 mg/kg/h	Bradycardia, myocardial depression, hypotension	Hepatic and thyroid toxicity, GI disorders, neutropenia, anaemia	Avoid solutions containing co-solvents benzyl alcohol and polysorbate 80; anaphylactic reactions are common.
Atenolol	*Dogs*: 0.25–1 mg/kg q12h *Cats*: 6.25–12.5 mg/cat q12–24 h	Exacerbation of CHF (can be life-threatening in cats), bradycardia	Lethargy, depression	Withdraw gradually after chronic therapy.
Digoxin	*Dogs*: 2.5–3 µg/kg q12h **OR** 0.22 mg/m² in dogs >20 kg *Cats*: 1/8 to 1/4 of a 0.125 mg tablet q 48 h	AV block, ventricular arrhythmias	Diarrhoea, vomiting, anorexia	Recommended trough level in dogs (>6–8 h after administration): 0.8–1.2 ng/mL
Diltiazem	*Dogs*: 0.05–0.25 mg/kg slow IV; 2–6 µg/kg/min IV by CRI 1–4 mg/kg PO q8h (sustained-release form: 3–5 mg/kg q12h) *Cats*: 0.125–0.35 mg/kg slow IV in 2 minutes; 2–6 µg/kg/min IV by CRI; 1–2.5 mg/kg PO q8h	Bradycardia, AV block, hypotension, exacerbation of heart failure	Lethargy, GI signs are common in cats	Sustained release forms with highly variable pharmacokinetics in cats
Esmolol	*Dogs*: 0.05–0.5 mg/kg IV bolus 25–200 µg/kg/min as CRI, start low, titrate to effect	Hypotension, bradycardia		Use with caution, and avoid bolus with severe structural heart disease.
Lidocaine	*Dogs*: 2–4 mg/kg IV bolus, repeat up to cumulative dose of 8 mg/kg, followed by 25–100 µg/kg/min IV by CRI *Cats*: 0.25–2 mg/kg in 0.25–0.5 mg/kg boluses, followed by 0.01–0.04 mg/kg/min IV as CRI	Bradycardia, arrhythmia aggravation	Nausea, vomiting, depression, muscle tremors, seizures	Avoid or use with caution in cats.
Metoprolol	*Dogs*: 0.2–1 mg/kg q8–12h (titrate to effect)	Bradycardia, CHF exacerbation	Lethargy, depression	
Mexiletine	*Dogs*: 4–10 mg/kg q8h 8 mg/kg q8h (with Sotalol)	Bradycardia, arrhythmia aggravation	GI disturbances, muscle tremors, depression	Sotalol increases plasma concentration.
Procainamide	*Dogs*: 2–4 mg/kg IV, repeat up to 20 mg/kg CRI 20–50 µg/kg/min **OR** 7–10 mg/kg IM q6–8 h 20–30 mg/kg PO q8h (sustained-release form) *Cats*: 3–5 mg/kg PO q8–12h	Prolonged QRS and QT, AV block (IV), pro-arrhythmia	GI disturbances, depression, fever	If oral for is used, consider monitoring serum concentration (therapeutic range: 4–12 mcg/ml).
Propranolol	*Dogs*: 0.02–0.08 mg/kg IV (titrate to effect) 0.1–1.5 mg/kg PO q8–12h (titrate to effect) *Cats*: 0.02–0.06 mg/kg IV slowly and to effect; 2–5 mg/kg PO q12h	Bradycardia, AV block, exacerbation of heart failure	Bradycardia, lethargy, depression; may cause bronchoconstriction	Withdraw gradually after chronic therapy. Titrate dose carefully in cases with heart failure.
Sotalol	*Dogs*: 0.5–3 mg/kg q12h PO *Cats*: 2 mg/kg or 10–20 mg/cat 12h PO	Bradycardia, myocardial depression, hypotension	Lethargy, GI signs	Aggressive behaviour in dogs anecdotally reported
Verapamil	*Dogs*: 0.05 mg/kg IV over 5–10 min with ECG monitoring; may be repeated up to 4 times at 5–10 min intervals at dose of 0.025 mg/kg IV q5min followed by 2–10 µg/kg/min IV CRI 0.5–3 mg/kg PO q8h *Cats*: 0.025 mg/kg IV slowly over 5 min; can repeat q5min up to 8 times	Bradycardia, AV block, hypotension, exacerbation of CHF		Use with caution with other drugs that cause bradycardia or myocardial depression (e.g. β-blockers).

AV, Atrioventricular; CHF, congestive heart failure; CRI, continuous rate infusion; ECG, electrocardiography; GI, gastrointestinal; h, hour; IV, intravenous; IM, intramuscular; min, minute; PO, per os (orally); q, every.

Appendix 5

Sample ECG Reports

Date: __ /__ /____

Electrocardiographic Report
Feline

Patient identification:

ECG trace *Leads:* ____ mm/s ____ mm/mV *Quality:*

	Reference Range	Patient
Heart rate (bpm)	120–220	
Rhythm	Regular	
P wave (ms)	≤ 40	
P wave (mV)	≤ 0.2	
PR (ms)	50–90	
Q wave (mV)		
QRS (ms)	≤ 40	
QRS configuration		
R wave (mV)	≤ 0.9	
S wave (mV)		
ST segment	No depression/elevation	
QT (ms)	70 to 200	
QTc (ms)		
T wave (mV)	≤ 0.3 (most often positive)	
MEA (Frontal Plane)	0 to +160°	

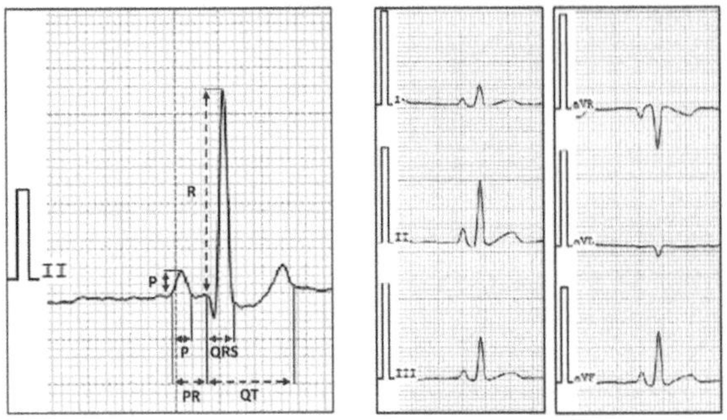

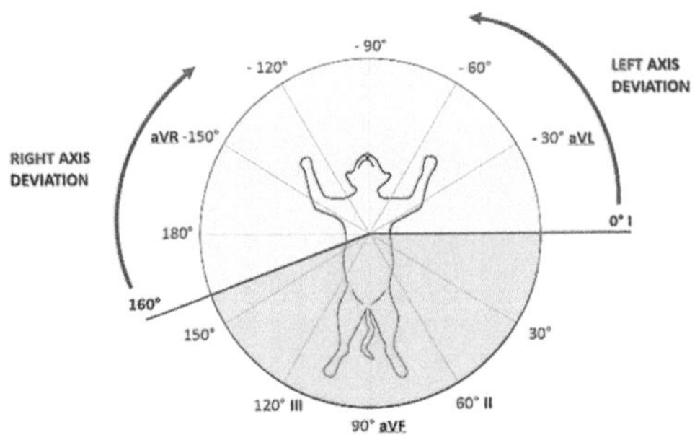

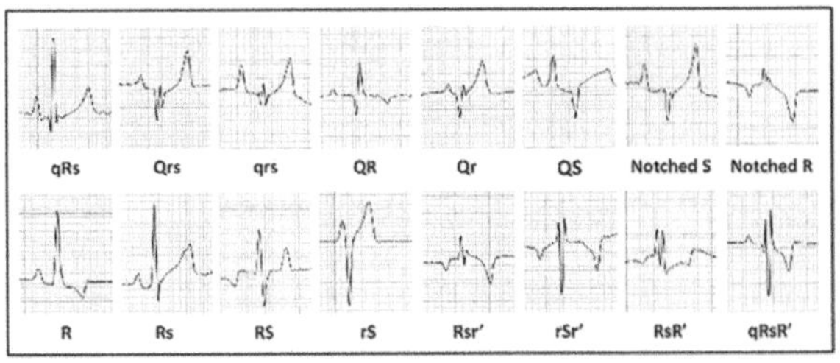

Interpretation:

Date: __ /__ /____

Electrocardiographic Report
Canine

Patient identification:

| **ECG trace** *Leads:* | ____ mm/s | ____ mm/mV | *Quality:* |

	Reference Range	Patient
Heart rate (bpm)	70–160	
Rhythm	Regular	
P wave (ms)	≤ 40; ≤ 50 (giant)	
P wave (mV)	≤ 0.4	
PR (s)	60 to 130	
Q wave (mV)		
QRS (ms)	≤ 70	
QRS configuration		
R wave (mV)	> 0.5 and ≤ 3.0	
S wave (mV)		
ST segment	≤ 0.2 mV depression/elevation	
QT (ms)	150–250	
QTc (ms)		
T wave (mV)	≤ ¼ of R	
MEA (Frontal Plane)	+40° to +100°	

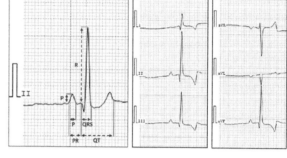

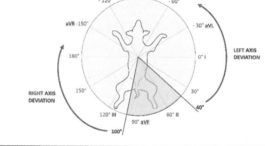

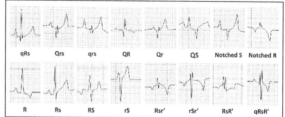

Interpretation:

Self-assessment

ECG Trace 1

Canine, 10-year-old, male, neutered French Bulldog

	Reference range	Patient	Interpretation:
Heart rate (bpm)	70–160		
Rhythm	Regular or sinus arrhythmia		
P wave (ms)	<40		
P wave (mV)	<0.4		
PR (s)	60–130		
QRS (ms)	<70		
R wave (mV)	>0.5 in leads II, III and aVF		
S wave (mV)			
ST segment	<0.2 mV below or above baseline		
QT (ms)			
QTc (ms)	150–240		
T wave (mV)			
MEA (frontal plane)	+40° to +100°		

Guide to Canine and Feline Electrocardiography, First Edition. Ruth Willis, Pedro Oliveira and Antonia Mavropoulou.
© 2018 John Wiley & Sons Ltd. Published 2018 by John Wiley & Sons Ltd.
Companion website: www.wiley.com/go/willis/electrocardiography

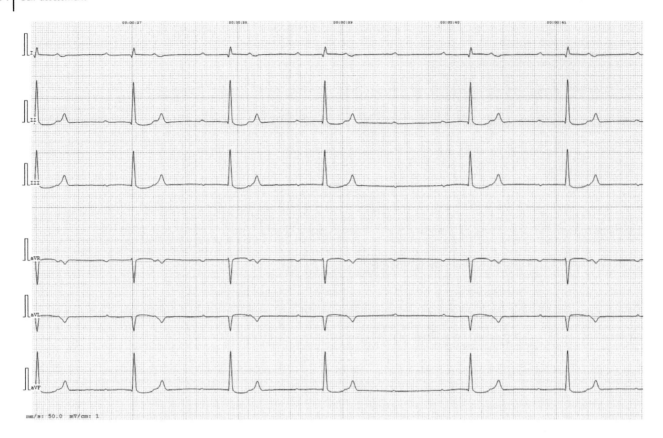

ECG Trace 1: Interpretation

The underlying rhythm is an irregular narrow-QRS rhythm (QRS, 60 ms; normal, <70 ms) with a rate of approximately 60 bpm. The QRS has a normal appearance with a main positive deflection in leads I, II, III and aVF, and a main negative deflection in leads aVR and AVL. The estimated mean electrical axis is approximately 80°, which is within the expected range (+40° to +100°). The QRS duration (60 ms; normal, <70 ms) and amplitude (R wave in lead II, 1.4 mV; normal, >0.5 mV) are also within the expected range. Given these findings, we can conclude that ventricular depolarisation is occurring normally. P waves are seen preceding each QRS with a constant PR interval, although it is longer than normal (260 ms; normal, 60–130 ms), indicating the presence of first-degree atrioventricular block. Additionally, a non-conducted P wave may be seen after the fourth QRS, accounting for the rhythm irregularity and indicating the presence of second-degree atrioventricular block. Closer inspection of the trace reveals the presence of small waves in the beginning of the T wave most visible in lead aVR, with a similar appearance to the P waves. The interval between these deflections and the P

waves is consistent throughout the trace (440–460 ms), and is also the same as the interval between the non-conducted P wave after the fourth QRS and the following P. This suggests that these small deflections are in fact non-conducted P waves. The P wave characteristics suggest an origin in the floor of the right atrium with a positive deflection in leads I, II, aVL and aVF; biphasic in lead III; and negative in aVR corresponding to an estimated electrical axis of −30°. This may be due to an ectopic atrial rhythm, the activity of a subsidiary pacemaker further down the conduction system along the internodal pathways or a sinus rhythm with abnormal intra-atrial conduction. The P wave duration is normal (40 ms; normal, <40 ms), suggesting normal inter-atrial conduction. The atrial rate is 125–130 bpm, and the ventricular rate is 60 bpm. The QT interval is 320 ms and therefore prolonged. In conclusion, the underlying rhythm is either sinus or an ectopic atrial rhythm with first-degree atrioventricular block as well as second-degree atrioventricular block with a 2:1 and 3:1 atrioventricular conduction pattern. These findings suggest abnormal function of the conduction system. Echocardiography revealed an intracardiac mass, and the arrhythmias were attributed to cardiac neoplasia in this case.

ECG Trace 2

Canine, 10-year-old, female Bernese Mountain Dog

	Reference range	Patient	Interpretation:
Heart rate (bpm)	70–160		
Rhythm	Regular or sinus arrhythmia		
P wave (ms)	<40		
P wave (mV)	<0.4		
PR (s)	60–130		
QRS (ms)	<70		
R wave (mV)	>0.5 in leads II, III and aVF		
S wave (mV)			
ST segment	<0.2 mV below or above baseline		
QT (ms)			
QTc (ms)	150–240		
T wave (mV)			
MEA (frontal plane)	+40° to +100°		

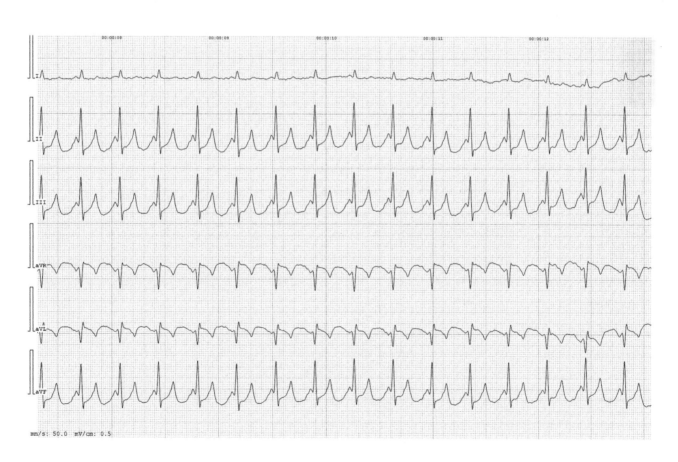

mm/s: 50.0 mV/cm: 0.5

ECG Trace 2: Interpretation

The underlying rhythm is a regular narrow-QRS rhythm (QRS, ≈50 ms; normal, <70 ms) with a rate of approximately 160–180 bpm. The QRS has a normal appearance with a main positive deflection in leads I, II, III and aVF, and a main negative deflection in leads aVR and aVL. The estimated mean electrical axis is approximately 80°, which is within the expected range (+40° to +100°). The QRS duration (≈50 ms; normal, <70 ms) and amplitude (R wave in lead II, ≈0.9 mV; normal, >0.5 mV) are also within the expected range. Given these findings, we can conclude that ventricular depolarisation is occurring normally and that this is a supraventricular rhythm. Two deflections are seen between each QRS, and it is logical to assume that the first is the T with a QT interval within the normal limits (QT, 200–210 ms; QTc, 203–213 ms; normal, 150–240 ms). The second wave is likely the consequence of atrial depolarisation (P or F wave) and occurs very close to the QRS without an obvious return to baseline. This presentation is very suspicious of an atrial flutter, and it is likely that an F wave is also present within the T wave with a 2:1 atrioventricular conduction pattern, as the distance between the peak of these waves is the same (180 ms corresponding to an atrial depolarisation rate of 333 bpm). To ascertain this fact, it is necessary to compare this trace to a period of sinus rhythm if documented or reduce the heart rate to reveal underlying F waves and separate them from the T waves. Differential diagnoses could include focal junctional tachycardia with type II isorhythmic atrioventricular dissociation accounting for the position of the P in relation to the QRS. In this case, the administration of oral sotalol revealed F waves by enhancing atrioventricular block, confirming the presence of a *typical atrial flutter* (see Figure 8.16).

ECG Trace 3

Canine, 8-year-old, female, neutered English Bulldog

	Reference range	Patient	Interpretation:
Heart rate (bpm)	70–160		
Rhythm	Regular or sinus arrhythmia		
P wave (ms)	<40		
P wave (mV)	<0.4		
PR (s)	60–130		
QRS (ms)	<70		
R wave (mV)	>0.5 in leads II, III and aVF		
S wave (mV)			
ST segment	<0.2 mV below or above baseline		
QT (ms)			
QTc (ms)	150–240		
T wave (mV)			
MEA (frontal plane)	+40° to +100°		

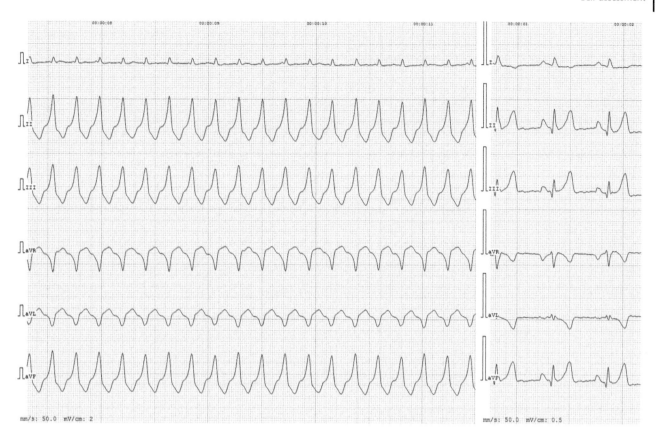

ECG Trace 3: Interpretation

The trace on the left shows a regular wide-QRS rhythm (80–100 ms; normal, <70 ms) with a rate of approximately 260–280 bpm. The QRS displays a main positive deflection in leads I, II, III and aVF, and a main negative deflection in leads aVR and aVL. These characteristics would suggest either a supraventricular rhythm with a left bundle branch block or a ventricular rhythm possibly originating from the right ventricle. Obvious P waves are not seen in any of the leads. Analysis of the trace on the right during sinus rhythm reveals the absence of a bundle branch block with a QRS of normal duration (60 ms; normal, <70 ms) and MEA (≈70°; normal, +40° to +100°). A P wave precedes each QRS with a normal PR interval (100 ms; normal, 60–130 ms). The characteristics of the P wave are consistent with a sinus rhythm (positive in leads I, II, III and aVF; negative in leads aVR and aVL) with a normal amplitude (0.2 mV; normal, <0.4 mV) but prolonged duration (60 ms; normal, <40 ms), suggesting possible atrial enlargement or delayed interatrial conduction. The main differential diagnosis in this case is a rapid monomorphic ventricular tachycardia. A rapid supraventricular rhythm with left bundle branch block is unlikely given the absence of bundle branch block during sinus rhythm, although it is possible in cases of tachycardia-dependent (phase 3) block. Analyses of additional sections of ECG recording in this patient after treatment with intravenous lidocaine revealed frequent ventricular ectopic complexes and fusion complexes, confirming the diagnosis of *ventricular tachycardia*. This patient was diagnosed with arrhythmogenic right ventricular cardiomyopathy with marked right ventricular and atrial enlargement.

ECG Trace 4

Feline, 9-year-old, male, neutered Domestic Longhair

	Reference range	Patient	Interpretation:
Heart rate (bpm)	140–220		
Rhythm	Regular		
P wave (ms)	<40		
P wave (mV)	<0.2		
PR (s)	50–90		
QRS (ms)	<40		
R wave (mV)	<0.9 in lead II		
S wave (mV)			
ST segment	Isoelectric		
QT (ms)	70–200		
QTc (ms)			
T wave (mV)			
MEA (frontal plane)	+0° to +160°		

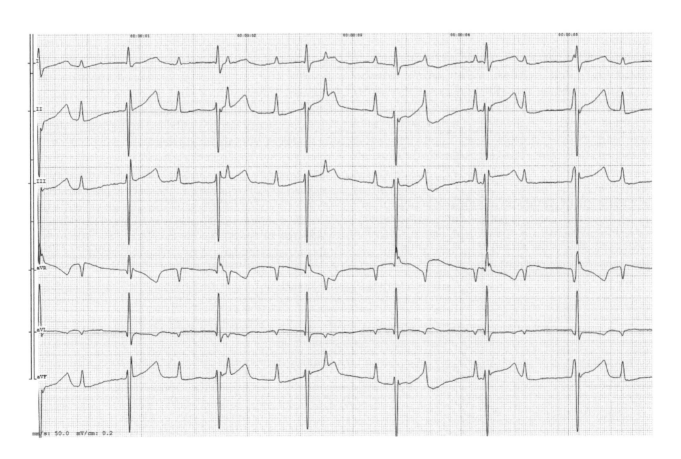

ECG Trace 4: Interpretation

The underlying rhythm is a regular wide-QRS rhythm (QRS, 60 ms; normal, <40 ms) with a rate of approximately 70 bpm. The QRS displays a main negative deflection in leads II, III and aVF, and a main positive deflection in leads I, aVR and aVL. The mean electrical axis is deviated to the right (approximately −80°). These characteristics would suggest either a supraventricular rhythm with a right bundle branch block or a ventricular rhythm possibly originating from the right ventricle. P waves are seen throughout the trace in all leads but are not associated with the QRS, as indicated by a varying PR interval and the fact that some P waves are superimposed on the QRS complex (e.g. second and last QRS) or the ST segment. The characteristics of the P waves are consistent with a sinus rhythm (positive in leads I, II, III and aVF; negative in leads aVR and aVL) with a normal amplitude (0.16 mV; normal, <0.2 mV) and duration (40 ms; normal, <40 ms). The P-P interval is regular (460 ms), corresponding to a sinus rhythm of approximately 130 bpm. These findings are consistent with *sinus bradycardia with third-degree atrioventricular block and an underlying ventricular escape rhythm.* This electrocardiographic trace was recorded during anaesthesia for a dental procedure, and there was no history of clinical signs potentially referable to this bradyarrhythmia, such as reduced activity or syncope.

ECG Trace 5

Canine, 10-year-old, male, neutered German Shepherd

	Reference range	Patient	Interpretation:
Heart rate (bpm)	70–160		
Rhythm	Regular or sinus arrhythmia		
P wave (ms)	<40		
P wave (mV)	<0.4		
PR (s)	60–130		
QRS (ms)	<70		
R wave (mV)	>0.5 in leads II, III and aVF		
S wave (mV)			
ST segment	<0.2 mV below or above baseline		
QT (ms)			
QTc (ms)	150–240		
T wave (mV)			
MEA (frontal plane)	+40° to +100°		

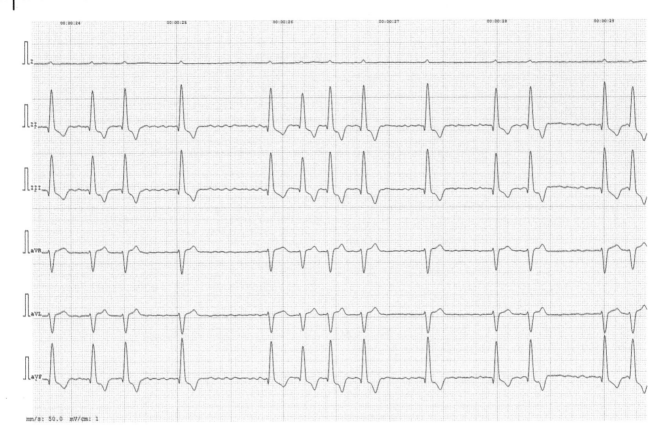

mm/s: 50.0 mV/cm: 1

ECG Trace 5: Interpretation

The underlying rhythm is an irregular wide-QRS rhythm (≈80 ms; normal, <70 ms) with a rate of approximately 140 bpm. The QRS has a normal appearance with a main positive deflection in leads I, II, III and aVF, and a main negative deflection in leads aVR and aVL. The estimated mean electrical axis would be approximately 86°, which is within the expected range (+40° to +100°). The QRS duration is increased (≈80 ms; normal, <70 ms), and the amplitude is within the expected range (R wave in lead II, ≈1.9 mV; normal, >0.5 mV and <3 mV). These findings suggest either a supraventricular rhythm with ventricular enlargement/hypertrophy or left bundle branch block, or a ventricular rhythm possibly originating in the right ventricle. The QTc interval is approximately 200 ms

and therefore within the expected range (150–240). Obvious P waves are not seen throughout the trace, and instead small deflections may be seen in the sections of trace where the baseline is seen. These deflections are suggestive of fibrillation (f) waves that, in conjunction with the irregularity of the rhythm, strongly suggest atrial fibrillation. Whilst a ventricular rhythm merits consideration in view of the wide-QRS complexes, ventricular rhythms are generally regular with the exception of polymorphic ventricular rhythms. This dog was diagnosed with myocardial disease consistent with dilated cardiomyopathy and *atrial fibrillation*. At the time of this recording, he was under rate control treatment with a combination of digoxin and diltiazem, explaining the observed heart rate. The wide QRS was attributed to marked cardiomegaly.

ECG Trace 6

Canine, 16-year-old, male, neutered Jack Russell Terrier

	Reference range	Patient	Interpretation:
Heart rate (bpm)	70–160		
Rhythm	Regular or sinus arrhythmia		
P wave (ms)	<40		
P wave (mV)	<0.4		
PR (s)	60–130		
QRS (ms)	<70		
R wave (mV)	>0.5 in leads II, III and aVF		
S wave (mV)			
ST segment	<0.2 mV below or above baseline		
QT (ms)			
QTc (ms)	150–240		
T wave (mV)			
MEA (frontal plane)	+40° to +100°		

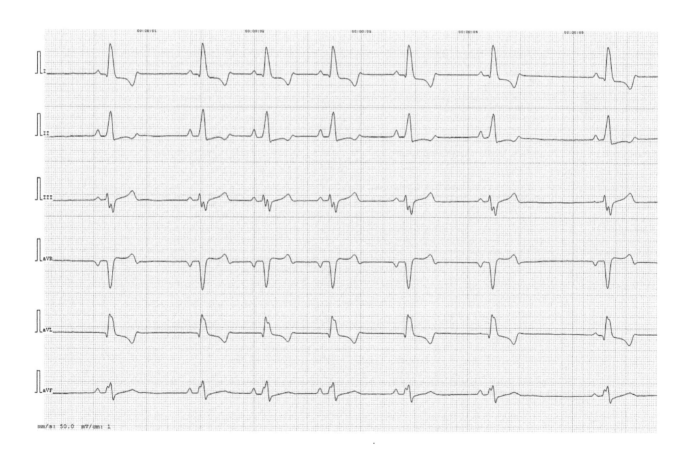

mm/s: 50.0   mV/cm: 1

ECG Trace 6: Interpretation

The underlying rhythm is a slightly irregular wide-QRS rhythm (≈100 ms; normal, <70 ms) with a rate of approximately 70–80 bpm. The QRS displays a main positive deflection in leads I, II, aVL and aVF; an rsr'S' conformation in lead III; and a main negative deflection in lead aVR. The estimated mean electrical axis would be approximately +20° and is therefore deviated to the left (normal, +40° to +100°). The QRS duration is increased (≈100 ms; normal, <70 ms), and the amplitude (R wave in lead II, ≈1.3 mV; normal, >0.5 mV and <3 mV) is within the expected range. These findings would suggest either a supraventricular rhythm with a bundle branch block/aberrant ventricular conduction or a ventricular rhythm possibly originating in the right ventricle. The QTc interval is approximately 300 ms, which is above the expected range (150–240), suggesting a ventricular repolarisation abnormality that would also fit with abnormal ventricular conduction. A P wave precedes each QRS with a normal PR interval (100 ms; normal, 60–130 ms). The characteristics of the P wave are consistent with a sinus rhythm (positive in leads I, II, III and aVF; negative in lead aVR) with a normal amplitude (0.2 mV; normal, <0.4 mV) but slightly prolonged duration (≈50 ms; normal, <40 ms), suggesting possible atrial enlargement or delayed intra-/interatrial conduction. These findings are consistent with a *sinus rhythm with abnormal ventricular conduction*.

ECG Trace 7

Canine, 7-month-old, male Boxer

	Reference range	Patient	Interpretation:
Heart rate (bpm)	70–200		
Rhythm	Regular or sinus arrhythmia		
P wave (ms)	<40		
P wave (mV)	<0.4		
PR (s)	60–130		
QRS (ms)	<70		
R wave (mV)	>0.5 in leads II, III and aVF		
S wave (mV)			
ST segment	<0.2 mV below or above baseline		
QT (ms)			
QTc (ms)	150–240		
T wave (mV)			
MEA (frontal plane)	+40° to +100°		

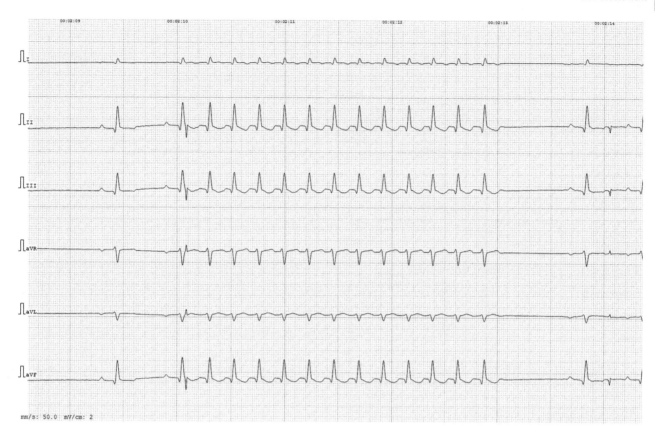

ECG Trace 7: Interpretation

The first, second and last complexes are sinus beats. A QRS with normal duration (60 ms; <70 ms) and amplitude (2.0 mV; normal, >0.5 mV and <3.0 mV) is seen preceded by a P wave of normal duration (40 ms; normal, <40 ms), amplitude (0.4 mV; normal, <0.4 mV) and morphology (positive in leads I, II, III and aVF; negative in leads aVR and aVL) and a PR interval at the upper limit of the normal range (≈130 ms; normal, 60 to 130). The second sinus complex is followed by a short run of narrow-QRS tachycardia (12 complexes at 260 bpm) with sudden onset and offset. The QRS characteristics are the same as those of the QRS of the sinus complexes, indicating a supraventricular rhythm with normal ventricular depolarisation. Obvious P or P' waves are not seen preceding the QRS during tachycardia; however, a small deflection may be seen on the ST segment of all the tachycardia complexes and the sinus complex at the beginning of tachycardia. This deflection is negative in leads II, III and aVF and positive in leads I, aVR and aVL, suggesting a possible retroconducted P'. The start of the retrograde P' is too indistinct to calculate the RP'/P'R, although it is clear that the RP' is shorter than the P'R. These findings are suggestive of orthodromic atrioventricular reciprocating tachycardia. Differential diagnoses should include focal atrial tachycardia, focal junctional tachycardia and atypical atrial flutter. This dog also showed signs of pre-excitation via an accessory pathway in other sections of the ECG trace, supporting the diagnosis of *orthodromic atrioventricular reciprocating tachycardia*.

ECG Trace 8

Canine, 12-year-old, female, neutered Labrador Retriever

	Reference range	Patient	Interpretation:
Heart rate (bpm)	70–200		
Rhythm	Regular or sinus arrhythmia		
P wave (ms)	<40		
P wave (mV)	<0.4		
PR (s)	60–130		
QRS (ms)	<70		
R wave (mV)	>0.5 in leads II, III and aVF		
S wave (mV)			
ST segment	<0.2 mV below or above baseline		
QT (ms)			
QTc (ms)	150–240		
T wave (mV)			
MEA (frontal plane)	+40° to +100°		

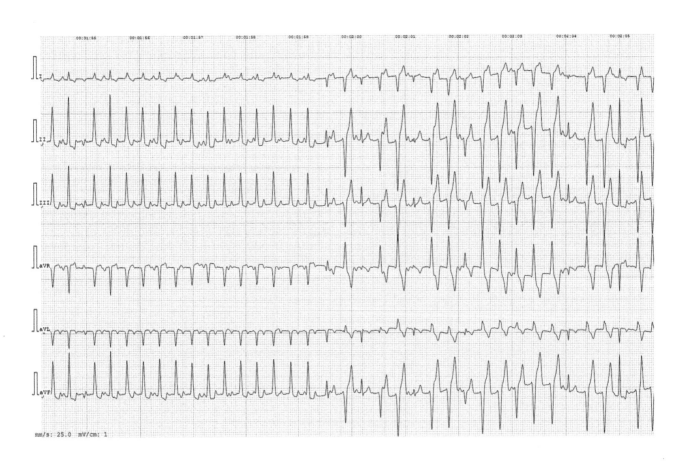

mm/s: 25.0 mV/cm: 1

ECG Trace 8: Interpretation

On the left half of this trace, a wide-QRS (80 ms; normal, <70 ms) rhythm is seen with a heart rate of 200 bpm and a regular rhythm, except for the second complex that is premature and followed by a short pause. The QRS morphology displays a left bundle branch block morphology (positive in leads I, II, III and aVF; negative in leads aVR and aVL). The T wave is easily identified after each QRS, with a QTc of approximately 215–220 ms (normal, 150–240). Deflections that could represent P waves may be seen between QRS complexes with two different morphologies: (1) one appears negative in lead I, positive in aVR and biphasic in the other leads (an example may be seen between complexes 2 and 3); and (2) the other is consistent with sinus P waves and may be seen preceding the second, fourth and seventh QRS and others throughout the trace. The first deflection would suggest either an ectopic atrial focus or possibly interatrial block considering its long duration (80 ms) and biphasic conformation; none of these seem to result in a QRS, as the PR is variable, suggesting atrioventricular dissociation. Differential diagnoses include ventricular tachycardia, or focal junctional tachycardia with atrioventricular dissociation and abnormal ventricular conduction. The sinus P waves precede the QRS of some of the complexes with a consistent PR of 80–100 ms (normal, 60–130), suggesting that they result in ventricular activation. This may be seen in complexes 2 and 4 that also display a different QRS morphology with a taller R wave and a shorter QRS closer to 70 ms, suggestive of fusion complexes. This is highly suggestive of ventricular tachycardia. Analysis of the rest of the trace allows identification of two sinus complexes (19 and 30) with a normal QRS (70 ms in duration, and preceded by a sinus P wave with a consistent PR interval of approximately 90 ms). This finding is useful as it allows comparison of the P-QRS-T with the abnormal complexes and suspected fusion complexes, also supporting a diagnosis of ventricular tachycardia. The rest of the trace is dominated by a different wide-QRS (120 ms) rhythm with a right bundle branch morphology (main negative deflection in leads I, II, III and aVF; main positive deflection in leads aVR and aVL) and a rate of 180–200 bpm. Additional fusion complexes (17, 22, 25 and 34) and the above-mentioned sinus complexes may be seen accounting for the rhythm irregularity. In conclusion, this patient was diagnosed with a *polymorphic ventricular tachycardia* attributed to myocarditis.

ECG Trace 9

Canine, 13-year-old, male, neutered Staffordshire Bull Terrier

	Reference range	Patient	Interpretation:
Heart rate (bpm)	70–160		
Rhythm	Regular or sinus arrhythmia		
P wave (ms)	<40		
P wave (mV)	<0.4		
PR (s)	60–130		
QRS (ms)	<70		
R wave (mV)	>0.5 in leads II, III and aVF		
S wave (mV)			
ST segment	<0.2 mV below or above baseline		
QT (ms)			
QTc (ms)	150–240		
T wave (mV)			
MEA (frontal plane)	+40° to +100°		

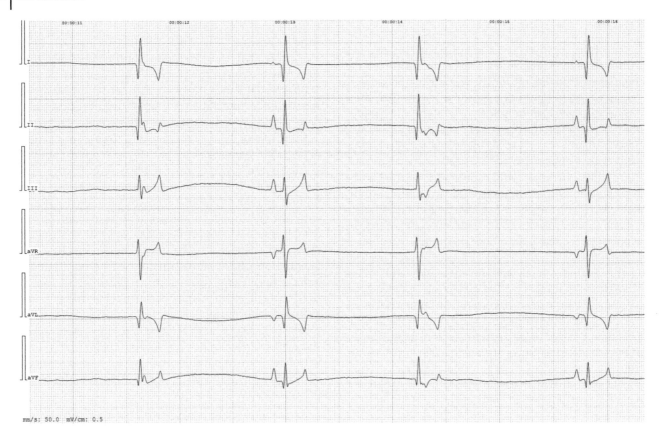

mm/s: 50.0 mV/cm: 0.5

ECG Trace 9: Interpretation

The underlying rhythm is a regular wide-QRS rhythm (QRS, 80 ms; normal, <70 ms) with a rate of approximately 40 bpm consistent with bradycardia. The QRS appearance is similar in all leads with a main positive deflection in leads I, II, aVR and aVF; isobiphasic in lead III; and a main negative deflection in lead aVR. The estimated mean electrical axis is between +25 and +30°, indicating a deviation to the left. These findings would suggest either a supraventricular rhythm conducted with a left bundle branch block/aberrancy, or a ventricular rhythm. The appearance of the T wave is consistent with a QTc interval within the expected range (214 ms; normal, 150–240). A P wave consistent with a sinus P may be seen preceding the second and fourth complexes with a slightly different PR interval (120 ms for complex 2 and 100 ms for complex 4), although both are within the expected range (60–130 ms). The P wave morphology is normal with a positive deflection in leads I, II, III and aVF, and negative in leads aVR and aVL; its amplitude is normal (0.3 mV; normal, <0.4 mV), and its duration is longer than normal (50 ms; normal, <40 ms),

suggesting possible atrial enlargement or abnormal intra-/interatrial conduction. A similar wave may be seen in the descending branch of the R of the first QRS. Additionally, a deflection may be seen in the ST segment of the third complex that is negative in leads II, III and aVF and positive in leads I, aVR and aVF. This deflection is consistent with a P' that reaches the atria retrogradely via the atrioventricular junction, causing concentric retrograde atrial activation. As the QRS morphology is consistent, but the relationship between the P or P' waves and QRS complexes is variable, it is logical to assume that the predominant rhythm is a *ventricular escape rhythm* and that the sinus P waves seen preceding complexes 2 and 4 are dissociated from the QRS despite a PR interval within the expected range. The slight variation in PR interval between complexes would also support this assumption. Alternatively, complexes 1 and 3 could be junctional complexes conducted with a bundle branch block/aberrancy, and complexes 2 and 4 could be sinus complexes also conducted with a bundle branch block/aberrancy. This dog was diagnosed with sick sinus syndrome and was treated successfully with an artificial pacemaker.

ECG Trace 10

Canine, 11-year-old, male, neutered Norfolk Terrier

	Reference range	Patient	Interpretation:
Heart rate (bpm)	70–160		
Rhythm	Regular or sinus arrhythmia		
P wave (ms)	<40		
P wave (mV)	<0.4		
PR (s)	60–130		
QRS (ms)	<70		
R wave (mV)	>0.5 in leads II, III and aVF		
S wave (mV)			
ST segment	<0.2 mV below or above baseline		
QT (ms)			
QTc (ms)	150–240		
T wave (mV)			
MEA (frontal plane)	+40° to +100°		

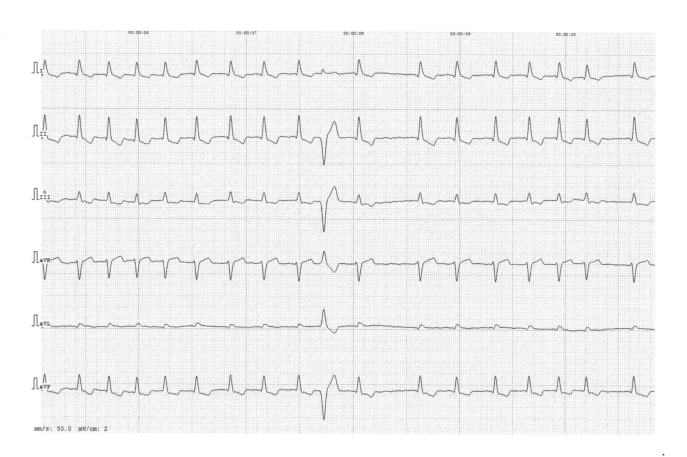

mm/s: 50.0 mV/cm: 2

ECG Trace 10: Interpretation

The underlying rhythm is an irregular narrow-QRS rhythm (QRS, 60 ms; normal, <70 ms) with a heart rate of 180–200 bpm consistent with tachycardia. Obvious P waves are not seen preceding the QRS, and instead very slight undulations of the baseline are seen in the sections of trace where the baseline is more easily seen. These findings are suggestive of *atrial fibrillation*. In the middle of the trace, a wide-QRS complex is seen (QRS duration, 90–100 ms) with a right bundle branch block morphology (main negative deflection in leads I, II, III and aVF; main positive deflection in leads aVR and aVL) that is not preceded by a P. This is a *ventricular ectopic complex*. This patient suffered from chronic valvular degenerative disease with congestive heart failure, concomitant atrial fibrillation and ventricular ectopy.

ECG Trace 11

Feline, 17-year-old, male, neutered Persian

	Reference range	Patient	Interpretation:
Heart rate (bpm)	140–220		
Rhythm	Regular		
P wave (ms)	<40		
P wave (mV)	<0.2		
PR (s)	50–90		
QRS (ms)	<40		
R wave (mV)	<0.9 in lead II		
S wave (mV)			
ST segment	Isoelectric		
QT (ms)	70–200		
QTc (ms)			
T wave (mV)			
MEA (frontal plane)	+0° to +160°		

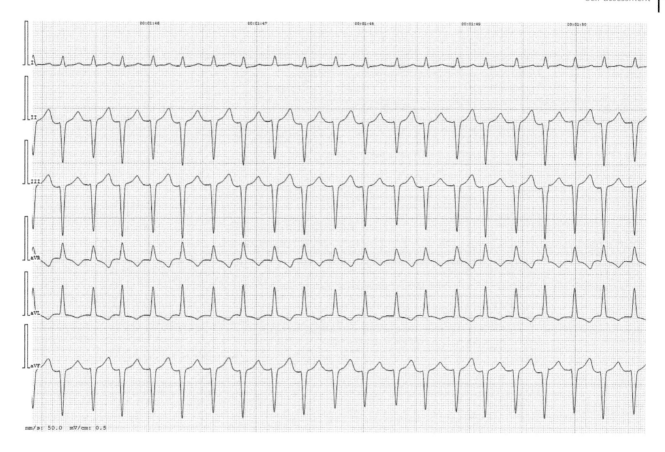

ECG Trace 11: Interpretation

The underlying rhythm is a regular wide-QRS rhythm (QRS, 60 ms; normal, <40 ms) with a rate of approximately 220 bpm consistent with tachycardia. The QRS displays a right bundle branch block morphology (main negative deflections in leads II, III and aVF; main positive deflections in leads aVR and aVL). P waves are not visible, which may be because they are absent or superimposed on the ST segment or T wave of the preceding complex; however, these areas of the trace are uniform in appearance and therefore do not display obvious signs suggestive of hidden P waves. The most likely diagnosis is *ventricular tachycardia*. Alternatively, a supraventricular tachycardia (sinus, atrial or junctional) with a right bundle branch block could be a potential differential diagnosis, although this is unlikely given the absence of P:QRS coupling in all leads.

ECG Trace 12

Canine, 4-year-old, male, neutered Labrador Retriever

	Reference range	Patient	Interpretation:
Heart rate (bpm)	70–160		
Rhythm	Regular or sinus arrhythmia		
P wave (ms)	<40		
P wave (mV)	<0.4		
PR (s)	60–130		
QRS (ms)	<70		
R wave (mV)	>0.5 in leads II, III and aVF		
S wave (mV)			
ST segment	<0.2 mV below or above baseline		
QT (ms)			
QTc (ms)	150–240		
T wave (mV)			
MEA (frontal plane)	+40° to +100°		

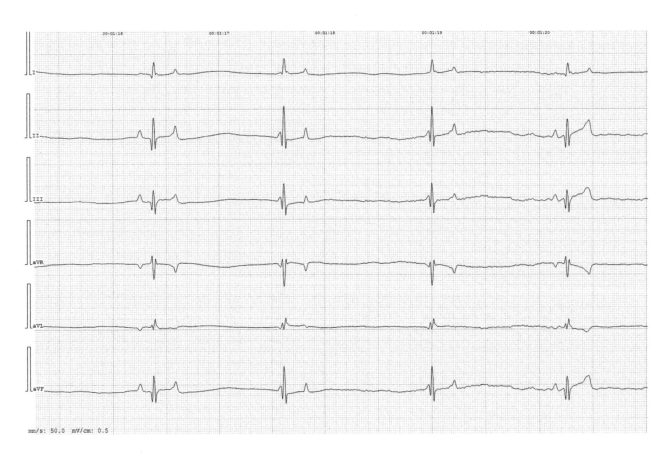

mm/s: 50.0   mV/cm: 0.5

ECG Trace 12: Interpretation

A relatively regular narrow-QRS rhythm (QRS, 60 ms; normal, <70 ms) is seen with a rate of approximately 60 bpm, suggesting bradycardia. The QRS amplitude is normal (R, 0.9–1.2 mV; normal, >0.5 mV and <3 mV in lead II) but is slightly aberrant, with an estimated mean electrical axis deviated to the left (MEA, −30°; normal, +40° to +100°) suggestive of abnormal ventricular conduction. The QTc is similar for all complexes at 230 ms (normal, 150–240 ms). The first and fourth QRS complexes are preceded by a P wave with the characteristics of a sinus P (main positive deflection in leads I, II, III and aVF; main negative deflection in leads aVR and aVL) and a slightly different PR interval but within the expected range (130 ms for the first complex and 100 ms for the fourth complex; normal, 60–130 ms). These two complexes are suspected to be sinus complexes with some degree of aberrant ventricular conduction. The second and third complexes are not preceded by a P, although a deflection with the same characteristics as the P wave may be partially buried in the beginning of the QRS. The QRS of complexes 2 and 3 is otherwise similar to the sinus complexes (1 and 4), except for a slightly higher amplitude of the R wave (or S in aVR) visible in all leads except I and aVL. Therefore, complexes 2 and 3 are likely to be junctional in origin. These findings suggest two concomitant rhythms: *a sinus rhythm with a rate of 60 bpm and a junctional rhythm with a similar rate*. This rhythm was observed during general anaesthesia for a MRI scan in a dog with suspicion of trigeminal nerve disease. Sinus bradycardia was likely to be a consequence of the anaesthetic drugs causing suppression of the sinus node discharge rate, thereby allowing a subsidiary pacemaker in the junctional area to compete with the sinus rhythm.

ECG Trace 13

Canine, 15-year-old, male, neutered Yorkshire Terrier

	Reference range	Patient	Interpretation:
Heart rate (bpm)	70–160		
Rhythm	Regular or sinus arrhythmia		
P wave (ms)	<40		
P wave (mV)	<0.4		
PR (s)	60–130		
QRS (ms)	<70		
R wave (mV)	>0.5 in leads II, III and aVF		
S wave (mV)			
ST segment	<0.2 mV below or above baseline		
QT (ms)			
QTc (ms)	150–240		
T wave (mV)			
MEA (frontal plane)	+40° to +100°		

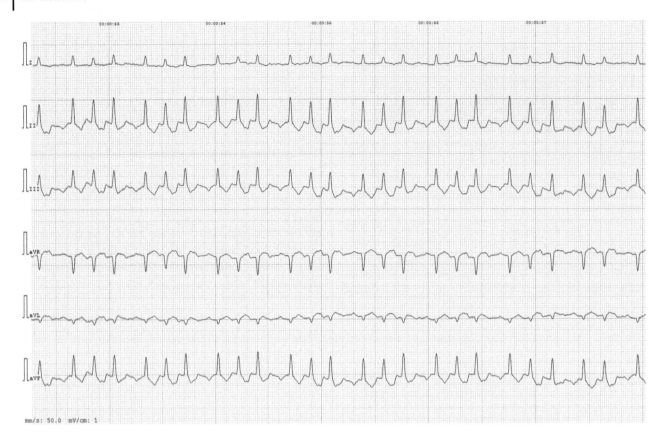

mm/s: 50.0 mV/cm: 1

ECG Trace 13: Interpretation

The underlying rhythm is an irregular narrow-QRS rhythm (QRS, 40–50 ms; normal, <70 ms) with a ventricular rate of approximately 260 bpm. The QRS duration, amplitude (R, 1.2 mV; normal, >0.5 mV and <3.0 mV in lead II), morphology (main positive deflection in leads I, II, III and aVF; main negative deflection in leads aVR and aVL) and mean electrical axis (MEA, ≈70°; normal, +40° to +100°) are all normal. This indicates a normal ventricular activation and is suggestive of a supraventricular rhythm. QRS alternans is seen and is most obvious in leads I, II, aVR and aVF. The QTc interval is within the expected range (170 ms; normal, 150–240 ms). The rhythm irregularity seems to be due to occasional dropped beats, as the RR interval for most complexes seems constant at 180–200 ms and then occasionally is 320 ms. Deflections consistent with P' waves may be seen during these periods, supporting this hypothesis. The morphology of these P' waves is consistent with an origin in the floor of the left atrium (negative in leads I, II, III and aVF; positive in leads aVR and aVL; MEA, –120°), and this is suggestive of an *ectopic atrial tachycardia*. P' waves buried in the ST are suspected, and the dropped beats are consistent with occasional 2:1 atrioventricular conduction due to atrioventricular block without termination of the arrhythmia. Atypical atrial flutter would be a differential diagnosis. Atrioventricular reciprocating tachycardia may be ruled out, as atrioventricular block did not influence the underlying arrhythmia. This patient suffered from advanced chronic valvular degenerative disease. Sotalol was used successfully to reduce heart rate and suppress the arrhythmia.

ECG Trace 14

Canine, 10-year-old, male, neutered Border Terrier

	Reference range	Patient	Interpretation:
Heart rate (bpm)	70–160		
Rhythm	Regular or sinus arrhythmia		
P wave (ms)	<40		
P wave (mV)	<0.4		
PR (s)	60–130		
QRS (ms)	<70		
R wave (mV)	>0.5 in leads II, III and aVF		
S wave (mV)			
ST segment	<0.2 mV below or above baseline		
QT (ms)			
QTc (ms)	150–240		
T wave (mV)			
MEA (frontal plane)	+40° to +100°		

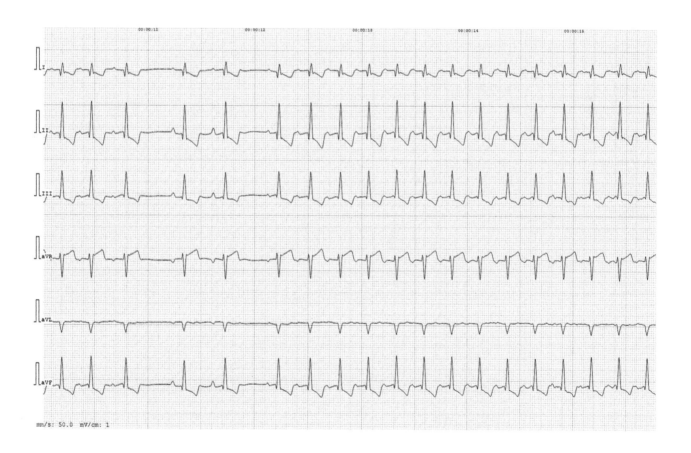

ECG Trace 14: Interpretation

A narrow-QRS rhythm is seen (QRS, 60 ms; normal, <70 ms). All QRS have the same appearance with normal duration, amplitude (R, 1.3 mV; normal, >0.5 mV and <3.0 mV in lead II), morphology (main positive deflection in leads I, II, III and aVF; main negative deflection in leads aVR and aVL) and mean electrical axis (MEA, ≈88°; normal, +40° to +100°), indicating a supraventricular rhythm with normal ventricular conduction. The fourth and fifth complexes are sinus beats. The QRS is preceded by a P wave of normal duration (40 ms; normal, <40 ms), amplitude (0.3 mV; normal, <0.4 mV) and morphology (positive deflection in leads I, II, III and aVF; negative deflection in leads aVR and aVL), and a normal PR interval (100–110 ms; normal, 60–130 ms). The other complexes are preceded by a P wave that is slightly different (smaller amplitude, biphasic in lead III and positive in aVL) with an estimated electrical axis of +30°, suggestive of an origin in the floor of the right atrium. This is suggestive of an *ectopic atrial tachycardia* given that the rate is approximately 210 bpm. During tachycardia, the P' may be seen at the end of the T wave with a slightly variable position (compare the T during tachycardia with the T from the sinus complexes). This patient was presented with atrial tachycardia, and further imaging revealed an adrenal mass, raising suspicion of pheochromocytoma.

ECG Trace 15

Canine, 9-year-old, male, neutered Jack Russell Terrier

	Reference range	Patient	Interpretation:
Heart rate (bpm)	70–160		
Rhythm	Regular or sinus arrhythmia		
P wave (ms)	<40		
P wave (mV)	<0.4		
PR (s)	60–130		
QRS (ms)	<70		
R wave (mV)	>0.5 in leads II, III and aVF		
S wave (mV)			
ST segment	<0.2 mV below or above baseline		
QT (ms)			
QTc (ms)	150–240		
T wave (mV)			
MEA (frontal plane)	+40° to +100°		

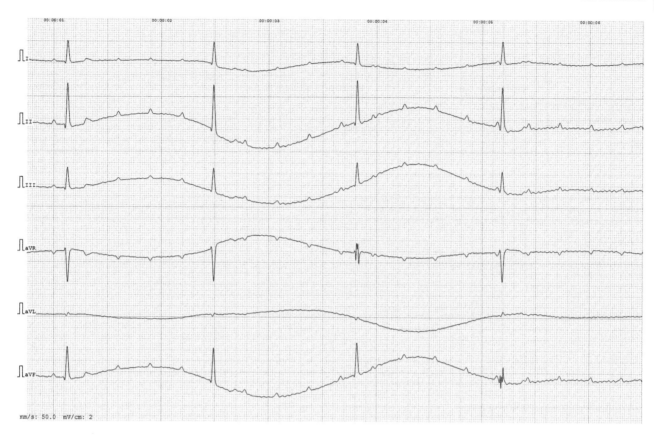

ECG Trace 15: Interpretation

The underlying rhythm is a regular narrow-QRS rhythm (QRS, 60 ms; normal, <70 ms) with a rate of approximately 50–60 bpm consistent with bradycardia in this patient. The normal QRS duration and estimated mean electrical axis (MEA, +60°; normal, +40° to +100°) indicate a supraventricular rhythm with normal ventricular conduction. The QRS amplitude is above normal (R, 4.0 mV; normal, >0.5 mV or <3.0 mV in lead II) and suggestive of possible ventricular enlargement. P waves are seen throughout the trace with normal duration (40 ms; normal, <40 ms), amplitude (0.4 mV; normal, <0.4 mV) and morphology (positive in leads I, II, III and aVF; negative in leads aVR and aVL), consistent with a sinus rhythm. The sinus rate is approximately 200 bpm and therefore sinus tachycardia. The P waves are dissociated from the QRS complexes with a variable PR interval. These findings indicate *sinus tachycardia with third-degree atrioventricular block and a junctional escape rhythm*. This patient was presented for investigation of intermittent syncope and was successfully treated by implantation of an artificial pacemaker.

ECG Trace 16

Canine, 11-year-old, male, neutered Cavalier King Charles Spaniel

	Reference range	Patient	Interpretation:
Heart rate (bpm)	70–160		
Rhythm	Regular or sinus arrhythmia		
P wave (ms)	<40		
P wave (mV)	<0.4		
PR (s)	60–130		
QRS (ms)	<70		
R wave (mV)	>0.5 in leads II, III and aVF		
S wave (mV)			
ST segment	<0.2 mV below or above baseline		
QT (ms)			
QTc (ms)	150–240		
T wave (mV)			
MEA (frontal plane)	+40° to +100°		

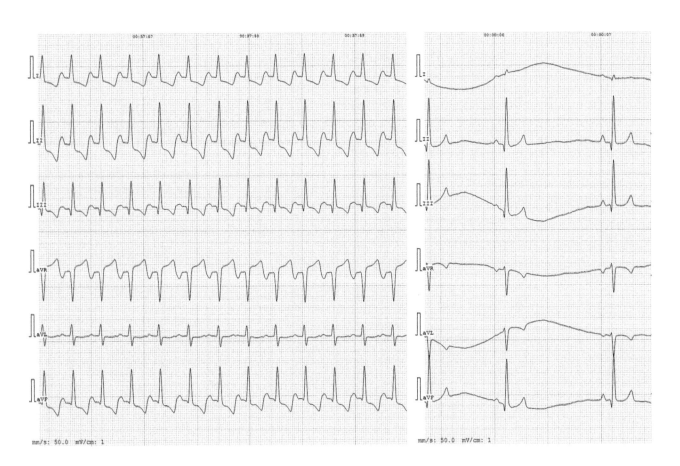

ECG Trace 16: Interpretation

The trace on the left shows a regular narrow-QRS rhythm (QRS, 40 ms; normal, <70 ms) with a rate of approximately 220 bpm and therefore tachycardia. The normal QRS duration and estimated mean electrical axis (+64°; normal, +40° to +100°) indicate a supraventricular rhythm with normal ventricular conduction. The trace on the right shows two sinus complexes from the same patient. This is useful for comparison of the ST segment and T waves to identify possible superimposed atrial depolarisation waves (P, P' or F waves) during periods of tachycardia. In this case, during sinus rhythm the ST is isoelectric and the T appears as a positive deflection in leads II, III and aVF with a QTc of 222 ms (normal, 150–240 ms); during tachycardia, the T wave appears biphasic with a QTc of 238 ms. The appearance of the T wave during tachycardia differs from that of the sinus rhythm, raising the possibility that one of its deflections is a P' or F wave. Close examination of lead aVL reveals two distinct positive deflections supporting this hypothesis. The first deflection is negative in leads I, II, III and aVF and positive in leads aVR and aVL. This would be consistent with a P' originating in the floor of the right atrium/atrioventricular junction or a retrograde P' following the QRS. The second deflection is similar to the T wave in sinus rhythm, and therefore it is likely that this is the T wave. Assuming this is correct, the RP' (100 ms) is shorter than the P'R (160 ms) with a RP'/P'R of 0.625 (<0.7). Based on these findings, the differential diagnoses should include orthodromic atrioventricular reciprocating tachycardia, focal junctional tachycardia with a 1:1 retrograde P', focal atrial tachycardia and atypical flutter. In this case, a diagnosis of *focal atrial tachycardia* was thought most likely, based on the identification of isolated ectopic complexes where the QRS was preceded by a P' with the same characteristics of the suspected P' during tachycardia.

ECG Trace 17

Canine, 7-year-old, male Siberian Husky

	Reference range	Patient	Interpretation:
Heart rate (bpm)	70–160		
Rhythm	Regular or sinus arrhythmia		
P wave (ms)	<40		
P wave (mV)	<0.4		
PR (s)	60–130		
QRS (ms)	<70		
R wave (mV)	>0.5 in leads II, III and aVF		
S wave (mV)			
ST segment	<0.2 mV below or above baseline		
QT (ms)			
QTc (ms)	150–240		
T wave (mV)			
MEA (frontal plane)	+40° to +100°		

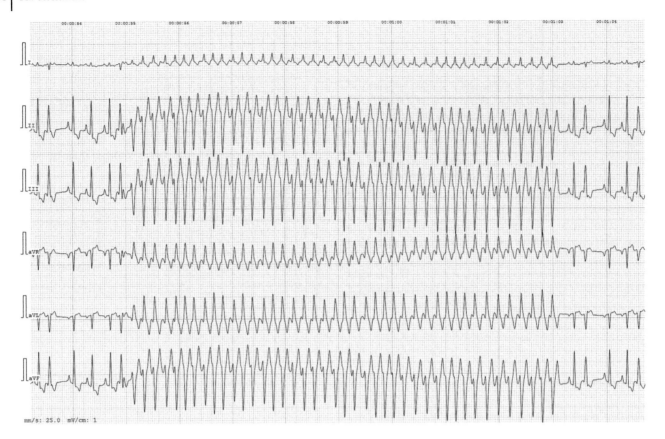

mm/s: 25.0 mV/cm: 1

ECG Trace 17: Interpretation

The beginning and end of this trace show sinus rhythm with QRS complexes of normal duration (40 ms; normal, <70 ms), amplitude (R, 1.4 mV; normal, >0.5 mV and <3.0 mV in lead II) and morphology (main positive deflection in leads I, II, III and aVF; main negative deflection in leads aVR and aVL), preceded by a normal P wave with a normal PR interval (80–90 ms; normal, 60–130 ms). The sinus P have a normal duration (40 ms; normal, <40 ms), amplitude (0.3 mV; normal, <0.4 mV) and morphology (positive deflection in leads I, II, III and aVF; negative deflection in leads aVR and aVL). From complexes 7 to 47, a regular wide-QRS rhythm (QRS, 80–100 ms; normal, <70 ms) is seen with a rate of approximately 280 bpm and therefore tachycardia. The QRS displays a right bundle branch block morphology (main negative deflections in leads II, III and aVF; main positive deflections in leads aVR and aVL), and all QRS have a similar appearance. P waves are not discernible during this rhythm. These characteristics are suggestive of a monomorphic ventricular tachycardia with possible origin in the left ventricle. Alternatively, a supraventricular rhythm conducted with a tachycardia-dependent (phase 3) bundle branch block could be possible but less likely. Additionally, some complexes are premature with a wide QRS (80 ms) that has a different morphology (complexes 2, 6, 49 and 52). These complexes are likely ventricular premature complexes with a different origin, rather than fusion complexes, as the morphology does not appear to be a fusion of the sinus and other ectopic QRS (notice the polarity in lead I that is negative for these complexes but positive for both the sinus QRS and QRS during tachycardia).

This patient was diagnosed with a myocardial disease with frequent *multifocal ventricular tachycardia*. The differential diagnoses included dilated cardiomyopathy, tachycardia-induced cardiomyopathy and myocarditis. This rhythm was successfully controlled with oral sotalol.

ECG Trace 18

Feline, 2-year-old, female, neutered Domestic Shorthair

	Reference range	Patient	Interpretation:
Heart rate (bpm)	140–220		
Rhythm	Regular		
P wave (ms)	<40		
P wave (mV)	<0.2		
PR (s)	50–90		
QRS (ms)	<40		
R wave (mV)	<0.9 in lead II		
S wave (mV)			
ST segment	Isoelectric		
QT (ms)	70–200		
QTc (ms)			
T wave (mV)			
MEA (frontal plane)	+0° to +160°		

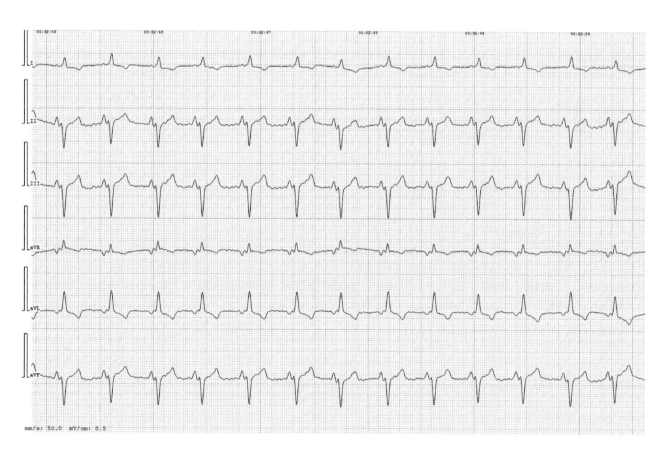

mm/s: 50.0   mV/cm: 0.5

ECG Trace 18: Interpretation

The underlying rhythm is a regular wide-QRS rhythm (QRS, 60 ms; normal, <40 ms) with a rate of approximately 150. The QRS morphology is suggestive of a right bundle branch block (main negative deflection in leads II, III and aVF; main positive deflection in leads aVR and aVL; MEA, −77°). All QRS are preceded by a P wave with a normal morphology (positive deflection in leads I, II, III and aVF; negative deflection in leads aVR and aVL) and a consistent PR interval at the lower limit of normal (50 ms; normal, 50–90 ms). These findings are suggestive of a sinus rhythm conducted with a right bundle branch block. The P wave duration (40 ms; normal, <40 ms) and amplitude (0.2 mV;

normal, <0.2 mV) are within the expected range. It is interesting to see such a short PR interval at this ventricular rate, although it is still within the expected range for a cat. Curiously, the QT interval is at the higher range of normal, as expected at this ventricular rate (200 ms; normal, 70–200 ms). An alternative for a short PR interval and wide QRS could be the presence of pre-excitation via an accessory pathway. In fact, this patient was referred for suspicion of a narrow-QRS tachycardia that had characteristics consistent with orthodromic atrioventricular reciprocating tachycardia, and periods of sinus rhythm with a normal QRS and a longer PR interval were also present, supporting this hypothesis.

ECG Trace 19

Canine, 12-year-old, male Labrador Retriever

	Reference range	Patient	Interpretation:
Heart rate (bpm)	70–160		
Rhythm	Regular or sinus arrhythmia		
P wave (ms)	<40		
P wave (mV)	<0.4		
PR (s)	60–130		
QRS (ms)	<70		
R wave (mV)	>0.5 in leads II, III and aVF		
S wave (mV)			
ST segment	<0.2 mV below or above baseline		
QT (ms)			
QTc (ms)	150–240		
T wave (mV)			
MEA (frontal plane)	+40° to +100°		

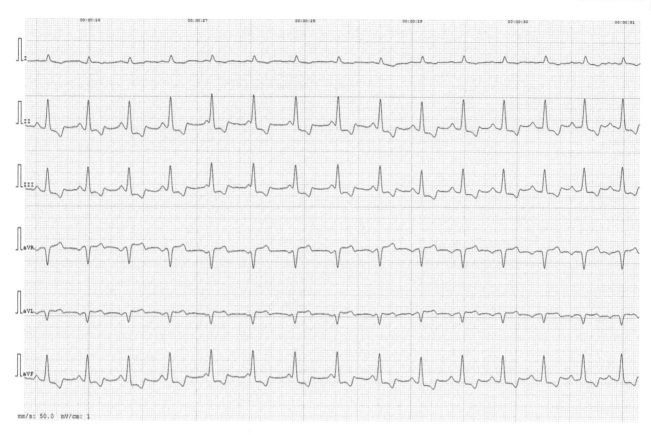

ECG Trace 19: Interpretation

The underlying rhythm is a regular narrow-QRS rhythm (QRS, 60 ms; normal, <70 ms) with a rate of approximately 160 bpm. The QRS morphology is normal (main positive deflection in leads I, II, III and aVF; main negative deflection in leads aVR and aVL) with a normal mean electrical axis (MEA, +77°; normal, +40° to +100°). These findings suggest a supraventricular rhythm with normal ventricular conduction. The QRS are preceded by a P wave with normal morphology (positive deflection in leads I, II, III and aVF; negative deflection in leads aVR and aVL) consistent with sinus P waves. However, the PR interval is variable, with the P waves becoming progressively closer to the QRS and then apart. This is suggestive of a concomitant *junctional tachycardia*, and a sinus rhythm with *type I isorhythmic atrioventricular dissociation*. Additionally, the P wave duration is prolonged (50–60 ms; normal, <40 ms), suggesting possible atrial enlargement that was confirmed by echocardiography.

ECG Trace 20

Canine, 9-year-old, male Bernese Mountain Dog

	Reference range	Patient	Interpretation:
Heart rate (bpm)	70–160		
Rhythm	Regular or sinus arrhythmia		
P wave (ms)	<40		
P wave (mV)	<0.4		
PR (s)	60–130		
QRS (ms)	<70		
R wave (mV)	>0.5 in leads II, III and aVF		
S wave (mV)			
ST segment	<0.2 mV below or above baseline		
QT (ms)			
QTc (ms)	150–240		
T wave (mV)			
MEA (frontal plane)	+40° to +100°		

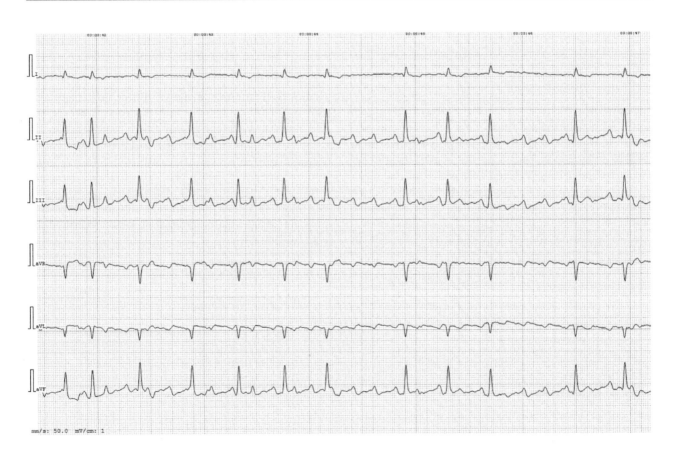

mm/s: 50.0   mV/cm: 1

ECG Trace 20: Interpretation

The underlying rhythm is an irregular narrow-QRS rhythm (QRS, ≈60 ms; normal, <70 ms) with a rate of approximately 120 bpm. The QRS has a normal appearance with a main positive deflection in leads I, II, III and aVF and a main negative deflection in leads aVR and aVL. The estimated mean electrical axis is approximately 78°, which is within the expected range (+40° to +100°). The QRS duration (≈60 ms; normal, <70 ms) and amplitude (R wave in lead II, ≈0.9 mV; normal, >0.5 mV) are also within the expected range. Given these findings, we can conclude that ventricular depolarisation is occurring normally and that this is a supraventricular rhythm. Atrial depolarisation waves (P' or F) are seen between the QRS complexes, with variable atrioventricular conduction accounting for the rhythm irregularity. The atrial depolarisation rate is regular with a rate of approximately 300 bpm. These findings are suggestive of *atrial flutter* or, alternatively, focal atrial tachycardia. This electrocardiogram was recorded after treatment with sotalol that successfully controlled the heart rate.

Index

Note: Page numbers in *italic* indicate Figures and those in **bold** indicate Tables.